Pediatric Swallowing and Feeding
Assessment and Management

SECOND EDITION

Dedication

■

To my family members of long standing
Gerald, Frieda, Peter, Stephen, and Mark
And those who have become part of my family in recent years
Jeanne, Matthew, Jonathan, Jason, and Tara
You all know how special you are to me.
Joan C. Arvedson, PhD

To my parents Zelda (of blessed memory) and Milton Brodsky
Who "nourished" me so well
and
to Saul, Jeremy, Dana, and Rebecca Greenfield
Who were so supportive during the time
I took from them to complete this book.
Linda Brodsky, MD
(aka Linda Greenfield)

Pediatric Swallowing and Feeding
Assessment and Management
SECOND EDITION

Joan C. Arvedson, PhD
Linda Brodsky, MD

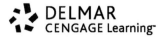

Australia • Brazil • Japan • Korea • Mexico • Singapore • Spain • United Kingdom • United States

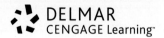
DELMAR
CENGAGE Learning™

Pediatric Swallowing and Feeding: Assessment and Management,
Second Edition

By Joan C. Arvedson, PhD.
and Linda Brodsky, MD

Health Care Publishing Director:
William Brottmiller

Acquisitions Editor:
Candice Janco

Developmental Editor:
Kristin Banach

Executive Marketing Manager:
Dawn F. Gerrain

Production Editor:
James Zayicek

Editorial Assistant:
Maria D'Angelico

For product information and technology assistance, contact us at
Cengage Learning Customer & Sales Support, 1-800-354-9706

For permission to use material from this text or product, submit all requests online at **cengage.com/permissions**
Further permissions questions can be emailed to

Library of Congress Control Number: 20011020110

ISBN-13: 978-0-7693-0076-4

ISBN-10: 0-7693-0076-6

Delmar Cengage Learning
5 Maxwell Drive
Clifton Park, NY 12065-2919
USA

Cengage Learning products are represented in Canada by Nelson Education, Ltd.

For your lifelong learning solutions, visit
delmar.cengage.com

Visit our corporate website at **www.cengage.com**

Notice to the Reader

Publisher does not warrant or guarantee any of the products described herein or perform any independent analysis in connection with any of the product information contained herein. Publisher does not assume, and expressly disclaims, any obligation to obtain and include information other than that provided to it by the manufacturer. The reader is expressly warned to consider and adopt all safety precautions that might be indicated by the activities described herein and to avoid all potential hazards. By following the instructions contained herein, the reader willingly assumes all risks in connection with such instructions. The publisher makes no representations or warranties of any kind, including but not limited to, the warranties of fitness for particular purpose or merchantability, nor are any such representations implied with respect to the material set forth herein, and the publisher takes no responsibility with respect to such material. The publisher shall not be liable for any special, consequential, or exemplary damages resulting, in whole or part, from the readers' use of, or reliance upon, this material.

Printed in Canada
11 12 13 14 12 11 10 09

Contents

About the Authors

■

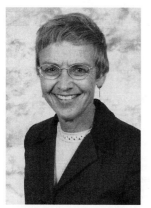

JOAN C. ARVEDSON, PhD

Joan C. Arvedson, PhD is Director of Speech-Language and Hearing at the Center for Pediatric Otolaryngology and Communicative Disorders and the General Mills Swallow/Speech Center, Children's Hospital of Buffalo/ Kaleida Health, in Buffalo, NY. She is also Clinical Associate Professor in the Department of Otolaryngology, School of Medicine and Biomedical Sciences, and Adjunct Associate Professor in the Department of Communicative Disorders and Sciences, at the State University of New York at Buffalo. She received her BS, MS, and PhD degrees from the University of Wisconsin–Madison. She has authored numerous scientific publications and book chapters in the field of pediatric feeding and swallowing. She is co-author of *Pediatric Videofluoroscopic Swallow Studies: A Professional Manual with Caregiver Guidelines,* 1998 (with M. Lefton-Greif, PhD). She is on the editorial board of *Dysphagia.* Dr. Arvedson has presented many workshops and seminars on swallowing and feeding disorders in infants and children throughout the United States, Canada, Europe, and Asia. Her teaching and research endeavors are focused in these areas. Patient care focuses include swallowing and motor speech disorders in varied pediatric populations.

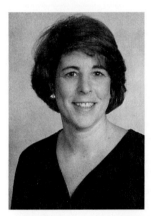

LINDA BRODSKY, MD

Linda Brodsky, MD is the chief of Pediatric Otolaryngology at the Center for Pediatric Otolaryngology and Communicative Disorders and the General Mills Swallow/Speech Center, Children's Hospital of Buffalo/Kaleida Health in Buffalo, New York. She is Professor of Otolaryngology and Pediatrics, and Adjunct Professor of Communication Sciences at the State University of New York at Buffalo, School of Medicine and Biomedical Sciences. She is also director of the Center for Integrated Outcomes in Healthcare, the Women's and Children's Research Foundation/Children's Hospital of Buffalo. She has authored over 100 scientific publications and book chapters in the field of pediatric otolaryngology. She is on the editorial boards of the *International Journal of Pediatric Otolaryngology, Acta Otolaryngologica,* and *Journal of Pediatric Respiratory Diseases.* Dr. Brodsky is active in numerous national societies, recently serving two terms as treasurer for the American Society of Pediatric Otolaryngology. She is listed in the Best Doctors in America Series and Who's Who in Science and Engineering. As an entrepreneur, she is president of the Institute for Integrated Outcomes, a consulting firm that provides frontline, data-driven support to organizations and individuals interested in rapid cycle health care improvement. She is married to Saul P. Greenfield, MD, and has three children, Jeremy, Dana and Rebecca.

Contributors

■

Bruce Bleichfeld, PhD
Clinical Psychologist
Private Practice
Feeding Disorders Clinic
Robert Warner Rehabilitation Center
Children's Hospital of Buffalo/Kaleida
  Health
Buffalo, NY

Steven Christensen, MD
Director of Nuclear Medicine
Children's Hospital of Buffalo
Assistant Professor, Department of
  Radiology
School of Medicne and Biomedical
  Sciences
State University of New York at
  Buffalo
Buffalo, NY

**Nancy Claxton, MS, Registered
  Dietician**
Department of Gastroenterology
Children's Hospital of Buffalo/Kaleida
  Health
Buffalo, NY

**Donna Reigstad, MA, Licensed
  Occupational Therapist**
Lecturer, Occupational Therapy
  Department
State University of New York at
  Buffalo
Coordinator, Feeding Disorders Clinic
Robert Warner Rehabilitation Center
Children's Hospital of Buffalo/Kaleida
  Health
Buffalo, NY

Brian Rogers, MD
Associate Professor of Pediatrics
State University of New York at
  Buffalo
School of Medicine and Biomedical
  Sciences
Medical Director of the Robert
  Warner Rehabilitation Center
Children's Hospital of Buffalo/Kaleida
  Health
Buffalo, NY

Thomas Rossi, MD
Professor of Pediatrics, University of
  Rochester
School of Medicine
Division of Gastroenterology and
  Nutrition, Children's Hospital at
  Strong Memorial Hospital
Rochester, NY

Preface to the Second Edition

■

The area of pediatric swallowing and feeding disorders is one of the most rapidly evolving patient care areas for physicians and other health care professionals, particularly hospital-based speech–language pathologists, occupational therapists, psychologists, dietitians, and nurses. In addition, as an increasing number of high-risk infants survive to pre-school and school age, medical knowledge and new skills must be acquired by school-based nurses, occupational and physical therapists, educational-based speech–language pathologists, and teachers of children with special needs. This second edition is focused on providing information to the practitioner interested in and involved with children who face these problems. Reorganization of the basic science information, expansion of diagnostic and therapeutic approaches, and the addition of new chapters make this an exciting new undertaking.

Simply stated, breathing and eating are the most important functions for survival of any living being. Breathing should be automatic and usually does not require active effort by the infant. Eating, on the other hand, requires that food be given or sought. Eating also provides the first opportunity for the human infant to communicate with other human beings. As the infant grows and develops, the seeking of food becomes one of the major foundations for the development of key cognitive processes on which a lifetime of learning will continue to grow.

Although basic to survival, eating is not a simple process. Food must be found, ingested, swallowed, and finally, digested. If any step in the process in disrupted, the child may demonstrate malnutrition, poor growth, delayed development, poor academic achievement, psychologic problems, and loss of general good health and well-being. Thus, at the risk of stating the obvious, the development of normal eating is extraordinarily important.

Recent advances in medicine have provided many children and their families with enhanced survival and improved clinical outcomes. One by-product of this situation is that many surviving infants suffer neurologic damage and hence require alternative strategies for the management of such basic physiologic processes as eating, breathing, and communicating.

Since the first edition of this text 8 years ago, the need to address these issues has increased enormously.

Oral sensorimotor function and swallowing encompass most of the processes that relate to the development of normal feeding, eating, and speech/language patterns. Oral sensorimotor dysfunction is often an early and specific marker of future neurologic challenges ranging from mild learning disabilities to severe mental retardation and cerebral palsy. The Introduction sets feeding and swallowing into a framework of a *multi*disciplinary problem that needs to be handled with an *inter*disciplinary approach. It is in this philosophical and practical setting that the medical, social, and ethical concerns come together. This book is divided into two parts. Part I focuses on the assessment and management issues of feeding and swallowing problems. Relevant anatomy, embryology, and physiology are consolidated into Chapter 2 and provide the background for the in-depth study of this subject. The pediatric neurodevelopmental, gastroenterology, and airway assessments are treated separately.

Clinical oral sensorimotor and feeding assessment, including posture and tone, is described. The chapter on instrumental measures is expanded to include videofluoroscopic swallow studies (VFSS) and flexible endoscopic examination of swallowing (FEES). This section concludes with a chapter on oral sensorimotor management of children with feeding and swallowing disorders.

Part II covers special topics that include an update of drooling and the feeding of children with craniofacial anomalies. New chapters on chronic aspiration and psychologic and behavioral problems associated with feeding have been added. Case studies throughout the book highlight salient points.

We would like to acknowledge the many people who made this book possible. First, a special thanks to all the authors who worked so hard and kept to their deadlines. Next are the members of the Department of Speech-Language Pathology and the Pediatric Center for Otolaryngology and Communicative Disorders/General Mills Swallow Voice Center at the Childrens' Hospital of Buffalo/Kaleida Health. Without their input, suggestions, and understanding, this book could not have been completed. A special thanks to Marilyn Smistek, Laurie Beth Giza, Michelle Stallworth, Nancy Garrison, Jung Kim, and Joanne Matteliano for their technical assistance. Medical photography was expertly provided by Brian Smistek. the medical illustrations were done by Rachel Byron-Moore of Biographics, Inc. The children, their families, and other caregivers require special mention. These courageous people have continued to simultaneously challenge and delight us. And, of course, appreciation must be given to our families, to whom this book is dedicated.

■ PART I ■

Diagnosis and Treatment

■ CHAPTER 1

Introduction

Linda Brodsky and Joan Arvedson

Breathing and eating are the most basic physiologic functions that define life's beginning outside of the mother's womb for newborn infants. Breathing is reflexive and life sustaining but provides no other intrinsic pleasure. Eating, on the other hand, is partly instinct and partly a learned response. It requires the ingestion of food, which in the newborn must be provided by an outside source. Sucking and swallowing require a complex series of events and coordination of the neurologic, respiratory, and gastrointestinal (GI) systems. Normal GI function must occur in digestion of foods to provide nutrients. All of these functions occur within the framework of developing physical and emotional maturity. The pleasure of eating extends beyond the feeling of satiety to the pleasure gained through food ingested by the infant and provided by the mother, who is most often the primary caregiver. This interactive primary relationship is the first for the newborn. It serves as a foundation for normal development, somatic growth, communication skills, and psychosocial well-being. Thus, feeding of the newborn infant, young child, and rapidly growing teen is an activity with far-reaching consequences. When disrupted, the sequelae can include malnutrition, behavioral abnormalities, and severe distress for family and child alike. Interruption of growth and development sometimes cannot be reversed if it occurs at a critical time during the early months and years of a child's life (Chapter 3). Lifelong disabilities may result.

Medical and technological progress over the past 4 decades has resulted in the survival of many infants and children who previously would not have lived. The range and complexity of their problems will continue to challenge the medical profession because many of these children are now living longer, remaining healthier, and having greater expectations for a normal and productive life. Although many children and their families have benefited greatly, the increasing number of children born prematurely at low birth weight (less than 2,500 g), very low birth weight (less than 1,500 g), and with genetic abnormalities are confronted with multiple complex medical problems. Early recognition and intervention have been invaluable despite the mental retardation, cerebral palsy, chronic pulmonary problems, structural deficits, and neurologic impairments endured. Feeding and swallowing problems compound most of these conditions.

After the establishment of adequate respiration, the highest priority for caregivers is to meet the nutritional needs of newborns. To achieve this successfully, children require a well-functioning oral sensorimotor swallowing mechanism, overall adequate health (including respiratory, gastrointestinal, and neurologic), appropriate nutrition, central nervous system integration, and adequate musculoskeletal tone. In addition, the successful emergence of communication, an often-overlooked process, depends heavily on successful feeding and swallowing. Normal feeding patterns are reflected in the early developmental pathways that sequentially and rapidly emerge during the first several months and years of life. Communication is one of the most important of those pathways. The interrelationship between feeding, shared by all biologic creatures, and language based, verbal communication, unique to humans, cannot be overemphasized. The comparative anatomy of the upper aerodigestive tract and its implication for the development of human communication has been established (Laitman & Reidenberg, 1993; Madriples & Laitman, 1987).

Children who are born prematurely with very low birth weight or with neurologic impairment are fairly commonly found to have feeding and swallowing problems. Other high-risk children are those experiencing birth trauma, pre- and perinatal asphyxia, and a multitude of genetic syndromes with accompanying structural and neurologic impairment (Chapters 3 and 12). The presence of cardiac, pulmonary, and GI disease often creates additional difficulty in sorting out primary and secondary etiologies. Diagnosis and management in these patients present even greater challenges (Table 1–1).

The ability to feed successfully and thereby nurture an infant is imprinted early on the maternal–infant relationship. Characteristic of normal oral, sensorimotor development is establishing: (a) stability and mobility of the ingestive system, (b) rhythmicity, (c) sensation, and (d) oral-motor efficiency and economy (Gisel, Birnbaum, & Schwartz, 1998). Optimally, maternal– (or paternal–) infant bonding begins at the outset by providing nutrition simultaneously with the visual and auditory stimulation of a loving and concerned parent. Thus, feeding and swallowing disorders impact not only on the physical but also on the psychosocial well-being of the infant and child.

The epidemiology of oral sensorimotor dysfunction in the general population and in the population of neurologically impaired children is not well defined. Precise incidence and prevalence data are hard to ascertain, but estimates are that 85–90% of children with cerebral palsy (CP) are believed to have swallowing difficulties at some time during their lives.

Table 1–1. Major Diagnostic Categories Associated with Feeding and Swallowing Disorders in Infants and Children

Neurologic
- Encephalopathies (e.g., cerebral palsy, perinatal asphyxia)
- Traumatic brain injury
- Neoplasms
- Mental retardation
- Developmental delay

Anatomic and Structural
- Congenital (e.g., tracheoesophageal fistula, cleft palate)
- Acquired

Genetic
- Chromosomal (e.g., Down syndrome)
- Syndromic (e.g., Pierre Robin sequence, Treacher Collins syndrome)
- Inborn errors of metabolism

Secondary to Systemic Illness
- Respiratory (e.g., chronic lung disease, bronchopulmonary dysplasia)
- Gastrointestinal (e.g., GI dysmotility, constipation)
- Congenital cardiac anomalies

Psychosocial and Behavioral
- Oral deprivation

Secondary to Resolved Medical Condition
- Iatrogenic

During the 1st year of life of all children with CP, 57% are estimated to have problems with suck, 38% with swallow, and 33% with malnutrition (Reilly, Skuse, & Poblete, 1996). As the severity of the CP increases, not surprisingly the severity of the oral sensorimotor dysfunction increases. The most severely affected are children with spastic quadriparesis, 90% of whom have problems (Stallings, Charney, Davies, & Cronk, 1993).

Feeding and swallowing difficulties manifest in many different ways. Resistance to accepting foods, lack of energy for the work of eating and digestion, and oral sensorimotor disabilities broadly encompass most problems (Gisel et al., 1998). Effective management of these medically complex children depends on the expertise of many specialists, working independently and as a team. An interdisciplinary approach offers the benefit of coordinated consultation and problem solving for multiply coincident and interrelated problems. Case coordination is often intensive and necessary to optimize the child's health and development, as well as the family's ability to synthesize and cope with multiple, sometimes disparate opinions. An *interdisciplinary* approach refers to interaction of a group of professionals. Each one brings expertise that is useful in the solution of a complex medical problem. Interdisciplinary management is based on the desire and ability to communicate in a collegial fashion with other interested practitioners to solve these complex medical problems (Table 1–2). This process is aided by the development of a group philosophy for both evaluation and treatment, which then engenders respect for other team members' expertise. An organized structure with a clearly defined leader is also necessary. Finally, a shared fund of knowledge is critical and results in creative problem solving and fruitful research. An interdisciplinary approach should be adopted at institutions where professionals evaluate and treat children with complex feeding and swallowing problems (Table 1–3; Figure 1–1).

In a pediatric medical center, several types of models and settings accommodate interdisciplinary team assessment and treatment. Most teams function in an outpatient setting and serve a transitional purpose between the inpatient and outpatient setting. Names for such teams can include Feeding Clinic, Feeding Disorders Clinic, Nutrition Clinic, or

Table 1–2. Success Factors for an Interdisciplinary Approach

- Collegial interaction among relevant specialists
- Shared group philosophy for diagnostic approaches and treatment protocols
- Team leadership with organization for evaluation and information sharing
- Willingness to engage in creative problem solving and research
- Time commitment for the labor-intensive nature of such work

Table 1–3. Swallowing Team Members and Their Function

Team Member	Function
Speech–Language Pathologist	Team co-leader (active in feeding clinic, coordinates bimonthly complex dysphagia conference)
	Clinic/inpatient feeding and swallowing evaluation
	Video fluoroscopic swallow study (w/ radiologist)
	Flexible endoscopic examination of swallow (w/ otolaryngologist)
	Oral sensorimotor habilitation program
Developmental Pediatrician	Team co-leader
	Pediatric and neurodevelopmental diagnosis and management

(continues)

Table 1–3. *(continued)* Swallowing Team Members and Their Function

Team Member	Function
Otolaryngologist	Physical examination of the upper aerodigestive tract
	Detailed airway assessment including flexible fiberoptic nasopharyngolaryngoscopy[a]
	Flexible endoscopic evaluation of swallow w/ sensory testing (w/ speech–language pathologist)
	Medical and surgical treatment of related issues of drooling, aspiration, and gastroesophageal reflux/extraesophageal reflux disease[b]
Gastroenterologist	Evaluation and management of gastrointestinal (GI) disease
	Endoscopy of the GI tract
	Nutritional issues (w/ nutritionist)
Nutritionist/Dietitian	Nutritional needs and assessment
	Methods for feeding
Occupational Therapist	Posture, tone, and sensory evaluation/treatment
Social Worker or Nurse	Coordinates home care and other appointments
Pediatric Surgeon[c]	Surgical management of GI disease
Psychologist[c]	Identifies and treats psychological and behavioral problems
Neurologist/Neurosurgeon[c]	Identifies and treats neurologic problems
Pulmonologist[c]	Lower airway disease—evaluation and management

Note. This is a suggested list based on the team as it has evolved at the Children's Hospital of Buffalo over the past 10 years. Depending on the expertise and interest at your institution, the team members may emerge from different disciplines; however, their functions should approximate those listed in the table.

[a]The terms *flexible fiberoptic nasopharyngosopy* and *laryngoscopy* are used interchangeably throughout the literature. All procedures use a flexible endoscope to view the nose, nasopharynx, pharynx, and larynx in the awake patient.

[b]Gastroesophageal reflux disease refers to the regurgitation of acid and other stomach contents from the stomach into the esophagus. When it causes symptoms, it is deemed pathologic and is in need of treatment. Extraesophageal reflux disease refers to the regurgitation of acid out of the esophagus into the pharynx, larynx, and oral cavity.

[c]As needed.

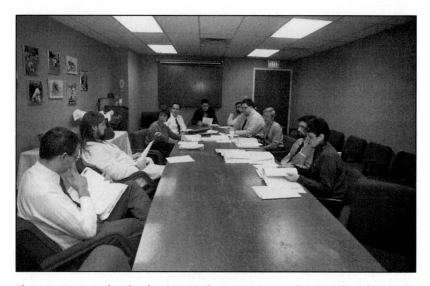

Figure 1–1. Complex dysphagia team that meets every other month to discuss the most difficult multiply-involved patients. Patients are presented and discussed among the various team members. Included here are the team leader, (speech–language pathologist), developmental pediatricians, otolaryngologists, pulmonologists, pediatric surgeon, and, for this meeting, the child's school-based speech–language pathologist. Primary care physicians and treating therapists are often interested in attending such conferences. They are other sources of important information, as well as a conduit for recommendation reinforcement at school.

Dysphagia Clinic. An inpatient feeding and swallowing team is also helpful both as a consultative and management service. The core team members usually include a developmental pediatrician (or pediatric neurologist), nutritionist, occupational therapist, nurse, social worker, and an oral sensorimotor specialist, such as a speech–language pathologist. Other consultants for specific problems may include a gastroenterologist, pulmonologist, otolaryngologist, radiologist, a psychologist, or any combination of these (Table 1–3). The interdisciplinary team leader, in most instances, is a physician with significant interest in neurologic or upper GI problems. The primary oral sensorimotor swallow therapist can be either a speech–language pathologist or occupational therapist, and all teams benefit from the ideal of having both. In the best of circumstances, these teams provide the interface between the sick hospitalized child and a healing, home-based child in need of ongoing services.

Oral sensorimotor and swallowing specialists may need to function outside of the inpatient hospital setting and outpatient clinic. Children with complex feeding and other medical problems are now found more commonly in a variety of educational (school-based) and residential (home-based) settings. Working knowledge of the challenges faced by infants and children with a wide variety of swallowing problems is mandatory. Families may be followed through a center or home-based educational program. These services have been mandated by federal legislation that guarantees a free and appropriate educational program for all handicapped children. The amendment, known as Public Law #99-457, to the original Education for All Handicapped Children Act of 1975 has added the mandate for service of children who are at-risk for developmental problems from birth to 3 years of age. The initial 1975 law guaranteed appropriate education for all handicapped children aged 3–21 years. The children from birth to age 3 years represent a category of special children who now must be serviced in programs by special educators, early childhood educators, developmental and school psychologists, social workers, nurses, speech–language pathologists, and occupational and physical therapists. All of these professionals will benefit from information about and an understanding of problems they may encounter related to oral sensorimotor function, feeding, swallowing, and ultimately to communication.

A comprehensive, interdisciplinary approach to children with swallowing and oral sensorimotor function problems is hampered by the lack of a shared fund of knowledge. A clearly defined set of terms related to this rapidly expanding field is necessary. A glossary of terms is included at the end of the book; however, several will be defined at the outset. *Deglutition*[1] is the act of swallowing and is just one process in the broader context of feeding. Swallowing begins at the lips and ends in the stomach. Sucking, chewing, and swallowing are three physiologically distinct processes occurring during deglutition (Kennedy & Kent, 1985). *Feeding* is the process for intake of food, including both its gathering and preparation. This is accomplished by sucking, chewing and swallowing. *Dysphagia* means difficulty in swallowing. *Oral sensorimotor function* covers all aspects of motor and sensory function of the structures in the oral cavity and pharynx related to swallowing from the lips until the onset of the pharyngeal phase of the swallow (Chapter 2). Finally, *nutrition* is the process by which a living organism obtains nutrients to sustain life, growth, and development.

Estimates of the frequency of swallowing have ranged from 600 to 1,000 times per day for children, and up to 2,400 times per day for adults (Lear, Flanagan, & Morres, 1965). The highest frequency is during food

---

[1]Swallowing and deglutition are used interchangeably. The former is the common usage, and the latter is the technical. The term swallowing will be preferred throughout the text.

intake, and the lowest is during sleep. Aside from feeding, swallowing accomplishes other purposes, such as the removal of saliva and mucous secretions from the oral, nasal, and pharyngeal cavities. A decrease in swallowing frequency may be coupled with oral sensorimotor dysfunction and thereby may result in severe drooling.

To care for children with swallowing disorders, a broad knowledge base must be supplemented by a thoughtful and often creative problem-solving approach. The steps to such an approach are universal to the diagnosis and treatment of any illness. Their importance to the approach of a medically complex child cannot be overemphasized and they are listed in Table 1–4. Interdisciplinary care is most effective in developing alternate strategies when normal swallowing and nutrition are absent or severely compromised.

This book provides a fund of knowledge, as well as a clinical approach that the reader will find useful in the evaluation and management of infants and children with oral sensorimotor dysfunction and swallowing problems. The first nine chapters emphasize the anatomy, embryology, physiology, and pathophysiology of the upper aerodigestive tract and other relevant areas. This information provides a basis for understanding the common problems associated with swallowing and feeding disorders. Neurodevelopment, airway, GI and nutrition, and oral sensorimotor and feeding evaluations are addressed in separate chapters. Instrumental assessment and management strategies complete this section.

Chapters 10–13 highlight special situations including aspiration, drooling, and problems in children with craniofacial anomalies. The final chapter about psychologic and behavioral issues has relevance to all aspects of feeding and swallowing disorders. Throughout the book interdisciplinary evaluation and management are stressed and demonstrated using clinical case studies, which are found at the end of most chapters. Flow charts for both evaluation and treatment are included whenever the problem at hand and the scientific literature support consideration of a "pathways" approach. Medical, psychosocial, and satisfaction outcomes are

Table 1–4. Process Steps for Diagnosis and Treatment of Pediatric Feeding and Swallowing Problems

- Define problem feeding and swallowing
- Identify etiology(ies)
- Determine appropriate diagnostic tests
- Plan approach to patient/family
- Teach about problem, implement treatment
- Monitor progress
- Evaluate progress (outcomes focused)

reported when available, although the literature in still sparse in the areas of pediatric feeding and swallowing.

It cannot be emphasized strongly enough that diagnosis based on etiology of disease must precede treatment and that infant and early childhood professionals must have appropriate knowledge and training to assess and treat infants and children with dysphagia and related conditions. The overall importance of an appropriate fund of knowledge and shared experience employing an interdisciplinary approach is emphasized throughout the book.

■ REFERENCES

Gisel, E. G., Birnbaum, R., & Schwartz, S. (1998). Feeding impairments in children: Diagnosis and effective intervention. *International Journal of Orofacial Myology, 24,* 27–33.

Kennedy, J. G., & Kent, R. D. (1985). Anatomy and physiology of deglutition and related functions. *Seminars in Speech and Language, 6,* 257–273.

Laitman, J., & Reidenberg, J. (1993). Specializations of the human upper respiratory and upper digestive systems as seen through comparative and developmental anatomy. *Dysphagia, 8,* 318–325.

Lear, C. S. C., Flanagan, J. B. J., & Morres, C. F. A. (1965). The frequency of deglutition in man. *Archives of Oral Biology, 10,* 83–100.

Madriples, U., & Laitman, J. (1987). Developmental change in the position of the fetal human larynx. *American Journal of Physical Anthropology, 72,* 463–472.

Reilly, S., Skuse, D., & Poblete, X. (1996). Prevalence of feeding problems and oral motor dysfunction in children with cerebral palsy: A community survey. *Journal of Pediatrics, 129,* 877–872.

Stallings, V. A., Charney, E., Davies, J. C., & Cronk, C. E. (1993). Nutritional-related growth failure of children with quadriplegic cerebral palsy. *Developmental Medicine and Child Neurology, 35,* 126–138.

CHAPTER 2

Anatomy, Embryology, Physiology, and Normal Development

Linda Brodsky and Joan Arvedson

■ SUMMARY

The human upper aerodigestive tract is the most complex neuromuscular unit in the body. It is the unlikely intersection of the digestive, respiratory, and phonatory systems. Normal swallowing requires precise integration of the important functions of breathing, eating, and speaking. A thorough understanding of the anatomy, embryology, and physiology of these systems is necessary to appreciate the etiology, diagnosis, and treatment of feeding and swallowing disorders in infants and children.

Attention to functional anatomy provides a basis for discussion of clinically relevant embryologic development. The physiology of swallowing, with emphasis on neurophysiology, posture, and muscle tone, is discussed in detail in this chapter. The challenges of developmental change beginning with premature infants and extending through adolescents are nowhere more apparent than for feeding and swallowing. Feeding and swallowing are explained in the context of normal oral sensorimotor development of the infant and child. Special focus on the anatomy and physiology of the airway and gastrointestinal tract will help to enhance the reader's understanding of the clinical manifestations, diagnosis, and treatment of feeding and swallowing problems in children.

■ INTRODUCTION

Deglutition, more commonly referred to as swallowing,[1] is defined as the semiautomatic motor action of the muscles of the respiratory and gastrointestinal tracts that propels food from the oral cavity into the stomach (Miller, 1986). Swallowing results not only in transporting food to the stomach but also in clearing the mouth and pharynx of secretions, mucous, and regurgitated stomach contents. Thus, the function of swallowing is nutritive as well as protective of the lower airways.

The act of swallowing is complex because respiration, swallowing, and phonation all occur at one anatomic location—the region of the pharynx and larynx. To be successful, normal swallowing requires the coordination of 31 muscles, 6 cranial nerves, and multiple levels of the central nervous system, including the brain stem and cerebral cortex (Bosma, 1986). Thus, understanding the anatomy, embryology, physiology, and normal development of this functional neuromuscular unit is of paramount importance to the proper diagnosis and treatment of feeding and swallowing disorders in children.

■ ANATOMY

The upper aerodigestive tract consists of the nose, oral cavity, pharynx, larynx, and esophagus. The trachea, bronchi, and pulmonary parenchyma are considered the lower airways. The upper digestive tract ends at the entrance to the stomach. Each area will be discussed separately.

Nose

The nose is important for respiration throughout life, but particularly in the neonatal and young infant (up to 6 months), when preferential nasal breathing is present. The nose also cleans, warms, and humidifies inspired air. As the nasal passage continues posteriorly, it opens at the bilateral posterior nasal choanae into a chamber called the nasopharynx, which is important anatomically as a resonator for speech production. In addition, the nasopharynx serves as one of the two airway conduits into the pharynx (Figure 2–1). The lateral nasal walls are comprised of three bones covered with a highly reactive mucosa—the nasal turbinates. The nose is separated

---

[1]The common usage term, "swallowing," will be used throughout this textbook for ease of reading. Similarly, ingestion, the taking in of food, will be referred to as feeding or eating (as age appropriate) throughout.

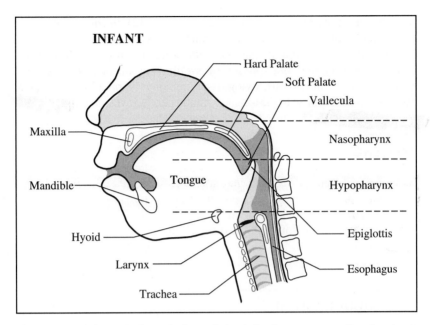

Figure 2–1. Schematic lateral view of the infant's upper aerodigestive tract. Structures and boundaries of the oral cavity, pharynx, and larynx are noted. The soft palate is in close approximation to the vallecula. This anatomic proximity effectively separates the oral route for ingestion from the preferred nasal route for respiration.

into two nasal cavities by the midline septum, which is cartilage anteriorly and bone posteriorly. Septal deviation in the newborn may occur from birth trauma and result in severe nasal obstruction leading to perinatal feeding difficulties (Emami, Brodsky, & Pizzuto, 1996; Chapter 4).

Oral Cavity (Mouth)

The structures of the oral cavity include the lips, mandible, maxilla, floor of the mouth, cheeks, tongue, hard palate, soft palate, and anterior surfaces of the anterior tonsillar pillars. Older infants and children also have teeth for chewing. The lateral sulci are spaces between the mandible or maxilla and the cheeks. The anterior sulci are spaces between the mandible or maxilla and the lip muscles.

The structures in the mouth are important for the oral preparatory (bolus formation) and oral phase of swallow (described in detail below). In infants, the cheeks are important for sucking. When anatomic defects of the lips, palate, maxilla, mandible, cheeks or tongue are present, normal sucking and swallowing are compromised (see Chapters 4 and 12). In children with oral sensorimotor problems, food or liquid can be lodged in both the anterior and lateral sulci, making bolus preparation quite difficult. Muscles involved in the oral preparatory and oral phases of swallowing include the digastric, palatoglossus, genioglossus, styloglossus, geniohyoid, mylohyoid, buccinators, and those intrinsic to the tongue. Cranial nerves involved include V, VII, IX, X, XI, and XII (Bosma, 1986; Derkay & Schechter, 1998).

Pharynx

The pharynx consists of three anatomic areas (Figures 2–1 and 2–2): the nasopharynx, the oropharynx, and the hypopharynx. In the infant, the nasopharynx and hypopharnx blend into one structure, and thus there is no true oropharynx as is found in the older child.

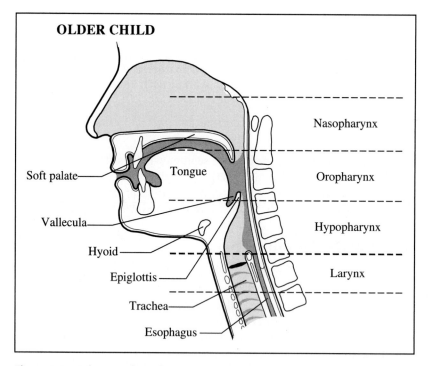

Figure 2–2. Schematic lateral view of the older child's upper aerodigestive tract. Note the wide distance between the soft palate and the larynx. The elongated pharynx is unique to humans and has allowed the development of human speech production.

As growth and development occur, two important anatomic changes emerge: (a) the angle of the nasopharynx at the skull base becomes more acute and approaches 90°, and (b) the pharynx elongates so that an oropharynx is created. The oropharynx begins at the posterior tonsillar pillars and ends at the superior tip of the epiglottis. The vertical enlargement of this space enables the development of human speech. Phonation of a wide variety of speech sounds can thus occur. However, this elongation challenges simultaneous swallowing and breathing as a common, large intersection of the respiratory and digestive tracts is created (Laitman & Reidenberg, 1993).

The walls of the pharynx consist of three pairs of constrictor muscles—the superior, medial, and inferior constrictors. These striated muscle fibers arise from a median raphe in the midline of the posterior pharyngeal wall. They extend laterally and attach to bony and soft tissue structures located anteriorly. Onset of pharyngeal phase is under voluntary neural control and becomes involuntary under the control of cranial nerves (CN) V, IX, and X, which synapse in the swallowing center located in the medulla.

Nasopharynx

The nasopharynx is a boxlike structure located at the base of the skull. It connects the nasal cavity above with the oropharynx below and serves as a conduit for air, a drainage area for the nose and paranasal sinuses and eustachian tube/middle ear complex, and as a resonator for speech production. The boundaries of the nasopharynx are the posterior nasal choanae (anteriorly), the soft palate (anterior-inferior), the skull base (posteriorly), and the hypopharynx in infants and oropharynx in children and adults (inferiorly). During the act of swallowing, posterior tongue propulsion assists in the elevation of the soft palate and closes off the nasopharyx from the rest of the pharynx. Anatomic or functional defects of the soft palate may result in nasopharyngeal reflux during feeds (Chapters 4 and 12).

The adenoids are located on the roof of the nasopharynx. During the first years of life, the adenoids increase in size. Involution begins at about age 8 years and extends through puberty. Excessive enlargement of the adenoids may cause nasal obstruction and feeding difficulties, even in older children.

Oropharynx

The oropharynx is the posterior extension of the oral cavity. The oropharynx begins at the posterior surface of the anterior tonsillar pillars and extends to the posterior pharyngeal wall. The palatine tonsils are attached to the lateral pharyngeal walls between the anterior and posterior tonsillar pillars. The superior boundary of the oropharynx is parallel to the pharyngeal aspect of the soft palate in a line extending back to the posterior pharyngeal wall. The inferior boundary of the oropharynx is at the base of the tongue and the tip of the epiglottis. The vallecula is a wedge-shaped space between the base of the tongue and the epiglottis. At the base of the tongue are the lingual tonsils, which, when enlarged, can encroach on the vallecula and cause significant airway, feeding, and swallowing problems as seen when severe GERD/EERD[2] is present (Figures 4–4 and 4–5; Chapters 4 and 5). The lateral and posterior walls of the oropharynx are formed by the middle and part of the inferior pharyngeal constrictor muscles. The greater cornuae of the hyoid bone are included in the lateral pharyngeal walls (Donner, Bosma, & Robertson, 1985). The body of the hyoid bone, located in the deep musculature of the neck, attaches to the base of the tongue. The base of the tongue and the larynx descend inferiorly during the first 4 years of life. By age 4, the base of the tongue is anatomically separated from the larynx in the vertical plane and thus becomes the anterior border of the oropharynx (Caruso & Sauerland, 1990). Because the larynx is "tucked under" the base of the tongue in the infant, no true oropharynx exists (Figures 2–1 and 2–2). Thus, in neonates and young infants, a single line of breathing is created from the nasopharynx to the hypopharynx that allows infants to coordinate sucking, swallowing, and breathing.

Hypopharynx

The hypopharynx extends from the tip of the epiglottis at the level of the hyoid bone down to the cricopharyngeus muscle. Anteriorly it ends above the larynx at the level of the false vocal folds. Posteriorly, the hypopharynx ends at the level of the entrance to the esophagus, which is guarded by the cricopharyngeus muscle. This muscle has no median raphe, in contrast to the pharyngeal constrictors. Except during a swallow, the cricopharyngeus is in a state of tonic contraction functioning as the pharyngoesophageal sphincter or upper esophageal sphincter [UES][3] (Caruso & Sauerland, 1990). The fibers of the inferior constrictors attach to the sides of the thyroid cartilage anteriorly forming a space between the fibers and each side of the thyroid cartilage. These spaces are known as the pyriform sinuses, and they extend down to the cricopharyngeus muscle (Figure 2–3). The

---

[2]Gastroesophageal reflux disease (GERD) refers to the abnormal regurgitation of acid into the esophagus causing symptoms. When acid and other stomach contents emerge from the esophagus into the pharynx, larynx, mouth, and nasal cavities, the most commonly accepted term is extra-esophageal reflux disease (EERD) (Sasaki & Toohill, 2000).

[3]Terminology is rapidly changing in this field. For purposes of this book, the more familiar term *upper esophageal sphincter* (UES) will be used.

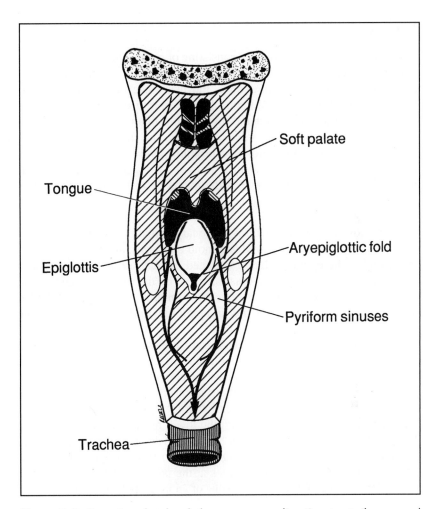

Figure 2–3. Posterior sketch of the upper aerodigestive tract (larynx and pharynx). Pathway for food bolus is around the larynx and down the channels made by the pyriform sinuses, which elongate during the act of swallowing. The bolus is guided through the relaxed cricopharyngeus while the larynx is closed and protected high in the neck, under the tongue base.

oblique fibers of the inferior constrictor muscles end where the horizontal fibers of the cricopharyngeus muscle begin. The lateral and posterior walls of the hypopharynx are supported by the middle and inferior constrictors. The anterior boundary of the hypopharynx is the larynx.

Larynx

The larynx is a complex structure consisting of cartilages, muscles, and ligaments. The cartilages include the epiglottis, thyroid, cricoid, and paired arytenoid, cuneiform and corniculate. Intrinsic muscles of the larynx form the vocal folds (true and false), muscles of respiration, and other muscles of phonation. The thyrohyoid and thyrocricoid ligaments aid in laryngeal suspension and stability. In order of priority, the three functions of the human larynx are protection, respiration, and phonation. Detailed anatomic description of the intrinsic muscles of the larynx (involved primarily with phonation) is beyond the scope of this chapter. Structures important in swallow production and in airway protection during swallowing are described in detail.

The most important structures of the larynx that protect against aspiration are the epiglottis, the paired arytenoid cartilages, and the two pairs of vocal folds. The epiglottis has a flattened lingual surface, which acts to direct food laterally into the recesses formed by the pyriform sinuses. The movement of food is directed away from the midline and the laryngeal inlet. The arytenoid cartilages and the aryepiglottic folds, reinforced by the smaller cuneiform and corniculate cartilages, move medially to further buttress the larynx from penetration. The larynx is elevated anteriorly under the tongue and mandible by the hyoid bone and attached musculature.

The valvelike function provided by the paired false and true vocal folds is the next and most critical level of laryngeal structures involved in airway protection. The false vocal folds (ventricular folds) are primarily involved in regulating the expiration of air from the lower respiratory tract (Sasaki & Isaacson, 1988). In contrast, the true vocal folds do not resist expired air but can prevent inspired air (and foreign material) from entering the larynx. Thus, specific anatomic abnormalities at the laryngeal level must be precisely defined to avoid serious sequelae of an incompetent larynx.

Neuroanatomy of the Larynx

This multilevel sphincteric closure of the upper airway is under control of the recurrent laryngeal nerves. The aryepiglottic folds, made up of the superior part of the thyroarytenoid muscles, approximate to cover the superior inlet of the larynx. The anterior gap is protected by the posteriorly displaced epiglottis, the posterior gap closed by the arytenoid cartilages (Figure 2–4). The false vocal folds form the roof of the laryngeal ventricles and are the second level of protection within the larynx itself. The thyroarytenoid muscles aid in adduction of the false vocal folds. The third level of protection is the true vocal folds, with the inferior part of the thyroarytenoid muscles providing the bulk of these folds. The true vocal folds

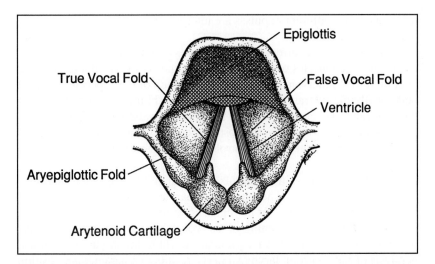

Figure 2–4. Superior view of the larynx showing the intrinsic structures of the larynx. The laryngeal ventricle is the space between the false and true vocal folds.

attach to the vocal processes of the arytenoid cartilages posteriorly, to the inside surface of the thyroid lamina laterally, and to the thyroid notch anteriorly. Muscular pull by the arytenoid cartilages controls movement of the true vocal folds during both swallowing and phonation.

Innervation of the laryngeal protective and respiratory functions is centrally located in the brain stem. This control relies on fine sensory and motor innervation to the region. Sensory innervation of the supraglottic and glottic areas is provided by the internal branch of the superior laryngeal nerve, a branch of the vagus nerve (CN X). The recurrent laryngeal nerve (also from CN X) provides sensory innervation to the subglottic mucosa. The posterior part of the true vocal folds and the superior surface of the epiglottis appear to be the most densely innervated part of the larynx (Sasaki & Isaacson, 1988). Chemical and thermal receptors are also found in the supraglottic larynx and are sensitive to a variety of stimuli. In particular, receptors sensitive to water in infants and young children may explain the favorable response to cool mist in children with laryngotracheitis, also known as "croup." The effect of the mist slows the rate of respiration while increasing tidal volume, resulting in an overall positive effect on the respiratory status (Sasaki, Suzuki, Horiuchi, & Kirchner, 1979). Other sensory receptors of the larynx include joint, aortic, baroreceptors, and stretch receptors. These afferent impulses are interpreted at the brain-stem level in the tractus solitarius.

The ipsilateral recurrent laryngeal nerves (vagus—CN X) innervate all of the intrinsic muscles of the larynx except the cricothyroid muscles. The cricothyroid is innervated by the external branch of the superior laryngeal nerve. Only the interarytenoid muscles receive bilateral innervation from the recurrent laryngeal nerves. All the intrinsic muscles of the larynx are involved in adduction except the posterior cricoarytenoid muscles, the only abductors of the vocal folds. Control at the brain-stem level is within the nucleus ambiguus.

Anatomic changes in the larynx are evident when superior laryngeal nerve paralysis occurs. The lateral cricoarytenoid muscle, a laryngeal adductor, rotates the posterior laryngeal commissure to the paralyzed side. This results in a foreshortening of the vocal fold on the ipsilateral side, which gives an appearance of asymmetry or tilt to the larynx. In contrast, paralysis of the recurrent laryngeal nerve results in a paramedian position of that vocal fold, caused by the unopposed adductor action of the ipsilateral cricothyroid muscle, innervated by an intact external branch of the superior laryngeal nerve.

Esophagus

The esophagus is a muscular tube lined with mucosa that propels food from the hypopharynx to the stomach. The cricopharyngeus is the major muscle of the UES and forms the junction between the hypopharynx and the esophagus. The mucosa just above the cricopharyngeus muscle is thin and vulnerable to injury such as perforation from foreign bodies (Caruso & Sauerland, 1990). The gastroesophageal or lower esophageal sphincter (LES) forms the juction between the esophagus and the stomach. These two sphincters are normally in tonic contraction and keep the esophagus empty between swallows (Derkay & Schechter, 1998).

The esophagus is in close proximity to other structures in the neck and thorax. In the neck, it lies anterior to the cervical vertebrae, posterior to the trachea, and between the carotid arteries. The recurrent laryngeal nerves are located on either side of the esophagus in the tracheoesophageal groove. Other important structures in the posterior mediastinum related to breathing, feeding, and swallowing are the left main stem bronchus, the aortic arch, the pericardium, and the nerves and blood vessels to the esophagus.

The wall of the esophagus is composed of four layers: the mucosa, submucosa, muscularis, and adventitia. The mucosa of the esophagus is stratified squamous, continuous with the epithelium in the pharynx. Intrinsic muscles of the esophagus are found in an outer longitudinal layer and an inner circular layer. The posterior and lateral portions of the longitudinal muscle encircle the inner muscle layer in a spiral pattern. The upper third of the esophagus is composed of striated muscle similar to the constrictors in the pharynx; the lower two thirds is made up of smooth muscle fibers. The pharynx and proximal esophagus are the only regions in the body where striated muscle is not under voluntary neural control. Both sympathetic and parasympathetic fibers innervate the esophagus, although the cricopharyngeus muscle seems to be primarily under parasympathetic control (Derkay & Schechter, 1998).

Anatomic Differences Between Infants and Older Children

Significant anatomic differences are found between the infant and older child/adult (Figures 2–1 and 2–2). These are listed by anatomic location in Table 2–1.

Table 2–1. Anatomic Differences in the Infant's and Older Child's Upper Aerodigestive Tract

Anatomic Location	Infant	Older Child
Oral Cavity	• Tongue fills mouth • Edentulous • Tongue rests between lips and sits against palate • Cheeks have sucking pads (fatty tissue within buccinators) • Relatively smaller mandible • Sulci important in sucking	• Mouth is larger, tongue rests on floor of mouth • Dentulous • Tongue rests behind the teeth and is not against palate • Buccinators are muscles for chewing only • Mandibular–maxillary relationship relatively normal • Sulci have little functional benefit
Pharynx	• No definite/distinct oropharynx • Obtuse angle at skull base in nasopharynx	• Elongated pharynx, so distinct oropharynx exists • 90° angle at skull base
Larynx	• One third adult size • Half true vocal fold of cartilage • Narrow, vertical epiglottis	• Less than one third true vocal fold of cartilage • Flat, wide epiglottis

■ EMBRYOLOGY

Embryology is the study of prenatal development, including the embryo and the fetus. The anatomy of the oral cavity, pharynx, larynx, and esophagus is the result of embryologic processes that begin at fertilization of the ovum and continue through infancy, childhood, and even into adulthood. In this section, the development of the head and neck, respiratory system, digestive system, and pertinent parts of the central nervous system will be described in detail. Salient features of the related cardiovascular and musculoskeletal systems will also be reviewed. The interested student is referred to texts on embryology for further detail (Brookes & Zietman, 1998; Carlson, 1998; Larsen, 1998). Normal embryologic development related to oral sensorimotor function and swallowing will be discussed here, followed by a brief description of some of the congenital abnormalities that present with swallowing problems.

Embryonic Period (Weeks 1–8)

Human prenatal development begins at fertilization with formation of a zygote. The zygote is a diploid cell containing 46 chromosomes with half from the mother and half from the father. Fertilization of the egg is completed within 24 hours of ovulation. Repeated mitotic divisions of the zygote result in a rapid increase in the number of cells. By the 3rd week, three germ layers (ectoderm, mesoderm, and endoderm) are formed from which all tissues and organs of the embryo develop. The ectoderm gives rise to the epidermis and the nervous system. The mesoderm gives rise to smooth muscle, connective tissue, and blood vessels. The endoderm gives rise to the epithelial linings of respiratory and digestive systems.

During the 3rd week, the central nervous system and the cardiovascular system begin to form. The neural plate, which is the origin of the central nervous system, gives rise to the neural folds and the beginning of the neural tube. The neural crest consists of neuroectodermal cells that form a mass between the neural tube and the overlying surface ectoderm. The neural crest gives rise to the sensory ganglia of the cranial and spinal nerves, as well as to several skeletal and muscular components in the head and neck region.

All major organ systems are formed during the 4th to 8th weeks of development. During the 4th week, the trilaminar embryonic disc forms into a C-shaped cylindrical embryo, which later becomes the head, tail, and lateral folds. The dorsal part of the yolk sac becomes incorporated into the embryo and gives rise to the primitive gut (Moore, 1988). Infolding at the head region yields the oropharyngeal membrane. The heart is carried ventrally, and the developing brain is at the most cranial part of the embryo. By the end of the 8th week, the embryo begins to have a human appearance.

Fetal Period (Week 9 to Birth)

The fetal period begins in the 9th week and is primarily marked by rapid body growth, with relatively slower head growth compared with the rest of the body. Differentiation of tissues and organs continues during this time. A brief description of major embryologic changes is followed by more detailed information regarding systems directly involved in swallowing.

9 to 12 Weeks

At the beginning of the 9th week, the head makes up half the length of the fetus, measured from the crown to the rump (Caruso & Sauerland, 1990). At 9 weeks, the face is broad, with widely separated eyes, fused eyelids, and low-set ears. The legs are short with relatively small thighs. By the end of 12 weeks, the upper limbs will have almost reached the final relative lengths, although lower limbs are still slightly shorter than the final relative lengths.

13 to 16 Weeks

By the 13th week, body length has more than doubled. Body growth occurs so rapidly that by the 16th week, the head is relatively small compared with the end of the 12th week. Ossification of the skeleton begins during this period.

17 to 20 Weeks

Somatic growth slows down, but length continues to increase. Fetal movements are beginning to be felt by the mother. Eyebrows and head hair become visible at 20 weeks.

21 to 25 Weeks

Substantial weight gain occurs during this time. By 24 weeks, the lungs begin producing surfactant, which is a surface-active lipid that maintains the patency of the developing alveoli of the lungs. However, the respiratory system is still very immature and unable to sustain life independently. If born at this premature stage, however, surfactant replacement therapy has allowed some of these premature infants to survive.

26 to 29 Weeks

The lungs are capable of breathing air, but with some difficulty. The central nervous system is beginning to mature, and rhythmic breathing movements are possible although not present in all infants. Control of body temperature begins. The eyes are open at the beginning of this period.

30 to 34 Weeks

By 30 weeks, the pupillary light reflex of the eyes can be elicited. By 34 weeks, white fat in the body makes up about 8% of body weight. The presence of white fat is a developmental milestone for normal feeding potential because the infant then begins to show some nutritional reserves. Body temperature regulation is more stable by 34 to 35 weeks.

35 to 40 Weeks

At 36 weeks, the circumferences of the head and the abdomen are approximately equal. After 36 weeks, the abdomen circumference may be greater than that of the head. Although at full term the head is much smaller relative to the rest of the body than it was during early fetal life, it is still one of the largest components of the newborn.

The expected time of birth is 38 weeks after fertilization (gestational age or postconceptual age) or 40 weeks after the last menstrual period. By full term, the amount of white body fat should be about 16% of body weight.

Head and Neck Development

Branchial Apparatus Development

The head and neck are developed from the branchial apparatus, which consists of branchial arches, pharyngeal pouches, branchial grooves, and branchial membranes. Branchial arches are derived from the neural crest cells and begin to develop early in the 4th week, as the neural crest cells migrate into the future head and neck region. By the end of the 4th week, four pairs of branchial arches are visible (Figure 2–5). The fifth and sixth pairs are too small to be seen on the surface of the embryo. The branchial arches are separated by the branchial grooves, which are seen as prominent clefts in the embryo.

The branchial arches contribute to formation of the face, neck, nasal cavities, mouth, larynx, and pharynx, with the muscular components forming striated muscles in the head and neck. The cranial nerve supply for each branchial arch, along with the skeletal structures and muscles derived from the branchial arch components are described in Table 2–2.

Facial Development

The mandible is the first structure to form by the merging of the medial ends of the two mandibular prominences of the first branchial arch during the 4th week. Maxillary prominences of the first branchial arch grow medially

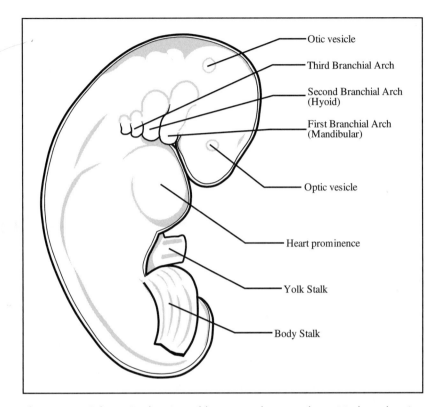

Figure 2–5. Schematic drawing of human embryo at about 28 days showing early branchial apparatus relationships. Four pairs of branchial arches can be seen with their respective branchial grooves.

toward each other, as do the medial nasal prominences soon thereafter. The auricles of the external ear begin to develop by the end of the 5th week. As the brain enlarges, a prominent forehead is noted, the eyes move medially, and the external ears ascend. At 16 weeks, the eyes begin to migrate and are situated anteriorly rather than laterally. The ears are closer to their final position at the sides of the head.

The medial and lateral nasal prominences are formed by growth of the surrounding mesenchyme, which results in formation of primitive nasal sacs. The nasal cavity is separated from the oral cavity by the oronasal membrane (Figure 2–6), which ruptures at about 6 weeks. This rupture that forms the primitive choanae brings the nasal and oral cavities into direct communication. If the oronasal membrane does not rupture, a choanal atresia will

Table 2–2. Skeletal Structures and Muscles Derived From Branchial Arch Components

Arch	Cranial Nerves	Structures	Muscles
First (mandibular)	Trigeminal (V)	• Mandible • Maxilla • Malleus, incus • Zygomatic bone • Temporal bone (squamous portion)	• Muscles of mastication • Mylohyoid and anterior belly of digastric • Tensor tympani • Tensor veli palatini

Second (hyoid)	Facial (VII)	• Stapes
		• Styloid process
		• Hyoid bone
		  (Lesser cornu)
		  (Upper body)
			• Muscles of facial expression
			• Stapedius
			• Stylohyoid
			• Posterior belly of digastric

Third	Glossopharyngeal (IX)
	Hypoglossal (XII)
		• Hyoid bone
		  (Greater cornu)
		  (Inferior body)
		• Posterior one third of tongue
		• Epiglottis
			• Stylopharyngeus

Fourth & Sixth	Vagus (X) SLN RLN	• Tongue • Laryngeal cartilages • Epiglottis (fourth)	• Palatoglossus • Cricothyroid • Levator veli palatini • Pharyngeal constrictors • Intrinsic muscles of larynx • Striated muscles of esophagus

Note. Adapted from The Branchial Apparatus and the Head and Neck. In *The Developing Human* (4th ed., p. 173), by K. L. Moore. Philadelphia: W. B. Saunders, 1988.

SLN = superior laryngeal nerve; RLN = recurrent laryngeal nerve.

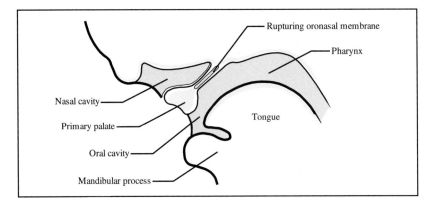

Figure 2–6. Schematic sagittal section showing oronasal membrane, which separates the nasal and oral cavities. At about 6 weeks, the oronasal membrane ruptures to form the primitive choanae. This brings the nasal and oral cavities into direct communication.

make it impossible for an infant to suck, swallow, and breathe synchronously (Chapter 4). The posterior nasal choanae are located at the junction of the nasal cavity and the nasopharynx once the development of the palate is completed.

Palatal development begins toward the end of the 5th week and is completed in the 12th week (Figure 2–7). Development occurs from the anterior to the posterior direction, as mesenchymal masses merge toward the midline. The primary palate, or medial palatine process, develops at the end of the 5th week and is fused by the end of the 6th week to become the premaxillary part of the maxilla. The primary palate gives rise to a very small part of the adult hard palate, the portion anterior to the incisive foramen. The secondary palate develops from two horizontal lateral palatine processes that fuse over the course of a few weeks from the incisive foramen posterior to the soft palate and uvula. The hard palate is fused by 9 weeks, and the soft palate is completed by the 12th week.

The nasal septum develops downward from the merged medial nasal prominences. During the 9th week, the fusion between the nasal septum and the palatine processes begins anteriorly and is completed at the posterior portion of the soft palate by the 12th week. This process occurs in conjunction with the fusion of the lateral palatine processes. The palatine processes fuse about a week later in female than in male fetuses, which may explain why isolated cleft palate is more common in female infants (Burdi, 1969). As the jaws and the neck develop, the tongue descends and occupies

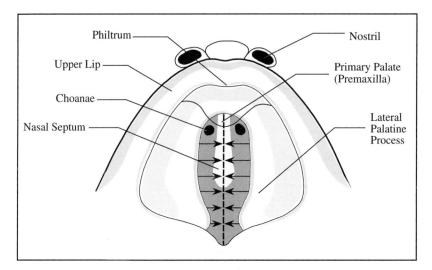

Figure 2–7. Schematic drawing showing palatal development from anterior to posterior. The lateral processes fuse to form most of the hard and soft palate, completed by 9 and 12 weeks respectively.

a relatively smaller space in the oral cavity. The tongue also develops from the third and fourth branchial arches.

Suck and Swallow Development

The pharyngeal swallow is one of the first motor responses in the pharynx, and it is seen beginning in the 10th to 11th weeks of fetal life. Pharyngeal swallows have been observed in delivered fetuses at 12.5 weeks gestation (Humphry, 1967). A suckling response may be elicited at this stage because stroking the lips has been found to yield suckling responses in spontaneously aborted fetuses (Moore, 1988), although true suckling begins around the 18th to the 24th week. Suckling, the earliest intake phase for liquids, is characterized by a definite backward and forward movement of the tongue, with the backward phase more pronounced (Figure 2–8). Tongue protrusion does not extend beyond the border of the lips (Morris & Klein, 1987). By the 34th week, most healthy fetuses, if born at that time, can suckle and swallow well enough to sustain nutritional needs via the oral route. Some infants appear coordinated enough to begin oral feedings by 32 to 33 weeks gestation (Cagan, 1995). Decreased rates of fetal suckling are

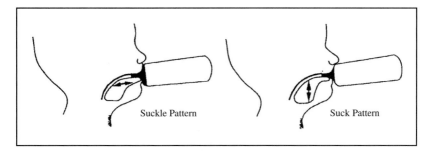

Figure 2–8. Sketch showing suckling and sucking comparisons of tongue and mandibular action. Suckling is characterized by in–out tongue movements and some jaw opening and closing; sucking is characterized by up–down tongue movements and less vertical jaw action.

associated with alimentary tract obstruction or neurologic damage, the latter of which manifests as intrauterine growth retardation (Derkay & Schechter, 1998). It is estimated that 450 ml of the total 850 ml of amniotic fluid produced daily is swallowed in utero (Bosma, 1986).

Ultrasound has shown that suckling motions increase in frequency in the later months of fetal life. The frequency of the suckling motions can be modified by taste. Taste buds are evident at 7 weeks gestation, with distinctively mature receptors noted at 12 weeks (Miller, 1982).

Digestive System Development

The endoderm of the primitive gut, which forms in the 4th week, gives rise to most of the epithelium and glands of the digestive tract. The muscles, connective tissue, and other layers comprising the wall of the digestive tract are derived from the splanchnic mesenchyme (loosely organized connective tissue) surrounding the endodermal primitive gut. The foregut, midgut, and hindgut make up the primitive gut.

The derivatives of the foregut include the pharynx and its derivatives, respiratory system, esophagus, stomach, duodenum (up to the opening of the bile duct), liver, pancreas, and the biliary apparatus (gallbladder and biliary duct system). The celiac artery supplies all derivatives except the pharynx, respiratory tract, and most of the esophagus.

The esophagus elongates rapidly and reaches its final relative length by the 7th week. Although the upper third of the esophagus is made up of striated muscle and the lower two thirds of smooth or nonstriated muscle, there is a transition region between the cervical and thoracic levels where striated and smooth muscle fibers intermingle. Both types of muscle are inner-vated by branches of the vagus nerve (CN X).

Respiratory System Development

The respiratory system begins to develop during the 4th week by formation of a median laryngotracheal groove in the caudal end of the ventral wall of the primitive pharynx. This laryngotracheal groove develops into a laryngo-tracheal diverticulum that then becomes separated from the primitive pharynx (cranial part of the foregut) by longitudinal tracheoesophageal folds. During the 4th and 5th weeks, these folds fuse and form the tracheo-esophageal septum, which is a partition dividing the foregut into a ventral and a dorsal portion. The ventral portion is the laryngotracheal tube that eventually becomes the larynx, trachea, bronchi, and lungs. The dorsal por-tion becomes the esophagus. It is clear from these early embryologic changes that the airway and digestive systems are inextricably related because they initially develop from the same embryonic structure.

Laryngeal Development

The opening of the laryngotracheal tube into the pharynx becomes the prim-itive glottis. The laryngeal cartilages and muscles are derived from the fourth and sixth pairs of branchial arches (Table 2–2). The epithelium of the mucous membrane lining of the larynx develops from the endoderm of the cranial end of the laryngotracheal tube. The mesenchyme proliferates rap-idly at the cranial end of the laryngotracheal tube to produce paired ary-tenoid swellings at 5 weeks (Figure 2–9A). The primitive glottis (Figure 2–9B), a slitlike opening, is converted into a T-shaped opening as the ary-tenoid swellings grow toward the tongue (Figure 2–9C). This action reduces the developing laryngeal lumen again to a narrow slit. The laryngeal lumen is temporarily occluded by rapid proliferation of the laryngeal epithelium. By the 10th week, recanalization of the larynx occurs (Figure 2–9D). The epiglottis develops from the caudal part of the hypobranchial eminence. This eminence is produced by proliferation of mesenchyme in the ventral parts of the third and fourth branchial arches.

Tracheobronchial and Pulmonary Development

The laryngotracheal tube distal to the larynx gives rise to the epithelium and glands of the trachea and lungs. The tracheal cartilages, connective tissue, and muscles are derived from the surrounding splanchnic mesenchyme. The cartilage is in the form of C-shaped rings in the trachea and major bronchi. In more peripheral airways the cartilage becomes more irregular and less prominent. The subglottic space is defined by the cricoid cartilage, the

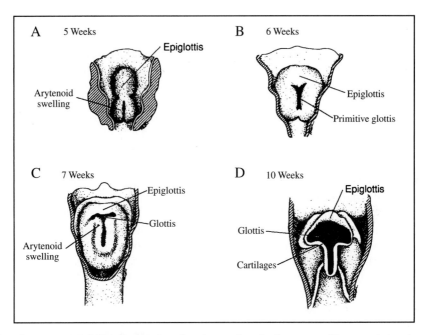

Figure 2–9. Schematic drawing showing embryologic stages of laryngeal development. **A.** At 5 weeks, paired arytenoid swellings develop at cranial end of the laryngotracheal tube. **B.** At 6 weeks, the primitive glottis can be seen. **C.** At 7 weeks, T-shaped opening is evident in the glottis as arytenoid swellings grow toward the tongue. **D.** At 10 weeks, recanalization of the larynx occurs.

only cartilage that forms a complete ring. The respiratory system develops so that it is capable of immediate function at birth. The lungs must have sufficiently thin alveolocapillary membranes and an adequate amount of surfactant for normal respiration to occur.

Cardiovascular System Development

The cardiovascular system is the first organ system to function in the embryo. By the end of the 3rd week, blood begins to circulate, and the first heart beat occurs at 21 to 22 days. The heart develops from splanchnic mesenchyme as paired endocardial heart tubes form and fuse into a single heart tube, which is the primitive heart. From the 4th to the 7th week, the four chambers of the heart are formed. The critical period of heart development is from day 20 to day 50 after fertilization. The partitioning of the primitive heart results from complex processes, and defects of the cardiac septa are relatively common.

Fetal blood is oxgenated in the placenta. The lungs are nonfunctional as organs of respiration during prenatal life. Adequate respiration in the newborn infant is dependent on normal circulatory changes occurring at birth. The modifications that establish postnatal circulatory patterns at birth are gradual and continue for the first several months of life.

Central Nervous System Development

The central nervous system develops from the neural plate, which appears about the middle of the 3rd week. This then becomes the neural tube. The cranial end of the neural tube forms the brain, which consists of the forebrain, midbrain, and hindbrain. The forebrain is the basis for the cerebral hemispheres and the diencephalon. The midbrain becomes the adult midbrain. The hindbrain becomes the pons, cerebellum, and medulla oblongata. The spinal cord is formed from the rest of the neural tube.

The ventricles of the brain and the central spinal canal are derived from the lumen of the neural tube. Proliferation of neuroepithelial cells causes the walls of the neural tube to thicken. These cells give rise to all nerve and macroglial cells in the central nervous system. Twelve pairs of cranial nerves are formed during the 5th and 6th weeks of development. The cranial nerves of the branchial arches, described earlier, are particularly important for normal swallowing. The central nervous system regulates the buccal, lingual, and pharyngeal movements necessary for sucking and swallowing. Further description of central nervous system development is found in Chapter 3. The neural control of deglutition is discussed in more detail in the physiology section in this chapter.

■ EMBRYOLOGIC ABNORMALITIES AFFECTING SWALLOWING AND FEEDING

Congenital malformations result from both genetic factors (e.g., chromosomal abnormalities) and environmental factors, with some malformations caused by these factors acting together. Central nervous system damage from congenital malformations is a major underlying cause of swallowing and feeding problems in infants. Additionally, there may be upper airway anomalies or other anatomic defects. It is estimated that 5 to 7% of human developmental abnormalities result from the in utero action of drugs, viruses, and other environmental factors (Persaud, Chudley, & Skalko, 1985). Exposure of the embryo to teratogens (agents that produce or raise the incidence of congenital malformations, such as drugs and viruses) have their effect during the stage of active differentiation of an organ or a tissue (Moore, 1988). Certain stages of embryonic development are more vulnerable than others (Persaud et al.). Teratogenic potential for major malformations is greatest during the embryologic period before the 8th week, thus it is not unusual for multiple congenital anomalies to be present in the infant who is exposed to a teratogen.

Injuries early in gestation are generally more severe for two reasons. First, little or no barrier exists between blood and brain, so chemicals enter the brain easily. After birth, the blood–brain barrier is more effective. Second, a small injury in the early developing brain will be magnified by the effect on the total remaining sequence of development which is dependent on the injured area (Lenn, 1991). Patterns of malformation occur in recognizable ways because the parts of the brain that arise from a region of early injury are malformed after the injury.

Low birth weight and prematurity are other potential complicating factors. Survival is unlikely with a birthweight of less than 500 g and a gestational age of less than 22 to 23 weeks. By 28 weeks gestational age, survival is more common because significant development occurs in the respiratory and central nervous systems from 24 to 32 weeks. The following discussion will illustrate some of the congenital abnormalities that can result in swallowing and feeding difficulties.

Central Nervous System Abnormalities

Central nervous system (CNS) congenital malformations are common and occur in about 3 per 1,000 births. Most CNS malformations are caused by a combination of genetic and environmental factors. About 85% of these malformations can be accounted for by defects in the closure of the neural tube, such as spina bifida cystica and anencephaly (an absence of a major part of the brain) (Moore, 1988). The incidence of neural tube defects appears to be decreasing in certain populations. The use of folic acid in pregnant women has been cited as helpful, but the evidence continues to be questioned (Rosano et al., 1999). Congenital malformations of the ventricular system of the brain may result in hydrocephalus.

One of the most common conditions in childhood resulting from neurologic impairment is cerebral palsy. The neurologic impairment may occur during prenatal development or at birth (Warkany, 1971). One example of specific etiology for cerebral palsy is bilateral cystic periventricular leukomalacia. Defects from perinatal or postnatal events may become evident within the first 2 years of life. The relationships of CNS problems to swallowing and feeding are discussed in detail in Chapter 3.

Branchial Arch Abnormalities

Most congenital malformations of the head and neck originate during transformation of the branchial apparatus into its adult derivatives (Moore, 1988). These malformations usually represent remnants of the branchial apparatus that should disappear as adult structures develop. First and second branchial arch abnormalities are manifest in such conditions as the Treacher Collins syndrome or the Pierre Robin sequence.

Treacher Collins syndrome (mandibulofacial dysostosis) is transmitted through an autosomal dominant inheritance pattern. Major characteristics include malar hypoplasia (underdevelopment of the zygomatic bones), downslanting palpebral fissures, defects of the lower eyelids, deformed external ears, and abnormalities of the external and middle ears (Behrman & Vaughan, 1987). The Pierre Robin sequence is characterized by mandibular hypoplasia, glossoptosis, and posterior U-shaped cleft of the palate (Goodman & Gorlin, 1970) (Chapters 4 and 12; Figure 4–1).

Cleft palate with or without cleft lip occurs as a result of failure of the mesenchymal masses to merge toward the midline. The critical period of development is from the 6th week until about the end of the 12th week. In the majority of cases, multifactorial inheritance is implicated and can be secondary to both genetic and nongenetic factors. A cleft palate with or without a cleft lip has implications for oral–motor function and feeding because these infants do not develop sufficient negative pressure while sucking for adequate oral intake (Chapter 12). Some infants with craniofacial anomalies demonstrate upper airway obstruction, which further complicates the oral feeding potential in the newborn period (Chapter 4).

Tongue Abnormalities

Tongue malformations are relatively uncommon, although there are a few abnormalities that can interfere with feeding and swallowing. Beckwith-Wiedemann syndrome is an abnormality of somatic growth in which an exceptionally large tongue may interfere with effective sucking and swallowing at birth. Children with Down syndrome may have fissures of the tongue and hypertrophy of the lingual papillae (Goodman & Gorlin, 1970). This usually does not interfere with feeding and swallowing. The more common feeding difficulty with Down syndrome relates to oral sensorimotor coordination rather than a structural problem.

Ankyloglossia (tongue tie), which is seen in about 1 in 300 North American infants, rarely interferes with nipple feeding and occasionally with breast feeding (Berg, 1990; Marmet, Shell, & Marmet, 1990). This condition occurs when the lingual frenulum, which connects the inferior surface of the anterior part of the tongue to the floor of the mouth, is short and thus interferes with tongue protrusion and elevation. The frenulum usually stretches as the infant grows. Oral feeding and speech production skills most often develop appropriately. Surgical correction is needed relatively infrequently.

Respiratory Tract Abnormalities

The most common malformation of the respiratory tract is tracheo-esophageal fistula (TEF). This is associated with esophageal atresia in about 90% of cases. TEF is an abnormal communication between the trachea and the esophagus. The incidence is 1 in 2,500 births, with the majority seen in male infants. A TEF occurs during the 4th week of development because of incomplete division of the cranial part of the foregut into respiratory and digestive portions. Chapters 4 and 5 elaborate on the clinical presentations and management strategies for TEF and esophageal atresia.

Diaphragmatic hernia is the only common congenital abnormality of the diaphragm. The incidence is 1 in 2,000 births (Moore, 1988). This defect is usually unilateral, and it is 5 times more common on the left side than on the right. A diaphragmatic hernia occurs when the pleuroperitoneal membrane on the affected side fails to fuse with other parts of the diaphragm. This then leads to herniation of abdominal contents into the thoracic cavity resulting in severe respiratory distress at birth and eventually leading to severe gastroesophageal reflux. The lungs are frequently hypoplastic (reduced in size) at birth. With severe lung hypoplasia, air may enter the pleural cavity (pneumothorax) because of rupture of some primitive alveoli. These infants tend to need extended time for recovery to reach full oral feedings.

Esophageal Abnormalities

Esophageal atresia usually occurs with tracheoesophageal fistula, although it can occur as a separate malformation (Figure 4–11B). This failure of recanalization of the esophagus occurs during the 8th week. With esophageal atresia, the fetus is unable to swallow amniotic fluid. Polyhydramnios then occurs in the mother and intrauterine growth retardation in the infant (Derkay & Schechter, 1998). Immediately after birth, the infant seems healthy and the first one or two swallows appear normal. Soon thereafter, however, ingested liquids are regurgitated through the nose and mouth, and respiratory distress occurs. Esophageal atresia may be confirmed by passing a fine radiopaque catheter through the nose into the esophagus. The catheter will not pass into the stomach in the presence of esophageal atresia. A chest and abdominal radiograph showing the presence of air in the stomach also is characteristic of esophageal atresia.

Incomplete recanalization of the esophagus during the 8th week of development can result in esophageal stenosis. This congenital narrowing usually occurs in the distal third of the esophagus, either as a web or a long segment of esophagus with only a threadlike lumen (Moore, 1988).

Stomach Abnormalities

Hypertrophic pyloric stenosis is the only common malformation of the stomach. The incidence is 1 in 150 male infants as compared with 1 in 750 female infants. A marked thickening of the pylorus (distal sphincteric region of the stomach as it becomes the duodenum) is noted. Both the circular and longitudinal muscles in the pyloric region are hypertrophied. The severe narrowing of the pyloric canal results in obstruction to the passage of food. The infant presents with projectile vomiting. Although the exact cause of congenital pyloric stenosis is unknown, the high incidence in monozygotic twins suggests a role for genetic factors.

Cardiac Malformations

Heart malformations constitute about 25% of all congenital malformations. Cardiac defects in themselves do not cause oral-motor feeding problems; however, infants with cardiac anomalies have increased work of breathing and usually fatigue easily during oral feedings. Hypercapnia may interfere with oral and pharyngeal phases indicating that respiration inhibits swallowing (Timms, DiFiore, Martin, & Miller, 1993). Cyanosis and hypoxia may indicate severe cardiac conditions. Neurologic deficits may further complicate the infant's status with weakness or incoordination of the suck/swallow/breathe pattern.

■ PHYSIOLOGY OF SWALLOWING

The swallowing process depends on a highly complex and integrated sensorimotor system. Swallowing is considered one of the most complex functions because it includes several anatomic areas, has voluntary and involuntary components, and requires simultaneous inhibition of respiration. Neuromuscular coordination must engage the central nervous system, afferent sensory input, motor responses of voluntary and involuntary muscles, the brain stem, and the enteric nervous system. Hormonal factors also play a critical, although poorly understood, role.

The integration of several normal functions further complicates the act of swallowing. These include chewing and swallowing, respiration and chewing, and the pharyngeal phase of swallowing and respiration (Miller,

1999). These functions, along with the entire act of swallowing, are controlled by pattern generators in the brain stem that are modulated by the cerebral cortex as well as through sensory input (Miller, 1999).

The interest in adult dysphagia has provided a rich and detailed understanding of the swallowing process in that age group. Although much of the information may be applicable to the older child, preterm infants, neonates, infants, and young children have additional factors of normal and abnormal development (see below) to consider. For the student interested in the neurophysiology of swallowing, recent publications by Miller and co-workers are highly recommended (Miller, 1999; Miller, Bieger, & Conklin, 1997).

Swallow Phases

For descriptive purposes, swallowing is described in four phases:

1. oral preparatory (also known as bolus formation),
2. oral,
3. pharyngeal, and
4. esophageal.

The first two phases are under voluntary neural control. The pharyngeal phase has both voluntary and involuntary control. The esophageal phase is under involuntary control. The sequence of movements is diagrammed in Figure 2–10.

Oral Preparatory Phase (Bolus Formation Phase)

The oral preparatory phase is voluntary and requires someone to feed the infant or child when age or neurologic impairment precludes self-feeding. This phase begins with the intake of food into the mouth and the formation of a bolus. In a normal infant, bolus formation per se is minimal, and this phase is characterized by latching onto the nipple. Once foods are added, duration of the oral preparatory phase varies considerably, depending on the texture of the food. As children begin to handle thicker, chunkier textures, the bolus formation may last for several seconds. The more chewing that is required, the longer this phase lasts. Oral manipulation of liquid presented via cup varies significantly from one child to another, but usually liquid is held in the oral cavity for less than 2 sec.

Lip closure is needed once the material is placed into the mouth so that no liquid will be dribbled down the chin. Some children may move the liquid around in the mouth before they form a cohesive bolus. The material is then held between the elevated tongue and hard palate. The digastric, genioglossus, geniohyoid, and mylohyoid muscles aid in tongue elevation. The bolus is held in a median groove in the tongue created by the movement

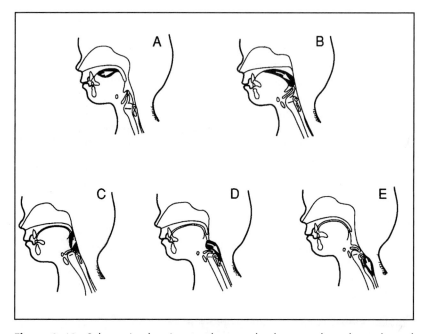

Figure 2–10. Schematic drawing to show oral, pharyngeal, and esophageal phases of normal swallow in a young child. **A.** Oral phase showing formed bolus moving posteriorly through the oral cavity. **B.** Beginning of pharyngeal phase. **C.** Bolus moving through the pharynx with adequate airway protection. **D.** End of pharyngeal phase as cricopharyngeus opens. **E.** Esophageal phase with bolus in the cervical esophagus.

of the intrinsic muscles of the tongue and the lateral borders of the tongue abutting the hard palate (e.g., Derkay & Schechter, 1998). The buccinator muscles help to generate suction in neonates and hold food between the teeth in older infants and children. During this phase, the soft palate is in a lowered position and resting against the tongue base. This position helps to prevent a bolus of liquid from entering the pharynx before the swallow is produced. This active lowering of the soft palate occurs by contraction of the palatoglossus muscle. The airway remains open and nasal breathing continues until a pharyngeal swallow is initiated.

Oral Phase

The oral phase, also under voluntary neural control, begins with the posterior propulsion of the food bolus by the tongue and ends with the onset of a pharyngeal swallow. The voluntary actions in manipulating a bolus of food or liquid include elevation and posterior movement of the tongue, aided in part by the styloglossus muscle. Sequential contact of the tongue to the hard and soft palate occurs. Propulsion of the bolus into the pharynx then results. Elevation of the soft palate against the posterior pharyngeal wall seals the nasopharynx and prevents nasopharyngeal reflux. The oral phase timing does not vary according to texture and is minimal in infants and less than 1 sec in normal children. The precise anatomic location of the pharyngeal trigger has not been determined but may be at the anterior tonsillar pillars, base of tongue, vallecula, or the pyriform sinuses (Derkay & Schechter, 1998).

Sensory input and feedback during the bolus formation and oral phases are critical to normal swallowing. The rich and diverse sensors include mechanoreceptors (touch, pressure), pain receptors, proprioceptive receptors (shape, location), chemical receptors, and special receptors for taste, smell, and temperature. Interestingly, water is perceived differently than other liquids, particularly in the oropharynx (Miller, 1999). Mechanoreceptors located in the tongue, teeth, soft palate, and hard palate help to modulate the muscles of mastication through brain-stem integrative pathways.

Pharyngeal Phase

Pharyngeal phase function is critical because the potential for aspiration is greatest in this phase of the swallow. Tongue base propulsion is an important basis for pharyngeal swallow onset. The pharyngeal phase begins with the voluntary production of a swallow and the elevation of the soft palate to close off the nasopharynx. Pharyngeal constrictors contract to propel the bolus through the pharynx. Simultaneously, the larynx is closed to protect the airway. There is no interruption of the posterior bolus movement with normal swallowing.

From a biomechanical perspective, the pharyngeal phase of swallowing can be divided into six steps (Miller, 1999):

1. elevation and retraction of the soft palate that results in closure of the nasopharynx,
2. opening of the UES (relaxation and passive opening with anterior laryngeal movement),
3. laryngeal closure at the level of the laryngeal vestibule,
4. tongue loading or ramping,
5. tongue propulsion, and
6. pharyngeal clearance.

It was thought that the mylohyoid muscle initiates this series of steps; however, the genioglossus may be the first tongue muscle to start the pharyngeal swallow (Miller, 1999).

As the swallow occurs, the larynx engages several mechanisms to provide protection:

1. respiration ceases;
2. laryngeal elevation and anterior movement supported by the hyoid bone bring the larynx under the base of the tongue;
3. the epiglottis diverts food laterally into the pyriform sinuses, which open into the esophageal inlet during simultaneous cricopharyngeal (UES) opening;
4. aryepiglottic folds move in an anterior and medial direction to cover the glottis;
5. false vocal folds adduct; and
6. true vocal folds adduct.

The most important protection is the complete and automatic closure of the larynx during swallowing. Contrary to popular belief, the epiglottis is not absolutely essential for glottic closure or for the prevention of aspiration; however, it does play an important and active role. The epiglottis is brought down over the glottis during swallowing and deflects the bolus of swallowed material laterally and posteriorly toward the esophagus.

High-speed cineradiography has been used to distinguish two steps in closure of the laryngeal vestibule (as opposed to the glottis) during swallowing. The first step observed was closure of the supraglottic space of the laryngeal vestibule. Apposition of the lateral walls seemed to be caused by contraction and thickening of the superior portion of the thyroarytenoid muscles (Ekberg, 1982). The second step was compression of the subepiglottic space from above as the posterior tongue movement brought the epiglottis down over the laryngeal vestibule. This sequence of events supported the observation that a peristaltic-like motion can clear the vestibule of bolus material. Therefore, when the vestibule is open after a swallow, it is free from any residue of foreign particles.

Normally an infant swallows about six times per minute while awake and six times per hour while asleep. However, in infants a safe swallow is aided by the apnea-induced sustained laryngeal closure. This mechanism is very effective in protecting the larynx from aspiration. During an apnea event, the swallowing rate increases, presumably to clear secretions from the airway before another breath is drawn (Loughlin & Lefton-Greif, 1994).

The second major protective mechanism for the airway is the cough reflex. Cough is triggered by sensation receptors stimulated in both the larynx and the subglottic space and transmitted to the brain stem by the vagus nerve (CN X). Immediately upon stimulation of these receptors, the glottis is closed and an explosive cough follows. The glottic closure reflex also aids in protecting the larynx from noxious stimuli (Chapter 4).

During swallowing, as the epiglottis moves posteriorly and inferiorly, contraction of intrinsic laryngeal muscles brings together the arytenoids, epiglottis, and the false and true vocal folds. Simultaneously, the larynx is elevated and pulled forward, away from the path of the bolus. Laryngeal function during swallow has been examined in healthy young adults via frame-by-frame analysis of concurrent transnasal videoendoscopy, video-fluoroscopy, pharyngeal intraluminal manometry, and submental surface electromyography (Shaker, Dodds, Dantas, Hogan, & Arndorfer, 1990). Four sequential events associated with laryngeal closure were noted: (a) adduction of the true vocal folds associated with the horizontal approximation of arytenoid cartilages, (b) vertical approximation of the arytenoids to the base of the epiglottis, (c) laryngeal elevation, and (d) epiglottal descent. The onset of vocal fold adduction was the first event to occur in the oropharyngeal swallow sequence. Shaker and colleagues (1990) noted that the mere introduction of liquid into the mouth frequently caused the vocal folds to adduct partially, suggesting that there may be sensory afferent fibers within the oral cavity that trigger the laryngeal closure protective mechanism. A simple oroglottal reflex or higher brain-stem function may be involved.

Maximal vocal fold adduction preceded the appearance of the peristaltic wave in the oropharynx. The most striking finding by Shaker et al. (1990) was that true vocal fold closure was the first event to occur in the oropharyngeal swallow sequence and that it persisted throughout the sequence. The vocal fold closure results primarily from contraction of the intrinsic laryngeal adductor muscles, specifically the thyroarytenoids, lateral cricoarytenoids, interarytenoids, and cricothyroids. Previous studies (Barclay, 1930; Sasaki & Isaacson, 1988; Sasaki & Masafumi, 1976) showed that the false vocal folds closed during swallowing, but Shaker et al. (1990) found that the false vocal folds generally remained open. More recently published work reported in infants and children confirm that cessation of breathing with laryngeal closure precedes posterior bolus propulsion (Derkay & Schechter, 1998; Loughlin & Lefton-Greif, 1994).

■ AIRWAY PHYSIOLOGY

Coordination and regulation of breathing and eating occur during the first several weeks after birth. During nutritive sucking in the first week of life, normal preterm and full-term infants often experience decreases in minute ventilation, respiratory rate, and tidal volume (Durand et al., 1981; Guilleminault & Coons, 1984; Mathew, Clark, Pronske, Luna-Solazano, & Peterson, 1985; Shivpuri, Martin, Carlo, & Fanaroff, 1983; Wilson, Thach, Brouillette, & Abu, 1981). Shortly after birth, these physiologic aberrations disappear except in neurologically compromised children (Rosen, Glaze, & Frost, 1984).

Normally throughout oral feeds, infants take from 1 to 3 sucks before a swallow. A short apnea may precede such a run. Although full-term infants tolerate apnea reasonably well, preterm infants may not and therefore experience hypoxia more readily, especially if they have bronchopulmonary dysplasia (Garg, Kurzner, Bautista, & Keens, 1988). As the infant grows, suck and swallow occur in a 1:1 ratio, and the infant takes a breath after a burst of suck and swallow sequences (e.g., 10–30 sucks and swallows, then a breath). Mathew et al. (1985) found decreased minute ventilation secondary to a slower respiratory rate in 19 healthy term infants during continuous nutritive sucking. The mechanism of the decreased respiratory rate was thought to be from the inhibitory effects of liquid in the pharynx. Minute ventilation was found to decrease during continuous sucking, with return to baseline during rest (Shivpuri et al., 1983). Infant maturation leads to a reduction in the degree of hypoventilation.

Ten percent of the 150 infants studied by Rosen and co-workers (1984) experienced an episode of hypoxia (sometimes associated with bradycardia). These 16 children were more likely to have CNS abnormalities on computed tomography (CT) and increased end tidal CO_2 during normal respiration. Inhibition of breathing by laryngeal chemoreceptors was implicated because the oxygen levels normalized when the sucking stopped. In contrast, nonnutritive sucking in 32- to 35-week preterm infants has been shown to improve blood oxygenation. It is suggested that children who undergo tube feedings, which tend to reduce oxygenation by mechanisms as yet unknown, engage in nonnutritive sucking during those feeds (Paludetto, Hack, Robertson, Martin, & Shivpuri, 1984).

A normal pharyngeal swallow requires complete bolus transport through the pharynx and through the cricopharyngeus, or UES. This must occur while the body insures protection of the airway from aspiration of the swallowed material. Posterior transport through the pharynx is achieved via coordinated posterior tongue movement, effective pharyngeal constriction, and UES opening by inhibition of tonic contraction (Cook et al., 1989; Dodds, 1989; Loughlin & Lefton-Greif, 1994; Shapiro & Kelly, 1994). Safe transport through the upper esophagus is achieved through precise coordination between bolus transport and anterior superior elevation of the larynx that assists in airway protection (Derkay & Schechter, 1998; Loughlin & Lefton-Greif, 1994; Martin, Logemann, Shaker, & Dodds, 1994; Rogers, Arvedson, Msall, & Demerath, 1993; Shaker et al., 1990). During swallowing, normal subjects occasionally show transient barium spillover into the laryngeal vestibule above the level of the true vocal folds. Aspiration does not occur as long as vocal fold closure is maintained throughout the swallow.

In the young infant, the airway may be compromised by neck flexion, intrinsic hypotonia of pharyngeal muscles, posterior displacement of the mandible, and hyoid bone compression. Airway patency is critical to the infant and is helped by appropriate positioning and muscle tone.

Elevation of the entire larynx occurs by shortening of the thyrohyoid and suprahyoid muscles. The arytenoids come together by contraction of the thyroarytenoids. The epiglottis closes off the vestibule by a vertical-to-horizontal movement achieved primarily by thyrohyoid shortening. These multiple levels of sphincteric action are capable of closing off the trachea completely from the pharynx and may prevent food or liquid from penetrating into the trachea during swallowing. As the bolus moves through the pharynx, it usually divides so that approximately half moves through the pyriform sinus at each side of the pharynx (Figure 2–3). These two portions of the bolus rejoin just above the level of the opening into the esophagus.

The cricopharyngeus is closed during quiet respiration. During swallowing the UES opens as anterior–superior motion of the larynx occurs with contraction of the genioglossus and other muscles of the larynx (Derkay & Schechter, 1998; Shapiro & Kelly, 1994). The resting tonic contraction of the cricopharyngeus is initially inhibited by the swallowing center through CN X parasympathetic fibers (Derkay & Schechter; Doty, 1968). During inspiration, the closed UES assures that no air enters into the esophagus. At the instant of swallowing, inhibition of tonic contraction of the cricopharyngeus muscle allows a bolus of food or liquid to pass from the pharynx into the esophagus. It then closes immediately after the bolus has passed through the opening into the esophagus.

Elevated UES pressure at rest is necessary to protect the pharynx from reflux of esophageal or gastric contents. The innervation of the cricopharyngeus muscle remains controversial. According to Schechter (1990), parasympathetic innervation enters the muscle via CN X, as the source of both contraction and relaxation. Previous work suggested that the constant state of contraction of this muscle resulted from sympathetic innervation and that its relaxation was secondary to increased parasympathetic tone. Schechter gave an alternative scenario and described relaxation beginning when the larynx moves anteriorly and superiorly by the genioglossus and suprahyoid muscles. The bolus is then carried into the esophagus by a series of contraction waves, a continuation of the pharyngeal stripping action.

Esophageal Phase

The esophageal phase consists of an automatic peristaltic wave, which carries the bolus to the stomach. The process of peristalsis moves the bolus through the esophagus and ends when the food passes through the gastroesophageal junction. The skeletal muscle in the cervical esophagus propels the food more quickly than the smooth muscle in the thoracic esophagus. The primary wave goes from the UES to the LES in one contraction. Secondary waves occur and start at the mid-esophagus and extend to the stomach.

An esophageal phase promptly follows each separate pharyngeal phase of the swallow when there is a definite time delay between swallows. As long as the bolus remains in the striated segment, inhibition of the esophageal phase occurs. When the bolus is in the smooth muscle segment, delay in esophageal transit of the initial bolus will occur. An inactive, distended esophagus and continuous LES relaxation may result from rapid sequence swallowing seen during feeding and the risk of gastroesophageal reflux (GER) is thus present. Some infants may have an esophageal phase of the swallow after four or more pharyngeal swallows. The esophageal phase may be delayed until the end of an active burst of suckling. Swallow-induced peristalsis normally propagates at about 2 to 4 cm/sec and traverses the entire body of the esophagus in 6 to 10 sec in children (Arvedson & Lefton-Greif, 1998; Dodds, Hogan, Reid, & Stewart, 1973).

Solids have been shown to increase the probability that a primary peristaltic wave will progress through the entire esophagus (Miller, 1982). LES function is dependent on bolus size in adults with an increased opening diameter and prolongation of the interval of sphincter relaxation seen with larger bolus volumes (Kahrilas, Dodds, Dent, Logemann, & Shaker, 1988).

LES pressure is decreased by various pharmacologic and hormonal influences. Anticholinergics, theophylline, caffeine, nicotine, alcohol, dopaminergics, epinephrine, and prostaglandins lower LES pressure. GI hormones that lower LES pressure include glucagon, secretin, cholecystokinen, progesterone, and estrogen (Boeck, Buckley, & Schiff, 1997).

Mechanisms involved in normal acid clearance include salivation, swallowing, and peristalsis. All are significantly impaired in patients with swallowing disorders. The sequence of events for acid clearance is disrupted by drooling, decreased numbers of swallows, and abnormal peristalsis, all seen frequently in children with oral sensorimotor dysfunction. Delay in acid clearance sets the stage for a vicious cycle of reflux esophagitis.

Normal function of the GI tract is necessary for normal feeding in infants and children. Esophageal motility and esophageal and gastric competence are necessary for a healthy upper digestive tract. Feeding and swallowing problems are caused by and contribute to the development of GI disease in children. Less obvious may be the role that proper intestinal absorption and lower GI tract motility play in the development of dysphagia. For example, the cycle of dysphagia can result in decreased fluid intake. Reduced fluid intake leads to under-hydration or dehydration. The chronically low fluid intake, when combined with relative immobility often seen in the neurologically impaired child, can lead to chronic constipation, resulting in significant irritability during or after feedings and in early satiety.

Prevention of excessive gastric contents from returning to the esophagus and continuing upward beyond the esophagus, into the pharynx, larynx, nose, and oral cavity, is extremely important for the prevention and maintenance of normal swallowing in many infants and children. Thus, the physiology of sphincters, mucosal protection, and the role of swallowing in prevention of regurgitation of gastric contents are described in detail.

The lower esophageal (or gastroesophageal) sphincter (LES) at the distal end of the esophagus normally prevents free reflux of gastric contents into the esophagus. A definite, anatomically defined sphincter, such as that which exists at the pylorus, has not yet been identified. However, a zone of increased intraluminal pressure in the most distal 1 to 3 cm of esophagus does exist. During swallowing, a momentary relaxation of the LES allows swallowed food to enter the stomach.

The LES muscle is an extension of the esophageal circular muscle of the body of the esophagus. Although anatomically indistinguishable, the area of the LES muscle differs from the circular muscle of the body of the esophagus in that the LES demonstrates a greater responsiveness to cholinergic stimulation and more impressive length–tension characteristics. Pressure generated by the LES is important in maintaining sphincter competence. Several ligaments connect the LES to the diaphragm and may aid in maintaining sphincter function. The closed lumen of the distal esophagus is collapsed into an H-shape and is surrounded by a collection of loose areolar tissue, providing many of the attributes of a choke valve. The angled entrance of the esophagus into the stomach aids LES competence. This angle produces function similar to that of a flap valve. Intraluminal gastric pressure, aided by the presence of gastric contents, may also apply pressure on the esophageal lumen and aid in sphincter competence.

The normal location of the LES is partially in the abdomen. The pressure differential between the abdominal esophagus (high pressure) and thoracic esophagus (low pressure) helps to prevent the reflux of gastric contents into the esophagus. The stomach has a positive resting pressure of 6 to 10 mmHg, and the thoracic esophagus has a resting pressure of –6 to +10 mmHg. A pressure barrier of approximately 15 to 60 mmHg must be generated to overcome the LES and for stomach contents to reach the esophagus. The important effects of abdominal pressure on the LES are illustrated by the existence of a hiatal hernia. A hiatal hernia exists when the abdominal esophagus and part of the stomach rise up through the diaphragm into the chest cavity. The LES is then surrounded by negative intrathoracic pressure. The intraabdominal esophageal pressure differential is gone, and the LES is surrounded by a negative (instead of positive) pressure. Free reflux of gastric

contents into the esophagus occurs because of absence of this pressure differential (Heine & Mittal, 1991; Sondheimer, 1988).

To review, several anatomic and physiologic mechanisms help, in
combination, to prevent reflux into the esophagus: sphincter pressure, the
mucosal choke mechanism, a flap valve, intraabdominal position, and the
anchoring by phrenoesophageal ligaments, especially by the right crus of
the diaphragm. The relative importance of each of these mechanisms is not
clear at this time. Thus, GERD/EERD is prevented by several mechanisms
relative to the esophagus. At birth, the greater pressure in the esophagus is
the principle mechanism of preventing reflux of stomach contents (Boix-
Ochoa & Canals, 1976). In the first few weeks after a term birth, the LES
at the gastroesophageal junction matures rapidly and contributes to the
prevention of reflux. Thereafter, the pattern of esophageal swallow peristalsis is essentially the same in infants, children, and adults.

Gastrointestinal (GI) Physiology

The normal pattern of gastric motility and gastric emptying represents the
end result of a variety of complex interactions. Stomach function is influenced by myenteric neural and hormonal factors. Food volume, physical
state (solid or liquid), and specific food content all affect gastric emptying
(Siegel & Lebenthal, 1981). For example, the stomach empties breast milk
faster than cow's milk (Cavell, 1979). Increased concentrations of carbohydrates and proteins slow gastric emptying. This effect appears to be
mediated by osmoreceptors because gastric emptying is delayed when
higher concentrations of glucose are present (Barker, Cochrans, Corbett, &
Hunt, 1974; Cooke & Moulang, 1972). The ability of starches and most
proteins to delay emptying as effectively as isocaloric solutions of glucose
and amino acids implies that starches and proteins are broken down into
component glucose and amino acids before affecting gastric emptying.
Selective perfusion of the jejunum and duodenum with hyperosmotic solutions has localized osmoreceptors to the duodenum, because perfusion of
the duodenum slows gastric emptying while perfusion of the jejunum does
not (Meeroff, Go, & Phillips, 1975).

Gastric emptying is also responsive to fats. Long-chain fatty acids
have a greater retarding effect on emptying than do medium-chain fatty
acids when equal molar concentrations are compared (Siegel, Krantz, &
Lebenthal, 1985). The mechanisms by which small bowel receptors control
emptying is not established. Both neural and hormonal mechanisms are
possible.

Experimental animal and also human clinical studies have indicated that
when a small amount of acid is instilled in the distal esophagus, nearly all
of the acid material is cleared following the initiation of a single swallow

(Helm, Dodds, Pelc, Palmer, & Teeter, 1984). The low pH is not returned to normal until successive swallows occur, when saliva is delivered to the distal esophagus. Saliva clings to the esophageal mucosa and has an important role in mucosal protection. Saliva diverted by oral suction can prevent return to baseline esophageal pH. Awake adults with GERD/EERD have the same salivary volume and buffering capacity as those without reflux. During sleep, however, the mean resting salivary flow is very low in those who have GERD/EERD. Decreased swallowing frequency during sleep may also be responsible for prolongation of acid clearance time.

Esophageal acid clearance is delayed and requires greater number of sequences in the supine than in the erect position (Maddern, Slavotinek, Collins, & Jamieson, 1985). Subjects with reduced amplitude of peristaltic contractions may require one or two additional swallows initially to clear out an acid bolus placed in the distal esophagus. Esophageal peristaltic waves are sometimes abnormal in patients with GERD/EERD, particularly those with esophagitis. The most common abnormalities detected are reductions in amplitude of esophageal peristalsis followed by abnormalities of transmission, that is, failure of the wave to propagate and the presence of nonperistaltic, simultaneous contractions (Kahrilas, Dodds, Hogan, Kern, Arndorfer, & Reece, 1986).

Patients with oral sensorimotor problems may be particularly prone to the development of esophagitis by the mechanisms explained above. Excessive drooling limits the amount of saliva to the esophagus. Decreased rates and effectiveness of swallowing impair esophageal clearance frequency. All of these situations may interrupt normal acid clearance and predispose to GERD/EERD.

■ NEURAL CONTROL OF SWALLOWING

Neural control of swallowing has been studied by use of electromyography, through lesion studies of central nervous system pathways and peripheral nerves, by removal of specific muscles, and by electrical stimulation (Miller, 1986). The neural control of swallowing involves four major components (Dodds, 1989; Dodds, Stewart, & Logemann, 1990):

1. afferent sensory fibers contained in cranial nerves,
2. cerebral, midbrain, and cerebellar fibers that synapse with the brain-stem swallowing centers,
3. the paired swallowing centers in the brain stem, and
4. efferent motor fibers contained in cranial nerves (Figure 2–11).

Swallowing can be evoked by many different central pathways, even after removal of the entire cortical and subcortical regions above the brain stem.

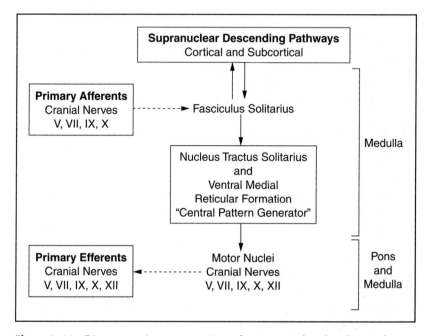

Figure 2–11. Diagrammatic representation of major peripheral and central nervous system pathways for deglutition. Significant afferents that include cranial nerves and subcortical pathways send input through fasciculus solitarius to the nucleus tractus solitarius (NTS) and the ventral medial reticular formation (VMRF) (central pattern generator). Efferent nerves synapse with motor nuclei primarily of cranial nerves V, VII, IX, X, and XII.

This indicates that the cerebral cortex is not essential to the pharyngeal and esophageal phases (Miller, 1972), although the cerebral cortex appears to facilitate the oral phase and the initiation of the pharyngeal phase. Nonetheless, limited information is available regarding the cortical control of both swallowing and respiration (Martin & Sessle, 1993).

Central Nervous System

The relevance of the cerebral cortex to motor control may relate to dependence on the cortical region for the learning of motor responses. Bilateral movements of the face and tongue and repetitive jaw movements have been observed by stimulation of the prefrontal cortex with microelectrodes (Kubota, 1976). Stimulation with larger electrodes and more current over the same regions evokes swallowing (Miller & Bowman, 1977; Sumi, 1970).

Sensory (afferent) cranial nerve input to the brain-stem swallowing centers is provided mainly by the glossopharyngeal (CN IX) and vagus (CN X) nerves, with some contribution of the maxillary branch of the trigeminal (CN V_2) and facial (CN VII) nerves (Table 2–3). Stimuli that induce swallowing vary from one region to another. Taste stimulation alone is a weak stimulus for swallowing (Dodds, 1989), although the degree of sweetness of the fluid appears to be one type of sensory input for infants (Burke, 1977). Light touch is the most effective stimulus at the faucial pillars, heavy touch in the posterior pharynx, and water at the posterior larynx (Shinghai & Shimada, 1976; Storey, 1968). The faucial pillars, pharynx, and posterior larynx are thought of as the origin of the major sensory stimuli needed to elicit a swallow (Miller, 1986). Peripheral nerve stimulation to the posterior tongue and the oropharyngeal region innervated by the pharyngeal branches of the glossopharyngeal nerve (CN IX) or by two branches of the vagus nerve (CN X—superior laryngeal nerve and the recurrent laryngeal nerve) evokes swallowing. Sensory fibers of these two cranial nerves proceed centrally and synapse within the nucleus tractus solitarius (NTS). Microelectrode recordings indicate that stimulation of the sensory fibers evokes potentials within the NTS and in an adjacent region, the ventral medial reticular formation (VMRF) around the nucleus ambiguus, which is a vagal motor nucleus (Car & Roman, 1970; Jean, 1972; Miller, 1972, 1982;). A small lesion within the dorsomedial region of the NTS prevents the sequence of esophageal contractions (Jean, 1972), and led Miller (1986) to suggest that the core central pathway, which controls the peristaltic activity of the esophagus, partially resides near or in the NTS.

The brain stem contains the interneurons essential to the swallowing response. Each side of the brain stem has its own central pattern generator, which is a complete neural circuit capable of generating the pattern without peripheral feedback. Miller (1982) described two animal studies

Table 2–3. Sensory (Afferent) Cranial Nerve Input for Swallowing

Cranial Nerve	Function
Trigeminal (V_2)	General sensation, anterior two thirds tongue, soft palate, nasopharynx, mouth
Facial (VII)	Taste, anterior two thirds tongue, touch sensation to lips
Glossopharyngeal (IX)	Taste and general sensation of posterior third tongue. Sensation to tonsils, palate, soft palate
Vagus (X) – SLN	Pharynx, larynx, viscera, base of tongue

SLN = superior laryngeal nerve

(Roman, 1966; Roman & Tieffenbach, 1972) establishing that once deglutition is elicited by stimulation of an afferent pathway, the motor sequence of peristalsis will proceed in the pharynx and esophagus, even with esophageal transection or deviation of a bolus. In contrast, Miller suggested that peripheral feedback modifies the central pattern generator as noted by the decrease in the number of peristaltic waves by deviation of a bolus in the esophagus.

These central pattern generators or swallowing centers (NTS, VMRF, and interneurons in the medulla) use many of the same cranial motor fibers and cervical muscles that are needed for coughing, gagging, and vomiting functions (McBride & Danner, 1987). These swallowing centers are not discrete focal areas, but consist of ill-defined broad areas located lateral to the midline and ventral to the caudal portion of the fourth ventricle, incorporating the NTS and the VMRF. Sensory cranial nerve input to the swallowing centers provides taste and sensory information from the tongue and oral–pharyngeal mucosa, as well as proprioceptive information from the musculature involved. The swallowing centers also receive input from rostral brain-stem centers, cerebellum, basal ganglia, and higher cortical centers (McBride & Danner). Thus, bolus size, taste, temperature, location, and consistency have well-defined receptors and are sensed at many levels of the CNS.

The sequential semiautomatic discharge of neurons to groups of muscles of the oropharyngeal, laryngeal, and esophageal regions is the most characteristic property of swallowing (Doty & Bosma, 1956). Motor neurons leave the swallow center to synapse in cranial nerve nuclei on the ipsilateral side. The lower motor neurons to the muscles for swallowing reside in cranial nerves V, VII, IX, X, and XII and the ansa cervicalis (C_1–C_3), which joins to run with the hypoglossal nerve (CN XII). The ansa cervicalis innervates some of the muscles in the neck responsible in part for laryngeal elevation. The motor nerves and their respective muscle innervation are shown in Table 2–4. The swallowing centers insure the accuracy of bilateral motor activity and proper sequencing of the muscles involved in swallowing. Prevention of competing muscle activities, for example, speech and respiration, allows completion of the complex motor act of deglutition without interruption (Kennedy & Kent, 1985).

Two functionally distinct central pattern generators appear to be present for the pharyngeal and esophageal phases of swallowing, with the interneurons relevant to the pharyngeal and esophageal phases residing in different regions of the medulla. Stimulation of a peripheral nerve to evoke swallowing elicits activity in muscles ipsilateral to the input, except for the middle and inferior pharyngeal constrictor muscles, which are controlled by the contralateral brain stem. Animal studies have established that once swallowing is elicited by electrical stimulation of an afferent pathway or by

Table 2–4. Motor (Efferent) Controls for Normal Swallow

Phase of Swallow	Innervation
Oral	
Buccinator muscles of masticastion	VII – buccal branch
Lip sphincter and face muscles	Trigeminal (V_3) mandibular branch
	Facial (VII)
Tongue-intrinsic muscles	Hyoglossal (XII)
Extrinsic muscles	Ansa cervicalis (C_1-C_2)
Palatoglossus	Vagus (X)
Pharyngeal	
Stylopharyngeus	Glossopharyngeal (IX)
Palate, pharynx, and larynx	Vagus (X)
Tensor veli palatini	Trigeminal (V_3)
Hyoid and laryngeal movement	V_3, VII, C_1-C_2
Esophageal	
Opening of cricopharyngeus (UES)	VII (primary), V
Peristalsis	Vagus (X)

volition, the motor sequence of peristalsis will proceed (Miller, 1982; Miller, Bieger, & Conklin, 1997). The fact that peristalsis occurs without peripheral feedback from an accompanying bolus indicates that the mammalian neural control of peristalsis is governed by a central pattern generator. Protection of the laryngeal opening from aspiration appears to be carried out more effectively with stimulation of those receptive fields innervated by the superior laryngeal nerve (SLN of CN X). The role of peripheral feedback is not clearly understood. Some authors suggest that there may be both facilitative and inhibitory inputs (Miller & Sherrington, 1916; Sumi, 1970). Miller (1982) suggested that peripheral feedback modifies the dominant central control of swallowing.

Repetition rate of swallowing is modified by both the type of bolus and the presence of material within the pharynx, larynx, or esophagus. The intensity and duration of individual muscle activity in pharyngeal and esophageal sequences vary with the consistency of a bolus and ease of passage through the tract. The genioglossus and the geniohyoid muscles demonstrate a longer duration of discharge if the bolus is of a more dense consistency (Hrychshyn & Basmajian, 1972). Topical anesthesia to the mucosal regions of soft palate, faucial pillars, tonsils, base of the tongue, and the pharynx causes an increase in the time required to evoke repeated swallows (Mansson & Sandberg, 1975). Electromyographic (EMG) studies have shown that esophageal muscle activity is of longer duration and higher amplitude with a bolus of water compared with a bolus of saliva (Miller, 1986). As the bolus proceeds through the esophagus, continuous sensory feedback occurs. Thus, primary and secondary peristalsis can be modulated as swallowing occurs. Furthermore, bolus movement is affected by intrathoracic pressure associated with respiration (enhances movement) and expiration (slows movement) (Schechter, 1990).

Swallowing may depend on a central patterned program (central pattern generator) that is modulated or reinforced by feedback from sensory input, but it is not dependent on that sensory input. Sensory feedback modification of the oral and pharyngeal phases of swallowing may occur as a prepro-grammed modification governed by proprioreceptors in the tongue that sense the bolus size before the swallow. It is also possible that sensory feed-back modification might occur on-line during the swallowing sequence.

The neural control mechanism for esophageal peristalsis in smooth muscle differs significantly from that for esophageal striated muscle. It is generally agreed that peristalsis in esophageal striated muscle is deter-mined by a descending sequence of efferent neural discharges, generated by the central swallow program (Diamant & El-Sharkawy, 1977). Esophageal smooth muscle appears to be innervated by at least two types of nerves (Dodds, Dent, Hogan, & Arndorfer, 1981), although the precise control mechanisms are controversial. It is not clear whether a neural con-trol mechanism of esophageal peristalsis occurs as an "on" response elicited by cholinergic nerves or an "off" response mediated by nonadren-ergic, noncholinergic nerves (Dodds, 1989). Nerve fibers that innervate esophageal smooth muscle originate in the dorsal motor nucleus rather than in the nucleus ambiguus and synapse in the esophageal intramural neu-ral plexus, known as Auerbach's plexus (Ingelfinger, 1958). General agree-ment exists that peristalsis in the esophagus, as well as in the pharynx, occurs as a rapid wave of relaxation followed by a slower wave contraction. The rapidly descending wave of inhibition relaxes the pharynx, UES, esophageal body, and LES in a sequence to allow the structures to accom-modate an oncoming bolus advanced by the peristaltic contraction wave. Gravity assists peristalsis in persons who are in an upright position.

Taste and Smell

Clinical concerns related to feeding problems in infants and young children usually revolve around the motor mechanisms and failure to handle changes in physical characteristics of food, but the sense of taste and smell also have important roles in feeding. The addition of sucrose to fluid (water or formula) has been found to aid in eliciting suck-and-swallow patterns in infants (Weiffenbach & Thach, 1973) and to increase intake over a period of several weeks (Desor, Maller, & Turner, 1973; Foman, Ziegler, Nelson,

& Edwards, 1983). The increasing variety in taste and smell of foods offered to infants may be one of the prime factors in the success of transitional feeding (Bosma, 1986). The interactions of chemosensory cues and physical characteristics of food continue to be studied. This is an area of research that may aid in increased effectiveness of intervention with some types of problem feeders.

Reflexes Related to Swallowing

A number of reflexes relate to swallowing. Table 2–5 details these reflexes, their stimuli, the cranial nerves involved, and the age of disappearance. Some of these reflexes are more directly related to the act of swallowing than others. They include the gag reflex, phasic bite reflex, transverse tongue response, tongue protrusion, and rooting response.

The gag reflex consists of tongue protrusion, head and jaw protrusion, and pharyngeal contractions. A gag reflex is evident at 26 to 27 weeks gestation and is usually strong in the full-term infant. A hyperactive gag may be noted in some neurologically impaired children, although the gag may be difficult to elicit when profound motor dysfunction exists (Love & Webb, 1992). With ataxia, the gag may be hypoactive. There is no direct relationship between the presence or absence of a gag reflex and swallowing ability. The gag reflex may diminish somewhat at about 6 months of age, which is usually marked by the onset of chewing and swallowing of solids.

Table 2–5. Infant Oral Reflexes Present at Term

Reflex	Stimulus	Response	Cranial Nerve	Age of Disappearance
Gag	Touch posterior tongue or pharynx	Contraction of palate and pharynx	IX, X	Persists
Phasic bite	Pressure on gums	Rhythmic closing and opening of jaws	V	9–12 months
Tongue	Touch to tongue or lips		XII	
Protrusion		Tongue protrudes		4–6 months
Transverse		Lateral tongue motion		6–9 months
Rooting	Touch corner of mouth	Turns head toward touch	V, VII, XI, XII	3–6 months

Phasic bite and tongue reflexes are present by 28 weeks gestation. The phasic bite reflex is the rhythmic closing and opening of the jaws in response to stimulation of the gums. Tongue protrusion is noted in a full-term infant in response to touching the anterior tongue. This tongue protrusion begins to diminish by 4 to 6 months of age, permitting introduction of solids and a spoon. The transverse tongue response is movement of the tongue toward the side of stimulation when the lateral surface of the tongue has been touched.

The rooting response, observed as the head turns toward the side of stimulation of the cheeks or the corner of the mouth, is noted by 32 weeks gestation. It strengthens gradually until term, when it becomes more difficult to prevent an alert, hungry infant from turning. Higher cortical pathways cause inhibition by 3 to 6 months of age, when the rooting reflex disappears.

■ DEVELOPMENT OF FEEDING SKILLS

Suckling and Sucking

Physiologic flexion (a characteristic of full-term infants) is observed when the limbs are flexed, whether the infant is in prone or supine position. Thus both suckling and sucking often are referred to as flexor skills. During the 1st month after term birth, infants maintain much of the physiologic flexion as a result of the crowded space in utero during the final weeks before birth. This overall body flexion contributes to successful oral feeding by allowing for attainment of appropriate body positioning relatively easily. Two distinct phases of the suck occur in infant development, suckling and sucking (Figure 2–8 and Table 2–6). Suckling, the first pattern to develop, is acquired gradually in the 2nd and 3rd trimesters and involves definite backward and forward movements of the tongue (Bosma, 1986; Morris & Klein, 1987). Liquid is drawn into the mouth through a rhythmic licking action of the tongue, combined with pronounced opening and closing of the jaw. Lips may be loosely approximated. The tongue moves forward for half the suckle pattern, but the backward phase is more pronounced. Tongue protrusion does not extend beyond the border of the lips.

In contrast, sucking is the second intake pattern to develop at about 6 months. The body of the tongue raises and lowers with strong activity of its intrinsic muscles, and thus the jaw makes a smaller vertical excursion. Firmer approximation of the lips along with the pattern of tongue motion allows for a negative pressure to build up in the mouth. This combination of movements works to pull liquid and soft food into the mouth. Strength of lip closure is a major factor in the shift of tongue patterns from an in–out to an up–down direction. The tongue has more room for movement because of the

Table 2–6. Suckling and Sucking Comparisons

Characteristic	Suckling	Sucking
Tongue configuration	• Flat, thin, cupped, or bowl shaped	• Flat, thin, slightly cupped, or bowl shaped
Movement direction	• In–out movement horizontal	• Up–down movement vertical
Range of movement	• Extension or protrusion no further out than middle of lip.	• From mandible to the anterior hard palate
Lip approximation	• Loose	• Firm
Expected time frame	• Normal in early infancy	• Normal later infancy, childhood, and adult

downward and forward growth of the oral cavity. The action is sometimes referred to as "pump sucking" because it resembles the action of a pump handle (Morris & Klein, 1987).

Similarities and differences can be noted between the suckle and suck patterns. Both patterns reveal a raising and lowering of the jaw and tongue together to create the pressure required to express the liquid and to draw it into the mouth. In addition, the sides of the tongue move upward to form a central groove, helping in formation of the liquid bolus and in movement of the bolus posteriorly over the back of the tongue. The differences between suckling and sucking are noted primarily in the direction of tongue movement and in the degree of valving or closure of the lips (Morris & Klein, 1987). The developmental sequence from suckling to sucking is one of the steps in preparation for oral manipulation of thicker liquids and soft food that requires spoon feeding.

The term "sucking" tends to be the generic term and will be used to refer to the organized intake of a liquid or soft solid as described in the previous paragraphs. "Suckle" will be used when emphasis is placed on a specific developmental sequence of mouth movements. Otherwise suck or sucking will be used to describe those infants younger than 6 to 9 months of age in whom a mixture of suckle and suck may be seen.

Patterns of sleeping and waking usually determine the time intervals between feedings. The process of feeding at fairly regular intervals is a major factor in establishing and maintaining quiet arousal episodes, or homeostasis. On the other hand, arousal helps prepare the infant for feeding. Initially, arousal is noted when gross motions of head, face, trunk, and extremities occur. Respiratory irregularities and an increased respiratory rate are also noted. Incidental phonation is common before crying. Crying may then become prominent with delays in initiation of the feeding process.

Breast-Feeding

The normal suck–swallow sequence during breast-feeding is similar to other nipple-feeding options (McBride & Danner, 1987). The tip of the tongue stays behind the lower lip and over the lower gum, while the rest of the tongue cups around the areola of the breast. The mandible moves the tongue up, allowing the breast areola to be compressed against the infant's alveolar ridge. Milk is then expressed into the oral cavity from the lactiferous ducts. While the anterior portion of the tongue is raised, the posterior tongue is depressed and retracted. This forms a groove that channels the milk to the posterior oral cavity where receptors are stimulated to initiate a voluntary swallow. As the posterior tongue is depressed, the buccal mucosa, supported by the buccinator muscles and fat pads, moves inward slightly and then outward while the mandible and tongue are elevated during compression. This movement of the buccal mucosa allows for the maintenance of tongue approximation to the cheeks keeping milk within the tongue's groove (Smith, Erenberg, Nowak, & Franken, 1985). The jaw is then lowered, allowing the lactiferous ducts to refill, and the sequence is repeated. A rhythm is created by this sequence of vertical jaw movement and posterior tongue depression and elevation.

The suck–swallow sequence is repeated approximately once per second as long as milk is present and the infant is hungry. The infant may interrupt feeding for rest periods of various lengths. These interruptions may be part of the total sequence (e.g., a few seconds after every 8–12 suck–swallow sequences) or they may be at less predictable intervals. Although the vertical jaw movement is a normal part of the total sequence, excessive jaw movement may interfere with effective sucking.

Most infants show a gradual decrease in consistency of the rhythmic pattern of sucking and swallowing with reduction in force of the suck. Breast-feeding infants usually empty each breast in the first 4 min. They may continue to suck because of the pleasurable aspects of sucking, apart from nutritional needs being met. In contrast, bottle-fed infants can be observed more directly regarding the volume consumed in a given time period. Bubbles in the ingested liquid seen in some bottles are gross indicators of flow.

A variety of behaviors may be noted in the time immediately after feeding. Some infants continue to hold the nipple in the mouth and move it around with the tongue, but not with real sucking movements. Others actively resist attempts to remove the nipple by clamping the jaws together or other types of struggle behavior. Newborn infants tend to go to sleep directly after feeding. Some infants give attention to the environment, making this period an appropriate time for communication. Vocalizations can be imitated by the feeder, who can also use this time for talking or singing to the infant in a gentle voice, with the infant held in a comfortable position allowing for eye contact and touch in ways that yield pleasurable interactions. These interactions are an integral part of early communication development, which is an ongoing process beginning in utero.

Transitional Feeding

The transitional feeding period usually begins at 4 to 6 months of age in normal infants. The readiness for varied textures after several months of suckle feeding is primarily related to changes in the central nervous system, along with some anatomic changes. Growth in the upper aerodigestive tract occurs, but with relatively minimal change in proportion or form. There is an increase in intraoral space as the mandible grows downward and forward. The oral cavity also elongates in the vertical dimension. The hyoid bone and larynx shift downward so coordination of breathing and swallowing becomes a factor during feeding. Breathing and swallowing truly become reciprocal activities. The sucking pads are gradually absorbed.

Eruption of teeth may be the most notable change in the peripheral anatomic structures. Mandibular teeth usually erupt before the maxillary teeth, and girls' teeth usually erupt sooner than boys' teeth (Moore, 1988). Deciduous teeth erupt between 6 and 24 months after birth, with all 20 deciduous teeth usually present by the end of the 2nd year in most healthy children. Mandibular incisors usually erupt 6 to 8 months after birth, but the process may be as late as 12 to 13 months in some normal children. Molars erupt from 12 to 24 months and the canines from 16 to 20 months. The erupted teeth are probably more important as sensory receptors than for motor purposes, because biting and chewing during the transitional period can be accomplished effectively with no teeth on the "molar tables." Biting and chewing at this developmental stage is usually described as "munching." The sensory inputs of teeth may be significant in the development of central nervous system control of the feeding process (Bosma, 1986).

The resorption of the sucking pads, eruption of molars, and enlargement of the oral cavity all contribute to an increase in the buccal space. As this buccal space increases, food is manipulated between the tongue and the buccal wall. The crushing and grinding of food is assisted by the molars (when present) or that portion of the gums. Lateral tongue movements are basic to manipulation of food in the oral cavity as food is moved from midline to the lateral buccal walls. It is common for infants to approach their first spoon experiences with suckling movements of the tongue. The anteroposterior tongue movements result in some food being pushed out of the mouth. At times, these movements appear similar to tongue thrusting. Gradually the lateral tongue action becomes more consistent along with the rotary jaw action required for efficient oral phase functioning.

The tongue continues to be a primary contributor to normal oral feeding. Bosma (1986) suggested that smooth food that is homogeneous or with fine granular bits is mashed by tongue gestures focused on the midline of the tongue. As infants mature toward semifirm food, the tongue moves the food to the lateral buccal area, where it is mashed by vertical motions of the tongue and jaw. These manipulations probably are a prelude to molar chewing. The motions of chewing occur with or without erupted molars in young children. Initial chewing gestures are simple vertical mandibular movements. As children continue to develop, the vertical movements become associated with alternating lateral motions characteristic of mature mastication. Mastication coordination becomes fully mature between 3 and 6 years of age (Vitti & Basmajian, 1975). Although the precise developmental stages have not yet been well delineated, normal infants and young children demonstrate increasing competence in the oral manipulation and swallowing of varied food textures.

As the ability to manipulate varied food textures increases, parallel gains occur in speech development as well as in trunk, head, and neck stability (see below). As the brain develops throughout the first several months of life, sensory inputs pertinent to feeding extend into the midbrain, cerebellum, thalamus, and to the cerebral cortex. These developmental processes permit the older infant and young child to gain competence in the evaluation of the physical character of food and ability to manipulate and swallow it. Children who are in this transition stage of feeding may still have inconsistent suckle patterns, especially when they are sleepy, distressed, or ill.

Termination of Nipple-Feeding

Many factors are considered when one thinks about ending breast- or bottle-feeding. These include age, culture, and a maternal desire to maintain the bonding established with breast- or bottle-feeding. By approximately 12 months of age most children have several teeth, along with appropriate central nervous system timing and coordination capabilities to manage cup drinking. Prolonged nipple-feeding has been identified as a cause of dental caries, particularly when sweetened liquid is taken immediately before a sleeping period or intermittently during sleeping periods. It appears that prolonged bottle-feeding with sweetened formula and juice has a greater effect as a cause of dental caries compared with breast-feeding (Kotlow, 1977), although breast-feeding infants also can get dental caries. Prolonged use of bottles, pacifiers, and "sippy-cups" is associated with an increased incidence of otitis media (Niemela, Pihakari, Pokka, Uhari, & Uhari, 2000).

■ NORMAL DEVELOPMENT AND FEEDING AND SWALLOWING

The evolution of feeding experiences is just one aspect of a more generalized development of the growing child. Oral sensorimotor skills improve within general neurodevelopment, acquisition of muscle control (posture and tone), and psychosocial differentiation. Cultural patterns, along with social factors within a family, have effects on the feeding patterns. Feeding is a complex developmental process in which the infant or child and caregivers all play active roles. The role of overall development, including posture and muscle tone and psychosocial development, is described in the next section.

Normal Development of Feeding Skills

Acquisition of age-appropriate feeding skills is critical to the infant's and young child's development of self-regulation, eventually leading to independence. The development of independent, socially acceptable feeding processes begins at birth and progresses throughout the first few years of childhood (Pridham, Martin, Sondel, & Tluczek, 1989). Tremendous strides in sensorimotor integration of swallowing and respiration, hand-eye coordination, normal posture and tone development, and appropriate psychosocial maturation are all acquired during the critical first 3 years. Within an appropriate nurturing environment, high-quality normal feeding and eating skills emerge and assist the infant to develop physically, to acquire cognitive and linguistic competence, and to secure strong emotional attachments with major caregivers. These basic, early skills are requisite for normal physical growth and emotional maturity extending through the adult years. Normal developmental, position and posture, and psychosocial milestones for self-feeding skills from birth to 36 months are shown in Tables 2–7 and 2–8.

Neonatal and Early Infancy Period (0–3 months)

Infant feeding behavior begins with a hunger and satiety pattern interspersed with an irregular pattern of sleep and awake periods. During the first 2 to 3 months after birth, a more regular pattern is established. The infant thus takes the first steps toward self-regulation.

Coordination of breathing and eating takes time to regulate. During the 1st week of life, normal preterm and full-term infants often experience decreases in minute ventilation, respiratory rate, and tidal volume (Durand et al., 1981; Guilleminault & Coons, 1984; Mathew et al., 1985; Shivpuri et

Table 2–7. Development/Posture and Feeding/Oral Sensorimotor Milestones, Birth–36 Months

	Milestone	
Age/Stage	**Development/Posture**	**Feeding/Oral Sensorimotor**
0–1 month (Neonate)	• Learning to control body against gravity • Weight bearing in prone (allows head, neck and shoulders freedom of motion) • Head moves side to side in supine position • Head lag when pulled to sit • Physiologic flexion • Posture to maintain pharyngeal airway • Strong grasp reflex	• Suckle on nipple • Nasal respirations • Rooting reflex present • During feeding, hands fisted/flexed across chest • Incomplete lip closure • Unable to release nipple
2 months (Infancy, 2–6 months)	• Low tone/disorganized, asymmetric movement • Improving head control • Exploring environment • Shifting weight toward chest and moving arms forward in prone • Visual tracking • Sitting supported, head bobs • Preparing background movement for future use (upper extremities coming off surface to function in space; weight shifting to pelvis, and lower extremities move more freely) • Pelvis and lower extremities provide additional support for upper extremities	• Range of movement for jaw • Suckling pattern • Anteroposterior motion of tongue • Mouth opens in anticipation of food • Lip closure improved • Active lip movement with sucking

(continues)

Table 2–7. *(continued)* Development/Posture and Feeding/Oral Sensorimotor Milestones, Birth–36 Months

	Milestone	
Age/Stage	Development/Posture	Feeding/Oral Sensorimotor
3 months	• Lifting head to 90° in prone • Lifting chest off the floor in prone • Weight bearing on lower abdominal muscles and pelvis in prone • Playing in space with flexion and extension of neck in supine • Head participating in final half pull to sit with fixation on examiner • Tolerating weight in supported standing • Early reflexes begin to fade	• Nipple feeds continue • Neck flexion widens pharyngeal airway • Midline orientation • Liquids
4 months	• Gaining balance between flexor and extensor development • Freeing arms for function in supine and supported sitting • Controlling head in prone, sitting • Controlling head in midline through pull to sit • Head in midline in supported sitting • Pivoting in prone • Rolling from prone accidentally • Rolling from supine actively • Playing with knees in supine • Tactile awareness in hands	• Dissociating lip and tongue • Lip pursing • Blowing bubbles with saliva • Increased sound imitation • Voluntary control of mouth

(continues)

Table 2–7. *(continued)* Development/Posture and Feeding/Oral Sensorimotor Milestones, Birth–36 Months

Age/Stage	Milestone	
	Development/Posture	**Feeding/Oral Sensorimotor**
5 months	• Refining head and trunk control • Moving constantly • Rocking in prone • Opening hands • Playing with hands and feet in supine • Putting hands in mouth • Chin tuck to sit maneuver • Rolling actively from prone to supine	• Holding nipple with center portion of lips with balance and stability • Tongue with small range of up–down movement • Tongue reversal after spoon removed, ejecting food involuntarily • Sucking pattern emerging (uses during spoon feeding) • Liquids, eating pureed • Gags on new textures
6 months	• Moving in a variety of directions • Pushing backward in prone • Reaching for toys; transfers from one hand to another • Shows visual interest in small objects • Pulling up independently in pull to sit • Elongating of muscles increasing as infant moves • Increasing upward movement against gravity • Displaying good spinal mobility and ribcage expansion (necessary for adequate respiratory coordination for phonation and swallowing)	• Moving with a wide range of up–down, forward–back tongue and jaw movements • Pushing semisolid foods by spoon out of mouth by tongue • Teething • Increased active oral exploration, with toys, other objects, and fingers • Rooting reflex, automatic bite release are gone • Diminished gag reflex • Longer lip closure

(continues)

Table 2–7. *(continued)* Development/Posture and Feeding/Oral Sensorimotor Milestones, Birth–36 Months

	Milestone	
Age/Stage	**Development/Posture**	**Feeding/Oral Sensorimotor**
7–9 months (late infancy)	• Crawling on belly, creeping on all fours • Full trunk control • Initiating movement from pelvis and upper extremities • Changing position with lower extremities as a base of support for upper extremities • Moving smoothly • Development of extension, flexion, and rotation has expanded what infant can do in sitting • Pull to stand/hold on • Uses index finger to poke • Increased active head and neck to lean forward	• Gag reflex becomes protective • Mouth used for investigation of the environment • Coordinated lip, tongue, and jaw movements in all positions • Drooling only with teething • Cup drinking, lower lip as stabilizer at 9 months • Mouth closure around cup rim • Moving lateral tongue to touch solids while upper lip cleans off spoon
10–12 months	• Full range of motion of upper extremities • Changes position of lower extremities independent of upper body • Stands independently • Learning to walk (cruising) • Pincer grasp (thumb and forefinger) • Smooth release for large objects	• Self finger-feeding • Increasing coordinated jaw, tongue, and lip movements in all positions • Weaning from nipple as cup drinking increases • Easily closes lips on spoon and uses lips to remove food from spoon • Controlled sustained bite on cracker • Chews with up–down and diagonal rotary movements
13–18 months	• Walking alone • Using stairs • Grasp and release with precision • Scoops food to mouth	• Movement in lips • Fully coordinated phonating, swallowing, and breathing • All textures taken • Lateral tongue motion • Straw drinking

(continues)

Table 2–7. *(continued)* Development/Posture and Feeding/Oral Sensorimotor Milestones, Birth–36 Months

Age/Stage	Milestone	
	Development/Posture	Feeding/Oral Sensorimotor
19–24 months	• Equilibrium improving	• Swallows with lip closure • Up–down tongue movements precise • Self-feeding predominates • Chewable foods • Rotary chewing • Independent food intake
24–36 months	• Refinement of skills of 1st 24 months • Jumps in place • Pedals tricycle • Uses scissors	• Circulatory jaw rotations • Lip closure with chewing • One-handed cup holding and open cup drinking without spillage • Fills spoon with use of fingers • Solids • Total self-feeding; uses fork

al., 1983; Wilson, Thach, Brouillette, & Abu, 1981). Shortly after birth, these physiologic alterations disappear except in neurologically compromised children (Rosen et al., 1984).

The position of a normal newborn is characterized by passive or physiologic flexion (Figure 7–5). Alexander (1987) describes the position of the extremities, head, and ribcage. The upper extremities are flexed, adducted, and internally rotated, whereas the lower extremities are flexed, abducted, and externally rotated. The limbs appear basically symmetrical, but the head is maintained to one side with the chin contacting the chest wall. The rib cage is positioned high and elevated in relation to the trunk. Postural control and normal sensorimotor development involve the infant's progression from primitive mass patterns of movement to selective movement against gravity (Caruso & Sauerland, 1990) and the development of stability and mobility.

The single most important example of postural stability in the newborn is the maintenance of the pharyngeal airway. The muscles of the pharynx adjust their contraction to maintain a constant diameter of the pharynx, so gravity does not pull the tongue back into the airway when an infant is in

Table 2–8. Psychosocial Milestones, Birth–36 Months

Stage	Psychosocial Milestones
0–3 months (homeostasis)	• Cues for feeding: arousal, cry, rooting, sucking • Caregiver response leads to self-regulation • Quiets to voice • Hunger–satiety pattern develops • Interaction with primary caregiver becomes established with infant smile • Pleasurable feeding experiences lead to greater environmental interaction
3–6 months (attachment)	• "Falling in love" • Increased reciprocity of positive infant–caregiver interactions • Cues consistent • Anticipates feeding • Somatic functions stabilize • Pauses may be socialization (not necessarily satiety or for burping) • Laughing, smiling, alert, social • Parents are preferred feeders • Calls for attention (~ 6 months) • Means–end: repeats actions for toys, people, and things to evoke a response (6 months)
6–36 months (Separation/individuation)	• Copies movements • Responds to "no" • Play activity to explore environment (7–9 mos.) • Uses facial expressions for likes and dislikes • Follows simple directions • Begins independent problem solving • Self-feeding emerging • Meal times become more predictable • Further experimentation with environment • Speech emerging • Speech very important • Follows two-step commands • Meals are increasingly linked to family schedule • Rapid increase in language • Independence complete

the supine position. Similarly, the pharynx does not collapse when the head is forward and the chin is tucked down toward the chest. The infant learns to control body against gravity with the head moving side-to-side when supine and weight bearing in prone to allow the head, neck, and shoulders increased freedom of movement. Simultaneously, muscle tone begins to develop, upon which a base of stability develops.

Neurodevelopmental milestones relevant to normal feeding at this stage include visual fixation and tracking and balanced flexor and extensor tone of neck and trunk. The infant should be held in a fairly upright semi-flexed posture during feeding. Infant–caregiver interaction during feeds should begin to emerge with a smile response by the infant at about 3–6 weeks of age. The rooting reflex is present, along with sucking and swallowing activities.

The psychosocial interactions during feeding, which occur between the infant and caregiver (usually the mother) begin at birth. The give-and-take exchange is necessary for the emergence not only of adequate feeding skills, but also positive behavior and attitudes toward eating (Satter, 1999). The normal newborn readily provides a set of cues for the caregiver to recognize a need to be fed (e.g., arousal, cry, rooting, sucking). The infant should feed until satiety and then demonstrate positive signs of fullness. Responsive and attentive early feeding is important in helping infants organize their behavior and to work toward the process of self-regulation (Satter, 1990, 1995).

During the first 2 to 3 months of life, the infant's primary goal is to achieve homeotasis with his or her environment. Sleep regulation, regular eating schedules, and developmentally advantageous awake states are some of the goals. Increasing interaction with the environment allows the infant to develop emotional attachment to the primary caregiver and others. Greater nipple control, reaching, smiling, and social play are all fostered by pleasurable and successful feeding experiences. Feeding gradually becomes a social time (Greenspan & Lourie, 1981; Pridham, 1990). Pauses between sucking bursts become more apparent and should not be interpreted as a need for burping or early satiety. Incorrectly interrupted pauses are uncommonly associated with undernutrition (Whitten, Pettit, & Fischoff, 1969). If engagement between infant and caregiver fails to develop, the infant may indicate lack of pleasure, loss of appetite, and, in its most severe forms, vomiting and rumination.

Infancy (3–6 months)

Infants receive essentially all of their nourishment through nipple feedings for the first 4 to 6 months. Breast-fed and formula-fed infants do not require additional types of food through the 1st year. Most infants begin taking other food when they reach the first transitional feeding stage at 6 months in the normally developing infant. CNS maturation allows the graduation from nipple feeding to transitional feeding. Physical characteristics of the face and mouth (particularly teeth) are less important at this stage (Bosma, 1986).

Self-weaning from breast or bottle to a cup is related to the infant's move toward self-regulation. A decreased interest in sucking at the breast or from the bottle often begins at about 5 to 6 months of age. This coincides with developmental advances and increased visual interest in surroundings (Brazelton, 1969). Thus, by 4 to 6 months of age, considerations can be made for spoon-feeding and, usually about 1 month later, the introduction of cup drinking. Cultural variability needs to be considered.

A developmental "critical or sensitive period" has been suggested for introduction of chewable textures in humans (Illingworth & Lister, 1964) and in other animals (e.g., Denenberg, 1959). The term *critical period* is applied to a fairly well-delineated time period in which specific stimuli must be applied to produce a particular developmental advancement. After that critical time, the desired action can no longer be learned. This can result in faulty neurologic growth, resulting in long-lasting, far-reaching negative impacts on multiple systems. The term *sensitive period* is applied to an optimal time for the application of such stimuli, after which it is more difficult to learn a desired action or pattern of behavior. With both normal and developmentally delayed children, there is evidence that solid foods need to be introduced at appropriate times or those milestones of development will be missed. If introduced at a later time, rejection of solids may then occur. The longer the delay, the more difficult it is for many children to accept texture changes.

By 6 months of age, solid foods on the tongue elicit a posterior stripping action of the tongue, followed by a swallow (Schechter, 1990), coinciding with the time when healthy children begin to reach for objects. Children who have motor coordination problems as a part of cerebral palsy or other neuromotor conditions may not yet be ready for solid foods. Illingsworth and Lister (1964) posed that withholding solids at a time when a child should be able to chew (6 to 7 months developmental level) can result in food refusal and vomiting. As described below and in Chapter 13, psychosocial development, personality, and environmental factors may complicate feeding issues.

The introduction of chewable food to a child with developmental delay can be challenging. The time for introduction of solid foods is estimated based on a developmental quotient (DQ) that more or less correlates to a level of functioning. A comprehensive developmental examination should yield an estimated DQ that can be used to determine the expected age of development for chewing. The DQ can be estimated on the basis of a variety of developmental scales (Chapter 3). Most normal children with an average DQ of 100 are ready for chewing at approximately 6 months of age.

Developmental milestones include visual recognition of parents, the beginnings of recognition of small objects (5–7 months), and the beginning of extended reach and grasp. Parents are preferred for feeds, and the child is now ready to assume an upright posture during feeding.

The overall development of postural stability and movement throughout the body facilitates oral-motor development. Postural control develops within a range of muscle tension that is not static but allows for adaptation to demands of the environment (Langley, 1991). For example, by about age 4 to 6 months, increasing head control and midline postural stability enable the temporomandibular joint to control jaw opening. By that age, the infant can open the mouth wide in anticipation of a spoon or a nipple. The jaw remains open in extension until food has entered the mouth at which time the jaw flexors take over. The development of jaw flexor control occurs later than jaw extensor control. Extensor and flexor components gradually become balanced so postural stability of the jaw appears consistent by 24 months (Morris, 1985). The increasing jaw stability permits increased tongue and lip movements not only for feeding, but also "sound" play. Vocalizations occur in conjunction with oral structure movement. For example, as the infant adapts to changes in position or attempts to mold the body into a caregiver's arms, pleasurable cooing or babbling sounds are likely to be produced (Connor, Williamson, & Siepp, 1978).

Late Infancy (6 months to 1 year)

In the second 6 months of the 1st year, four categories of feeding skills develop. These skills include (a) taking food from a spoon, (b) handling thicker and lumpier foods that may require chewing, (c) self-feeding with fingers or a spoon, and (d) drinking from a cup and managing the bottle independently (Pridham, 1990). These feeding skills emerge within the broader context of oral sensorimotor development, hand-to-mouth and fine motor coordination, body positioning, and communication.

Infants communicate interest in feeding by their posture, head and mouth movements, and vocalizations. As noted above, readiness for spoon-feeding usually occurs around 4 to 6 months of age, when a reduction in the typical anteroposterior tongue action for suckling is seen. At age 5 to 7 months, the infant learns to get semisolid food from a spoon, and by about age 8 months, the infant can remove food from the spoon quickly and efficiently (Pridham, 1990). A forward head motion and the use of both upper and lower lips bring the spoon into the mouth. Improved trunk control and a stable sitting posture enable improved head control (see below). It is during the second 6 months of the 1st year of life that position and tone impact the most on the rapidly developing feeding skills. The ability to sit without support is basic to the ability to swallow thicker foods. At about 6 months of age, oral-motor activity is characterized by a kind of munching with vertical movements of the jaw. At approximately 7 months of age, coincident with a spurt in gross motor development, rotary jaw action begins for chewing. This is refined over the next 5 months. The tongue's increased flexibility, especially for lateral motion, allows for a greater range of bolus manipulation before swallowing. The ability to manage a thicker bolus makes feasible the introduction of soft food with a lumpy texture.

New textures should be introduced gradually. Mixed textures in the same bite tend to be confusing to all children, particularly to those with neurologic impairment. For example, commercially prepared baby food may contain chunky pieces in a liquid base. Some children find this difficult to handle. The infant appears unsure whether to swallow it like liquid or to chew (or munch) the lumpier texture. The risks for choking and aspiration are higher with a mixed texture than when a food given in a single bite has a homogeneous consistency. Illingworth and Lister (1964) stressed that it is critical to introduce lumpy textures at this stage of development if the infant is to learn to accept the consistency. Otherwise, as each month passes the probability increases that the infant will resist changes in texture to a much greater degree than a child who was introduced to lumpier textures within the critical or sensitive time periods.

Chewing skills have been shown to vary according to different textures. In 143 healthy children, not surprisingly, chewing time was found to be the longest for solids and shortest for pureed foods. The chewing time for viscous foods was in between the other two textures (Gisel, 1991). Even though the chewing time for solids was found to be longer than it was for other textures, children developed mature chewing skills for solid foods earlier than for viscous and pureed foods. As expected, as children get older, less chewing time is needed for all textures (Gisel & Patrick, 1988).

From 6 to 12 months, infants and their families enjoy a burst of progress relative to the development of posture and muscle tone. As the trunk gains stability, the extremities gain mobility, setting the stage for self-feeding activities. In addition, with neck and shoulder stability control, the respiratory muscles, the larynx, and the oral–pharyngeal structures gain stability.

Alexander (1987) summarized basic concepts that underscore the observation that postural control against gravity is necessary for all other movement functions to occur. These are the following:

1. The development of coordinated oral-motor function directly influences antigravity movements throughout the body. In turn, the development of antigravity movements throughout the body has a direct influence on the development of coordinated oral-motor function.

2. The development of abnormal compensatory oral-motor function and of abnormal movements in other parts of the body also occur in reciprocal ways as in normal development.
3. The repetition of both normal and abnormal sensorimotor information directly influences all motor development.
4. Habitual repetition of abnormal and compensatory movements precipitates the development of abnormal sensorimotor feedback system with negative functional consequences over time.

As positional (external) and postural (proximal and internal) stability emerges, an infant can successfully reach for an object. One arm may be held close to the body to stabilize the shoulder girdle and upper arm (by resting the elbow on the chest), providing external stability. The fingers can then open and reach for the object. As time passes, internal or postural stability emerges. The infant can now reach for an object without needing external support for the arm. Contraction of muscles around the shoulder joint provides postural stabilization necessary for movement of other muscles. This postural stability enables the child to perform distal movements more freely and precisely.

With newfound motor skills, infants begin to exert increasing control over their environment. Transition feeding, beginning at age 6 months with spoon-feeding of smooth purees, coincides with the beginning of the period of separation. As young children begin self-feeding, the mealtime experience broadens from an intimate relationship with a primary caregiver to participation in the social event of the family meal. Caregivers and children typically work toward scheduled feeding times that by the end of the 1st year should coincide with family meal times. Effective feeding includes selection of developmentally appropriate feeding methods, as well as types and quantities of food. Older infants need opportunities to achieve independence in the feeding process.

It is during this phase that self-control must be balanced with independence. Introducing "food rules" for caregivers applicable to children older than 6 months is elaborated in Table 13–2. Once this occurs, eating becomes less of a focus of the child's life, allowing intellectual and social development to prevail.

■ REFERENCES

Alexander, R. (1987). Oral-motor treatment for infants and young children with cerebral palsy. *Seminars in Speech and Language, 8,* 87–100.

Arvedson, J., & Lefton-Greif, M. A. (1998). *Pediatric videofluoroscopic swallow studies: A professional manual with caregiver guidelines.* San Antonio, TX: Communication Skill Builders.

Barclay, A. E. (1930). The normal mechanism of swallowing. *British Journal of Radiology, 3,* 534–546.

Barker, G. R., Cochrans, G. M., Corbett, G. A., & Hunt, J. N. (1974). Actions of glucose and potassium chloride osmoreceptors slowing gastric emptying. *Journal of Physiology, 237,* 183–186.

Behrman, R. E., & Vaughan, V. C. I. (1987). *Nelson textbook of pediatrics* (13th ed.). Philadelphia, PA: W. B. Saunders.

Berg, K. L. (1990). Tongue-tie (ankyloglossia) and breastfeeding: A review. *Journal of Human Lactation, 6,* 109–112.

Boeck, A., Buckley, R. H., & Schiff, R. I. (1997). Gastroesophageal reflux and severe combined immunodeficiency. *Journal Allergy Clinics Immunology, 99,* 420–424.

Boix-Ochoa, L., & Canals, J. (1976). Maturation of the lower esophagus. *Journal of Pediatric Surgery, 11,* 749–756.

Bosma, J. F. (1986). Development of feeding. *Clinical Nutrition, 5,* 210–218.

Brazelton, T. B. (1969). *Infants and mothers.* New York, NY: Dell.

Brookes, M., & Zietman, A. (1998). *Clinical embryology: A color atlas and text.* Boca Raton, FL: CRC Press.

Burdi, A. R. (1969). Sexual differences in closure of the human palatal shelves. *Cleft Palate Journal, 6,* 1–4.

Burke, P. M. (1977). Swallowing and the organization of sucking in the human newborn. *Child Development, 48,* 523–531.

Cagan, J. (1995). Feeding readiness behavior in preterm infants [Abstract]. *Neonatal Network, 14,* 82.

Car, A., & Roman, C. (1970). Deglutition and esophageal reflex contractions induced by stimulation of the medulla oblongata. *Experimental Brain Research, 11,* 75–92.

Carlson, B. (1998). *Human embryology and developmental biology.* St. Louis, MO: Mosby.

Caruso, V. G., & Sauerland, E. K. (1990). Embryology and anatomy. In C. D. Bluestone, S. E. Stool, (eds.), *Pediatric Otolaryngology* (2nd ed., 807–815). Philadelphia, PA: W. B. Saunders.

Cavell, B. (1979). Gastric emptying in preterm infants. *Acta Paediatrica Scandinavia, 68,* 725–730.

Connor, F., Williamson, G., & Siepp, J. (1978). *Program guide for infants and toddlers with neuromotor and other developmental disabilities.* New York, NY: Teachers College Press

Cook, I. J., Dodds, W. J., Dantas, R. O., Kern, M. K., Massey, B. T., Shaker, R., & Hogan, W. J. (1989). Timing of videofluoroscopic, manometric events and bolus transit during the oral and pharyngeal phases of swallowing. *Dysphagia, 4,* 8–15.

Cooke, A. R., & Moulang, J. (1972). Control of gastric emptying by amino acids. *Gastroenterology, 62,* 528–532.

Denenberg, V. H. (1959). Effects of differential infantile handling on weight gain and mortality in the rat and mouse. *Science, 130,* 169–173.

Derkay, C., & Schechter, G. (1998). Anatomy and physiology of pediatric swallowing disorders. *Dysphagia, 31,* 397–404.

Desor, J., Maller, O., & Turner, R. (1973). Taste in acceptance of sugars by human infants. *Journal of Comparative Psychology, 84,* 496–501.

Diamant, N. E., & El-Sharkawy, T. Y. (1977). Neural control of esophageal peristalsis. *Gastroenterology, 72,* 546–556.

Dodds, W. (1989). The physiology of swallowing. *Dyspahagia, 3,* 171–178.

Dodds, W. J., Dent, J., Hogan, E. J., & Arndorfer, R. C. (1981). Effect of atropine on esophageal motor function in humans. *American Journal of Physiology, 3,* G290–G296.

Dodds, W. J., Hogan, W. J., Reid, W. J., & Stewart, E. T. A. R. C. (1973). A comparison between primary esophageal perstalsis following wet and dry swallows. *Journal of Applied Physiology, 35,* 851–857.

Dodds, W. J., Stewart, E. T., & Logemann, J. A. (1990). Physiology and radiology of the normal oral and pharyngeal phases of swallowing. *American Journal of Radiology, 154,* 953–963.

Donner, M. W., Bosma, J. F., & Robertson, D. L. (1985). Anatomy and physiology of the pharynx. *Gastrointestinal Radiology, 10,* 196–212.

Doty, R. W. (1968). Neural organization of deglutition. In C. F. Code (Ed.), *Handbook of physiology. Alimentary canal, 4 (Sect 6),* 1861–1902.

Doty, R. W., & Bosma, J. F. (1956). An electromyographic analysis of reflex deglutition. *Journal of Neurophysiology, 19,* 44–60.

Durand, M., Leahy, F. N., Maccallum, M., Cates, D. B., Rigato, H., & Chermick, V. (1981). Effect of feeding on the chemical control of breathing in the newborn infant. *Pediatric Research, 15,* 1509–1512.

Ekberg, O. (1982). Closure of the laryngeal vestibule during deglutition. *Acta Oto-Laryngologica, 93,* 123–129.

Emami, A. J., Brodsky, L., & Pizzuto, M. (1996). Neonatal septoplasty: Case report and review of the literature. *International Journal of Pediatric Otorhinolaryngology, 35,* 271–275.

Foman, S. J., Ziegler, E. E., Nelson, S. E., & Edwards, B. B. (1983). Sweetness of diet and food consumption by infants. *Proceedings of the Society for Experimental Biology and Medicine, 173,* 190–193.

Garg, M., Kurzner, S. I., Bautista, D. B., & Keens, T. G. (1988). Clinically unsuspected hypoxia during sleep and feeding in infants with bronchopulmonary dysplasia. *Pediatrics, 81,* 635–642.

Gisel, E. G. (1991). Effect of food texture on the development of chewing of children between six months and two years of age. *Developmental Medicine & Child Neurology, 33,* 69–79.

Gisel, E. G., & Patrick, J. (1988). Identification of children with cerebral palsy unable to maintain a normal nutritional state. *The Lancet, 1,* 283–286.

Goodman, R. M., & Gorlin, R. J. (1970). *The face in genetic disorders.* St. Louis, MO: Mosby.

Greenspan, S., & Lourie, R. S. (1981). Developmental structuralist approach to the classification of adaptive and pathologic personality organizations: Infancy and early childhood. *American Journal of Psychiatry, 138,* 725–735.

Guilleminault, C., & Coons, S. (1984). Apnea and bradycardia during feeding in infants weighing >2000 gm. *The Journal of Pediatrics, 104,* 932–935.

Heine, K. J., & Mittal, R. (1991). Cural diaphragm and lower esophageal sphincter as anti-reflux barriers. *Viewpoints on Digestive Diseases, 23,* 1–6.

Helm, J. F., Dodds, W. F., Pelc, L. R., Palmer, D. W., & Teeter, B. C. (1984). Effect of esophageal emptying and saliva on clearance of acid from the esophagus. *New England Journal of Medicine, 310,* 284–288.

Hrychshyn, A. W., & Basmajian, J. V. (1972). Electromyography of the oral stage of swallowing in man. *American Journal of Anatomy, 133,* 335–340.

Humphry, T. (1967). Reflex activity in the oral and facial area of the human fetus. In J. F. Bosma (Ed.) *Second symposium on oral sensation and perception.* Springfield, IL: Charles C. Thomas.

Illingworth, R. S., & Lister, J. (1964). The critical or sensitive period, with special reference to certain feeding problems in infants and children. *Journal of Pediatrics, 65,* 840–848.

Ingelfinger, F. J. (1958). Esophageal motility. *Physiological review, 38,* 533–584.

Jean, A. (1972). Effect of localized lesions of the medulla oblongata on the esophageal stage of deglutition. *Journal De Physiologie, 64,* 507–516.

Kahrilas, P. J., Dodds, W. J., Dent, J., Logemann, J. A., & Shaker, R. (1988). Upper esophageal sphincter function during deglutition. *Gastroenterology, 95,* 52–62.

Kahrilas, P. J., Dodds, W. J., Hogan, W. J., Kern, M., Arndorfer, R. C., & Reece, A. (1986). Esopohageal peristaltic dysfunction in peptic esophagitis. *Gastroenterology, 91,* 897–904.

Kennedy, J. G., & Kent, R. D. (1985). Anatomy and physiology of deglutition and related functions. *Seminars in Speech and Language, 6,* 257–273.

Kotlow, L. A. (1977). Breast feeding: A cause of dental caries in children. *Journal of Dentistry in Children, 44,* 192–193.

Kubota, K. (1976). Motoneurone mechanism: Suprasegmental controls. In B. J. Sessle & A. G. Hannam (Eds.), *Mastication and swallowing: Biological and clinical correlates.* Toronto, Ont.: University of Toronto Press.

Laitman, J., & Reidenberg, J. (1993). Specializations of the human upper respiratory and upper digestive systems as seen through comparative and developmental anatomy. *Dysphagia, 8,* 318–325.

Langley, M. B. (1991). Assessment: A multidimensional process. In M. B. Langley & L. J. Lombardino (Eds.), *Neurodevelopmental strategies for managing communication disorders in children with severe motor dysfunction.* Austin,TX: PRO-ED, 199–250.

Larsen, W. (1998). *Essentials of human embryology.* New York, NY: Churchill Livingstone.

Lenn, N. J. (1991). The basis for brain development, learning, and recovery from injury. *Infants and Young Children, 3(3),* 39–48.

Loughlin, G. M., & Lefton-Greif, M. A. (1994). Dysfunctional swallowing and respiratory disease in children. *Advances in Pediatrics, 41,* 135–161.

Love, R. J., & Webb, W. G. (1992). *Neurology for the speech-language pathologist* (2nd ed.). Stoneham, MA: Butterworth-Heineman.

Maddern, G. J., Slavotinek, J. P., Collins, P. J., & Jamieson, G. G. (1985). Effect of posture and pH on solid and liquid esophageal emptying. *Clinical Physiology, 5,* 425–432.

Mansson, I., & Sandberg, N. (1975). Oro-pharyngeal sensitivity and elicitation of swallowing in man. *Acta Otolaryngologica, 79,* 140–145.

Marmet, C., Shell, E., & Marmet, R. (1990). Neonatal frenotomy may be necessary to correct breastfeeding problems. *Journal of Human Lactation, 6,* 117–121.

Martin, B. J. W., Logemann, J. A., Shaker, R., & Dodds, W. J. (1994). Coordination between respiration and swallowing: Respiratory phase relationships and temporal integration. *Journal of Applied Physiology, 76,* 714–723.

Martin, R. E., & Sessle, B. J. (1993). The role of the cerebral cortex in swallowing. *Dysphagia, 8,* 195–202.

Mathew, O. P., Clark, M. L., Pronske, M. L., Luna-Solazano, H. G., & Peterson, M. D. (1985). Breathing pattern and ventilation during oral feeding in term newborn infants. *The Journal of Pediatrics, 106,* 810–813.

McBride, M. E., & Danner, S. C. (1987). Sucking disorders in neurologically impaired infants: Assessment and facilitation of breastfeeding. *Clinics in Peri-natology, 14,* 109–130.

Meeroff, J. C., Go, V. L., & Phillips, S. F. (1975). Control of gastric emptying by osmolality of duodenal contents in man. *Gastroenterology, 68,* 1144–1151.

Miller, A. J. (1972). Characteristics of the swallowing reflex induced by peripheral nerve and brain stem stimulation. *Experimental Neurology, 34,* 210–222.

Miller, A. J. (1982). Deglutition. *Physiological Reviews, 62,* 129–184.

Miller, A. J. (1986). Neurophysiological basis of swallowing. *Dysphagia, 1,* 91–100.

Miller, A. J. (1999). *The neuroscientific principles of swallowing and dysphagia.* San Diego, CA: Singular Publishing Group.

Miller, A. J., Bieger, D., & Conklin, J. (1997). Functional controls of deglutition. In A. L. Perlman & K. Schulze-Delrieu (Eds.), *Deglutition and its disorders: Anatomy, physiology, clinical diagnosis, and management* (43–98). San Diego, CA: Singular Publishing Group.

Miller, A. J., & Bowman, J. P. (1977). Precentral cortical modulation of mastication and swallowing. *Journal of Dental Research, 56,* 1154.

Miller, F. R., & Sherrington, C. S. (1916). Some observations on the buccopharyngeal stage of reflex deglutition in the cat. *Quarterly Journal of Experimental Physiology, 9,* 147–186.

Moore, K. L. (1988). *The developing human: Clinically oriented embryology* (4th ed.). Philadelphia: W. B. Saunders.

Morris, S. (1985). Developmental implications for the management of feeding problems in neurologically impaired infants. *Seminars in Speech and Language, 6,* 293–315.

Morris, S. E., & Klein, M. D. (1987). *Pre-feeding skills: A comprehensive resource for feeding development.* Tucson, AZ: Therapy Skill Builders.

Niemela, M., Pihakari, O., Pokka, T., Uhari, M., & Uhari, M. (2000). Pacifier as a risk factor for acute otitis media: A randomized, controlled trial of parental counseling. *Pediatrics, 106,* 483–488.

Paludetto, R., Hack, M., Robertson, S., Martin, R., & Shivpuri, C. (1984). Transcutaneous oxygen tension during nonnutritive sucking in preterm infants. *Pediatrics, 74,* 539–542.

Persaud, T. V. N., Chudley, A. E., & Skalko, R. F. (1985). *Basic concepts in teratology.* New York, NY: Alan R. Liss.

Pridham, K. F. (1990). Feeding behavior of 6–12 month old infants: Assessment of sources of parental information. *Journal of Pediatric Nursing, 117,* S174–S180

Pridham, K. F., Martin, R., Sondel, S., & Tluczek, A. (1989). Parental issues in feeding young children with bronchopulmonary dysplasia. *Journal of Pediatric Nursing, 4,* 177–185.

Rogers, B., Arvedson, J., Msall, M., & Demerath, R. (1993). Hypoxemia during oral feeding of children with severe cerebral palsy. *Developmental Medicine and Child Neurology, 35,* 3–10.

Roman, C. (1966). Nervous control of esophageal peristalsis. *Journal De Physiologie, 58,* 79–108.

Roman, C., & Tieffenbach, L. (1972). Recording the unit activity of vagal motor fibers innervating the baboon esophagus. *Journal De Physiologie, 64,* 479–506.

Rosano, A., Smithells, D., Cacciani, L., Botting, B., Castilla, E., Cornel, M., Erickson, D., Goujard, J., Irgens, L., Merlob, P., Robert, E., Siffel, C., Stoll, C., & Sumiyoshi, Y. (1999). Time trends in neural tube defects prevalence in relation to preventive strategies: An international study. *Journal of Epidemiology and Community Health, 53,* 630–635.

Rosen, C. L., Glaze, D. G., & Frost, J. D. Jr. (1984). Hypoxemia associated with feeding in the preterm infant and full-term neonate. *American Journal Diseases Children, 138,* 623–628.

Sasaki, C. T., & Isaacson, G. (1988). Functional anatomy of the larynx. *Otolaryngology Clinics of North America, 21,* 196–199.

Sasaki, C. T., & Masafumi, S. (1976). Laryngeal reflexes in cat, dog and man. *Archives of Otolaryngology, 102,* 400–401.

Sasaki, C. T., Suzuki, M., Horiuchi, M., & Kirchner, F. (1979). The effect of tracheostomy on the laryngeal closure reflex. *The Laryngoscope, 87,* 1428–1433.

Sasaki, C. T., & Toohill, R. J. (2000). Ambulatory pH monitoring for extraesophageal reflux—introduction. *Annals of Otology, Rhinology, & Laryngology, 109 (Suppl.),* 2–3.

Satter, E. M. (1990). The feeding relationship: Problems and interventions. *The Journal of Pediatrics, 117,* 181–189.

Satter, E. M, (1995). Feeding dynamics: Helping children to eat well. *Journal of Pediatric Health Care, 9,* 178–184.

Satter, E. M. (1999) The feeding relationship. In P. Kessler & P. Dawson, (Eds.), *Failure to thrive and pediatric undernutrition: A transdisciplinary approach* (121–144). Baltimore, MD: Paul H. Brookes.

Schechter, G.L. (1990). Physiology of the mouth, pharynx, and esophagus. In C. Bluestone & S. Stool (eds.) *Pediatric Otolaryngology,* (2nd ed., 816–822). Philadelphia, PA: W. B. Saunders.

Shaker, R., Dodds, W. J., Dantas, R. O., Hogan, W. J., & Arndorfer, R. C. (1990). Coordination of deglutitive glottic closure with oropharyngeal swallowing. *Gastroenterology, 98,* 1478–1484.

Shapiro, J. & Kelly, J. H. (1994). Anatomy, histology, and clinical dysfunction of the cricopharyngeus muscle. *Current Opinions in Otolaryngology Head and Neck Surgery, 2,* 52–54.

Shinghai, T., & Shimada, K. (1976). Reflex swallowing elicited by water and chemical substances applied in the oral cavity, pharynx, and larynx of the rabbit. *Japanese Journal of Physiology, 26,* 455–469.

Shivpuri, C. R., Martin, R. J., Carlo, W. A., & Fanaroff, A. A. (1983). Decreased ventilation in preterm infants during oral feeding. *The Journal of Pediatrics, 103,* 285–289.

Siegel, M., Krantz, B., & Lebenthal, E. (1985). Effect of fats and carbohydrate composition on the gastric emptying of isocaloric feedings in premature infants. *Gastroenterology, 89,* 785–790.

Siegel, M., & Lebenthal, E. (1981). Development of gastrointestinal motility and gastric emptying during the fetal & newborn periods. In E. Lebenthal (Ed.), *Textbook of gastroenterology and nutrition in infancy,* (121–138). New York: Raven Press.

Smith, W. L., Erenberg, A., Nowak, A., & Franken, E. A. (1985). Physiology of sucking in the normal term infant using real-time US. *Radiology, 156,* 379–381.

Sondheimer, J. M. (1988). Gastroesophageal reflux: Update on pathogenesis and diagnosis. *Pediatric Clinics of North America, 35(1),* 103–116.

Storey, A. T. (1968). A functional analysis of sensory units innervating epiglottis and larynx. *Experimental Neurology, 20,* 366–383.

Sumi, T. (1970). Changes of hypoglossal nerve activity during inhibition of chewing and swallowing by lingual nerve stimulation. *Pflugers Achiv-European Journal of Physiology, 317,* 303–309.

Timms, B. J. M., DiFiore, J. M., Martin, R. J., & Miller, M. J. (1993). Increased respiratory drive as an inhibitor of oral feeding of preterm infants. *The Journal of Pediatrics, 123,* 127–131.

Vitti, M., & Basmajian, J. V. (1975). Muscles of mastication in small children: An electromyographic analysis. *American Journal of Orthodontics, 68,* 412–419.

Warkany, J. (1971). *Congential malformations: Notes and comments.* Chicago, IL: Year Book.

Weiffenbach, J. M., & Thach, B. T. (1973). Elicited tongue-movements: Touch and taste in the mouth of the neonate. *Symposium Oral Sensory Perception, 4,* 232–244.

Whitten, C. R., Pettit, M. G., & Fischoff, J. (1969). Evidence that growth failure from maternal deprivation is secondary to undereating. *Journal of the American Medical Association, 209,* 1675–1682.

Wilson, S. L., Thach, B. T., Brouillette, R. T., & Abu, O. Y. K. (1981). Coordination of breathing and swallowing in human infants. *Journal of Applied Physiology: Respiratory, Environmental and Exercise Physiology, 50,* 851–858.

CHAPTER 3

Pediatric and Neurodevelopmental Assessment

Brian Rogers, Linda Brodsky, and Joan Arvedson

■ SUMMARY

Feeding and swallowing can only be meaningfully understood in the context of each child's neurodevelopmental status. The neurologic and developmental processes controlling or influencing feeding and swallowing are complex and involve multiple levels of the central and peripheral nervous system (see Chapter 2). These processes undergo significant maturation during early childhood and encompass many "streams of development," including cognitive, communicative, and motor skills.

Disorders of feeding and swallowing in childhood are primarily neurologic in origin. The manifestation of neurogenic dysphagia in childhood is greatly influenced by developmental processes including neurodevelopmental status, airway development, general health, and the environment. The purpose of this chapter is to provide an overview of important neurodevelopmental aspects of feeding and swallowing. This overview will include a brief discussion of central nervous system (CNS) development and associated feeding and swallowing skills, neurodevelopmental history and examination methods, and a review of commonly associated medical disorders.

■ FUNCTIONAL DEVELOPMENT OF THE CENTRAL NERVOUS SYSTEM

Embryology

There are many common anatomic and maturational central nervous processes involved in normal feeding and development. A more detailed discussion of the CNS pathways involved in feeding and swallowing can be found in Chapter 2. Major events of brain development include primary neurulation, prosencephalic development, neuronal proliferation, neuronal migration, organization, and myelination (Volpe, 2000). Emphasis will be placed on normal and abnormal brain development and its relationship to feeding, swallowing, and general development. Malformations of the developing brain are significant causes of severe mental retardation and developmental disabilities which are commonly associated with feeding and swallowing disorders (Capone, 1996).

The process of neurulation refers to the inductive events that occur on the dorsal aspect of the embryo and result in the formation of the brain and spinal cord. This dorsal induction is nearly complete by the end of the 4th postconceptual week. The nervous system begins on the dorsal aspect of the embryo as a plate of differentiating tissue in the middle of the ectoderm. The underlying chordal mesoderm and the notochord induce the formation of the neural plate at 18 days of gestation. The lateral margins of the neural plate invaginate and close dorsally to form the neural tube. The neural tube gives rise to the nervous system. Interactions of the neural tube with the surrounding mesoderm give rise to the dura (covering of the brain and spinal cord) and the axial skeleton (skull and vertebrae). Disturbances of neurulation result in various errors of neural tube closure ranging from anencephaly (lack of forebrain development with variable anomalies of the upper brain stem that are incompatible with life), encephalocele (restricted closure of the anterior neural tube), and myelomeningocele (restricted closure of the posterior neural tube). Myelomeningocele is usually associated with other brain anomalies including Chiari type II malformation and hydrocephalus. The Chiari type II malformation can result in various cranial nerve deficits that may lead to significant feeding and swallowing problems (see discussion on cranial nerves).

Prosencephalic development refers to the inductive influences of the prechordal mesoderm that result in the formation of the face and the forebrain. The peak period of prosencephalic development occurs in the 2nd and 3rd months of gestation. Prosencephalic formation begins at the rostral end of the neural tube at the end of the 1st month of gestation. Prosencephalic cleavage occurs in the following 2 weeks and results in the development of paired optic vesicles, olfactory tracts, separation of the telencephalon from the diencephalon, and the sagital cleavage of the telencephalon to form the paired cerebral hemispheres, lateral ventricles, and basal ganglia. Midline prosencephalic development involves the formation of three thickenings of tissue including the commissural, the chiasmatic, and the hypothalamic plates. These structures are important in the formation, respectively, of the corpus callosum, septum pellucidum, optic chiasm, and the hypothalamic structures.

Disorders of prosencephalic development usually result in abnormalities of both face and brain development. Abnormalities of prosencephalic formation that are usually incompatible with life include aprosencephaly (lack of development of the telencephalon and diencephalon) and atelencephaly (lack of telencephalon). The holoprosencephalies result from failed prosencephalic cleavages in the horizontal, transverse, and saggital planes. A common anomaly includes the formation of a single sphered telencephalon and a less involved diencephalon. Common disorders of midline prosencephalic development include agensis of the corpus callosum, septum pellucidum, and septo-optic dysplasia. Common facial anomalies associated with these disturbances of midline brain development include hypotelorism, midline cleft lip and palate, and a single front incisor. Children with disorders of prosencephalic brain development are at higher risk for various developmental disabilities, including mental retardation, cerebral palsy, and communication disorders. Children commonly present with developmental delays, early feeding problems, and facial anomalies.

Cerebral Cortex Development

The development of the cerebral cortex is characterized by three major processes: neuronal proliferation (1–4 months gestation), neuronal migration (3–5 months gestation), and neuronal differentiation (6 months–3rd postnatal year). The peak period of neuronal proliferation is from the 2nd to the 4th month of gestation. Rapidly dividing neuronal and glial stem cell precursors can be found adjacent to the lumen of the neural tube. Cell proliferation in the human forebrain increases dramatically through the first half of gestation (20 weeks) and continues into the 3rd postnatal year. Abnormalities of cell proliferation result in diminished number of neurons and can result in microencephaly and macroencephaly. These conditions are commonly associated with multiple congenital anomalies and mental retardation.

Neuronal migration refers to the mass movement of neurons from the ventricular zone adjacent to the lumen of the neural tube to various layers of the cerebral cortex. This rapid influx of migrating neurons from the 3rd to the 5th month of gestation is associated with the development of cerebral convolutions. These events result in the development of the familiar six-layered cortex in adults. Abnormalities of early neuronal migration (2–4 months gestation) include agensis of the cerebral wall (schizencephaly), loss of gyri (lissencephaly), and microgyria. Late migrational abnormalities result in less severe abnormalities including focal defects (heterotopias). The more severe abnormalities, including schizencephaly and lissencephaly, are often associated with multiple disabilities in addition to feeding and swallowing disorders.

Neuronal differentiation and organization extends from the 6th month of gestation to the 3rd postnatal year. This period is characterized by axonal and dendritic outgrowth, dentritic arborization, synapse formation, and pruning and expression of neurotransmitters. These neuronal circuits form the functional systems that subserve higher cognitive processes, sensory integration, and motor output. It is believed that disorders of neuronal differentiation and organization can result in mental retardation and seizures (Capone, 1996).

Myelination

Myelination of the CNS begins as early as the 4th month of gestation and continues in some regions of the brain into the 3rd and 4th decades of life. Myelin is a lipoprotein outer cover for axons. Its function is to increase the rate and efficiency of electrochemical signaling down the axonal shaft. Oligodendroglial cells, which originate from the ventricular zone of the embryonic neural plate, lay down myelin membranes. Myelination is a marker of maturation in the developing brain.

Areas of the CNS may differ in the onset and rate of myelination (Kinney et al., 1988; Yakovlev and Lecours, 1967). There are however, reconizable patterns of myelination of the CNS. Proximal pathways myelinate earlier and faster than distal pathways. Sensory tracts myelinate before motor tracts. Cerebral myelination occurs in projection (e.g., thalamocortical) before associative pathways (e.g., occipito-temporal pathways). Myelination, in general, progresses from the central sulcus outward toward the occipital, frontal, and temporal poles. Neural tracts mediating general proprioceptive (position sense) and exteroceptive somatic experience (tactile and pain) including the medial lemniscus, outer division of the inferior cerebellar peduncle, and the brachium conjunctivum, myelinate beginning at 6 months gestation and extending to 1 year of age. Myelination of specific thalamic projection fibers to respective cortical areas appears to be synchronized with cycles of myelination of descending efferent corticospinal and corticobulbar tracts from these areas. Myelination of the corticospinal and corticobulbar tracts appears initially at term or 40 weeks gestation and increases steadily with a "burst" at 8 to 9 months of age. Myelination events are correlated with motor-skill acquisition and other neurodevelopmental milestones during the 1st year of life. As myelination proceeds, the loss of primitive or brain-stem-mediated reflexes occurs. The Moro, asymmetric tonic neck, and suckle reflexes are replaced by voluntary motor skills including rolling, sitting, crawling, mature sucking, and vertical chewing. The proximal to distal myelination pattern is manifested by the observed motor pattern that batting or reaching for objects appears before the development of a voluntary grasp.

Myelination of the brain stem initially appears at 5 months gestation. The myelination of the statoacoustic system (vestibular and cochlear) commences at 5 months gestation and is completed by 9 months gestation. At 5 to 6 months gestation, the roots of cranial nerves III (oculomotor), IV (trochlear), VI (abducens) and the intramedullary roots of cranial nerves VII (facial), IX (glossopharyngeal) and XII (hypoglossal) are myelinated. By 40 weeks gestation, myelination of the reticular formation around the nucleus ambiguous and the nucleus tractus solitarius (site of the central pattern generator for swallowing; see Chapter 2) commences and continues beyond 2 years of age. These myelination patterns coincide with the appearance of suckling at 18 to 24 weeks gestation and the continued development and refinement of the oral and pharyngeal phases of deglutition in the first few years of life (see Chapter 2 for further discussion of the neurophysiology of swallowing).

■ CLINICAL EVALUATION

Pediatric and Neurodevelopmental History

The basic principles involved in obtaining an accurate and useful neurodevelopmental history are also essential in the diagnosis and management of feeding and swallowing disorders in childhood. Abnormalities of the developing brain commonly result in a spectrum of cognitive, communicative, behavioral, and motor abnormalities that are often associated with feeding and swallowing disorders. Developmental disabilities and feeding and swallowing disorders share many important risk factors and are influenced by similiar health conditions. An accurate developmental history is dependent on the appreciation of both the strengths and potential weaknesses of caretakers reports. Finally, the concepts of developmental delay, dissociation, and deviancy and their usefulness in developmental diagnosis is reviewed below.

The prevalence of feeding and swallowing disorders is estimated to be in the range of 5 to 10% of children seen by general pediatricians (Reau, Senturia, Lebailly, & Christoffel, 1996). General population surveys have estimated the prevalence of food refusal or "picky eaters" to be up to 35% (Jenkins, Bax, Hart 1980; Richman, 1981). Infants with failure to thrive are particularly at risk for both feeding problems (60%) and developmental delays (55%) (Raynor & Rudolf, 1996; Wright & Birks, 2000). Children with cerebral palsy are also at high risk for feeding and swallowing problems. Most studies have found that the prevalence of feeding problems is less in children with hemiplegia and diplegia (25–30%) compared with children with spastic quadriplegia or extrapramidal cerebral palsy (60–90%) (Dahl

Thommessen, Rasmussen, & Selberg, 1996; Reilly, Skuse, Poblete, 1996; Stallings et al., 1993a, 1993b). Longitudinal growth analysis and ongoing developmental assessment are very helpful in identifying infants particularly at risk for feeding and swallowing disorders.

The use of historical risk factors for developmental disabilities is particularly helpful in identifying infants who may benefit from more intensive developmental monitoring. Table 3–1 outlines prenatal risk factors for cerebral palsy. Perinatal signs including perinatal distress (abnormalities of fetal heart monitoring), Apgar scores, and birth trauma have not been found predictive of subsequent cerebral palsy (Nelson, Dambrosia, Ting, & Grether, 1996; Nelson & Grether, 1999). More important perinatal risk factors for cerebral palsy that have been emphasized over the past decade include signs of maternal infection at the time of delivery (Grether & Nelson, 1997) and prematurity and multiple gestation (Nelson & Ellenberg, 1995).

The development of children is a process that optimally should be assessed over time. Arnold Gesell's description of the maturation of the four major "streams" of development—communication, visual problem solving,

Table 3–1. Prenatal Risk Factors for Cerebral Palsy

Recognizable at time of first prenatal visit
  Mother
    Thyroid disorder
    Menstrual cycle > 36 days
    Previous pregnancy loss or neonatal deaths
    Mental retardation
    Seizure disorder
  Prior born child
    < 2,000 g
    Motor deficit
    Mental retardation or sensory deficit

In current pregnancy
  Polyhydramnios
  Treatment with thyroid hormone or estrogen, progesterone
  Congenital malformations
  Multiple gestation
  Maternal seizure disorder
  Severe late proteinuria, hypertension
  Bleeding in third trimester

Note. From "Epidemiology and Etiology of Cerebral Palsy" (pp. 73–79, by Karin B. Nelson, 1996, Table 1). In A. J. Capute & P. J. Accardo (Eds), *Developmental Disabilities in Infancy and Childhood* (2nd edition) Baltimore: Paul H. Brooks Publishing Co. Copyright 1996. Reproduced by permission.

motor, and social/adaptive skills—helped establish the field of infant development (Gesell, 1940). Estimates of the quality and rate of the four major streams of development should be made over time, avoiding a "crossectional" approach to developmental assessment. Feeding is also a developmental skill and should be assessed longitudinally.

The CNS is the primary determinant for Gesell's maturational model for development. There are, however, significant health and environmental influences on the four major streams of development, and subsequently on feeding and swallowing abilities:

- Children with chronic lung disease or severe congenital heart disease may have motor delays that are often associated with hypotonia and muscular weakness. They usually have exercise intolerance, particularly during feeding. Motor development improves as their cardiac and pulmonary status improves (Majnemer et al., 2000; Samango-Sprouse & Suddaby, 1997; Stieh, Kramer, Harding, & Fischer, 1999).
- Children with malnutrition (undernutrition) or failure to thrive often have global developmental delays and usually have behavioral disturbances that may include apathy and irritability. Children often are hypotonic, weak, and lack stamina. If malnutrition is severe and long standing there may be permanent stunting of brain growth and evidence of developmental disabilities (Benefice, Fouere, & Malina, 1999; Grantham-McGregor, 1995; Meeks Gardner, Grantham-McGregor, Chang, Himes, & Powell, 1995).
- Technology dependence may be associated with developmental delays. Tracheotomy and feeding gastrostomy tubes often result in limited play activities in the prone position that appear to result in motor delays of head control, crawling, and pulling to stand. These delays are usually mild and of short duration.
- There are a variety of medications that may widely influence neurologic function, including motor development, cognition, and feeding abilities. Table 3–2 contains a list of medications and their actions on both the central and peripheral nervous systems (Buchholz, 1995). Commonly used anticonvulsants (including barbiturates, phenytoin, and valproic acid) may produce drowsiness. Benzodiazepines are used as anticonvulsants and occasionally for treatment of spasticity. In additon to their sedative effects, benzodiazepines may directly reduce activity in brain-stem centers that regulate swallowing (Wyllie, Wyllie, Cruse, Rothner, & Ehrenberg, 1986; Buchholz, 1995). Dopamine antagonists, including the neuroleptics, are often used for agitation and aggressive behavior in children with cognitive and communicative impairments. These

Table 3–2. Medications That Can Result in Dysphagia

Abnormalities	Medications
Central nervous system	
Arousal	Benzodiazepines
	Chloral hydrate
	Hydroxyzine
	Antihistamines
	Neuroleptics
	Anticonvulsants (barbiturates, valproate, phenytoin)
Suppression of brain-stem regulation of swallowing	Benzodiazepines
Movement disorders (e.g., tardive dyskinesia)	Dopamine antagonists (e.g., neuroleptics)
Peripheral nervous system	
Neuromuscular junction blockade	Aminoglycosides
Myopathy	Corticosteroids
Diminished salivation	Anticholinergics (e.g., tricyclic antidepressants and antihistamines)

Note. From *Pediatric Dysphagia: Management Challenges for School-Based Speech-Language Pathologist,* J. C. Arvedson and B. T. Rogers (Eds.) 1997, Rehabilitation Training Network Health Care Group. Copyright 1997. Reproduced with permission

medications have been associated with the development of laryngeopharyngeal dystonia and esophageal dysmotility (Moss & Green, 1982; Sokoloff & Pavlakovic, 1997).

• Children with musculoskeletal abnormalities may have motor delays that result from altered body mechanics or limitations of movements. Achondroplasia is an example in which there is disproportionately short stature, hypotonia, and motor delays. Head control is often a problem during the 1st year. Children with various forms of in utero constraint may be born with club feet or multiple joint contractures (arthrogyposis multiplex) that can lead to difficulty using the limbs.

The neurodevelopmental history should commence with asking parents their perceptions of their child's development and if they have any questions or concerns. These subjective questions have been found to be reasonably useful to professionals in screening general populations of children for various developmental delays. Certain parental concerns regarding motor, language, and global/cognitive skills have been found to have high levels of sensitivity, identifying up to 80% of children with disabilities (Glascoe, 1997, 2000). Nonetheless, the lack of parental concerns cannot be relied on to identify infants accurately who are developing normally in the general population or in high-risk preterm infants (Glascoe, 1997; Rogers et al., 1992).

Parent-reported current developmental milestones have proven to be more accurate developmental screening measures compared with parental concerns. Instruments including the Ages and Stages Questionaire (Squires, Potter, & Bricker, 1999), The Child Development Inventory (Ireton & Glascoe, 1995), the Clinical Linguistic and Auditiory Milestone Scale and the Motor Quotient (Capute et al., 1986; Capute & Shapiro, 1985) have proven to be useful developmental assessment measures. Most of these assessments have defined developmental delays through the use of standard deviations or developmental quotients. Capute has advocated the use of developmental quotients (Capute & Shapiro). Developmental quotients can be calculated for all four of the major streams of development. Accurate normalized population data with generated means and standard deviations for various developmental milestones are required for the construction of developmental quotients. A developmental quotient is defined as the ratio of the development age of the child divided by the chronologic age multiplied by 100. Table 3–3 contains normalized data for common motor milestones in the first 2 years of life (Capute, Shapiro, & Palmer, 1985). The motor quotient of a 24-month-old, full-term infant who has just started to walk independently is the motor age (12 months) divided by the chronologic age (24 months) multiplied by 100, which is 50. Motor quotients used between the ages of 8 and 18 months have been shown to have high degrees of sensitivity and specificity in identifying infants with continued motor delays at 24 months of age, including those with cerebral palsy (Capute & Shapiro).

The concept of developmental dissociation involves the comparison of the rates of the four major streams of development. The appreciation of the pattern of delays of these streams of development is essential in the diagnosis of neurodevelopmental disorders associated with feeding and swallowing abnormalities. Table 3–4 includes examples of the presentations of mental retardation, communication disorders, and cerebral palsy. Children with mental retardation generally present with significant delays in communication, visual problem solving, and social and adaptive skills. In contrast, children with communication disorders have significant delays in communication and possibly social and adaptive skills but generally normal visual problem solving skills.

Clinicians need to assess both the sequence and the quality of developmental milestones provided by parents or caregivers. All streams of development are generally sequential and orderly. Nonsequential development or "developmental deviancy" is commonly observed in children with

Table 3–3. Gross Motor Milestones to Be Used in Calculating the Gross Motor Quotient

Gross Motor Milestones	Age (months)
Head up in prone position	1
Chest up in prone position	2
Head control	3
Up on hands or wrists in prone position	4
Roll over (Prone → Supine)	4
Roll over (Supine → Prone)	5
Sit (anterior propping)	5
Sit (lateral propping)	7
Creep (belly crawl)	7
Crawl (on hands and knees)	8
Come to sit	8
Pull to stand	8
Sit (posterior propping)	9
Cruise (walk along furniture)	10
Walk (independently)	12
Walk backward	14
Run	15

Note. Adapted from "The infant neurodevelopmental assessment: A clinical interpretive manual for CAT-CLAMS in the first two years of life, part 2," by A. J. Capute and P. J. Accardo, 1996, *Current Problems in Pediatrics, 26,* 279–306.

Table 3–4. Dissociation of Streams of Development Observed in Various Developmental Disabilities

Stream of Development	Mental Retardation	Communication Disorder	Cerebral Palsy
Motor			
Gross	V	N	D
Fine	V	N	D
Problem Solving (Visual)	D	N	V
Language			
Expressive	D	D	V
Receptive	D	V	V
Social-Adaptive	D	N	D

Note. N-normal; D-delayed; V-variable.

Adapted from "A neurodevelopmental perspective on the continuum of developmental disabilities," by A. J. Capute, P. J. Accardo, 1996. In A. J. Capute and P. J. Accardo (Eds.), *Developmental Disabilities in Infancy and Childhood* (2nd ed., p.4). Baltimore: Paul H. Brooks Publishing Co.

developmental disabilities. Children with more severe forms of cerebral palsy often have excessive extensor arching of trunk and extremities during the first few months of life. This extensor arching often will lead to recurrent "flipping episodes" or early rolling before adequate head control in supportive sitting is achieved. True rolling in both directions usually follows the development of head control in normal infants. Similarly, prominent echolalia or the repetition of phrases or sentences by children and the careless history taking of a language milestone can result in deviant or nonsequential language histories. For example, a 36-month-old boy was reported by his parents to have a vocabulary of 20 words and used short sentences. Normal development of language is characterized by the expression of short 3 to 4 word sentences when a vocabulary of at least 50 to 100 words is achieved. This particular child was not speaking in original short 3 to 4 word sentences but was engaging in echolalia or "parroting speech." Further questioning revealed that the child was speaking in short phrases, which is consistent with a vocabulary of 20 words and a language age of approximately 16 to 18 months.

A developmental and health history is essential in identifying acute, chronic static, and chronic progressive neurologic and health disorders resulting in abnormal feeding and swallowing. Table 3–5 is a diagnostic summary of some of the more common conditions associated with dysphagia. Conditions producing dysphagia can be classified as acute or chronic. Acute and chronic CNS disorders are usually characterized by more widespread neurologic dysfunction in addition to dysphagia. Table 3–5 also illustrates that both central and peripheral nervous system diseases can be degenerative and therefore progressive. In these disorders, previously mastered developmental and feeding skills are lost. A detailed feeding history, particularly regarding the oral, pharyngeal, and esophageal phases of swallowing, may be suggestive of these disorders. More common pediatric, progressive CNS diseases producing dysphagia include the Arnold Chiari malformation (Hesz & Wolraich, 1985), intracranial tumors, and various leukodystrophies. Leukodystrophies are disorders marked by degeneration of the white matter of the brain and characterized by demyelination and glial reaction. These and other disorders that affect the mental status, upper extremity function, or posture can seriously impair the acquisition and delivery of food.

Various cardiopulmonary disorders can significantly compromise respiration during oral feedings. Chronic lung disease and congestive heart failure are commonly manifested by progressive tachypnea or fatigue during oral feedings (Harris, 1983). Parents often report that their infant does well for the first half of oral feedings, but then loses interest or refuses the rest of the feeding.

Table 3–5. Etiologies of Dysphagia in Childhood

Site of Pathology	Acute	Static (Chronic)	Progressive (Chronic)

Central nervous system	Hypoxic-ischemic encephalopathy
	Cerebral infarctions
	Intracranial hemorrhage
	Infections
	  – Meningitis
	  – Encephalitis
	  – Poliomyelitis
	  – Botulism
	  – Syphilis
	Acute bilirubin encephalopathy
	Metabolic encephalopathies
	  – Aminoacidopathies
	  – Disorders of carbohydrate metabolism
	Neonatal withdrawal syndrome (heroin, barbiturates)
		Arnold Chiari malformation
		Genetic disorders
		Familial dysautonomia (Riley Day)
		Mobius sequence
		Congenital anomalies of the brain
		Cerebral palsy
		Chronic postkernicteric bilirubin encephalopathy
			Arnold Chiari malformation
			Intracranial malignancies
			  – Tumors
			  – Leukemia
			  – Lymphoma
			Degenerative white and gray matter diseases
			  – Lysosomal storage diseases (e.g., Mucopolysaccharidoses, Niemann-Pick, Krabbe's, Metachromatic Leukodystrophy, Tay-Sachs)
			  – Peroxisomal disorders (e.g., Zellweger's, Leigh's syndrome, neuroaxonal dystrophy, adrenoleukodystrophy)
			  – Purine and pyrimidine disorders (e.g., Lesch-Nyhan)

(continues)

Table 3–5. *(continued)* Etiologies of Dysphagia in Childhood

Site of Pathology	Acute	Static	Chronic
			Progressive
Central nervous system *(continued)*	Traumatic encephalopathies and brain stem injuries		Disorders of metal metabolism (e.g., Wilson's disease, Menkes' disease) Hypersensitivity disorders (e.g., Cockayne's syndrome) Infections (e.g., HIV encephalopathy) Rett syndrome Spinocerebellar disorders Dystonia musculorum deformans Multiple sclerosis Amyotrophic lateral sclerosis Syringobulbia
Anterior horn cell			Infantile spinal muscular atrophy
Peripheral nervous system	Acute inflammatory polyradiculoneuropathy	Polyneuropathies	Polyneuropathies
Neuromuscular junction	Hypermagnesemia		Myasthenia gravis

(continues)

Table 3–5. *(continued)* Etiologies of Dysphagia in Childhood

Site of Pathology	Acute	Chronic	
		Static	Progressive
Muscles	Polymyositis Dermatomyostis	Congenital myopathies – Nemaline rod Myotonic dystrophy Congenital muscular dystrophy Infantile fasciocapulo-humeral dystrophy	Metabolic myopathies (e.g.,glycogen storage disease, mitochondrial disorders) Duchenne's muscular dystrophy
Respiratory tract	Otitis media Sinusitis Adenotonsillitis/pharyngitis	Severe chronic lung disease (e.g., bronchopulmonary dysplasia) Structural anomalies of upper respiratory tract	
Cardiovascular disorders		Congenital heart disease – Cyanotic – Congestive heart failure	Congenital heart disease
Gastrointestinal tract		Gastroesophageal reflux Peptic ulcer	Gastroesophageal reflux and esophagitis
Psychological		Disorders of caregiver–child interaction	

Gastroesophageal disease can also be manifested as progressive dysphagia. Worsening of gastroesophageal reflux disease, esophagitis, or the development of esophageal strictures are not uncommon in children with severe cerebral palsy and dysphagia (Byrne, Campbell, Ascraft, Seibert, & Euler, 1983; Mollitt, Golladay, & Seibert, 1985; Scharli, 1985; Sondheimer & Morris, 1979; Wilkinson, Dudgeon, & Sondheimer, 1981). The more recently recognized extraesophageal reflux disease (EERD) can have direct untoward effects on the pharynx and larynx, making swallowing difficult. This topic is discussed in further detail in Chapters 4 and 5.

A precise feeding and swallowing history is useful and important. Changes in oral feeding techniques can lead to new feeding problems in children with preexisting dysphagia. Swallowing efficiency is often dependent on food texture. Newly introduced foods with more than one consistency can result in increased coughing and gagging, particularly in children with neurogenic dysphagia. Changes in the delivery of oral feedings also can lead to problems. A persistently strong tongue protrusion reflex is commonly observed in children with cerebral palsy and dysphagia. This reflex alone rarely interferes with bottle feedings but can result in excessive oral loss of semisolids when presented on a spoon. These examples illustrate potential new feeding problems in children with nonprogressive dysphagia. The astute clinician should note, however, that these developments do not result in the loss of previously mastered feeding skills. Generally, the majority of conditions listed in Table 3–5 can be suspected by history and then confirmed by a careful physical examination.

Neurodevelopmental Examination

The performance of an accurate and complete physical examination of children at various developmental ages requires keen observational skills, good judgment, a sense of timing, flexibility, and patience. These skills are not easily mastered and should continue to be developed and refined throughout the careers of physicians, nurses, physical and occupational therapists, speech–language pathologists, educators, and other developmental professionals.

The performance of a health and developmental history is often an excellent opportunity for the child and examiner to get to know each other before any direct examination or contact takes place. It is often quite helpful to begin the physical examination with the neurodevelopmental assessment. Initially, parent–child interaction and reported developmental milestones can be observed directly. These observations will help guide more structured or standardized assessments of cognition and communication including the Capute Scales (Capute, 1996) and the Bayley Scales of Infant Development II (Bayley, 1993). Valid and reliable measures of general motor development of infants and toddlers include the Alberta Infant Motor Scale (AIMS) (Piper, Pinnell, Darrah, & Mahapatra, 1992) and the Peabody Developmental Motor Scales (PDMS) (Hinderer, Richardson, & Atwater, 1989). Standarized measures of functional or daily living skills (eating, grooming, dressing, mobility, toileting, and communication skills) include the Functional Independence Measure for Children (WeeFIM) (Msall, Rogers, Ripstein, Lyon, & Wilczenski, 1997) and the Pediatric Evaluation of Disability Inventory (PEDI) (Haley, Coster, Ludlow, Haltiwanger, & Andrellos, 1992).

An important part of a neurodevelopmental examination is the observation of the quality or the way in which a child performs various motor skills. Figure 3–1 depicts a 10-month-old boy with delays in both gross and fine motor skills. In a supported sitting position, significantly increased hip and knee flexion can be observed (Figure 3–1A). When he is pulled to a standing position, a moderate degree of extensor posturing and adduction of his legs can be seen (Figure 3–1B). Excessive finger "splaying" and adduction of his left thumb can be appreciated during attempts to pick up a small pellet (Figure 3–1C). Neurologic examination revealed mild spasticity of the arms and moderate spasticity of the legs. A diagnosis of mild cerebral palsy with spastic diplegia was made.

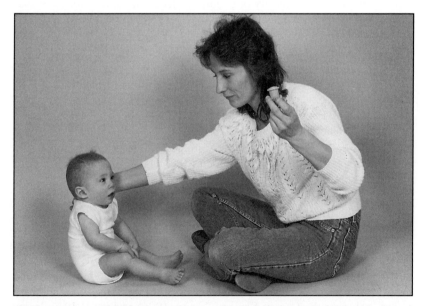

Figure 3–1A. A 10-month-old infant with cerebral palsy (spastic diplegia). In supported sitting, excessive hip and knee flexion can be seen.

The examination of muscle tone and resting posture is an essential part of a neurologic examination. Passive muscle tone is the amount of resistance that exists with movement of a relativily relaxed extremity and cannot be determined during active or voluntary movement of the trunk or extremities. Depending on the age and size of the child, passive muscle tone can be evaluated centrally (in trunk) as well as peripherally (in extremities). Truncal tone can be appreciated by suspending the infant in a prone position. The truncal resistance and posture during this maneuver can be observed. Axillary suspension is another measure of truncal tone. This assessment consists of holding the infant under the arms in upright vertical suspension and documenting whether the infant can support weight under the arms or whether the infant "slips through" the examiner's hands. Passive flexion and extension of shoulders, elbows, hips, knees, and ankles can be performed. Range of motion of various joints can be measured including the anterior scarf and popliteal angles (Amiel-Tison & Gremier, 1986). The anterior scarf is the position of the arm at the point of maximal resistance when it is pulled medially across the chest with the infant in

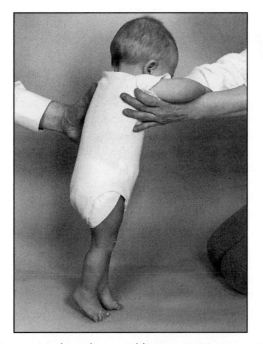

Figure 3–1B. In supported standing, an obligatory positive support reflex is present. Extensor posturing and adduction of the legs can be seen.

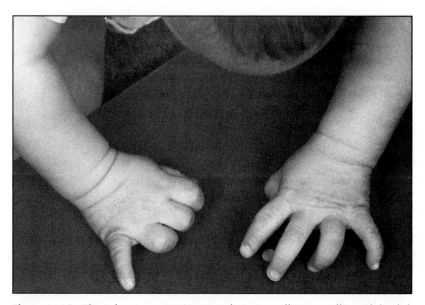

Figure 3–1C. The infant is attempting to pick up a small sugar pellet with his left hand. Excessive adduction of his left thumb and finger splaying can be appreciated.

supine position. The popliteal angle is formed when the lower leg is extended to the point of maximal resistance with the infant in supine position and the thigh fully flexed onto the abdomen. The popliteal angle is 0° when the thigh is fully flexed on the abdomen and the lower leg is fully extended. A 90° popliteal angle represents a right angle between the lower leg and thigh.

Muscle tone undergoes developmental maturation. Passive flexor tone, or resistance to passive extension of an extremity, develops in a caudal to cephalic fashion in preterm infants. It first appears in the legs of preterm infants at about 31 to 32 weeks postmenstrual age (PMA) (Allen & Capute, 1990). Flexor tone becomes equal in arms and legs by 35 to 37 weeks PMA, and this persists through 42 weeks PMA (Amiel-Tison & Gremier, 1986). A similar trend is seen in the popliteal angles. At 31 to 32 weeks PMA, the popliteal angles are usually 40 to 60°. By 35 to 42 weeks, the popliteal angles increase to 90°.

Once established, passive flexor tone gradually decreases during the 1st year of life in a cephalic to caudal pattern. By 4 months of age, full-term infants will have much less flexor tone in their arms compared with their legs. Eventually, by 9 months of age, passive flexor tone should be minimal in the arms and legs (Amiel-Tison & Gremier, 1986). By 9 months of age, popliteal angles have decreased to 30 to 40°. This reduction of passive tone in the legs is manifested by the typical "feet in the mouth" posture of normally developing infants at 9 to 12 months of age.

The resting posture of an infant or child, in general, reflects passive muscle tone. A typical posture of a premature infant at 30 to 32 weeks PMA is that of arms extended and legs semiflexed. By 35 to 37 weeks PMA, both arms and legs are equally semiflexed. Arms tend to be more extended than legs by 4 months of age; by 9 to 12 months of age, arms and legs tend to be more extended than flexed (Amiel-Tison & Gremier, 1986).

The development of truncal and axillary muscle tone follows a cranial to caudal progression in the immediate postnatal years. By 35 weeks PMA, there is an equal distribution of flexor and extensor tone of the trunk. This pattern continues throughout infancy and childhood. This can be most readily appreciated by observing resting posture and by the pull to sit maneuver. The pull to sit maneuver consists of pulling the infant from supine to a sitting position. Typically, when pulled to a sitting position, there is an equal tendency for an infant's head to either drop forward or backward. Another useful maneuver in assessing truncal tone involves the prone suspension of an infant over the examiner's hand. By 35 weeks PMA and throughout the first few years of life, infants will momentarily align their trunk in a parallel fashion with the examiner's hand while held in a prone position.

Muscle strength, or active muscle tone, is the amount of resistance the examiner "feels" when the infant or child actively resists or moves against gravity. Active or spontaneous extremity movements against gravity are often diminished in infants with significant reductions in muscle strength. Weakness of facial muscles can result in a "masked facies." Traction responses are also quite helpful in detecting significant weakness. A traction response represents the amount of active resistance an infant will use when a hand or foot is extended manually.

Observation of resting posture is extremely helpful in assessing muscle tone. The resting posture of equal extremity flexion in an infant at 36 weeks PMA demonstrates normal flexor extremity tone (Figure 3–2A). Arm and leg traction responses indicate normal muscle strength (Figure 3–2B). Prone suspension over the examiner's hand reveals momentary parallel alignment of the infant's trunk with the examiner's hand, indicating normal truncal tone (Figure 3–2C). Figures 3–2D–H demonstrate the degree of head control that can be expected at this age, as well as the balance of flexor and extensor tone of the trunk. In contrast, another preterm infant at 35 weeks PMA shows minimal flexion of extremities and excessive supination of arms (Figure 3–3A). This infant had a weak suck and

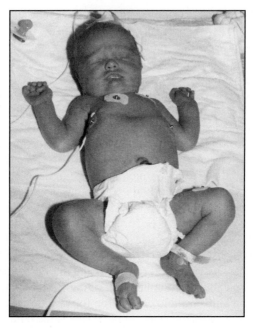

A

Figure 3–2A. A 36-week postmenstrual age infant in supine position demonstrating normal flexor posture of arms and legs. Arms and legs are about equally flexed.

swallowing problems. A computerized tomography scan revealed possible ischemic brain injury. Neurodevelopmental examination revealed central and peripheral hypotonia without significant weakness. In prone suspension, truncal "draping" over the examiner's hand and noticeable arm and leg extension are seen (Figure 3–3B). Figure 3–3C illustrates the marked increase in head lag of the infant when pulled to a sitting position. The initial reduction of passive flexor tone of the upper extremities during the first few postnatal months is demonstrated in Figure 3–4. This infant is a 26-week-gestation preterm infant at a corrected age of 3 months. Reassuring findings include midline position of the head, with legs semiflexed and arms extended. Examination was normal, revealing diminished passive flexor tone of the arms compared to the legs. This normal pattern of passive muscle tone and posture is in contrast to observations of a 3-month-old infant with known brain injury in Figure 3–5A, B. Figure 3–5A demonstrates excessive lateral turning of the head and equal flexor posture of the

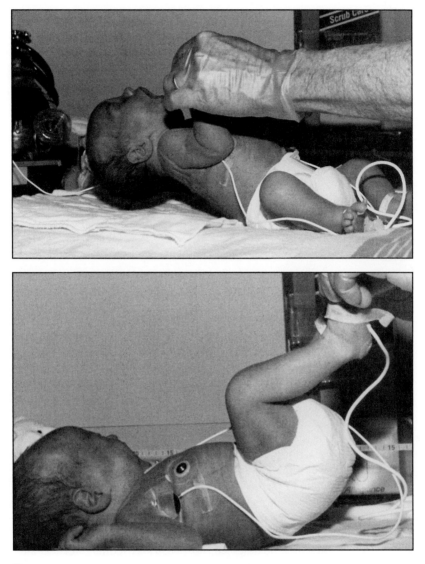

B

Figure 3–2B. The examiner is demonstrating the elicitation of the traction response. Gentle pulling or extension of the arm (upper photo) or leg (lower photo) results in active resistance or flexion of that extremity.

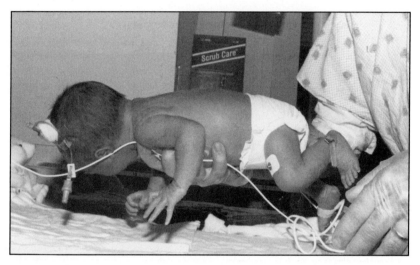

C

Figure 3–2C. The infant is suspended over the examiner's hand. Infants after 34 weeks postmentrual age have sufficient truncal muscle tone (active and passive) to briefly (2–3 seconds) maintain their trunk and occiput in line or parallel with the examiner's hand when placed in prone suspension.

arms and legs. Excessive extensor arching of the trunk is demonstrated in Figure 3–5B. Examination was abnormal and confirmed equal amounts of passive flexor tone of the arms and legs and extensor tone of the trunk and extremities. Increased truncal extensor tone can also be appreciated by the pull to sit maneuver. Figure 3–6A shows a 6-month-old infant with excessive extensor arching of the head and neck after being pulled to a sit. Typically, when a young infant is pulled to a sitting position from supine, the head will gently drop forward or stay in line with the trunk as the infant is pulled past an upright sitting posture (Figure 3–6B). As previously mentioned, axillary tone can be assessed most easily by axillary vertical suspension. Infants beyond 35 weeks PMA generally should not slip through the examiner's hands while being held under their arms in vertical suspension. Figure 3–7A shows a 1-month-old infant with good axillary tone without axillary "slip through." Axillary "slip through" is demonstrated in a 2-month-old with diffuse hypotonia without significant muscle weakness in Figure 3–7B.

The assessment of both passive muscle tone and muscle strength can help the clinician identify some of the more common etiologies of

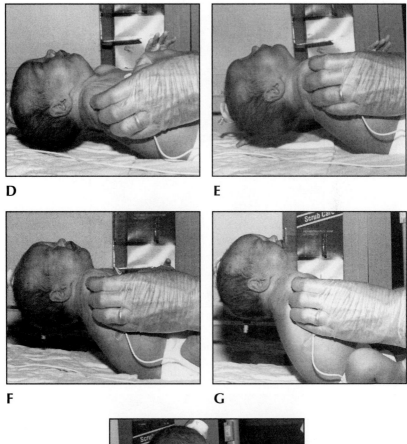

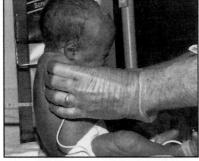

Figure 3–2D–H. This sequence demonstrates the pull to sit maneuver. The degree of head lag is within normal limits for infants from 35–42 weeks post-mentrual age. Once the infant is brought to a sitting position, the head drops forward easily, demonstrating a lack of excessive extensor tone of the trunk.

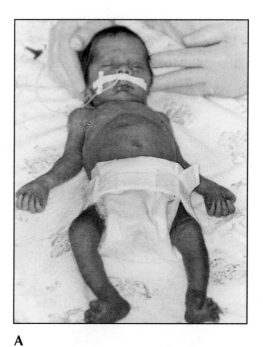

A

Figure 3–3A. The supine, resting posture of a 35-week postmentrual age infant with diffuse hypotonia (reduced passive muscle tone). Minimal flexion of the extremities is evident compared with posture of the infant in Figure 3–2A.

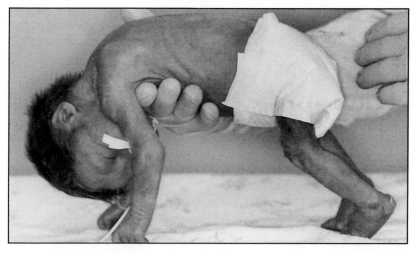

B

Figure 3–3B. In prone suspension, the infant's trunk is draped excessively over the examiner's hand.

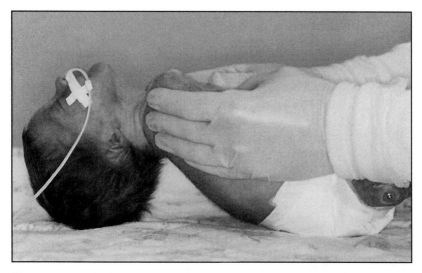

C

Figure 3–3C. Infant being pulled from supine to a sitting position, demonstrating excessive head lag.

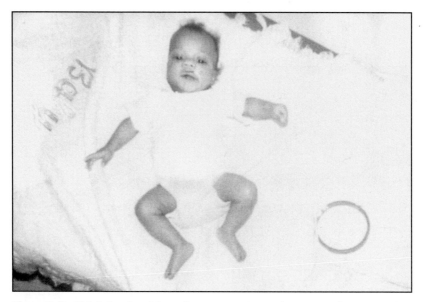

Figure 3–4. This infant is a 26-week preterm at 3 months corrected age. In supine position, this infant demonstrates a normal supine resting posture for a 3-month-old infant. Head is midline, arms are held in an extended position, and legs are still semiflexed.

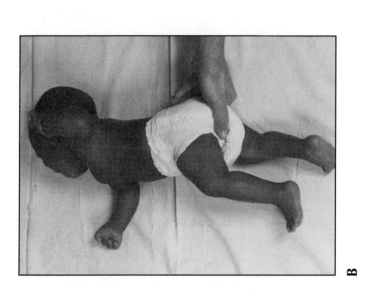

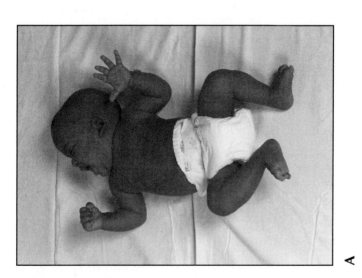

A

B

Figure 3–5A. A 3-month-old infant with known brain injury is viewed in supine position. Arms and legs are held in a flexed position, similar to a normal newborn posture. Excessive lateral head turning and truncal extensor arching can be appreciated.

Figure 3–5B. Excessive truncal extensor arching can be seen while the infant is lying on his side.

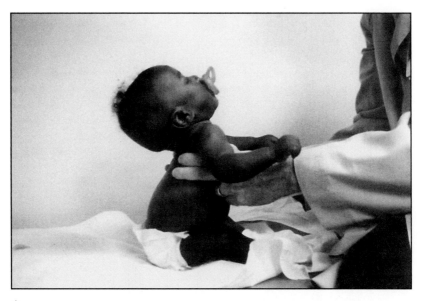

A

Figure 3–6A. A 6-month-old infant with excessive neck and trunk extensor tone has been brought up to a sitting position. Extensor posturing of the neck and trunk can be seen.

dysphagia in childhood (Table 3–5). Central nervous system disorders are usually characterized by abnormalities of muscle tone in the absence of significant muscle weakness (decreased active tone). Common abnormalities of passive muscle tone include early hypotonia, persistence of significant flexor tone of the extremities after 9 months of age, and the presence of excessive extensor tone of the trunk and extremities. Children with neuromuscular disorders including anterior horn cell diseases, myopathies, and muscular dystrophies generally have rather significant reductions in active muscle tone (muscle strength) and less striking reduction in passive muscle tone. Table 3–6 contains key physical examination findings that are useful in differentiating disorders of the CNS from neuromuscular conditions that result in feeding and swallowing problems

Cerebral palsy is a condition that results from a static nonprogressive cerebral lesion that occurs during the developmental period and is manifested by motor delays and abnormal neuromotor findings and a high prevalence of other CNS deficits in areas of cognition and neurobehavior. Cerebral palsy is one of the most common causes of neurogenic dysphagia. The resting posture of a 27-month-old girl with cerebral palsy reveals excessive flexion of her arms and predominant extensor posturing of her legs (Figure 3–8A).

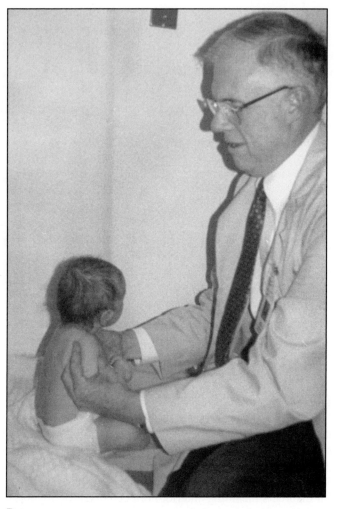

B

Figure 3–6B. A 1-month-old infant is brought up to a sitting position from supine. The appropriate posture of mild neck flexion in sitting can be appreciated.

These findings reflect increased passive flexor tone of the arms and passive extensor tone of the legs. Figure 3–8B illustrates the normal resting posture of children after the first 9 to 12 months of life. Typically, passive flexor tone of the arms and legs has significantly decreased, and the resulting posture consists of only minimal flexion of the extremities. Passive extensor tone and

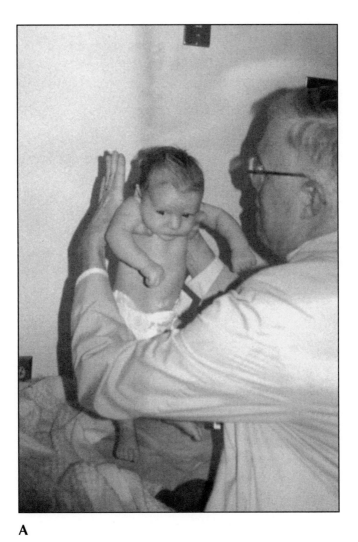

A

Figure 3–7A. This 1-month-old infant demonstrates normal axillary tone by successfully bearing weight while being suspended under the arms.

posture of the extremities should not be observed at any age. These abnormalities can also be appreciated by the pull to sit maneuver seen in Figure 3–8C. This type of extensor posturing can result in the child coming to a stand rather than to a sit. Abnormally increased passive muscle tone in the lower extremities usually results in popliteal angles of 90° or more (Figure 3–8D).

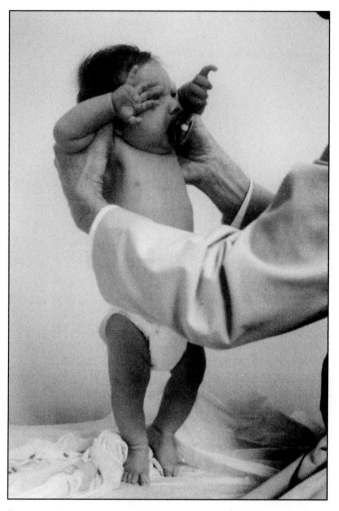

B

Figure 3–7B. Axillary vertical suspension of this 2-month-old results in axillary "slip through." This infant was diffusely hypotonic without significant muscle weakness.

A common finding in children with cerebral injuries including cerebral palsy is the "cortical thumb" (Figure 3–8E). This finding consists of the adduction of the thumb across the palm.

Figure 3–9A–C pictures an 8-month-old girl with myotonic dystrophy. She has a typical myopathic facies (inverted V posture of the mouth) and extension of the extremities (Figure 3–9A). In supported sitting, a collapsing

Table 3–6. Differentiation of Central Nervous System and Neuromuscular Causes of Dysphagia in Childhood

Neurologic Examination	Central Nervous System Disorders	Neuromuscular Disorders
Passive tone	Variable, hypertonia is common	Hypotonia
Active tone (strength)	Normal or mildly decreased	Significantly decreased
Deep tendon reflexes	Normal or increased	Decreased or absent
Primitive reflexes	Usually strong and persistent	May be absent or normal in degree and duration
Plantar response	Commonly up going (+ Babinski)	Plantar flexion
Cognitive	Cognitive deficits are common	Usually normal

kyphosis can be seen (Figure 3–9B). Physical examination revealed minimal spontaneous extremity movements against gravity. Active muscle tone was severely diminished compared with the reduction of passive muscle tone. Figure 3–9C is a computerized tomography scan of her brain revealing ventricular and extra-axial prominence, suggestive of cerebral atrophy. These brain anomalies are common in patients with myotonic dystrophy.

Spontaneous movements of infants refer to endogenously generated motor activities. These generalized movements (GMs) are sensitive indicators of brain function (Einspieler, Prechtl, Ferrari, Cioni, & Bos, 1997). GMs emerge during early fetal life (deVries, Visser, & Prechtl, 1982) and disappear around 3 to 4 months post-term when goal-directed motor behavior begins (Hadders-Algra & Prechtl, 1993; Hopkins & Prechtl, 1984). Normal GMs show age-dependent characteristics. Before 36 to 38 weeks PMA, GMs are characterized by an enormous variation in movement trajectory, speed, and amplitude (Hadders-Algra & Prechtl, 1993). Generalized movements develop a writhing character that is slower and more powerful than preterm GMs. At the end of the 2nd post-term month, writhing movements are replaced by GMs that have a fidgety character. Fidgety GMs consist of a continuous stream of tiny, elegant movements occurring irregularly over the entire body. Normal GMs at any age are characterized by their complexity, variability, and fluency. In contrast, abnormal GMs show a reduced complexity, variability, and fluency (Prechtl, 1990). In general, abnormal GMs are monotonous and predictable. Generalized movements have been shown to be one of the best predictors of neurologic outcomes in high-risk infants (Cioni et al., 1997).

Evaluation of deep tendon reflexes is helpful in children with dysphagia and abnormalities of motor development. Most children with CNS disorders

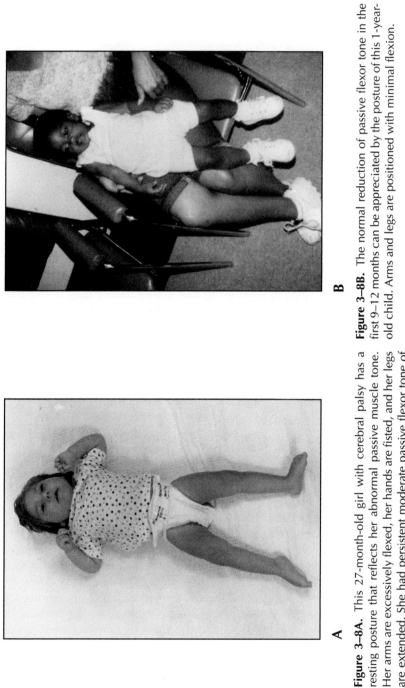

A

Figure 3–8A. This 27-month-old girl with cerebral palsy has a resting posture that reflects her abnormal passive muscle tone. Her arms are excessively flexed, her hands are fisted, and her legs are extended. She had persistent moderate passive flexor tone of her arms and extensor tone of her legs.

B

Figure 3–8B. The normal reduction of passive flexor tone in the first 9–12 months can be appreciated by the posture of this 1-year-old child. Arms and legs are positioned with minimal flexion.

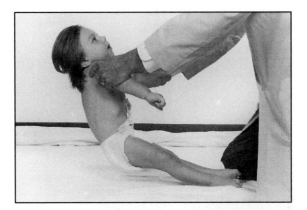

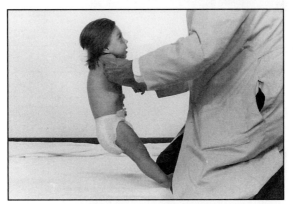

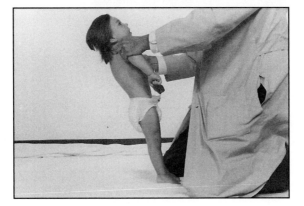

C

Figure 3–8C. Extensor tone of the trunk and legs can be appreciated by the pull to sit maneuver. Pulling this 27-month-old girl from supine to sitting results in extensor posturing of the trunk and legs and coming to stand rather than to sit.

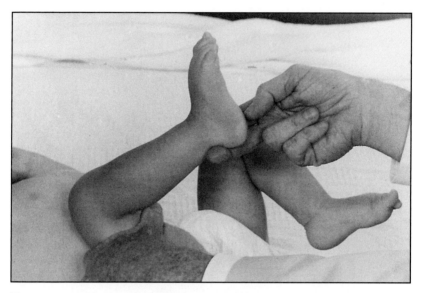

D

Figure 3–8D. This popliteal angle of approximately 90° indicates increased hamstring muscle tone.

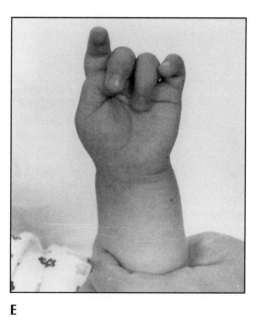

E

Figure 3–8E. The persistent adduction of the thumb across the palm (cortical thumb) is abnormal at any age.

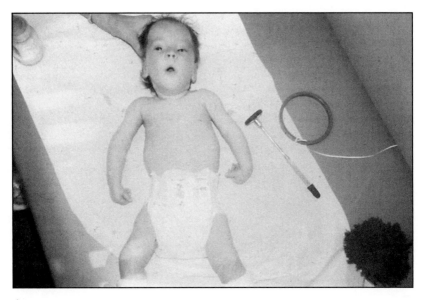

A

Figure 3–9A. An 8-month-old girl with myotonic dystrophy. In supine position, notable features include extension of arms and legs, and myopathic facies (inverted "V" shape of her mouth).

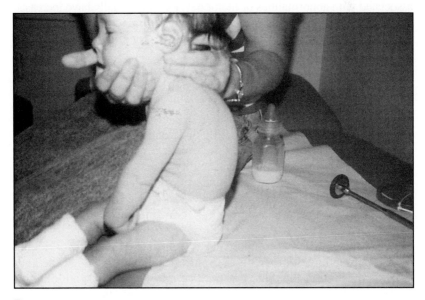

B

Figure 3–9B. In supported sitting, a collapsing kyphosis can be seen.

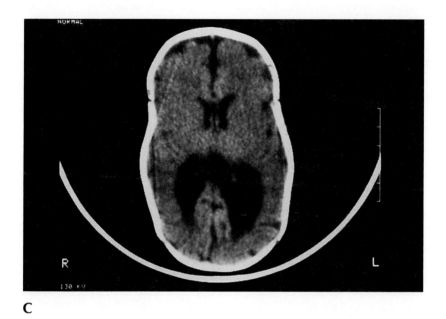

C

Figure 3–9C. A computerized tomography scan of her brain revealed ventricular and extra-axial prominence, suggestive of cerebral atrophy.

associated with abnormalities of motor development usually have increased or normal deep tendon reflexes. Neuromuscular disorders involving the anterior horn cells of the spinal cord, peripheral nerves, or muscles usually result in decreased or absent deep tendon reflexes.

Characteristic of central nervous system disorders, particularly cerebral palsy, is the persistence of strong primitive reflexes. A useful manual for the assessment of primitive reflexes has been compiled by Capute and colleagues (1978). These are brainstem–mediated reflexes that are most prominent in the first 3 months of life and generally disappear by 6 to 9 months of age. The most clinically useful reflexes include the Moro, tonic labyrinthine, asymmetric tonic neck, and positive support reflexes. These reflexes can be elicited by various maneuvers of the head and neck, and persistence of these reflexes generally precludes the development of higher voluntary motor skills including sitting, crawling, and walking. (Figure 3–10A–D.)

Primitive reflexes are important determinants of proper positioning during feeding in children with CNS disorder. Figure 3–11A, B demonstrates elicitation of the tonic labyrinthine reflex in a 27-month-old girl. Extension of her neck results in shoulder retraction and trunk and leg extension; when her neck is flexed, protraction of the shoulders and hip flexion result. Figure 3–11C illustrates the difficulties this child's mother

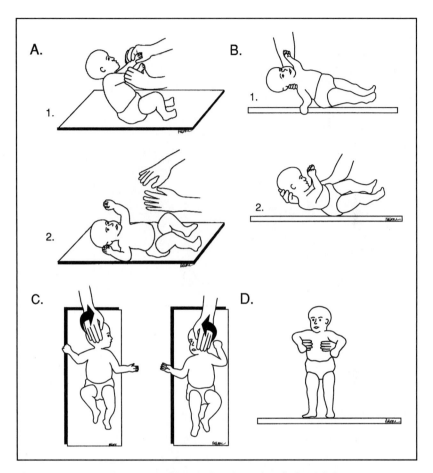

Figure 3–10. **(A)** The Moro reflex can be elicited with the infant in supine position. The infant's head is allowed to drop back suddenly from at least 3 cm off a padded surface (1). On extension of the neck, there is a quick symmetrical abduction and upward movement of the arms followed by opening of the hands (2). Adduction and flexion of the arms can then be noted. **(B)** The tonic labyrinthine reflex can be evaluated in supine or prone position. In supine, the infant's head is extended 45° below the horizontal and then flexed 45° above the horizontal. While the neck is extended 45°, the limbs are extended (1). With the neck flexed 45°, the limbs are flexed (2). **(C)** The asymmetric tonic neck reflex can be elicited by turning an infant's head laterally when in a supine position. Visible evidence includes extension of the extremities on the chin side or flexion on the occiput side. **(D)** A positive support reflex can be elicited by suspending the infant around the chest. The infant is bounced five times on the balls of his feet. The balls of the feet are then brought in contact with the table surface. Co-contraction of opposing muscle groups of the legs occurs, resulting in a position capable of supporting weight.

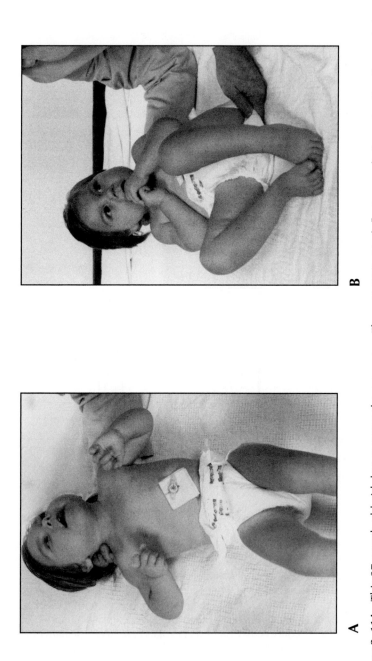

A

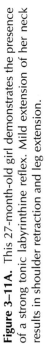

B

Figure 3–11A. This 27-month-old girl demonstrates the presence of a strong tonic labyrinthine reflex. Mild extension of her neck results in shoulder retraction and leg extension.

Figure 3–11B. Neck flexion results in protraction (forward placement) of her shoulders and arms and leg flexion. This posture is generally more conducive for oral feeding.

had trying to position her for feeding in the presence of a strong tonic labyrinthine reflex. Proper positioning techniques, including supportive neck and hip flexion, dramatically improved her positioning during feeding (Figure 3–11D). The asymmetric tonic neck reflex or the "fencer

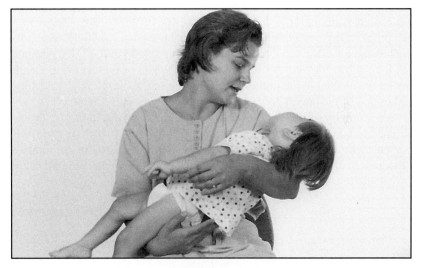

Figure 3–11C. This 27-month-old girl with cerebral palsy is being held on her mother's lap in preparation for an oral feeding. The strong tonic labyrinthine reflex results in excessive trunk and neck extension which may increase the risk for aspiration.

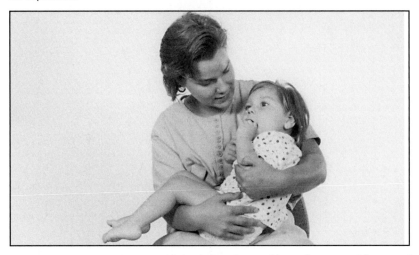

Figure 3–11D. Proper positioning including hip and knee flexion and flexion of the neck results in a more favorable position for feeding.

posture" can also have a deleterious effect on positioning during feeding. A strong or obligatory asymmetric tonic neck reflex often will result in asymmetric sitting posture during feeding (Figure 3–12).

Cranial Nerve (CN) Examination

A detailed examination of the cranial nerves involved with swallowing can be completed in most children. The trigeminal (CN V), facial (CN VII), glossopharyngeal (CN IX), vagus (CN X), and hypoglossal (CN XII) cranial nerves control the sensory and motor components of swallowing. Their nuclei are located in the pontomedullary area of the brain stem. A detailed discussion of the neural control of deglutition is given in Chapter 2.

A summary of physical examination findings useful in localizing the site of cranial nerve deficits that may be seen in patients with dysphagia is presented in Table 3–7. Supranuclear lesions are located in cerebral or descending efferent pathways above or proximal to the cranial nerve

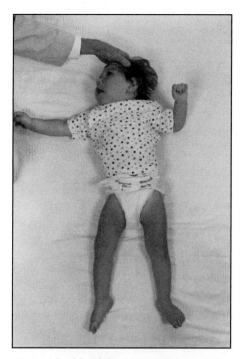

Figure 3–12. This 27-month-old girl demonstrates the presence of a strong asymmetric tonic neck reflex. Her arms and legs are extended in the direction in which her head is turned and flexed on the occiput side.

Table 3–7. Clinical Localization of Cranial Nerve Deficits Associated with Dysphagia

Cranial Nerve	Supranuclear	Nuclear or Peripheral
Trigeminal (CN V)	• Mandible movements are well preserved but often immature or poorly coordinated • Jaw reflex present or exaggerated • Tonic bite reflex may be t present	• Mandible movements are usually minimal or absent • Jaw reflex is usually absent • Tonic bite reflex is absen
Facial Nerve (CN VII)	• Paralysis of lower half of face. Paralysis is almost always unilateral	• Paralysis of upper (forehead) and lower half of face. Paralysis can be unilateral or bilateral
Glossopharyngeal (CN IX) and Vagus Nerves (CN X)	• Muscular palate has normal strength • Normal appearance of palatopharyngeal folds • Vocal fold movement preserved	• Weakness of muscular palate. Asymmetry of muscular palate movement is common • Flattening or asymmetry of palato-pharyngeal folds • Vocal fold paralysis
Hypoglossal Nerve (CN XII)	• Tongue movements are dysfunctional but present • Tongue protrusion reflex can be exaggerated and prolonged in duration	• Unilateral or bilateral absence of tongue movements • Tongue fasciculations • Tongue atrophy

nucleus in the brain stem. Nuclear or peripheral lesions are located in the cranial nerve nucleus in the brain stem or peripheral pathways from the brain stem to the target organ. Generally, supranuclear lesions can result in disordered movement without paralysis, atrophy, or signs of denervation including fasciculations. Nuclear or peripheral lesions, in contrast, result in significant paresis or paralysis, muscle atrophy, and fasciculations. Nuclear or peripheral cranial nerve deficits in patients with dysphagia usually result from acute traumatic or ischemic injuries, destructive lesions (tumors, syringobulbia), or infections (polio, acute inflammatory polyradiculoneuropathy) that in turn are of acute diagnostic significance to the clinician.

The trigeminal nerve (CN V) contains motor and sensory fibers important in the oral phase of swallowing. The third (mandibular) division of CN V innervates the muscles of mastication (temporalis, masseters, and pterygoids). Nuclear lesions of the trigeminal nerve will produce drooping or opening of the jaw and absence of the jaw reflex (jaw jerk). Atrophy of the temporalis and masseter muscles may be seen. Supranuclear lesions will result in poorly coordinated jaw movements and exaggerated jaw reflex. Sensory fibers for pinprick and light touch are provided to the mucous membranes of the nose and mouth; sensation is also provided to the face in a similarly complex manner.

The facial nerve (CN VII) innervates muscles of facial expression. The seventh nerve nuclei are located in the pons. The rostral part of the nucleus controls the ipsilateral forehead, and the caudal part controls the ipsilateral cheek. The rostral part of the facial nucleus is controlled by pyramidal tracts from both cerebral hemispheres, and bilateral supranuclear damage is required to produce paralysis of the forehead musculature. When paralysis is of central origin, however, weakness of the lower facial musculature is commonly found with contralateral pyramidal tract lesions superior to the facial nucleus. These types of lesions will be manifested by contralateral widening of the palpebral fissure and flattening of the nasolabial fold. The facial nerve also provides motor fibers to the stylohyoid muscle and posterior belly of the digastric muscle. Paralysis of the facial nerve may lead to abnormalities of the pharyngeal swallow resulting in delayed passage of food (Bass, 1988). Parasympathetic innervation to the salivary glands and mucous membranes travels with CN VII and controls production of saliva (Chapter 11). Sensory fibers provide taste sensation for the anterior two thirds of the tongue.

The glossopharyngeal nerve (CN IX) provides motor innervation to the stylopharyngeus muscle and sensory fibers to the mucous membranes of the inferior aspect of the muscular palate, mucosa of the tongue, and the posterior pharyngeal wall. The nuclei of the glossopharyngeal and vagus nerves are represented by the salivatory nuclei, the nucleus tractus solitarius, and the nucleus ambiguus of the medulla. The sensory component of the gag reflex is carried by CN IX, and the motor output for the gag reflex includes the vagus, hypoglossal, and trigeminal nerves. The most effective receptor regions for the elicitation of the pharyngeal phase of swallowing are innervated by fibers of CN IX carried through the pharyngeal plexus and by the superior laryngeal branch (SLN) of CN X. A delay in swallow initiation is one of the more common abnormalities in children with dysphagia and cerebral palsy (Logemann, 1983).

Motor nerve fibers are provided to the soft palate, pharynx, and larynx by CN X. The dorsal motor nucleus of the vagus nerve, located in the medulla, contributes to the sensorimotor integration of swallowing, respiration, phonation, cardiovascular responses, and emesis. An acute unilateral lesion of the vagus nerve or its nucleus in the dorsolateral part of the medulla may result in neurogenic dysphagia, with ipsilateral weakness of the muscular palate, asymmetry of the palatopharyngeal folds, and ipsilateral vocal fold paralysis.

The hypoglossal nerve (CN XII) is involved with complex movements of the tongue that have impact on the hyoid and larynx, all important for normal swallowing. Injury to the hypoglossal nerve or to its nucleus in the medulla leads to loss of muscle mass on the ipsilateral side of the tongue. Unilateral weakness of the extrinsic muscles of the tongue results in protrusion to the weak side. Supranuclear lesions characteristic of cerebral palsy result in weakness without muscle atrophy or fasciculations, as well as poorly coordinated tongue movements.

A 26-week-gestation, preterm male infant at 41 weeks post menstrual age is seen in Figure 3–13A, B. Perinatal history was significant for severe asphyxia. Prolonged mechanical ventilation and nasogastric feedings were required. A feeding gastrostomy tube was subsequently placed. In supine position while crying vigorously, a "mask-like" facies is seen, consistent with bilateral nuclear facial (CN VII) paralysis (Figure 3–13A). The jaw is wide open with no active movement, consistent with bilateral trigeminal

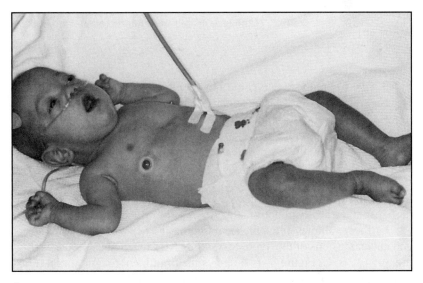

A

Figure 3–13A. A 26-week gestation preterm infant at 41 weeks PMA in supine position during a crying episode. "Mask-like" facies is evident.

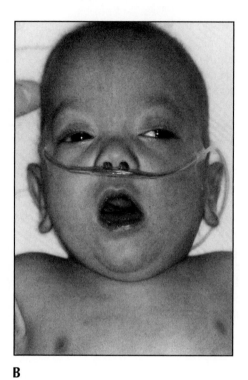

B

Figure 3–13B. A closer view of the face reveals asymmetric tongue atrophy.

nerve (CN V) paralysis. He could not suckle and had a very weak cry. A close-up facial view reveals no spontaneous movements of his tongue (Figure 3–13B). His tongue appeared atrophied and somewhat asymmetric. A subsequent laryngoscopy revealed bilateral vocal fold paralysis. Bilateral extensor tone was observed in his legs. Audiologic evaluation revealed bilateral sensorineural hearing loss. The etiology for the wide range of deficits was severe perinatal asphyxia with patchy ischemic necrosis of his brain stem involving cranial nerves V, VII, VIII, IX, X, and XII, as well as corticospinal tract dysfunction.

Further examples of the physical findings associated with supranuclear and nuclear lesions of the hypoglossal (CN XII) nerve can be found in Figure 3–14A, B, C. Figure 3–14A shows the prominent tongue thrust reflex in a 27-month-old girl with cerebral palsy. Reflexive protrusion of the tongue is spontaneous and on examination poorly controlled tongue movements are associated with normal tongue mass. A young boy with spina bifida is pictured in Figure 3–14B, C. He was diagnosed with an Arnold

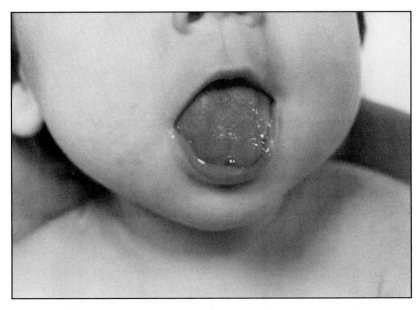

A

Figure 3–14A. Prominent tongue thrusting or protrusion is evident in this 27-month-old girl with cerebral palsy. Tongue mass is preserved. These findings are commonly found in suprabulbar or supranuclear palsy of the hypoglossal cranial nerve.

Chiari malformation and received a ventricular peritoneal shunt in the newborn period. The type II Arnold Chiari malformation consists of downward displacement or herniation of the brain stem (medulla) and cerebellar tonsils through the foramen magnum. This type of malformation is common in patients with spina bifida and can result in brain-stem dysfunction. Figure 3–14B demonstrates the patient's asymmetric tongue atrophy. Tongue fasciculations were also evident.

Somatic Growth

Measurements of weight, height, head circumference, and weight for height or body mass index, along with tricep skinfold thickness and midarm circumference, are helpful to assess nutritional status and trends. Accurate measurements of height may be difficult or impossible in children with scoliosis and joint contractures. Standardized values for upper arm and lower leg lengths are useful in assessing linear growth of children with severe cerebral palsy (Spender, Cronk, Charney, & Stallings, 1989; Stevenson, 1995).

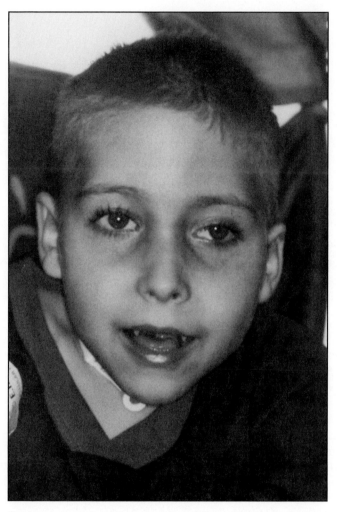

B

Figure 3–14B. This 6-year-old boy has asymmetric tongue atrophy resulting from an Arnold Chiari malformation with spina bifida. Tongue atrophy is most consistent with a bulbar nuclear lesion of the hypoglossal cranial nerve.

Stunted growth is a common complication in children with neurogenic dysphagia. Serial anthropometric measurements are preferable for the diagnosis of malnutrition and stunted growth. If previous growth data are limited, the interrelationship between height, weight, and head circumference measurements can still provide valuable information about nutritioinal

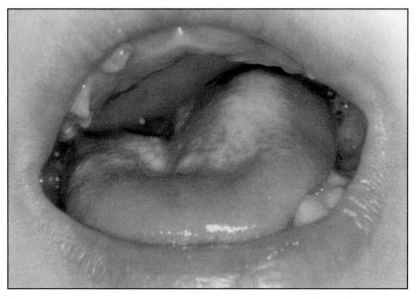

C

Figure 3–14C. Close-up of child in Figure 3–14B showing asymmetric tongue atrophy.

history. Signs of acute protein-calorie malnutrition include reduction of weight to below the 5th percentile for age and weight for height or body mass index less than the 10th percentile. Chronic protein-calorie malnutrition in children with cerebral palsy and dysphagia can result in reductions of fat stores, fat free mass (muscle area), and linear growth (Stallings, Charney, Davies, & Cronk, 1993a, 1993b). In high-risk groups, including children with cerebral palsy, tricep skinfold thickness less than the 10th percentile is far superior to U. S. National Center for Health Statistics weight-for-height ratios less than 10th percentile for identifying children with severely depleted fat stores (Samson-Fang & Stevenson, 2000). (See Chapter 6 for detailed discussion of nutrition.)

Dysmorphology Evaluation

Recognized genetic syndromes, particularly those associated with developmental disabilities, are important causes of neurogenic dysphagia. These conditions are generally recognized by a careful search for major or minor malformations. The more common genetic syndromes associated with dysphagia are listed in Table 3–8.

Table 3–8. Genetic Syndromes with Prominent Dysphagia

Diagnoses	Anomalies	Neurodevelopmental Profile	Feeding Abnormalities
Noonan	– Triangular facies, low-set ears, hypertelorism, epicanthus, ptosis, micrognathia, low posterior hairline, webbed neck – Cardiac anomalies (pulmonic stenosis) – Shield-like chest	– Mental retardation, articulation abnormalities, deafness	– Poor suck, food refusal – Gastroesophageal reflux, esophageal dysmotility, constipation, failure to thrive
Costello	– Low-set ears, large thick ear lobes, thick lips and macroglossia. Coarse facial features, hoarse voice – Loose skin of hands and feet, hyperkeratotic soles and palms – Nasal papillomas – Postnatal growth failure – Cardiac anomalies	– Mental retardation	– Reported feeding problems

(continues)

Table 3–8. *(continued)* Genetic Syndromes with Prominent Dysphagia

Diagnoses	Anomalies	Neurodevelopmental Profile	Feeding Abnormalities
Russell Silver	– Small for gestational age, normal head circumference – Dwarfism – Asymmetries (hemihypertrophy) – Triangular facies and cranial facial disproportionality – Generalized camptodactily – Hypospadias and other genital and urinary anomalies	– Learning disabilities requiring special education	– Severe feeding problems in more than 50% of cases
Kabuki	– Long palpebral fissures, eversion of the lateral third of the lower eyelid, large ear lobes, broad depressed nasal tip, cleft or high arched palate – Cardiac anomaly – Brachydactilly – Postnatal dwarfism	– Mental retardation	– Parent-reported feeding problems
Velocardiofacial	– Cleft palate, tubular nose, narrow palpebral fissures, recessed mandible, small open mouth – Cardiac anomalies	– Learning disabilities	– Velopharyngeal insufficiency, pharyngeal dysmotility

(continues)

Table 3–8. *(continued)* Genetic Syndromes with Prominent Dysphagia

Diagnoses	Anomalies	Neurodevelopmental Profile	Feeding Abnormalities
Opitz G/BBB	– Midline anomalies including cleft lip, laryngeal cleft, heart defects, hypospadias and agenesis of the corpus callosum	– Mental retardation in more than 25% of cases	– Esophageal dysmotilty
Prader Willi	– Narrow bifrontal diameter – Almond shaped palpebral fissures – Small hands and feet – Obesity after 1st year	– Mental retardation and hypotonia	– Dysphagia frequently observed in the 1st year
Coffin Siris	– Microcephaly, growth deficiency – Coarse facies, full lips, wide mouth – Sparse scalp hair – Hypoplastic or absent fifth digit	– Mental retardation and hypotonia	– Difficulty sucking, swallowing, and breathing
Oculo-mandibulo-facial syndrome (Hallermann Streiff)	– Short stature (proportionate) – Dyscephaly, frontal bossing – Mandibular and nasal cartilage hypoplasia – Microstomia, glossoptosis – Microphthalmia – Hypotrichosis	– Normal intelligence	– Feeding and respiratory problems common during infancy

(continues)

Table 3–8. *(continued)* Genetic Syndromes with Prominent Dysphagia

Diagnoses	Anomalies	Neurodevelopmental Profile	Feeding Abnormalities
Freeman-Sheldon	– Masklike "Whistling Facies" – Hypoplastic alae nasi – Club feet	– Hypotonia, facial paresis, ? myopathic arthrogryposis	– Feeding problems secondary to severe microstomia (small mouth)
Smith-Lemli-Opitz syndrome	– Microcephaly, narrow and high forehead, prominent metopic suture – Short nose, anteverted nose, ptosis – Broad maxillary–alveolar ridge – Syndactyly of second and third toes – Hypospadias, cryptorchidism	– Moderate to severe mental retardation – Hypotonia progressing to hypertonia	– Poor suck, gastroesophageal reflux
de Lange syndrome	– Hirsutism, synophrys – Microcephaly – Thin, down-turned upper lip – Micromelia, oligodactyly or phocomelia	– Mild to severe mental retardation – Spasticity, motor delays	– Poor suck, frequent respiratory infections

(continues)

Table 3–8. *(continued)* Genetic Syndromes with Prominent Dysphagia

Diagnoses	Anomalies	Neurodevelopmental Profile	Feeding Abnormalities
Dubowitz	– Low birthweight and post-natal growth retardation – Microcephaly – Hoarse cry – Small facies, shallow nasal bridge, telecanthus, ptosis – Micrognathia	– Mild mental retardation common	– Poor oral intake, frequent emesis and diarrhea during 1st year
Pierre Robin sequence	– Mandibular hypoplasia – Glossoptosis – U-shaped cleft palate	– Generally normal development	– Respiratory distress with feeding in infancy including coughing, grunting, and sputtering
Facio-auriculo-vertebral spectrum	– First and second branchial arch anomalies – Microtia – Maxillary and mandibular hypoplasia	– Normal development	– Respiratory distress with feeding in infancy
Klippel-Feil	– Short neck – Low hairline – Fusion of cervical vertebrae	– Syringomyelia may develop	– Cranial nerve deficits result in dysphagia
Mobius sequence	– "Masklike" facies at birth – Cranial nerve palsies		– Paralysis of cranial nerves VI, VII (usually permanent) – Dysphagia not usually severe unless other cranial nerves involved (CN V, IX, X, or XII) *continues*

Table 3–8. *(continued)* Genetic Syndromes with Prominent Dysphagia

Diagnoses	Anomalies	Neurodevelopmental Profile	Feeding Abnormalities
Rubinstein-Taybi	– Short stature – Downward slanting palpebral fissures – Hypoplastic maxilla and narrow palate – Broad thumbs and toes	– Mental retardation – Motor delays	– Infants have a weak suck – Swallowing is poorly coordinated – Frequent vomiting during infancy
Beckwith-Wiedemann	– Macroglossia – Omphalocele – Ear creases – Macrosomia	– Mild to moderate mental retardation has been reported – Development can be normal	– Feeding problems secondary to large tongue
Trisomy 18	– Growth deficiency – Prominent occiput – Low-set ears – Short sternum – Congenital heart defects – Micrognathia, narrow palate	– Profound mental retardation – Hypertonia	– High-pitched cry – Poor suck
Trisomy 21 (Down syndrome)	– Brachycephaly with relatively flat occiput – Upward slanting palpebral fissures – Small nose with flat nasal bridge – Small ears – Short metacarpals and phalanges – Single transverse palmar crease	– Hypotonia – Usually moderate mental retardation	– Weak suck – Feeding can be further compromised by cardiovascular anomalies

Dysphagia in children with genetic syndromes usually represents only one part of a much broader spectrum of neurologic dysfunction. Nonetheless, dysphagia may be the most easily recognized manifestation of these neurodevelopmental disorders because feeding is such an important and pervasive daily activity. An example follows. Prader-Willi syndrome can be recognized initially by a history of poor fetal movement in utero, significant hypotonia, and dysphagia in the neonatal period. Physical features are often subtle, particularly in the 1st year of life, and include prenatal or postnatal growth retardation, narrow bifrontal diameter, almond-shaped eyes, and hypogonadism (Figures 3–15A,B). Dysphagia is often severe in the neonatal period, commonly requiring nasogastric tube feeding; however, it is usually transient. Slowing of linear growth, obesity, mental retardation, behavioral problems, and hyperphagia are common problems in the preschool and school-age years. Karyotype with expanded banding of chromosome 15 may detect an interstitial deletion of the Q 11 to 13 region in more than 70% of patients (Robinson et al., 1991).

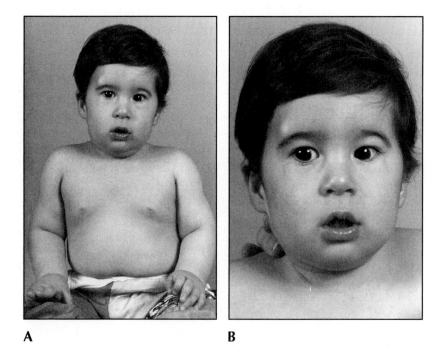

A   **B**

Figure 3–15A,B. A 1-year-old boy diagnosed with Prader-Willi syndrome. Narrow bifrontal diameter and abnormal shaped eyes can be appreciated.

Airway Assessment

In patients with clinically significant dysphagia, the coordination of swallowing with respiration requires careful review. It appears that the maintenance of respiration during swallowing undergoes some degree of developmental maturation. During the 1st week of life, normal preterm and full-term infants often experience decreases in minute ventilation, respiratory rate, and tidal volume during episodes of continuous nutritive sucking (Durand et al., 1981; Guilleminault & Coons, 1984; Mathew et al., 1985; Shivpuri, Martin, Carlo, & Fanaroff, 1983; Wilson, Thach, Brouillette, & Abu-Osbsa, 1981). Decreases in minute ventilation during oral feedings in term neonates appear to be proportional to swallowing frequency presumably as a consequence of neural inhibition of breathing and airway closure during swallowing (al-Sayed, Schrank, & Thach 1994). In neurologically compromised neonates, these occurrences can persist, and prolonged periods of bradycardia and hypoxemia may also occur during nutritive sucking (Rosen, Glaze, & Frost, 1984). Beyond the neonatal period, the relationship of respiration to feeding has been limited to studies performed in adults. In adults the onset of swallowing interrupts expiration. Normal respiratory function appears to be preserved during oral feedings in healthy adults (Nishino, Yonezawa, & Honda, 1985; Smith, Wolkove, Colacone, & Kreisman, 1989). Children with neurogenic dysphagia can have significant respiratory compromise during oral feedings. Pulse oximetry, a noninvasive measure of hemoglobin oxygen saturation (estimate of oxygen carrying capacity of the blood), has been used to detect significant degrees of hypoxemia during oral feedings in older children with cerebral palsy (Rogers, Arvedson, Msall, & Demerath, 1993).

Prior to oral feedings, the upper and lower respiratory tracts should be carefully examined. Respiratory and heart rates at rest and during oral feedings should be taken. The presence of audible pharyngeal secretions, stridor, and chest retractions should be noted before, during, and after oral feedings. Anatomic obstructions to airflow in the upper respiratory tract may be most noticeable during oral feedings. (See Case Study 1 and Chapter 4.) In children with neurologic impairments and dysphagia, pulmonary complications are well known. Aspiration during oral feedings has been linked with bronchospasm, pneumonia, and chronic lung disease (Loughlin, 1989). Auscultation of lung fields before and after oral feedings can be helpful. The presence of diminished breath sounds, inspiratory rales, and tachypnea after oral feeding may indicate tracheal–bronchial aspiration.

In young infants, a careful cardiac examination is especially important. Acute or chronic heart failure resulting primarily from congenital heart disease (e.g., ventricular septal defect, patent ductus arteriosus, aortic coarctation) can present with a variety of signs and symptoms, including failure to thrive and fatigue during oral feedings (Harris, 1983).

Gastrointestinal Evaluation

Gastroesophageal disorders are important causes of feeding problems in children. Esophageal dysmotility, gastroesophageal reflux, and esophagitis are commonly encountered problems in children with cerebral palsy (Byrne et al., 1983; Sondheimer & Morris, 1979). These conditions can lead not only to recurrent vomiting and failure to thrive, but also to significant food refusal and abnormal extensor arching of the trunk and extremities (Kinsbourne, 1964). A high index of suspicion and the appropriate use of sensitive diagnostic evaluations (endoscopy and esophageal PH monitoring) are often required. A more complete discussion of this topic is found in Chapter 5.

One of the more common complications of significant dysphagia in children is reduced fluid intake. Reduced intake leads to dehydration during various acute illnesses and is not uncommon in children with neurologic impairment and severe dysphagia. Chronically low fluid intake, particularly when combined with immobility, often directly leads or contributes to the development of chronic constipation. Severe chronic constipation can result in significant irritability during or after feedings. Chronic stool retention can be identified by a careful stool history. Palpable masses, particularly in the left lower abdominal quadrant, dullness on percussion, and masses on rectal examination can all be found (Antanitus, 1989).

■ INTERDISCIPLINARY STATEGIES

The health, neurodevelopmental, and emotional implications of feeding and swallowing disorders of children and their families are significant. Thus, pediatricians with appropriate training and experience should assume a leadership role in the initial evaluation and management of children with feeding and swallowing disorders.

It is also essential to recognize the increasing importance of other health and developmental professionals in the diagnosis and management of the wide variety of feeding disorders in children. In this chapter, the importance of the association between swallowing and respiration has been emphasized. Otolaryngologists should be consulted in the evaluation of children suspected of having upper airway compromise at rest or during oral feedings. Pediatric gastroenterologists can provide invaluable diagnostic and management strategies for children with complicated gastrointestinal disorders. Children with refractory gastroesophageal reflux, esophagitis, achalasia, peptic ulcer disease, intestinal motility disorders, and severe malnutrition may need to be evaluated by a pediatric gastroenterologist. Additionally, nutritionists can provide expertise in the evaluation and management of children with nutritional deficits. The value of accurate oral–motor and feeding assessments by occupational therapists and speech–language pathologists in children with significant feeding and swallowing disorders should be clearly recognized. Finally, the recent increase of interdisciplinary teams of professionals providing coordinated care for children with dysphagia is encouraging and should be supported and fostered by all professionals.

■ CASE STUDIES

The cases presented in this section emphasize the challenges of diagnosis and management of children with complex feeding and swallowing disorders.

Case Study 1

A full-term infant was born after an uncomplicated pregnancy except for poor progression of labor. Thus, a Caesarean section was performed; Apgars were 7 and 9 at 1 and 5 min respectively. "John's" birth weight was 3,530 g. He developed respiratory distress at 1 hour of age and was transferred to the neonatal intensive care nursery. He was diagnosed with transient tachypnea of the newborn, and he rapidly improved during the first 3 days of life. On day 2 of life, John developed right-sided tonic–clonic seizures lasting 30 sec. A computerized tomographic scan of his cranium and an electroencephalogram were both normal. At 1 week of age, a consultation was requested for evaluation of difficult oral feedings. John took up to 1 hour to consume 1 oz of formula from a bottle. He frequently gagged, choked, and at times "gasped for air" during oral feedings. At rest, his respirations were normal, and no stridor was observed. His cry was high pitched and somewhat muffled, however. A neurodevelopmental examination was normal. During a bottle-feeding, John had a good suck but quickly developed inspiratory stridor with moderate chest retractions. Supraglottic airway obstruction was suspected, and the pediatric otolaryngology service was consulted.

Lateral neck X-ray revealed a mass anterior to but separate from the epiglottis (Figure 3–16A). A bedside flexible fiberoptic nasopharyngo-laryngoscopic examination was performed. His vocal folds moved normally. A mass was noted in his vallecula that was partially occluding his supraglottic larynx, especially with swallowing (when the larynx was elevated). A computerized tomographic scan of his nasopharynx showed a 1 cm^2 soft tissue mass in his vallecula (Figure 3–16B). Surgical excision of the mass was completed; bronchoscopy revealed no further abnormalities.

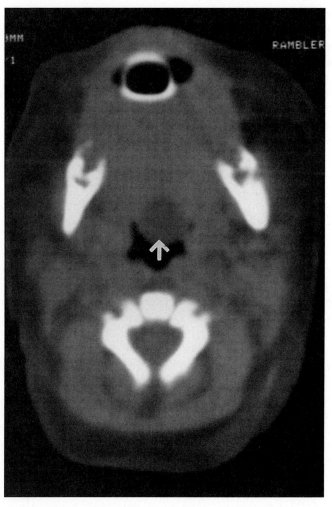

A

Figure 3–16A. A lateral neck X-ray reveals a mass in the vallecula (arrow).

Pathologic evaluation revealed a benign cyst. Postoperatively, John's oral feedings were normal, and at the time of discharge, he was bottling well.

Comment

This case illustrates that upper airway obstructions in infants and children can result in significant dysphagia. Occasionally these obstructions are more prominent during swallowing. Careful observation of a bottle-feeding suggested the diagnosis.

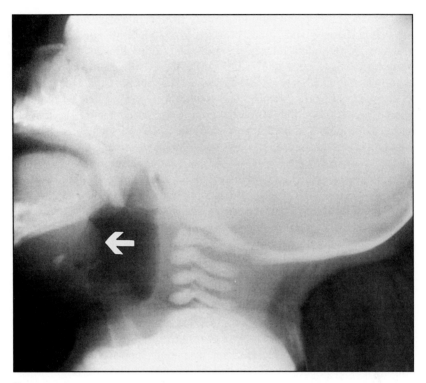

B

Figure 3–16B. A computerized tomographic scan of the nasopharynx (horizontal cross section) revealed a 1 cm^2 mass in the vallecula (arrow).

Case Study 2

"Michael," an 11-year-old boy, had a recent onset of excessive oral loss of food and fatigue during feedings. His oral feeds consisted of liquids, thickened liquids, and soft foods. His health was complicated by severe malnutrition. For the previous 5 years, his weight ranged from 12 to 13.6 kg. He was a 28-week-gestation premature infant. He developed severe bronchopulmonary dysplasia and had required a temporary tracheotomy. He was subsequently diagnosed with cerebral palsy and dysphagia requiring a feeding gastrostomy tube at 3 years of age. He was nonambulatory and had a severe expressive communication disorder.

Michael's resting respiratory rate was 34 breaths/min. Tongue lateralization was limited, and tongue thrust was strong. Lung fields were clear on auscultation. Pulse oximetry revealed a 3-min resting hemoglobin oxygen saturation (S_pO_2) of 95% and a heart rate of 57 to 60 beats/min. During oral feedings, he developed a mild inspiratory stridor; however, his respiratory rate was unchanged, and cyanosis was not observed. Consecutive 2- to 3-min oral feedings of liquids, thickened liquids, and soft foods were monitored by pulse oximetry. Average S_pO_2 values during these 2- to 3-min intervals were as follows: liquids (S_pO_2 = 84%, heart rate (HR) 84/min), thickened liquids (S_pO_2 = 92–93%, HR 84/min), and solids (S_pO_2 = 81%, HR 98/minute). Direct laryngoscopy and esophagoscopy revealed edematous arytenoids and a 40% stricture in the midportion of the trachea. Esophagitis was also noted. A videofluoroscopic swallow study (VFSS) using liquids, purees, and soft food was performed while Michael was in an upright sitting position. Food boluses were moved over his tongue in a piecemeal fashion. His pharyngeal swallow was delayed, with pooling in the valleculae and pyriform sinuses. Pharyngeal peristalsis was significantly reduced, and there was pharyngeal residue after swallows. Portions of boluses did enter the laryngeal vestibule, but no aspiration below the vocal folds was noted. All food textures were swallowed in a similar manner.

The esophagitis was treated with antacid and metoclopramide. No treatment was elected for the tracheal stricture. Because thickened liquids did not produce hypoxemia, oral feedings were limited to this texture. The presence of significant pharyngeal residue after swallows indicated the need to reduce the amount and rate of oral feedings and increase gastrostomy tube feedings. Four months later, his parents reported that he required 4 hours less sleep per day. He gained 4.1 kg in the following year.

Comment

Michael unfortunately experienced many of the long-term complications of dysphagia including malnutrition, pulmonary complications, and esophagitis. He had severe dysphagia that seriously compromised his food intake and necessitated the placement of a feeding gastrostomy. The utilization of pulse oximetry at rest and during oral feedings helped to estimate his respiratory compensation during oral feedings. This method used in conjunction with his VFSS allowed for development of a feeding program that avoided hypoxemia during oral feedings and improved his nutritional state. The observed hypoxemia during oral feedings of liquids or solid food most likely resulted from aspiration. Aspiration can result in the rapid development of distal airway closure and ventilation perfusion mismatches (Colebatch & Halmagyi, 1962; Conn & Barker, 1984; Lewis, Burgess, & Hampson, 1971; Schwartz, Wynne, Gibbs, Hood, & Kuck, 1980).

Michael also developed esophagitis and inflammation of his larynx from recurrent gastroesophageal reflux and extraesophageal reflux in the absence of frequent emesis. Gastroesophageal reflux is unfortunately a common complication in children with severe cerebral palsy.

Case Study 3

"Dunya" was a full-term, small-for-gestation infant with a birth weight of 4 lbs, 1 oz. Pregnancy was uncomplicated except for maternal emesis and diarrhea. Labor and delivery was uncomplicated, and Apgar scores were 9 and 9 at 1 and 5 min respectively. Transient hypoglycemia was treated with intravenous glucose. There were no reported feeding problems.

Dunya was admitted to the hospital for failure to thrive at 6 months of age. Oral feedings of a standard formula were frequent and of small volume. Oral motor examination did not reveal any abnormalities. A genetics evaluation revealed no abnormalities. There was no history of emesis or extensor arching during or after oral feedings. Oral feedings with a higher calorie formula went well, and she was discharged.

She started having frequent otitis media episodes, and oral feedings continued to be difficult. Weight gain continued to be poor, and Dunya was subsequently admitted to the hospital for failure to thrive at 1 and 2 years of age. Figures 3–17A,B outline Dunya's slow progressive weight gain during the first 2 years of life. Her linear growth was generally steady at slightly below the 5th percentile, but her cranial growth slowed between 24–27 months of age. Her weight-for-height ratios were below the 5th percentile, indicating a mild degree of undernutrition. Dunya was being fed by her mother every 1–2 hours throughout the day and night and was consuming about 24–30 ounces of Kindercal formula (30 calories/ounce) and 3–4 teaspoons of puree or soft food per day. She would generally be eager for feedings but seemed to lose her appetite quickly. There was no history of emesis or diarrhea, and her health was otherwise uncomplicated. An upper gastrointestinal UGI series was normal, a scintiscan (radioisotope assessment) revealed no gastroesophageal reflux, and gastric emptying was 26% after 1 hour. Blood studies including a complete blood count and electrolytes were all normal. A sweat chloride test was normal. Endomysial antibodies for celiac disease were negative. Neurodevelopmental examinations at 1 and 2 years of age were normal.

At 28 months of age, Dunya was evaluated for placement of a feeding gastrostomy tube (GT). An esophageal pH probe was performed to rule out gastroesophageal reflux prior to GT placement. Gastroesophageal reflux was detected on the esophageal pH probe. The GT placement was canceled, and Dunya was started on metoclopramide and ranitidine for treatment of her gastroesophageal reflux. Dunya's appetite, receptiveness to oral feedings, and amount of formula per feeding increased dramatically within 3 weeks of starting metoclopramide and ranitidine. Within 2 months, her mother reported that she seemed more energetic and that her expressive language improved. The rather abrupt increase in weight gain from 27 months to her last outpatient visit at 37 months of age can be seen in Figure 3–17A. Significant increases in linear and cranial growth also occurred between 27

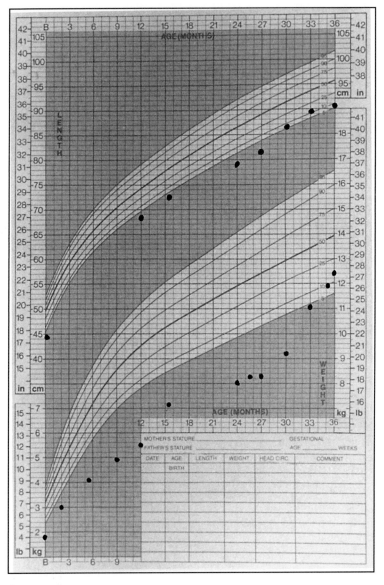

A

Figure 3–17A. The weight growth chart reveals a decrease of weight gain velocity between 6 and 12 months of age and again between 24 and 27 months of age. A rapid weight gain is evident between 27 and 36 months of age. Linear growth in the top graph remained consistent at slightly below the 5th percentile until 24 months of age. Linear growth velocity was diminished until 27 months and subsequently increased to 33 months.

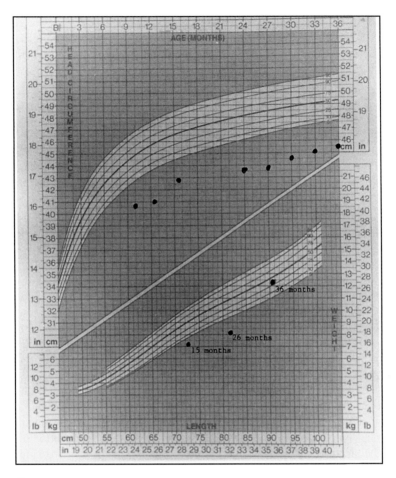

B

Figure 3–17B. The top graph reveals head circumferences consistently below the 5th percentile through 24 months. Head growth velocity increased between 27 and 33 months. Weight for height ratios were consistently below the 5th percentile but moved within the normal range after 30 months.

and 30 months (see Figure 3–17A,B). Weight for height ratios quickly climbed from below the 5th percentile to the 30th percentile.

Comment

This case emphasizes the need to consider gastroesophageal reflux in children who present with food refusal and small volume feeds especially in the context of undernutrition. Gastroesophageal reflux has a wide range of presentations and vomiting may not be prominent. This case also highlights the importance of nutritional status on growth and general development of children.

Case Study 4

"Timothy" is a 12-year-old boy with Trisomy 21 (Down syndrome). He was admitted for a 2-month history of persistent bilateral lower lobe pneumonia. Although he had received a number of courses of antibiotics, he had not improved clinically. Direct questioning of his mother revealed that during the previous 6 months, he had increasing difficulty in swallowing solid food, had poorer speech, and had begun drooling excessively. His past medical history was significant for C_1–C_2 vertebral instability that had led to a posterior cervical spinal fusion. He had previously been diagnosed with a neurogenic spastic bladder. He was on no medications at the time.

Physical examination revealed an alert, cooperative preteenage boy in no acute distress. Inspiratory rales were noted over both lower lung fields. He drooled excessively, and his speech reflected flaccid dysarthria. Jaw clonus was observed, and no gag reflex could be elicited. All four extremities were weak, his arms more so than his legs. Deep tendon reflexes were increased in the legs. Plantar responses were up going. Gait was mildly ataxic; mild dysmetria was noted. Romberg response was observed and cremasteric reflex was absent.

Recent chest X-rays revealed chronic bibasilar infiltrates. A VFSS showed aspiration of liquid barium during swallows. A cranial magnetic resonance image revealed marked C_1–occiput instability. Herniation of the cerebellar tonsils was noted. Additionally, the clivus was compressing the anterior medulla (Figure 3–18).

Timothy subsequently underwent an occiput to C_1–C_2 fusion and halo vest application. Oral feedings were discontinued, and a feeding gastrostomy tube was placed. His pneumonia subsequently cleared.

Timothy's neurologic status and swallowing gradually improved over the following year. One year after discharge, his gait was normal. A follow-up VFSS revealed mild pharyngeal dysmotility but no tracheal aspiration. Oral feedings were gradually resumed without difficulty.

Comment

Timothy's clinical course highlights the complexity of feeding and swallowing disorders and exemplifies the value of interdisciplinary evaluation. This case emphasizes the diagnostic importance of recognizing progressive dysphagia. Knowledge of the potential CNS complications of C_1–C_2

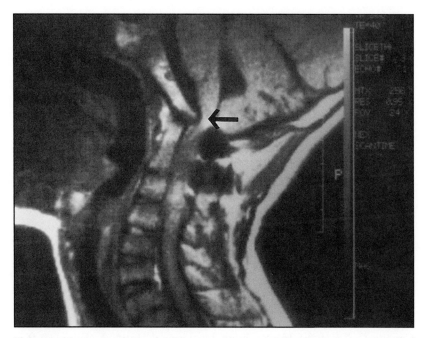

Figure 3–18. A cranial magnetic resonance image (midline sagittal view) revealed herniation of the cerebellar tonsils. The clivus (arrow) is shown to be compressing the medulla anteriorly.

vertebral instability in children with Down syndrome and a detailed feeding history were essential in his diagnosis. The compression of his medulla by the floor of his skull directly resulted in his dysphagia and chronic aspiration.

Timothy's follow-up care was maximized by the interdisciplinary team. Videofluroscopic swallow studies in conjunction with clinical oral–motor feeding assessments were essential for choosing safe and effective methods for his feeding.

■ REFERENCES

Allen, M. C., & Capute, A. J. (1990). Tone and reflex development before term. *Pediatrics 85* (Suppl. *March 1990)*, 393–399.

al-Sayed, L. E., Schrank, W. I., & Thach, B. T. (1994). Ventilatory sparing strategies and swallowing pattern during bottle feeding in human infants. *Journal of Applied Physiology, 77,* 78–83.

Amiel-Tison, C., & Gremier, A. (1986). *Neurologic assessment during the 1st year of life* (R. Boldberg, Trans.). New York: Oxford University Press. (Original work published 1984.)

Antanitus, D. (1989). Primary care physician. In I. L. Rubin and A. C. Crocer (Eds.), *Developmental disabilities: Delivery of medical care for children and adults* (437–438). Philadelphia: Lea and Febiger.

Bass, N. (1988). Neurogenic dysphagia: Diagnostic assessment and rehabilitation of feeding disorders in the neurologically impaired. In M. G. Eisenberg & R. C. Grzeiak (Eds.), *Advances in Clinical Rehabilitation* (Vol. 2; 186–228). New York: Springer.

Bayley, N. (1993). Bayley Scales of Infant Development II. San Antonio, TX: The Psychological Corporation.

Benefice, E., Fouere, T., & Malina, R. M. (1999). Early nutritional history and motor performance of Senegalese children, 4–6 years of age. *Annals of Human Biology, 26,* 443–455.

Buchholz, D. W. (1995). Oropharyngeal dysphagia due to iatrogenic neurological dysfunction. *Dysphagia, 10,* 248–254.

Byrne, W. J., Campbell, M., Ascraft, E., Seibert, J. J., & Euler, A. R. (1983). A diagnostic approach to vomiting in severely retarded patients. *American Journal of Diseases of Children, 137,* 259–262.

Capone, G. T. (1996). Human brain development. In: A. J. Capute, & P. J. Accardo, (Eds.), *Developmental disabilities in infancy and childhood* (2nd ed.; 25–75). Baltimore: Paul H. Brooks.

Capute, A. J., (1996) *The Capute Scales: The CAT-CLAMS project.* Baltimore: Kennedy Fellows Association.

Capute, A. J., & Accardo, P. J. (Eds.) (1996). *Developmental Disabilities in Infancy and Childhood* (2nd ed.). Baltimore: Paul H. Brookes.

Capute, A. J., & Accardo, P. J. (1996). The infant neurodevelopmental assessment: A clinical interpretive manual for CAT-CLAMS in the first two years of life, part 2. *Current Problems in Pediatrics, 26,* 299–306.

Capute, A. J., Accardo, P. J., Vining, E. P. G; Rubenstein, J. E., & Harryman, S. (1978). *Primitive reflex profile.* Baltimore: University Park Press.

Capute, A. J., Palmer, F. B., Shapiro, B. K., Wachtel, R. C., Schmidt, S., & Ross, A. (1986). A clinical linguistic and auditory milestone scale: Prediction of cognition in infancy. *Developmental Medicine and Child Neurology 28,* 762–771.

Capute, A. J., & Shapiro, B. K. (1985). The motor quotient: A method for the early detection of motor delay. *American Journal of Diseases of Childhood, 139,* 940–942.

Capute A. J., Shapiro B. K., & Palmer, F. B. (1985). Normal gross motor development: The influence of race, sex and socio-economic status. *Developmental Medicine and Child Neurology, 27,* 635–643.

Cioni, G., Prechtl, H. F., Ferrari, F., Paolicelli, P. B., Einspieler, C., & Roversi, M. F. (1997). Which better predicts later outcome in full-term infants: quality of general movements or neurological examination? *Early Human Development, 50,* 71–85.

Colebatch, H. J. H., & Halmagyi, D. F. J. (1962). Reflex airway reaction to fluid aspiration. *Journal of Applied Physiology, 17,* 787–794.

Conn, A. W., & Barker, G. A. (1984). Fresh water drowning and near drowning. *Canadian Anaesthetists Society Journal Toronto, 31,* 538–544.

Dahl, M., Thommessen, M., Rasmussen, M., & Selberg, T. (1996). Feeding and nutritional characteristics in children with moderate or severe cerebral palsy. *Acta Paediatrica, 85,* 697–701.

deVries, J. I. P., Visser, G. H. A., & Prechtl, H. F. R. (1982). The emergence of fetal behaviour. I. Qualitative aspects. *Early Human Development, 7,* 301–22.

Durand, M., Leahy, F. N., Maccallum, M., Cates, D. B., Rigato, H., & Chermick, V. (1981). Effect of feeding on the chemical control of breathing in the newborn infant. *Pediatric Research, 15,* 1509–1512.

Einspieler, C., Prechtl, H. F., Ferrari, F., Cioni, G., & Bos, A. F. (1997). The qualitative assessment of general movements in preterm, term and young infants—review of the methodology. *Early Human Development, 24,* 47–60.

Gesell, A. (1940). *The first five years of life.* New York: Harper & Row.

Glascoe, F. P. (1997). Parents' concerns about children's development: Pre-screening technique or screening test? *Pediatrics, 99,* 522–8.

Glascoe, F. P. (2000). Evidence-based approach to developmental and behavioural surveillance using parents' concerns. *Child Care Health Development, 26,* 137–49.

Grantham-McGregor, S. (1995). A review of studies of the effect of severe malnutrition on mental development. *Journal of Nutrition, 125*(Suppl. 8), 2233S-2238S.

Grether, J. K., & Nelson, K. D. (1997). Maternal infection and cerebral palsy in infants of normal birth weight. *Journal of the American Medical Association, 278,* 207–11.

Guilleminault, C., & Coons, S. (1984). Apnea and bradycardia during feeding in infants weighing >2000 gm. *The Journal of Pediatrics, 104,* 932–935.

Hadders-Algra, M., & Prechtl, H. F. R. (1993). EMG correlates of general movements in healthy preterm infants. *Journal of Physiology, 459,* 330 (Abstract).

Haley, S. M., Coster, W. J., Ludlow, L. H., Haltiwanger, J. T., & Andrellos, P. J. (1992). *Pediatric Evaluation of Disability Inventory (PEDI), Version I. Development, standardization and administration manual.* Boston: New England Medical Center-PEDI Research Group.

Harris, J. P. (1983). Heart failure. In M. Ziai (Ed.), *Bedside pediatrics: Diagnostic evaluation of the child* (313–319). Boston: Little, Brown.

Hesz, N., & Wolraich, M. (1985). Vocal cord paralysis and brainstem dysfunction in children with spina bifida. *Developmental Medicine and Child Neurology, 27,* 522–531.

Hinderer, K. A., Richardson, P. K., & Atwater, S. W. (1989). Clinical implications of the Peabody Developmental Motor Scales: A constructive review. *Physical and Occupational Therapy in Pediatrics, 9,* 81–106.

Hopkins, B., & Prechtl, H. F. R. (1984). A qualitative approach to the development of movements during early infancy. In H. F. T. Prechtl (Ed.), *Continuity of Neural Functions from Prenatal to Postnatal Life. Clinics in Developmental Medicine No. 94.* London: Spastics International Medical Publications. 179–197.

Ireton, H., & Glascoe, F. P. (1995). Assessing children's development using parents' reports. The Child Development Inventory. *Clinical Pediatrics (Phila), 34,* 248–255.

Jenkins, S., Bax, M., & Hart, H. (1980). Behavior problems in pre-school children. *Journal of Child Psychology and Psychiatry, 21,* 5–17.

Kinney, H. C., Brody B.A., Kloman A. S., et al. (1988). Sequence of central nervous system myelination in human infancy II. Patterns of myelination in autopsied infants. *Journal of Neuropathology Experimental Neurology, 47,* 217–234.

Kinsbourne, M. (1964). Hiatus hernia with contortions of neck. *The Lancet, 1,* 1058.

Lewis, R. T., Burgess, J.H., & Hampson, L. G. (1971). Cardiorespiratory studies in critical illness. Changes in aspiration pneumonitis. *Archives of Surgery, 103,* 335–340.

Logemann, J. A. (1983). *Evaluation and treatment of swallowing disorders* (216–217). Austin, TX: PRO-ED.

Loughlin, G. M. (1989). Respiratory consequences of dysfunctional swallowing and aspiration. *Dysphagia, 3,* 126–130.

Majnemer, A., Riley, P., Shevell, M., Birnbaum, R., Greenstone, H., & Coates, A. L. (2000). Severe bronchopulmonary dysplasia increases risk for later neurological and motor sequelae in preterm survivors. *Developmental Medicine and Child Neurology, 42,* 53–60.

Mathew, O. P., Clark, M. L., Pronske, M. L., Luna-Solazano, H. G., & Peterson, M. D. (1985). Breathing pattern and ventilation during oral feeding in term newborn infants. *The Journal of Pediatrics, 106,* 810–813.

Meeks Gardner, J., Grantham-McGregor, S. M., Chang, S. M., Himes, J. H., & Powell, C. A. (1995). Activity and behavioral development in stunted and nonstunted children and response to nutritional supplementation. *Child Development, 66,* 1785–1797.

Mollitt, D. L., Golladay, E. S., & Seibert, J. J. (1985). Symptomatic gastroesophageal reflux following gastrostomy in neurologically impaired patients. *Pediatrics, 75,* 1124–1126.

Moss, H. B., & Green, A. (1982). Neuroleptic-associated dysphagia confirmed by esophageal manometry. *American Journal of Psychiatry, 139,* 515–516.

Msall, M. E., Rogers, B. T., Ripstein, H., Lyon, N., & Wilczenski, F. (1997). Measurements of functional outcomes in children with cerebral palsy. *Mental Retardation and Developmental Disabilities Researh Reviews, 3,* 194–203.

Nelson, K. B., Dambrosia, J. M., Ting, T. Y., Grether, J. K. (1996). Uncertain value of electronic fetal monitoring in predicting cerebral palsy. *New England Journal of Medicine, 334,* 613–618.

Nelson, K. B., & Ellenberg, J. H. (1995). Childhood neurological disorders in twins. *Paediatric Perinatal Epidemiology, 9,* 135–145.

Nelson, K. B., & Grether, J. K. (1999). Causes of cerebral palsy. *Current Opinions in Pediatrics, 11,* 487–491.

Nishino, T., Yonezawa, T., & Honda, Y. (1985). Effects of swallowing on the pattern of continuous respiration in human adults. *American Review of Respiratory Distress, 132,* 1219–1222.

Piper, M. C., Pinnell, L., Darrah, J., & Mahapatra, A. K. (1992). Construction and validation of the Alberta Infant Motor Scale (AIMS). *Canadian Journal of Public Health, 83*(Suppl. 2): S46–S50.

Prechtl, H. F. R. (1990). Qualitative changes of spontaneous movements in fetus and preterm infant are a marker of neurological dysfunction (Editorial). *Early Human Development, 23,* 151–158.

Raynor, P., & Rudolf, M.C. (1996). What do we know about children who fail to thrive? *Child Care Health Development, 22,* 241–50.

Reau, N. R., Senturia, Y. D., Lebailly, S. A., & Christoffel, K. K. (1996). Infant and toddler feeding patterns and problems: Normative data and a new direction. Pediatric Practice Research Group. *Journal of Developmental and Behavioral Pediatrics, 17,* 149–153.

Reilly, S., Skuse, D., & Poblete, X. (1996). Prevalence of feeding problems and oral motor dysfunction in children with cerebral palsy: A community survey. *Journal of Pediatrics, 219,* 877–82.

Richman, N. (1981). A community survey of characteristics of one to two year olds with sleep disturbances. *Journal of American Academy of Child Adolescent Psychiatry, 20,* 281–291.

Robinson, W. P. Bottani, A., Xie, Y. G., Balakrishman, J., Binkert, F., Machler, M., Prader, A., & Schinzel, A. (1991). Molecular, cytogenetic, and clinical investigations of Prader-Willi syndrome patients. *American Journal Human Genetics, 49,* 1219–1234.

Rogers, B. T., Arvedson, J., Msall, M., & Demerath, R. R. (1993). Hypoxemia during oral feeding of children with severe cerebral palsy. *Developmental Medicine and Child Neurology, 35,* 3–10.

Rogers, B. T., Booth, L., Duffy, L. C., Hassan, M. B., McCormick, P., Snitzer, J., & Zorn, W. (1992). Parents developmental perceptions and expectations for their high risk infants. *Journal of Developmental and Behavioral Pediatrics, 13,* 102–107.

Rosen, C. L., Glaze, D. G., & Frost, J. D. (1984). Hypoxemia associated with feeding in the preterm infant and full term neonate. *American Journal of Diseases of Children, 138,* 623–628.

Samango-Sprouse, C., & Suddaby, E.C. (1997). Developmental concerns in children with congenital heart disease. *Current Opinions in Cardiology, 12,* 91–98.

Samson-Fang, L. J., & Stevenson, R. D. (2000). Identification of malnutrition in children with cerebral palsy: Poor performance of weight-for-height centiles. *Developmental Medicine and Child Neurology, 42,* 162–168.

Scharli, A. F. (1985). Gastroesophageal reflux and severe retardation. In P. Wurnig (Ed.), *Progress in pediatric surgery* (84–90). Berlin: Springer-Verlag.

Schwartz, D. J., Wynne, J. W., Gibbs, C. T., Hood, C. I., & Kuck, E. J. (1980). The pulmonary consequences of aspiration of gastric contents at pH values greater than 2.5. *American Review of Respiratory Disease, 121,* 119–126.

Shivpuri, C. R., Martin, R. J., Carlo, W. A., & Fanaroff, A. A. (1983). Decreased ventilation in preterm infants during oral feeding. *The Journal of Pediatrics, 103,* 285–289.

Smith, J., Wolkove, N., Colacone, A., & Kreisman, H. (1989). Coordination of eating, drinking and breathing in adults. *Chest, 96,* 578–582.

Sokoloff, L. G., & Pavlakovic, R. (1997). Neuroleptic-induced dysphagia. *Dysphagia, 12,* 177–179.

Sondheimer, J. M., & Morris, B. A. (1979). Gastroesophageal reflux among severely retarded children. *Journal of Pediatrics, 94,* 710–714.

Spender, Q. W., Cronk, C. E., Charney, E. B., & Stallings, V. A. (1989). Assessment of linear growth of children with cerebral palsy: Use of alternative measures to height or length. *Developmental Medicine and Child Neurology, 31,* 206–214.

Squires, F., Potter, L., & Bricker, D. (1999). *Ages and Stages Questionnaire* (2nd ed.) Baltimore: Paul H. Brookes.

Stallings, V. A., Charney, E. B., Davies, J. C., & Cronk, E. E. (1993a). Nutrition-related growth failure of children with quadriplegic cerebral palsy. *Developmental Medicine and Child Neurology, 35,* 126–138.

Stallings, V. A., Charney, E. B., Davies, J. C., & Cronk, E. E. (1993b). Nutritional status and growth of children with diplegic or hemiplegic cerebral palsy. *Developmental Medicine and Child Neurology, 35,* 997–1006.

Stevenson, R. D. (1995). Use of segmental measures to estimate stature in children with cerebral palsy. *Archives of Pediatrics and Adolescent Medicine, 149,* 658–662.

Stieh, J., Kramer, H. H., Harding, P., & Fischer, G. (1999). Gross and fine motor development is impaired in children with cyanotic congenital heart disease. *Neuropediatrics, 30,* 77–82.

Volpe J. J. (2000). Overview: Normal and abnormal human brain development. *Mental Retardation and Developmental Disabilities Research Reviews, 6,* 1–5.

Wilkinson, J. D., Dudgeon, D. L., & Sondheimer, J. M. (1981). A comparison of medical and surgical treatment of gastroesophageal reflux in severely retarded children. *Journal of Pediatrics, 99,* 202–205.

Wilson, S. L., Thach, B. T., Brouillette, R. T., & Abu-Osbsa, Y. K. (1981). Coordination of breathing and swallowing in human infants. *Journal of Applied Physiology: Respiratory Environmental and Exercise Physiology, 50,* 851–858.

Wright, C., & Birks, E. (2000). Risk factors for failure to thrive: A population-based survey. *Child Care Health Development, 26,* 5–16.

Wyllie, E., Wyllie, R., Cruse, R. P., Rothner, A. D., & Erenberg, G. (1986). The mechanism of nitrazepam induced drooling and aspiration. *New England Journal of Medicine, 314,* 35–38.

Yakovlev P. I., & Lecours A. R. (1967). The myelogenetic cycles of regional maturation of the brain. In A. Minkowski (Ed.), *Regional development of the brain in early life* (3–70). Oxford, England: Blackwell.

■ CHAPTER 4

The Airway and Swallowing

Linda Brodsky and Joan Arvedson

■ SUMMARY

The intimate anatomic relationship of the upper airway to the upper digestive tract structures involved in swallowing necessitates precise coordination of breathing, swallowing, and laryngeal closure. Maintaining an
effective and efficient airway to provide adequate ventilation and prevent
aspiration is an important concern in infants and children who present with
feeding and swallowing problems. Problems of dysphagia can be secondary to both upper and lower airway problems. Sequelae of dysphagia also
can contribute to airway disease.

    The evaluation of the pediatric airway requires a thorough knowledge
of the relevant upper airway anatomy, particularly the larynx (Chapter 2).
Clinical examination of the child is often supplemented with appropriate
diagnostic studies, especially direct visualization of the larynx, trachea, and
esophagus. The diagnosis and treatment of airway problems, which are
associated with swallowing difficulties in children with specific airway
abnormalities, craniofacial anomalies, and tracheotomy, are also discussed.
Clinical case studies are used to highlight salient points.

■ INTRODUCTION

Establishing and maintaining an adequate airway are the first and most
important physiologic functions for the newborn infant. After airway maintenance, the ingestion and digestion of adequate nutrients is necessary to
provide energy for optimal growth and development. Human beings are the
only mammals in which a shared conduit for both breathing and swallowing exists. Although this seems an unlikely evolutionary development, the

unique ability of humans to communicate using voice and language is made possible precisely because of the development of these anatomic relationships (Laitman & Reidenberg, 1993a). To gain this communication advantage, humans have successfully confronted the challenges of anatomic proximity for swallowing, breathing, and vocalizing functions.

Feeding or swallowing problems may first present with airway symptoms alone. Conversely, an airway problem may lead to difficulty with feeding and swallowing. The occurrence of airway and feeding problems is increased when head and neck structural abnormalities, neurologic impairment, inflammatory or infectious disease, and metabolic disorders coexist.

Swallowing problems that present initially as airway problems often occur in children with structural or functional airway problems or gastrointestinal (GI) disease, most often gastroesophageal/extra-esophageal reflux disease (GERD/EERD).[1] The protean manifestations of GERD/EERD are becoming increasingly apparent to the pediatric otolaryngologist.

An evaluation of a feeding or swallowing difficulty associated with airway distress must also include evaluations of the cardiac, GI tract, and neurologic systems, as well as the ear, nose, throat, head, and neck. An effective and safe airway is the most important life-sustaining function. Recognition of a compromised airway during feeding and swallowing is essential when establishing an accurate diagnosis and optimal treatment plan.

■ CLINICAL EVALUATION

History

The clinical evaluation always begins with a detailed history. Prenatal, perinatal, and postnatal events may reveal prenatal infections (e.g., cytomegalovirus), intrauterine toxin exposures (e.g., medications, alcohol, or drugs), or perinatal or postnatal trauma (e.g., perinatal asphyxia from fetal distress or intubation for meconium aspiration). Neonatal nasal obstruction has been associated with the use of antihypertensives in the mother. Polyhydramnios during pregnancy may alert the clinician to functional (usually neurologic) or structural esophageal abnormalities, both of which are associated with airway problems. Family history should be

---

[1]Gastroesophageal reflux disease (GERD) refers to the abnormal regurgitation of acid into the esophagus causing symptoms. When the acid and other stomach contents emerge from the esophagus into the pharynx, larynx, mouth, and nasal cavities, the most commonly accepted term is extra-esophageal reflux disease (EERD) (Sasaki & Toohill, 2000).

explored for the presence of relatives with cleft lip or palate, other cranio-facial anomalies, GERD/EERD (Hu et al., 2000), and neurodevelopmental abnormalities.

In the older child, past medical history might reveal severe neonatal GERD, which can herald the development of EERD later in childhood. Repeated bouts of asthma, bronchitis, nonspecific reactive airway disease, croup, and pneumonia may all indicate particular airway problems or a faulty GI tract, particularly swallowing function. Knowledge of previous surgeries will help to establish any prior manipulations of the airway or cor-rective surgery performed for other problems, such as a tracheoesophageal fistula.

The environmental history provides information about potentiating irritants, such as tobacco smoke or contributory dietary habits. Social his-tory will help to establish the caregiver support available to the patient. Homecare airway support often requires enormous resources including round-the-clock nursing, supplies, and special equipment. Single parents, group homes, traditional nuclear families, and the presence of siblings with other health problems may influence treatment recommendations.

The review of systems should be thorough but particularly focused on the child's airway, GI tract, and neurodevelopment including speech and language acquisition. For neonates and infants, questions must be asked regarding breathing patterns, with the infant in quiet repose, in multiple positions, while both crying and feeding. The parent's or primary care-giver's description of respiratory difficulty and airway noises often provides invaluable information. Associated symptoms such as cough, wheezing, gurgling with respiration, cyanosis, apnea (cessation of breathing), snoring, hoarseness, opisthotonus (back arching), and food refusal are all sought.

Establishing a diagnosis and etiology is helped by using symptoms and signs to localize a problem to a specific anatomic localization (Table 4–1). Stridor, the term used to describe a high-pitched turbulent airflow through the larynx or trachea, may be present during inspiration, expiration, or both. Stridor is not a diagnosis itself but rather an indication of an airway abnormality. Sometimes stridor is mistakenly characterized as wheezing, often resulting in inappropriate and unsuccessful treatment directed at the lower airways and, therefore, ineffective in the upper airways. Other upper-airway sounds to note are nasal congestion, particularly when snorting (or stertor[2]) is present. Stertor is a low-pitched snorting or grunting sound that

---

[2]The terms "snorting" and "stertor" have been used interchangeably. Some clinicians include both under the general heading of stridor. However, stridor and stertor are dif-ferent sounds emanating from different anatomic locations in the upper airway. Implications for diagnosis and treatment also may be different.

Table 4–1. Abnormalities of Upper Aerodigestive Tract With Airway Presentation

Location	Abnormality	Clinical Presentation
Nose/nasopharynx	Choanal stenosis/atresia	• Nasal obstruction/discharge • Stridor and cyanosis with feeding • Relieved by crying
	Tumors	• Nasal obstruction • Stertor with feeding
	Deviated septum	• Traumatic birth • Nasal obstruction • Stertor with feeding
	Midface hypoplasias	• Craniofacial anomalies—Crouzon and Apert • Stertor increased with feeding
Oral cavity/ oropharynx	Cleft lip, palate, or both	• Air gulping, snorting, choking • Nasopharyngeal regurgitation • Ineffective suck
	Mandibular hypoplasias	• Craniofacial anomalies—Robin sequence, hemifacial microsomias, Treacher Collins (Chapter 12) • Choking and grunting that increase with feeding
	Adenotonsillar hyperplasia	• Obstructive sleep apnea with dysphagia • Failure to thrive/ malnutrition
Hypopharynx	Muscular hypotonia	• Stertor • Nasopharyngeal/ hypopharyngeal collapse on FFNL

(continues)

Table 4–1. *(continued)* Abnormalities of Upper Aerodigestive Tract with Airway Presentation

Location	Abnormality	Clinical Presentation
Laryngeal	Laryngeal/subglottic stenosis	• Stridor at rest that increases with feeding • Hoarseness and sometimes cough
	Laryngeal clefts	• Coughing with feeding • Stridor may be present at rest or increased with feeds
	Vocal fold paralysis	• Hoarseness • Stridor • Choking on feeds
	Laryngomalacia	• Stridor at rest and with feeds • Symptoms of EERD (Chapter 5)
	Tracheobronchomalacia	• Stridor • Apnea • Cyanosis • Increased work of breathing during feeds
	Supraglottic edema (secondary to EERD)	• Stridor • Hoarseness • Food refusal • Difficult and slow feeds
Esophagus	Tracheoesophageal fistula	• Cough, cyanosis, and choking with feeding • Recurrent pneumonia
	Esophageal mass	• Dysphagia • Stridor
Mediastinum	Vascular anomalies (aberrant right subclavian, double aortic arch, right aortic arch with left ligamentum)	• Feeding difficulties • Stridor
	Mediastinal tumors/cysts	• Dysphagia • Stridor

usually indicates a partial obstruction at the nose—nasopharyngeal, oropharyngeal, or hypopharyngeal level. Gurgling with respiration is associated with pooling of secretions in the hypopharynx, pyriform sinuses, and laryngeal inlet, often seen in children with focal or global neurodevelopmental delay or EERD. Cough can be indicative of aspiration occurring with, immediately after, or during a swallow (Chapter 10). The absence of a cough should not mislead the clinician into eliminating aspiration as operant in the feeding and swallowing problem. A weak or hoarse cry most often indicates laryngeal involvement—inflammatory disease such as EERD or anatomic–physiologic problems such as vocal fold paralysis. Apnea, the cessation of breathing for 8 seconds or more, may be associated with central nervous system (CNS) abnormalities, GERD, or anatomic obstruction.

Physical Examination

The physical examination of the pediatric airway begins with an overall assessment of the infant or child for neurologic abnormalities such as poor muscle tone, abnormal posture, and poor head control. Craniofacial or other congenital anomalies are noted and, if present, should prompt consultation with a geneticist or dysmorphologist.

When oral feeding is associated with significant airway distress, such as coughing, cyanosis, apnea, bradycardia, or choking, oral feedings should cease until the problem is well defined and the airway is deemed safe for feeding. Airway assessment begins with observation of the patterns of respiration, including resting respiratory rate and the presence of abnormal upper airway noises. An obstruction may occur at the level of the nasal cavity, nasopharynx, oral cavity, oropharynx, hypopharynx, larynx (supraglottic, glottic, or subglottic), tracheobronchial tree, or esophagus. Esophageal abnormalities can extrinsically compress the airway and present with stridor. Stertor and stridor, the most common respiratory signs with feeding and swallowing problems, may be accompanied by suprasternal, substernal, and intercostal retractions. Retractions indicate severe respiratory distress and indicate that the work of breathing is increased dramatically. In such instances adequate caloric intake for size may be inadequate for normal growth and development because of the increased caloric expenditure that occurs from the work of breathing (Case Study 1).

Evaluation of the infant's cry may help to localize the obstruction to level of the larynx if the cry is hoarse or weak. The presence of cough may indicate aspiration or an esophageal–airway connection. An assortment of primary cardiac and pulmonary diseases may also cause increased work of breathing with feeding problems and malnutrition.

It cannot be overemphasized that firsthand observation of the patient at rest, in multiple positions, and during feeding must be performed by the clinician evaluating the airway. The presence of overt airway obstruction should prompt immediate examination of the airway. Signs of airway distress are often absent until feeds are introduced, however. Several patterns may then emerge. Snorting, grunting, and frequent pauses between swallows may indicate a concomitant airway problem. Airway compromise may result in an increased respiratory rate due to the increased work of breathing needed during feeding. Cough during or immediately after eating is another warning sign of laryngeal distress or incompetence.

The triad of choking, cough, and cyanosis that begins after a feed is in progress is most commonly seen in unrecognized tracheoesophageal fistula (TEF), particularly in a patient who has had recurrent pneumonia during the first few months of life. Stertor, difficulty with feeding, and hoarseness comprise a symptom complex familiarly seen in a newborn or young infant with EERD. When a high-pitched stridor exists with this triad, laryngomalacia should be considered as well.

A thorough head and neck examination may reveal craniofacial anomalies such as mandibular hypoplasia (Figure 4–1A, B) or asymmetry seen in hemifacial microsomia, indicating abnormal soft tissue structures or tongue position that may interfere with feeding. Feeding difficulties can occur with various degrees of palatal clefting (Chapter 12). Identification of a submucous cleft palate (Figure 4–2) requires intraoral examination for bifid uvula, a zona pellucida (submucosal absence of the muscularis uvulae) and notching of the hard palate. However, all of these physical findings may be absent with nasopharyngeal regurgitation during feeding occurring as the only sign of an occult submucous cleft palate. Identification of an occult submucous cleft palate requires visualization of the nasal side of the palate where one sees a groove in the soft palate rather than the usual bulge in the soft palate normally created by contraction of the muscularis uvulae during palatal elevation.

Instrumental Evaluation

Flexible fiberoptic nasopharyngolaryngoscopy (FFNL[3]) is essential to complete an examination of the upper aerodigestive tract in infants and children

---

[3]The terms "flexible fiberoptic nasopharyngoscopy," "flexible fiberoptic nasopharyngolaryngoscopy," and "flexible fiberoptic laryngoscopy" are used interchangeably.

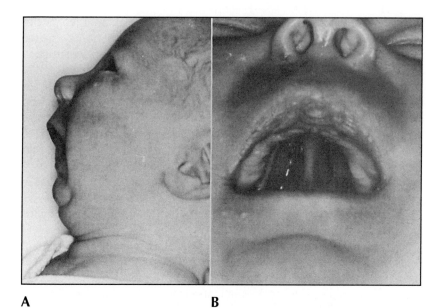

A   **B**

Figure 4–1. A. Infant with hypoplastic mandible from an isolated Pierre Robin sequence. **B.** U-shaped cleft palate also characteristic of Pierre Robin sequence. (From "Otolaryngology and Audiology" by M. S. Volk, S. Arnold, & L. Brodsky. In L. Brodsky, L. Holt, & D. H. Ritter-Schmidt (Eds.), *Craniofacial Anomalies: An Interdisciplinary Approach* (p. 169), 1992. St. Louis: Mosby-Year Book. Copyright 1992 by Mosby-Year Book. Reprinted by permission.)

with feeding and swallowing disorders (Figure 4–3). Visualization of structures from the anterior nares, posteriorly through the nasal cavity into the nasopharynx, and inferiorly into the hypopharynx and the larynx provides both structural and functional information regarding the upper airway. FFNL is particularly useful in determining functional aspects of airway dynamics, such as vocal fold function, tongue placement during inspiration and expiration, and the presence and degree of collapse of the nasopharynx or hypopharynx (Table 4–1). Videotape documentation is invaluable for monitoring children who require long-term care or in whom treatment for airway problems secondary to EERD must be reevaluated periodically. Functional assessment of the motor and sensory components of swallowing while visualizing the hypopharynx and larynx is termed flexible endoscopic examination of swallow with sensory testing—FEEST. This is described in detail under instrumental assessment (Chapter 8).

Radiologic evaluation of the airway may include a PA and lateral radiographs of the airway, performed with high KV filter so as to highlight

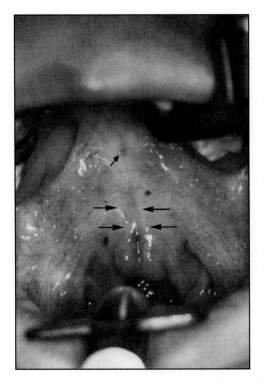

Figure 4–2. Intraoral view of a submucous cleft palate. Note bifid uvula; zona pellucida (large arrows); and notched, V-shaped, hard palate (small arrow).

soft-tissue/airway interfaces. Chest X-ray, barium esophagram, and ultra-fast dynamic and static computerized tomographic (CT) scans of the chest may provide further information valuable in diagnosis and treatment (Brody, Kuhn, Seidel, & Brodsky, 1991).

When an abnormality of the endolarynx, subglottis, trachea, bronchi, or esophagus is suspected, evaluation using a rigid laryngoscope, bronchoscope, or esophagascope under a general anesthesia is performed. In the airway, rigid endoscopy is necessary to evaluate for subglottic stenosis, laryngotracheal clefts, tracheoesophageal fistulae, chronic tracheitis from EERD, and tracheobronchomalacia.

Masses in the mediastinum, neck, and esophagus, as well as vascular anomalies of the great vessels, can also present with simultaneous feeding and breathing problems. Computerized tomographic scan with contrast, magnetic resonance imaging, echocardiography, or angiography may be indicated in select cases.

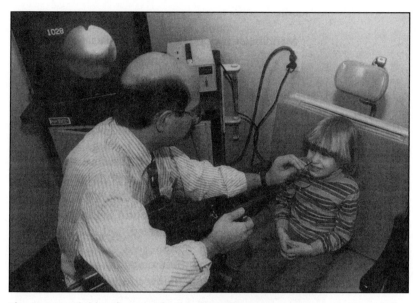

Figure 4–3. Child undergoing flexible fiberoptic laryngoscopy to evaluate stridor. Digital video recording allows storage and retrieval of multiple images from examinations performed at different times.

■ SPECIFIC AIRWAY AND FEEDING PROBLEMS

Gastroesophageal Reflux Disease and Extra-Esophageal Reflux Disease

Infants and older children who have airway distress when feeding or eating are often suffering from GERD/EERD.[4] Regurgitation of feeds is common in the young infant and is not necessarily regarded as pathologic, that is, requiring evaluation and treatment, unless it causes other symptoms that negatively impact on the health and well-being of the child. When GERD/EERD alter normal feeding and eating patterns or contribute to

---

[4]GERD/EERD is not necessarily a diagnosis in and of itself but may indicate an underlying disease process. Making a specific diagnosis is important if successful treatment is to occur.

airway distress or other otolaryngologic problems, then by definition the reflux is considered pathologic and requires evaluation and treatment. Airway symptoms are present in approximately 43% of children with GERD/EERD (Andze, Brandt, St. Vil, Bensoussan, & Blanchard, 1991). Conversely, the percentage of children with GERD/EERD induced respiratory problems is about 30% (Bauman, Sandler, & Smith, 1996). The children at greatest risk include those who have neurologic impairment, anatomic abnormalities (TEF and hiatal hernia), motility disorders, and hyperactive airways.

The anatomic and physiologic protective mechanisms that play a role in preventing GERD/EERD are described in Chapters 2 and 5 (Laitman & Reidenberg, 1997). Complications from GERD, such as erosive esophagitis, stricture formation, undernutrition, and malnutrition are well known and occur in about 15% of untreated cases (Bauman, et al., 1996). Refluxate, which contains acid, enzymes, bacteria, and partially digested food, has an unpredictable effect on the upper esophagus, larynx, and lower airways.

Two mechanisms appear to be operant: direct acid exposure and a reflex-mediated airway closure. Several reflexes are involved in the development of both upper and lower airway symptoms (Orenstein, 1988). The esophagolaryngeal reflex occurs when laryngospasm results after acid is introduced into the distal esophagus. The laryngeal chemoreflex occurs when acid directly stimulates the larynx. Reflex bronchospasm may also occur with direct acid stimulation of the esophagus, larynx, trachea, or bronchi. Apnea, bradycardia, and hypotension can all result. These reflexes are more active in infants, particularly premature infants. It is entirely possible that EERD can exist in the absence of GERD. Small amounts of acid may have no significant effect on the distal esophagus (GER); however, acid regurgitated into the larynx or trachea several times a day may have devastating effects on the less-well-protected respiratory mucosa. Indeed, GERD/EERD may present with stridor or apnea without any other signs or symptoms (Nielson, Heldt, & Tooley, 1990).

Animal studies have demonstrated that even small, intermittent exposures of refluxate to injured upper airway mucosa once every other day, can have severe symptoms and deleterious long-term effects (Little, Koufman, Kohut, & Marshall, 2000). The esophageal mucosa, particularly the distal portion, is able to withstand a certain amount of refluxate without irreparable harm. The mucosa of the larynx, pharynx, nasopharynx, nose/paranasal sinus passages, and the tracheobronchial tree are less well suited to these insults. In the older child, the untoward effects of EERD are potentiated by the low position of the larynx in the neck and the unprotected posterior larynx (Laitman & Reidenberg, 1993a,b).

Respiratory diseases may exacerbate or cause GERD/EERD (Orenstein, 1988). Reactive airway disease, asthma, bronchopulmonary dysplasia, recurrent bronchitis, cystic fibrosis, and central alveolar hypoventilation syndrome are all associated with GERD/EERD (Andze et al., 1991; Bauman et al., 1996; Halstead, 1999; Orenstein, 1988). Alterations in thoracoabdominal pressure relationships occur secondary to both forced expiration (cough, wheeze) and forced inspiration (stridor, stertor, hiccups). The associated increase in intra-abdominal pressure delays gastric emptying and increases the potential for gastric contents to flow into the esophagus. Both mechanisms result in refluxate being drawn from the stomach into the esophagus and upper airway.

Conversely, GERD/EERD can cause or worsen respiratory disease (Carr, Nguyen, Nagy, Poje, Pizzuto, & Brodsky, 2000). Airway symptoms can be nonspecific; however, when taken in combination, they will often point to the diagnosis of GERD/EERD (Table 4–2). Hoarseness, often described as a raspy or gravelly voice quality that is worse in the morning than in the evening, associated with morning nasal congestion and a throaty and wet cough, is a strong indicator that refluxate is entering the larynx during sleep. Symptoms of throat clearing, stomach aches, chest pain and pressure, hiccups, and frequent burping, especially between meals, all may be described. A feeling of something caught in the throat (globus sensation) and complaints of chronic sore throats are also common. This is particularly so when a normal tonsil examination is present or the sore throat is the initial symptom of recurrent or chronic sinusitis. Halitosis, frequent swallow with gurgling (particularly in the neurologically impaired child), food refusal (at any age), early satiety, and being a "picky, slow eater" are not infrequent in individuals with GERD/EERD.

Intractable cough, uncontrollable reactive airway disease, recurrent airway distress, and recurrent airway infections are all harbingers of GERD/EERD. It is estimated that up to 80% of children with asthma have temporally related GERD/EERD to wheezing episodes (Orenstein, 1988). A high index of suspicion is necessary because the symptoms and signs for reflux may be occult or atypical. The airway protective mechanism may become defective because of the effects of prior refluxate exposure, neurologic impairment, or anatomic changes in the larynx itself.

Apnea with feeding can be caused by GERD/EERD (Bauman et al., 1996; Orenstein, 1988). A large body of literature exists implicating reflux in acute life-threatening events, the best known of which is sudden infant death syndrome (SIDS). The mechanisms proposed include direct acid exposure to the upper airway, especially potent in the young infant in whom a prolonged laryngospasm may be fatal. Vagal afferents causing reflex central apnea and reflex bradycardia may also contribute (Orenstein, 1988). Snoring and other manifestations of obstructive apnea (both awake and asleep) may be secondary to reflux.

Table 4–2. Signs and Symptoms of GERD/EERD

Typical (gastrointestinal)
    Frequent emesis
    Burping
    Abdominal pain
    Heartburn
    Difficulty swallowing
    Failure to thrive/malnutrition (undernutrition)
    Chest pain
    Regurgitation of food
    Rumination
    Frequent swallowing
    Picky or slow eater
    Food refusal

Atypical (airway)
    Hoarseness
    Cough
    Throat clearing
    Recurrent croup
    Recurrent pneumonia
    Asthma exacerbations
    Stridor/stertor
    Apnea
    Obstructive or central sleep apnea
    Hiccups
    Gurgly respirations
    Acute life threatening events

Atypical (Other)
    Halitosis
    Torticollis (Sandifer's syndrome)
    Opisthotonis (back arching)
    Drooling
    Chronic sore throat
    Globus sensation
    Morning nasal congestion/cough
    Frequent nocturnal awakenings
    Otalgia
    Tooth enamel erosion
    Intractable rhinosinusitis
    Chronic otitis media
    Hypogusia (loss of taste)

Several unusual presentations that have an effect on swallowing and eating include food refusal (Dellert, Hyams, Treem, & Geertsma, 1993; Hyman, 1994), drooling (even in a child without neurologic impairment) (Mandel & Tamari, 1995), loss of taste, chronic halitosis, recurrent rhino-sinusitis, nasal congestion, and chronic otitis media. Occasionally dental erosions are seen secondary to the untoward effects of the acid on the tooth enamel.

Physical examination in the infant may reveal back arching, hoarse cry, stridor and stertor, and excessive nasal secretions. Soft palatal swelling, pharyngeal erythema, and posterior pharyngeal cobblestoning (islands of hyperplastic lymphoid tissue on the posterior pharyngeal wall) are commonly seen in these children.

Direct visualization of the larynx and tracheobronchial tree is the best way to diagnose EERD. The triad of lingual tonsillar hyperplasia, posterior glottic swelling, and loss of arytenoid architecture is pathognomonic of chronic laryngitis from EERD (Carr, Nguyen, Poje, Pizzuto, Nagy, & Brodsky, 2000; Figure 4–4). Tracheal mucosa may reveal cobblestoning, blunt carina, and loss of tracheal ring architecture, all potential indicators of chronic aspiration (Figure 4–5) (Carr, Nguyen, Nagy, et al., 2000). Bronchoalveolar lavage to assess for the presence of high levels of amylase or lipid laden macrophages (Colombo & Hallbert, 1987; Nussbaum, Maggi, Mathis, & Galant, 1987) is also useful to help establish the diagnosis of aspiration, but these findings are not specific for GERD/EERD.

When airway and upper digestive symptoms are present, aggressive medical management of the GERD/EERD is implemented. Dietary alterations including elimination of carbonated beverages, caffeine, spicy foods, chocolate, fried and fatty foods are recommended, especially in the older child and adolescent. Erratic eating schedules, frequent snacking, eating late into the night, reclining soon after eating (to watch television), and a sedentary or overly active lifestyle can all contribute to the development of GERD/EERD. The effects of nicotine from environmental tobacco smoke are not to be underestimated. Medications aimed at increasing the rate of gastric emptying, increasing lower esophageal sphincter pressures, and decreasing acid secretion or acidity may be used. In severe cases where life-threatening airway symptoms exist or when medical therapy fails, fundoplication should be considered (Chapter 5) (Andze et al., 1991).

Choanal Atresia and Nasal Stenosis

Choanal Atresia

Bilateral choanal atresia affects approximately 1 in 50,000 newborns and usually presents with the first feeding. Almost all infants are, if not obligate,

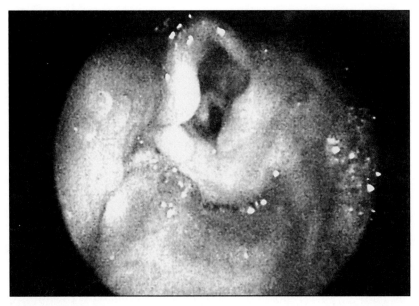

Figure 4–4. Direct laryngoscopy with magnification demonstrating severe posterior glottic swelling and loss of arytenoid architecture. Note short aryepiglottic folds.

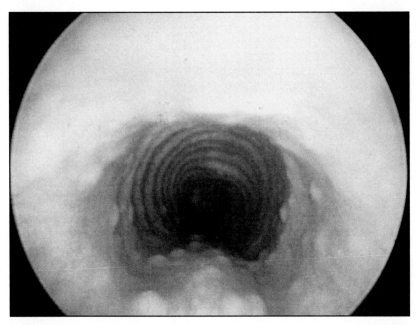

Figure 4–5. Severe tracheal cobblestoning associated with reflux induced chronic aspiration and presenting as chronic cough.

at least primarily nasal breathers for about the first 6 months of life. Classically, infants with bilateral choanal atresia have cyclical periods of cyanosis at rest, which are relieved when the child becomes agitated, begins to cry, and breathes through the mouth, thus relieving the airway obstruction. A return to the resting, noncrying state ensues, and the cycle begins anew. Surprisingly, some of these infants may have little or no respiratory distress at rest but become severely compromised (with cyanosis) at the onset of feedings. Nasal patency is first evaluated by inspection of the anterior nares. Checking for airflow using a wisp of cotton created at the end of a cotton-tipped applicator readily provides information regarding airflow. Passing catheters through the nose into the nasopharynx can help to evaluate nasal patency; however, with this technique, subtle forms of nasal or choanal stenosis may be missed.

Nasal Stenosis

Stenosis or obstruction from a deviated nasal septum secondary to birth trauma should be ruled out (Emami, Brodsky, & Pizzuto, 1996). Anterior and posterior rhinoscopy may be accomplished using an otoscope with nasal speculum attachment (Figure 4–6). Edema of the nasal mucosa is common in children who are nasally suctioned at birth. This resolves with cessation of suctioning. Topical decongestants such as neosynephrine 1/8% may be used for a few days, and sometimes prolonged use of steroid nose

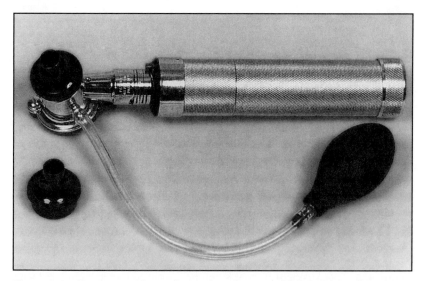

Figure 4–6. Otoscope with nasal speculum that is useful for anterior rhinoscopy.

drops will be useful (Derkay & Grundfast, 1991). Midnasal stenosis and anterior or nasal aperture stenosis may also cause obstructive symptoms and associated feeding problems (Knegt-Junk, Bos, & Berkovits, 1988).

Inspection of both posterior nasal choanae using FFNL with a 2mm or 3mm endoscope or a 2.7mm rigid telescope is most helpful. Direct visualization, combined with axial computerized tomographic scan of the nose and nasopharynx, will determine the type (membranous vs. bony) and the extent of the lesion (Figure 4–7, A–C). Surgical repair of bilateral choanal atresia is usually performed in the neonatal period. The transnasal approach is preferred in this age group by most (Lantz & Birck, 1981; Richardson & Osguthorpe, 1988). Transpalatal repair with long-term stenting may be indicated for revision surgery or in other cases where the anatomy is not favorable for the transasal approach (Maniglia & Goodwin, 1981). Nasal aperture stenosis is also amenable to surgical correction followed by long-term stenting. Severe midnasal stenosis often requires tracheotomy to bypass the obstruction until the child grows enough to support the airway orally.

Some children have choanal atresia as part of an association of multiple congential anomalies known as the CHARGE association. CHARGE stands for Coloboma, Heart, Atresia choanae, Retardation, Genitourinary, and Ear abnormalities. Children with CHARGE association almost always have neurodevelopmental delays associated with decreased neuromuscular tone and incoordination, all further complicating feeding. Tracheotomy offers the most effective means for managing the airway in these children (Asher, McGill, Kaplan, Friedman, & Healy, 1990).

Craniofacial Anomalies

Midface Hypoplasias

The most common midface hypoplasias are the craniosynostoses of Crouzon and Apert. Phenotypic presentation is highly variable for these autosomal, dominantly inherited craniofacial anomalies. Typically they are characterized by cranial synostosis (premature closure of the cranial sutures), midface hypoplasia, ocular proptosis due to shallow orbits, cleft palate, and, in the case of the Apert syndrome, finger and hand abnormalities (Figure 4–8A, B). In the more severe forms, especially when a cleft palate is not present, stridor at rest will occur. Lateral neck radiographs may reveal a maxilla that is literally impacted against the skull base (Figure 4–9). In less severe forms of maxillary retrusion, oral feeding may stress a marginally compensated airway. Management often requires tracheotomy until the diameter of the airway increases with growth. The airway may be improved with midface advancement, a procedure that has been performed in some cases as early as age 3 years, but is best deferred until after puberty.

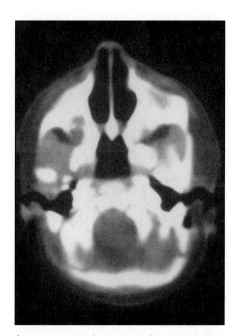

Figure 4–7A. Axial computerized tomographic scan showing bilateral bony choanal atresia. (From "Otolaryngology and Audiology" by M. S. Volk, S. Arnold, & L. Brodsky. In L. Brodsky, L. Holt, & D. H. Ritter-Schmidt [Eds.], *Craniofacial Anomalies: An Interdisciplinary Approach* (p. 172). St. Louis: Mosby-Year Book. Copyright 1992 by Mosby-Year Book. Reprinted by permission.)

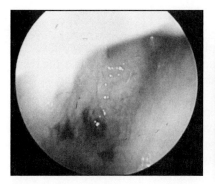

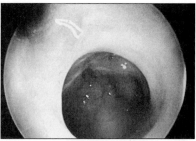

Figure 4–7B. Nasal telescopic view of a blind pouch at the posterior nasal choana, consistent with choanal atresia.

Figure 4–7C. Nasal telescopic view of repaired choanal atresia.

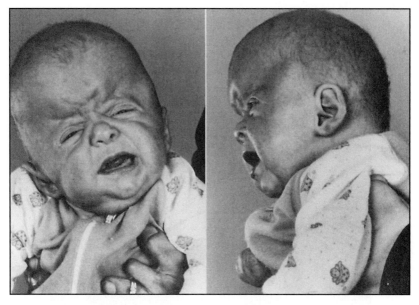

A   B

Figure 4–8. A. Frontal view of an infant with Apert syndrome. Note midface hypoplasia in the infant and syndactyly of the affected parent holding the child. **B.** Lateral view of infant with Apert syndrome. (From "Otolaryngology and Audiology" by M. S. Volk, S. Arnold, & L. Brodsky. In L. Brodsky, L. Holt, & D. H. Ritter-Schmidt [Eds.], *Craniofacial Anomalies: An Interdisciplinary Approach* (p. 172). St. Louis: Mosby-Year Book. Copyright 1992 by Mosby-Year Book. Reprinted by permission.)

Mandibular Hypoplasias

The Pierre Robin sequence classically presents with mandibular hypoplasia, glossoptosis (a retroplaced tongue), and a U-shaped cleft palate (Figure 4–1A, B). Some children have airway obstruction at rest, but the obstruction may be subtle in its presentation and not manifest until feeds are introduced. Grunting, choking, and coughing with prolonged, difficult feeds may indicate airway compromise. The mechanisms can vary among patients, but three basic mechanisms have been described and can be identified using FFNL. The most common mechanism for obstruction is glossoptosis at the level of the hypopharynx during inspiration. On occasion, the palatal shelves of the cleft may be drawn medially to obstruct the airway. At other times, lateral pharyngeal wall hypotonia may cause pharyngeal/

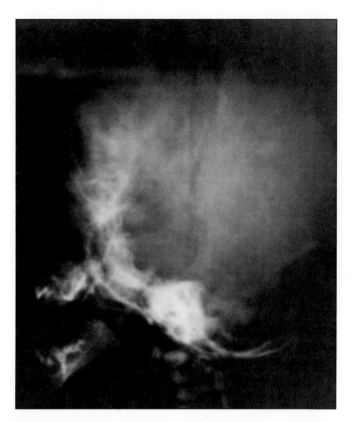

Figure 4–9. Lateral neck radiograph of infant in figures 4–8A, B. Note maxilla impacted on skull base and the absence of a nasopharynx. (From "Otolaryngology and Audiology" by M. S. Volk, S. Arnold, & L. Brodsky. In L. Brodsky, L. Holt, & D. H. Ritter-Schmidt [Eds.], *Craniofacial Anomalies: An Interdisciplinary Approach* (p. 172). St. Louis: Mosby-Year Book. Copyright 1992 by Mosby-Year Book. Reprinted by permission.)

hypopharyngeal collapse (Shprintzen, 1988). Concurrent GERD/EERD may further complicate the picture and argues for early treatment of the obstruction (Dudkiewicz, Sekula, & Nielepiec-Jalosinska, 2000).

Treatment of the airway obstruction in nonsyndromic Pierre Robin sequence depends on the anatomic location of the obstruction. Treatment options include watchful waiting for growth and development in mildly affected cases, nasopharyngeal tubes, stenting, subperiosteal tongue release (Delorme, Laroque, & Caouette-Laberge, 1989), glossopexy (lip–tongue fusion) (Figure 4–10; Argamaso, 1992), and tracheotomy. It is important to note that not all mandibular hypoplasias are manifestations of the Pierre Robin sequence. Accurate diagnosis is essential for the development of

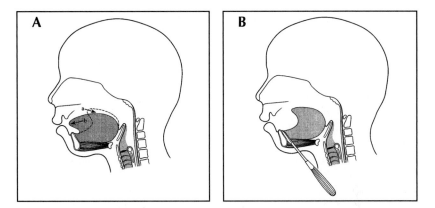

Figure 4–10A. Note position of tongue when glossoptosis occurs (a). Surgical procedures to bring tongue into normal position (b) are noted in B and C. **B.** Subperiosteal tongue release releases the tongue muscles from the mandible and allows the tongue to resume its normal position (Delorme, Laroque, & Caouette-Laberge, 1989).

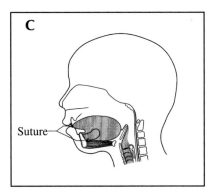

Figure 4–10C. Glossopexy prevents glossoptosis by bringing the tongue anteriorly, fusing it to the lip, and securing it in place with a circum-mandibular suture through the tongue base.

long-term treatment plans and for predicting prognosis. A genetics or dysmorphology evaluation is necessary in every case. Treatment depends on etiology and may vary considerably among patients (Case Study 2).

Infants with other craniofacial anomalies, such as cleft palate and Down syndrome, often present with, or encounter, feeding difficulties. These are discussed in depth in Chapter 12.

Tracheoesophageal Fistula

Tracheoesophageal fistula (TEF) may be either congenital or acquired. The acquired forms follows trauma, foreign body ingestion, or as a complication of surgery, such as tracheotomy. As mentioned previously, the triad of cough, choking, and cyanosis is common. Recurrent pneumonia, particularly in the first 6 months of life, is another presenting symptom. Several types of tracheoesophageal fistulae are described (Figure 4–11A–C). Those presenting with esophageal atresia tend to present with polyhydramnios in the mother and total inability of the infant to swallow during the first days of life (Figure 4–11A, B). In an H-type fistula, barium esophagram may reveal a tract from the esophagus into the trachea (Figures 4–11C and 4–12); however, rigid endoscopic evaluation of the esophagus and tracheobronchial tree usually is required to evaluate this type of TEF comprehensively. Surgical repair is required, but esophageal stenosis at the operative site may cause continued dysphagia and necessitate adjustment of diet and repeated esophageal dilatations. Tracheomalacia may also be present after repair of the TEF. This may result in or contribute to continued feeding difficulty, stridor, and respiratory distress (Case Study 3).

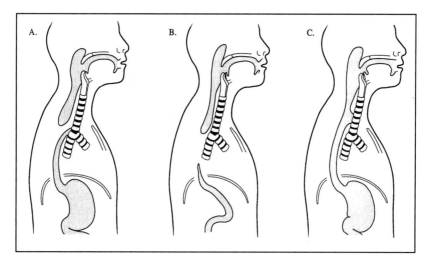

Figure 4–11. A. Distal tracheoesophageal fistulae are most commonly associated with proximal esophageal atresia. **B.** Esophageal atresia without tracheal connection. **C.** Of this group of anomalies, tracheoesophageal fistula alone, known as an H-type fistula, is the least common.

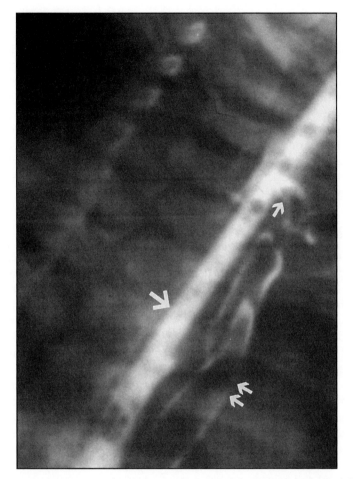

Figure 4–12. Barium esophogram reveals an H-type tracheoesophageal fistula with contrast in both the esophagus (large arrow) and trachea (double arrow) with a well-defined connection (small single arrow).

Laryngeal Anomalies

A wide variety of laryngeal abnormalities may present with stridor and feeding problems. Supraglottic cyst, epiglottic structural abnormalities (absent epiglottis) (Bonilla, Pizzuto, Brodsky, & Brody, 1998; Reyes, Arnold, & Brooks, 1994), and posterior laryngeal clefts all can lead to feeding difficulties associated with airway obstruction as the initial clinical presentation. Choking and cough soon after a feed is initiated may occur, and these conditions can mimic TEF. Infants with vocal fold paralysis, chronic reflux laryngitis (with or without laryngomalacia), and subglottic stenosis may have significant difficulty with both breathing and feeding. FFNL and rigid direct laryngoscopy provide different sets of information needed to arrive at an accurate diagnosis. The diagnosis of laryngeal cleft requires examination of the interarytenoid and postcricoid areas. Palpation of the arytenoid cartilages and interarytenoid area can only be accomplished by rigid direct laryngoscopy. Therapy for laryngeal anomalies will be determined by the underlying etiology but often requires some type of surgical intervention.

Sleep Disturbances

Sleep disturbances include a wide variety of sleep disorders including obstructive sleep apnea and frequent night awakenings. Obstructive sleep apnea is defined as the cessation of breathing during sleep for more than 8 seconds. In the neurologically normal pediatric population, it presents in both infants and young children and is almost always accompanied by hyperplasia of the nasopharyngeal tonsils (adenoids), pharyngeal tonsils (tonsils), or lingual tonsils. Young infants and children with swallowing and feeding difficulties may present with failure to thrive or undernutrition. Decreased caloric intake and increased caloric demands from increased work of breathing during sleep may both be operant. Alterations in growth hormone secretion during sleep may also be responsible (Goldstein et al., 1987). Dysphagia, especially for meats, may be present in older children. Tonsillectomy, adenoidectomy, or both will almost always relieve the obstruction, except in those instances when accompanying neurologic compromise is present. Pharyngeal and hypopharyngeal muscular hypotonia may then have a significant role. Enlargement of the lingual tonsils and swelling of the soft palate may present with obstructive sleep apnea and odynophagia and dysphagia. Elimination of GERD/EERD is most important in this subset of patients. When airway obstruction does not respond to appropriate medical therapy or tonsillectomy and adenoidectomy, alternative treatments to be considered include continuous positive oral or nasal pressure at night or tracheotomy.

Children with recurrent, very frequent (greater than 8–10) nocturnal arousals often wake up irritable and demand a drink. Daytime eating patterns are often erratic. These sleep disturbances are often difficult to diagnose and treat because of clinician skepticism and parental blame. Careful history, physical examination, and in-depth laboratory testing may reveal severe EERD (Carr & Brodsky, 1999).

Tracheotomy and Swallowing

Tracheotomy is a surgical procedure resulting in the formation of a direct passage between the trachea and skin to provide an alternate pathway for respiration (Figure 4–13A, B). The hole is maintained by a tracheotomy tube, which requires constant care and monitoring to prevent serious complications, some of which can result in death (Rosingh & Peek, 1999). Tracheotomies are performed for a variety of conditions in the pediatric population. These conditions most often include upper airway obstruction, neurologic impairment, chronic aspiration, and chronic pulmonary disease. When tracheotomy is recommended for chronic aspiration, the problem of the aspiration is seldom solved and may even be made worse. However, some believe that management of tracheal secretions may improve because of improved access for suctioning. Short-term tracheotomy with cessation of oral feeds in select patients with aspiration may prove to be beneficial (Chapter 10).

Swallowing problems are ubiquitous in the pediatric tracheotomy population, particularly because an increased number of these patients have multiple handicaps (Rosingh & Peek, 1999). The pharyngeal phase of swallowing is most affected by the presence of a tracheotomy. As described in Chapter 2, during a normal swallow, the bolus passes through the pharynx when elevation and anterior movement of the larynx occur. The epiglottis depresses and forms the first level of the three-tiered laryngeal closure. Alterations in swallowing efficiency, particularly a delayed swallow response in children with tracheotomy, have been described (Abraham & Wolf, 2000). Mechanical fixation of the larynx in the neck by the tracheotomy tube prevents superior excursion of the entire larynx, especially

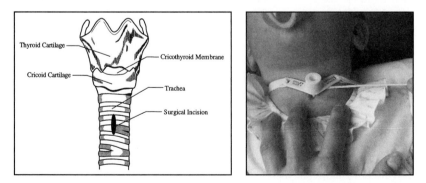

Figure 4–13. A. Diagrammatic representation of tracheotomy. **B.** Photograph of tracheotomy tube in infant's neck.

the arytenoids and epiglottis. Closure of the laryngeal vestibule is then delayed, sometimes resulting in laryngeal penetration. Laryngeal closure may be delayed until after the relaxation of the upper esophageal sphincter. Furthermore, in adults and some older children, in whom a cuffed tracheotomy tube is required for tight seal of the airway to maintain ventilation, cuff pressure transmitted to the esophagus may also interfere with swallowing. When cuffed tracheotomy tubes are deflated, secretions and food pooled above the cuff may enter into the lower airway.

The cough reflex is often blunted or absent in patients with tracheotomy. The inability to generate adequate intrathoracic pressure is the major contributor. Fitting patients with a Passy-Muir speaking valve increases subglottic pressure and has proven to be most effective in improving cough and pulmonary function in these patients (Eibling & Gross, 1996). Neurophysiologic mechanisms for laryngeal dysfunction have also been proposed. An uncoordinated laryngeal closure reflex has been described in dogs with chronic tracheotomy. Diversion of air through the tracheotomy may further desensitize the larynx and result in a blunted cough reflex (Sasaki, Suzuki, Horiuchi, & Kirchner, 1979).

■ CASE STUDY 1

"Betsy" was a 2-month-old infant who presented to the emergency department with a chief complaint of breathing difficulties and inability to gain weight. Her parents reported that the breathing became noisy approximately 1 week after birth. It was constant, present in all positions, and low pitched. The baby fed well with a bottle and eagerly took all feeds but became blue around the lips while feeding. The parents denied a history of emesis, diarrhea, chronic cough, or choking on feeds. She had gained only 9 ounces since birth. The practitioner following her at a local clinic told the family that her breathing was from a floppy larynx and that she would "grow out of it."

Betsy was the product of a normal vaginal delivery. Birth weight was 8 pounds, 1 ounce. She had received her immunizations. No other significant past medical, surgical, social, or family history contributed.

Physical examination revealed a markedly malnourished infant in moderate respiratory distress. Respirations were at 30 per minute. She weighed 8 pounds 10 ounces. A low-pitched stridor was noted. The voice was very hoarse and her cry was weak. She had suprasternal, intercostal, and substernal retracations. When she was given bottle feeds, her respiration did not change; however, she developed circumoral cyanosis and pulse oximetry indicated 88% saturation. The remainder of the neurologic, head and neck, and heart and lung examinations was normal.

Cardiac consult and echocardiogram failed to reveal any cardiac abnormalities. A FFNL was performed and showed severe swelling of the posterior glottis with collapse of the redundant arytenoid mucosa in the larynx. Her aryepiglottic folds were very short, and the lingual tonsils were prominent although not obstructing the vallecula. Hypopharyngeal collapse with glossoptosis was also seen. The infant was admitted to the intensive care unit and immediately begun on metoclopropamide (0.2 mg/kg/dose, 4 times daily) and ranitidine (2 mg/kg/dose, 2 times daily). The next day she underwent direct laryngoscopy, bronchoscopy, and tracheotomy. Severe laryngeal edema, posterior glottic swelling, loss of arytenoid architecture, and short aryepiglottic folds were found (Figure 4–4). Subglottic inflammation and narrowing were also present and thought to be contributing to the airway distress and likely secondary to the GERD/ EERD.

Postoperatively, a nutrition consult confirmed malnutrition and recommended increasing caloric intake to 24 kcal per ounce, 78 cc every 3 hours. Feeding evaluation by the speech–language pathologist revealed a normal suck–swallow pattern. A developmental pediatrician was asked to see the infant to evaluate for neurodevelopmental impairment to account for the severe hypopharyngeal collapse, usually seen with hypopharyngeal hypotonia and neurologic disease. The examination was normal. The child began to gain weight on the second postoperative day. The reflux medications were temporarily stopped while a 24-hour dual-channel pH probe was completed. Severe GERD/EERD was demonstrated with 47 acid episodes to the upper probe, and the pH was less than 4.0 6.2% of the time. The lower probe revealed 143 acid reflux episodes, and the pH was less than 4.0 8.2% of the time.

The reflux medications were restarted, soy formula begun, and the patient was discharged after tracheotomy teaching and after home-care nursing was obtained. Four months later, repeat endoscopy revealed a much improved larynx with normalization of the subglottis. FFNL, with the tracheotomy temporarily removed and the stoma obstructed, showed resolution of the glossoptosis and laryngomalacia. She was decannulated 1 month later but continued on reflux medications. Betsy will be followed closely for her reflux, growth, development, and airway.

Comment

This patient demonstrates how an airway problem can present with a severe feeding disorder (malnutrition), which is secondary to GERD/EERD. Although the child appeared to be taking adequate calories, the increased work of breathing quickly depleted those calories, and the infant developed a severe nutrition problem.

■ CASE STUDY 2

"Jane" was a 1-day-old infant born at 36 weeks gestation via normal vaginal delivery. The pregnancy was complicated by polyhydramnios. At birth, the child's Apgars were 2 and 5, for which she required oxygen and assisted ventilation. In addition to the respiratory distress, she was noted to have a small jaw (micrognathia) and a U-shaped cleft palate (Figure 4–1A, B). In the first day of life, she was transferred to the Children's Hospital of Buffalo for evaluation and management of continued respiratory distress. Intubation during transport was reported to be difficult.

When first seen by the pediatric otolaryngology service, she was intubated. She was small for weight but had good muscular movement; no focal neurologic problems were noted. Otolaryngologic examination revealed low-set ears and otitis media with effusion. There was no nasal obstruction. Intraoral examination revealed a large U-shaped cleft palate. She had a small tongue that was situated posteriorly in the pharynx. Her cranial nerves were otherwise intact; a left clubfoot was noted. Dysmorphologic diagnosis revealed an isolated Pierre Robin sequence and an isolated club foot deformity.

Jane was extubated on day 2 of life without respiratory distress. Oral feeds were introduced on day 3. Her first several days of feeding were uneventful with a Haberman feeder. However, by day 3, she began to have significant grunting and choking during feeds. Positional changes and feeding alterations suggested by the oral-motor feeding specialist did not result in improvement. Airway evaluation using a nasopharyngoscope revealed glossoptosis of the tongue to the posterior pharynx with no evidence of lateral pharyngeal wall or palatal shelf obstruction.

It was recommended that she have a nasopharyngeal tube placed and that she continue her oral gastric feedings. The increased growth and neurologic development were expected to be helpful for this child. At the end of 2 to 3 weeks of a nasopharyngeal tube with oral feedings supplemented by oral–gastric tube feedings, the child had reached a weight of 3.0 kg. The nasopharyngeal tube was removed. She continued to obstruct her airway, and a glossopexy was recommended and performed at approximately 3 weeks of life (Figure 4–10). The nasopharyngeal tube, placed at the time of surgery, was removed on the 2nd postoperative day, and the infant did well. She began to bottle feed on the 4th postoperative day. She went home from the hospital approximately 1 week later weighing 3.2 kg.

Jane was followed at the Craniofacial Center of Western New York. Approximately 9 months after birth, she underwent palatal closure and takedown of her glossopexy. Prior to this surgery, the airway was evaluated and thought to be adequate as expected in children with isolated Pierre

Robin sequence without an underlying genetic abnormality. Her nasopharyngeal tube was removed on postoperative day 2. No further respiratory distress occurred. Follow-up at 2 years of age revealed she was developing appropriate speech and had mandible growth and overall normal development.

Comment

Accurate diagnosis and interdisciplinary care were implemented in a timely fashion to maintain this infant's airway, nutrition, and normal growth and development.

■ CASE STUDY 3

"Jeremy" was a 5½-week-old boy who was born at 36 weeks gestation via normal vaginal delivery. Birth weight was 3.2 kg. At birth an orogastric tube was unable to pass into the stomach, and abdominal X-ray showed the tube at the level of the clavicles and a stomach filled with air. A proximal esophageal atresia with distal tracheoesophageal fistula was repaired (Figure 4–11A). Postoperatively, the infant had some difficulty in feeding, stridor, and a weak voice. The hospitalization was complicated by treatment for sepsis after prolonged rupture of membranes; seizures; Grade II intraventricular hemorrhage; venular malformation of shoulder, arm and chest; peripheral pulmonic stenosis; and coagulopathy. After 1 month, the infant weighed 1.82 kg and was discharged. Breast-feeding was supplemented with 27 kcal formula p.o., desired amount as needed.

Otolaryngologic follow-up 1 week after discharge revealed continued stridor that had worsened in the past week. Parents described "breath holding spells" between feeds and particularly when he was crying. The infant became agitated, tense, and then stopped breathing for 20–25 seconds. He would gasp and then recover. No vomiting, excessive burping, sour breath, or cyanosis was reported.

Because of the continued stridor, hoarseness, and complex medical history, Jeremy underwent FFNL, direct laryngoscopy, bronchoscopy, and esophagoscopy in the operating room. The FFNL was performed with the infant awake. A left vocal fold paralysis was noted; severe reflux laryngitis including mild subglottic inflammation with narrowing also was seen. Mild tracheomalacia at the TEF repair site was visualized. Postoperatively, this infant experienced continued apnea and bradycardia episodes that required intensive care monitoring postoperatively. He required oxygen and manual ventilation with ambu bag. A 24-hour dual-channel pH probe showed severe

GERD/EERD. Medical and positional treatment for reflux was begun; however, the family was advised that the child might need a tracheotomy because of the multiple levels of obstruction—the supraglottic swelling, the unilateral vocal fold paralysis, the subglottic swelling, and the mild tracheomalacia.

Over the next 3 weeks, the apnea–bradycardia episodes decreased. The stridor had diminished and the voice became much stronger. Repeat FFNL revealed a left vocal fold paresis and markedly diminished laryngeal swelling. Mother noted that Jeremy was calmer and ate without becoming agitated or tense. She continued to breast-feed, and supplements were added as needed. He was discharged weighing 3.2 kg.

Comment

TEF repair sometimes results in temporary or permanent vocal fold paralysis. In this case, mediastinal edema was the most likely cause of the paralysis that began to improve with time, indicating a reversible injury. Tracheomalacia to some degree is ubiquitous after TEF repair, as is gastroesophageal reflux. The vocal fold paralysis, laryngeal edema, and mild tracheomalacia all contributed to the stridor. In this case, the gastroesophageal reflux became pathologic and caused GERD/EERD. Once the laryngeal edema (supraglottic and subglottic) was treated, the stridor subsided.

The breath-holding spells with apnea and bradycardia were also due to GERD/EERD. One or both of the mechanisms described in the text above contributed. Jeremy is thriving, and the family is pleased with his eating, breathing, and growing. He will undergo laser treatments for his venular malformation. His GERD/EERD and airway status will also be followed regularly to identify relapse early if it occurs.

■ REFERENCES

Abraham, S. S., & Wolf, E. L. (2000). Swallowing physiology of toddlers with long-term tracheostomies: A preliminary study. *Dysphagia, 15,* 206–212.

Andze, G. O., Brandt, M. L., St. Vil, D., Bensoussan, A. L., & Blanchard, H. (1991). Diagnosis and treatment of gastroesophageal reflux in 500 children with respiratory symptoms: The value of pH monitoring. *Journal of Pediatric Surgery, 26,* 295–299.

Argamaso, R. (1992). Glossopexy for upper airway obstruction in Robin Sequence. *Cleft Palate Craniofacial Journal, 29,* 232–238.

Asher, B., McGill, T., Kaplan, L., Friedman, E., & Healy, G. (1990). Airway complications in CHARGE association. *Arch Otolaryngol Head Neck Surg, 116,* 594–596.

Bauman, N., Sandler, A., & Smith, R. (1996). Respiratory manifestations of gastroesophageal reflux disease in pediatric patients. *Annals of Otorhinol Laryngol, 105,* 23–32.

Bonilla, J. A., Pizzuto, M., Brodsky, L., & Brody, A. (1998). Aplasia of the epiglottis—A rare congenital anomaly. *Ear, Nose and Throat Journal. 77:1,* 51–55.

Brody, A., Kuhn, H., Seidel, F. G., & Brodsky, L. (1991). Ultrafast CT evaluation of the airway in children. *Pediatric Radiology, 178,* 181–184.

Carr, M., Nguyen, A., Nagy, M., Poje, C., Pizzuto, M., & Brodsky, L. (2000). Clinical presentation as a guide to the identification of GERD in children. *International Journal of Pediatric Otorhinolaryngology, 54,* 27–32.

Carr, M., Nguyen, A., Poje, C., Pizzuto, M., Nagy, M., & Brodsky, L. (2000). Correlation of findings on direct laryngoscopy and bronchoscopy with presence of extraesophageal reflux disease. *The Laryngoscope, 110,* 1560–1562.

Carr, M., & Brodsky, L. (1999). Severe non-obstructive sleep disturbance as an initial presentation of gastroesophageal reflux disease. *International Journal of Pediatric Otorhinolaryngology, 51,* 115–120.

Colombo, J., & Hallbert, T. (1987). Recurrent aspiration in children: Lipid laden aveolar macrophage quantitation. *Pediatric Pulmonology, 3,* 86–89.

Dellert, S. F., Hyams, J. S., Treem, W. R., & Geertsma, M. A. (1993). Feeding resistance and gastroesophageal reflux in infancy. *Journal of Pediatric Gastroenterology and Nutrition, 17,* 66–71.

Delorme, R., Laroque, Y., & Caouette-Laberge, L. (1989). Innovative surgical approach for the Pierre Robin anomalad: Subperiosteal release of the floor of the mouth musculature. *Plastic and Reconstructive Surgery, 83,* 960–964.

Derkay, C. S., & Grundfast, K. (1991). Airway compromise from nasal obstruction in neonates and infants. *International Journal of Pediatric Otorhinolaryngology, 21,* 255–257.

Dudkiewicz, Z., Sekula, E., & Nielepiec-Jalosinska, A. (2000). Gastroesophageal reflux in Pierre Robin sequence—early surgical treatment. *Cleft Palate-Craniofacial Journal, 37,* 205–208.

Eibling, D. E., & Gross, R. D. (1996). Subglottic air pressure: A key component of swallowing efficiency. *Annals of Otorhinol Laryngol, 105,* 253–258.

Emami, A. J., Brodsky, L., & Pizzuto, M. (1996). Neonatal septoplasty: Case report and review of the literature. *International Journal of Pediatric Otorhinolaryngology, 35,* 271–275.

Goldstein, S. J., Wu, R. H., Thorpy, M. J., Shprintzen, R. J., Marion, R. E., & Saenger, P. (1987). Reversibility of deficient sleep entrained growth hormone secretion in a boy with achondroplasia and obstructive sleep apnea [published erratum appears in *Acta Endocrinol (Copenh), 116,* 568]. *Acta Endocrinol. (Copenhagen), 116,* 95–101.

Halstead, L. (1999). Role of gastroesopahgeal reflux in pediatric upper airway disorders. *Head & Neck Surgery, 120,* 208–214.

Hu, F., Preston, R., Post, C., White, J. A., Kikuchi, L., Wang X., Leal, S., Levenstien, M., Ott, J., Self, T., Allen, G., Stiffler, R., McGraw, C., Pulsifer-Anderson, E., & Eibling, D. (2000). Mapping of a gene for severe pediatric gastroesophageal reflux to chromosome 13q14. *Journal of the American Medical Association, 284,* 325–334.

Hyman, P. E. (1994). Gastroesophageal reflux: One reason why baby won't eat. *The Journal of Pediatrics, 125(Suppl.),* S103–S109.

Knegt-Junk, K. J., Bos, C. E., & Berkovits, R. N. P. (1988). Congenital nasal stenosis in neonates. *The Journal of Laryngology and Otology, 102,* 500–502.

Laitman, J., & Reidenberg, J. (1993a). Specializations of the human upper respiratory and upper digestive systems as seen through comparative and developmental anatomy. *Dysphagia, 8,* 318–325.

Laitman, J., & Reidenberg, J. (1993b). Comparative and developmental anatomy of laryngeal position. *Head and Neck Surgery Otolarygnology, 1,* 36–43.

Laitman, J., & Reidenberg, J. (1997). The human aerodigestive tract and gastroesophageal reflux: An evolutionary perpective. *American Journal of Medicine, 109,* 2s–8s.

Lantz, H., & Birck, H. (1981). Surgical correction of choanal atresia in the neonate. *The Laryngoscope, 91,* 1629–1634.

Little, F. B., Koufman, J. A., Kohut, R. I., & Marshall, R. (2000). Effect of gastric acid on the pathogenesis of subglottic stenosis. *Oto Rhino Laryngology, 94,* 516–519.

Mandel, L., & Tamari, K. (1995). Sialorrhea and gastroesophageal reflux. *Journal American Dental Association, 126,* 1537–1541.

Maniglia, A., & Goodwin, W. (1981). Congenital choanal atresia. *Otolaryngologic Clinics of North America, 14,* 167–173.

Nielson, D., Heldt, G., & Tooley, W. (1990). Stridor and gastroesophageal reflux in infants. *Pediatrics, 85,* 1034–1039.

Nussbaum, E., Maggi, C., Mathis, R., & Galant, S. (1987). Association of lipid-laden alveolar macrophages and gastroesophageal reflux in children. *The Journal of Pediatrics, 110,* 190–194.

Orenstein, S. O. D. (1988). Gastroesophageal reflux and respiratory disease in children. *The Journal of Pediatrics, 112,* 847–858.

Reyes, B. G., Arnold, J. E., & Brooks, L. J. (1994). Congenital absence of the epiglottis and its potential role in obstructive sleep apnea. *International Journal of Pediatric Otorhinolaryngology, 30,* 223–226.

Richardson, M., & Osguthorpe, J. (1988). Surgical management of choanal atresia. *The Laryngoscope, 96,* 915–918.

Rosingh, H. J., & Peek, S. H. (1999). Swallowing and speech in infants following tracheotomy. *Acta Oto-Rhino-Laryngological Belgica, 53,* 59–63.

Sasaki, C. T., Suzuki, M., Horiuchi, M., & Kirchner, F. (1979). The effect of tracheostomy on the laryngeal closure reflex. *The Laryngoscope, 87,* 1428–1433.

Sasaki, C. T., & Toohill, R. J. (2000). Ambulatory pH monitoring for extraesophageal reflux—introduction. *Annals of Otology, Rhinology, & Laryngology, 109, (Suppl.),* 2–3.

Shprintzen, R. (1988). Pierre Robin, micrognathia and airway obstruction: The dependency of treatment on accurate diagnosis. *International Anesthesiology Clinics, 26,* 64–71.

■ CHAPTER 5

Pediatric Gastroenterology

Thomas Rossi, Linda Brodsky, and Joan Arvedson

■ SUMMARY

Gastrointestinal (GI) tract problems are commonly encountered in infants and children with swallowing and feeding difficulties. Nutritional needs are best met with a well-functioning GI tract.

Malnutrition (undernutrition) in neurologically impaired children is preventable and, if corrected, may lead to improved quality of life (Patrick, Boland, Stoski, & Murray, 1986). The pathogenesis of malnutrition may be due to GI problems compounded by poor nutritional intake (Chapter 6). Close attention therefore must be paid to GI disorders that lead to swallowing difficulties and malnutrition: oral sensorimotor dysfunction, gastroesophageal reflux disease and extraesophageal reflux disease[1] (GERD/EERD), gastrointestinal dysmotility, and constipation. Malnutrition and undernutrition are used interchangeably.

Understanding normal anatomy and physiology of swallowing is requisite to the study of GI problems (Chapter 2). The pathophysiology of malnutrition within the framework of the special situations of the neurologically impaired child is also important. Although growth failure is likely to be multifactorial (Sullivan, 1997), optimizing the function of the GI tract is important to restoring and maintaining optimal health in this increasingly complex group of children. Clinical case studies are used to highlight salient points.

---

[1]Gastroesophageal reflux disease (GERD) refers to the abnormal regurgitation of acid into the esophagus, causing symptoms. When the acid and other stomach contents emerge from the upper esophageal sphincter in the pharynx, larynx, mouth, and nasal cavities, the most commonly accepted term is extra-esophageal reflux disease (EERD) (Sasaki & Toohill, 2000).

■ INTRODUCTION

Advances in medicine have resulted in increased survival, longer life spans, and greater health for a wide variety of pediatric patients. Most notable are premature infants, those with genetic disorders, and neurologically impaired children, all of whom demonstrate a wide range of etiologies and severity. Normal GI tract function is of paramount importance in providing adequate nutrition in this diverse and challenging population.

The nutritionist (dietitian) is involved in determining nutrient requirements and planning appropriate intervention (Chapter 6). Issues of concern include route of intake (oral, tube, or parenteral), family dynamics, caregiver expectations and abilities, and the role of feeding as a primary source of communication and social interaction. The GI specialist must work closely with the nutritionist and keep abreast of the GI tract problems that result from or contribute to dysphagia.

It is estimated that 92% of children with cerebral palsy have clinically significant GI symptoms (Del Giudice et al., 1999), 63% of preterm infants (Marino, Assing, Carbone, Hiatt, Hegyi, & Graff, 1995), and an unknown number of other multiply-involved children. Swallowing disorders are common in cerebral palsy, involving approximately 60% of cases, 93% of which involve oral sensorimotor dysfunction. GERD/EERD is found in about 70% (Del Giudice et al., 1999). GI motility disorders, chronic constipation, structural problems (such as pyloric stenosis and tracheoesophageal fistula), and inflammation of the esophagus can also present with or exacerbate swallowing dysfunction in both normal and neurologically impaired children.

Normal GI anatomy, embryology, physiology, and the development of normal feeding are presented in Chapter 2. A more detailed presentation of undernutrition is found in Chapter 6. This chapter will briefly review the pathophysiology of malnutrition with special attention to the child with special needs. Methods of food delivery follow. A brief review of the other GI problems that contribute to dysphagia and feeding abnormalities will follow. The last section provides an in-depth discussion of GERD/EERD, including pathophysiology, diagnosis, and treatment.

■ MALNUTRITION

Problems with feeding or swallowing, if not recognized early, may rapidly result in malnutrition and growth failure in those infants and children who have little or no nutritional reserve. Malnutrition may be defined as a loss of body composition, particularly fat and proteins, which can be prevented or reversed by nutritional repletion. Primary and secondary types of malnutrition need to be differentiated. Primary protein energy malnutrition (PEM) results from a decrease in nutrient intake in the absence of an underlying organic disease process. PEM occurs when inadequate food supplies or the inability of the individual to gather or ingest nutrients is present. Inadequate nutrient intake leads to a significant decrease in linear growth, muscle strength, cough reflex, circulatory time, cerebral function, energy, motivation, and immunity.

Secondary malnutrition is caused by an underlying organic disease process, oftentimes malfunction of the GI tract. The energy provided by normal nutrient intake is overwhelmed by the body's inability to use the nutrients, by the unusual energy requirements of the illness, or by a failure of GI function. An increase in infectious illness, especially aspiration pneumonia (Chapter 10), emesis from GERD/EERD, food aversion, and behavioral problems (Chapter 13), challenge the infant and child to maintain adequate nutrition and growth.

In infants and children with swallowing and feeding difficulties, PEM is more common. However, these children have many other reasons for malnutrition to occur (see Table 6–1). Furthermore, as malnutrition develops, adverse affects on the GI and other organ systems compromise the child's nutritional status. Adverse effects of malnutrition on the GI tract include mucosal thinning, loss of absorptive surface area, alteration in motility, decreased levels of disaccharides, bacterial overgrowth, and reduced bile acid absorption. An associated protein-losing enteropathy may then occur with loss of immunoglobulins and other proteins into the intestinal lumen. Hence, the cycle of malnutrition–malabsorption is established (Rossi, 1986).

Attention to nutritional needs from birth is most advantageous (Cloud & Bergman, 1991); however, intervention at any stage is more likely to bring reversal of the anatomic, physiologic, and psychologic damage that results from malnutrition (Amundson, Sherbondy, Van Dyke, & Alexander, 1994; Sanders et al., 1990). Breaking the cycle of suboptimal growth and development secondary to malnutrition is obviously important. When aggressive gastrostomy tube feedings are instituted in children with swallowing problems, weight-for-length ratios improve (Shapiro, Green, Krick, Allen, & Capute, 1986). Despite aggressive nutritional support, growth failure and malnutrition are likely to be multifactorial and therefore difficult to overcome (Sullivan, 1997). The severity and degree of neurologic impairment, particularly in children with cerebral palsy, are often predictive of the degree of malnutrition (Stallings, Charney, Davies, & Cronk, 1993).

Adaptive Responses to Malnutrition

PEM is a dynamic condition that is a reflection of past and present nutritional status (Beghin & Viteri, 1973; Waterlow, 1973). The metabolic status of the child can change readily by changing the quantity or quality of nutrient intake, by encountering acute infections, and by acute or chronic GI dysfunction. Even for a short time (e.g., a few days), significant modifications in the metabolic profile of marginally nourished children can occur with diet alteration.

A great number of adaptive systemic mechanisms emerge. For example, in the dynamic process of starvation, the child mobilizes the primary energy source—adipose tissue. During this phase, muscles supply only a small portion of the energy by liberating amino acids that are necessary for gluconeogenesis. Protein mobilization is spared relative to adipose tissue consumption. As the energy deficit increases and internal fat sources become depleted, a more rapid mobilization of muscle protein takes place. Therefore, in chronic starvation, wasting of muscle mass is prominent. The degree of muscle wasting may be difficult to appreciate clinically in a small child. As protein and energy deficits increase, PEM becomes more evident (Viteri & Alvarado, 1970).

Severe protein deficiency is more often an acute process, generally superimposed on a marginally nourished child. Periods of "protein deficiency" can lead to decompensation from the chronic adaptation that a child with mild–moderate malnutrition achieves. These periods may be precipitated by an acute infectious episode, diarrhea, recurrent vomiting, or alterations in feeding patterns (Viteri, 1981).

These conditions are especially relevant to multiply involved children. They are often subjected to periods of fasting when admitted to hospitals for the treatment of infections or for the performance of diagnostic tests or surgical procedures. Although seldom realized, added attention to nutritional needs during these periods is critical.

Malabsorption

Malabsorption is defined as the inability of the intestinal mucosa to absorb nutrients from the gut. Generally, diseases of the GI tract lead to either a generalized malabsorption of all macronutrients or to a loss of specific micronutrients. For example, problems such as intestinal allergies, enteritis, celiac disease, and Crohn's disease may cause villus atrophy. This leads to a decrease in the content of all enzymes contained on the villus surface of the intestinal mucosa. Generalized malabsorption of all macronutrients then results. In contrast, conditions such as sucrase–isomaltase deficiency, glucose–galactose malabsorption, and intestinal lymphangiectasia result in specific losses in sugar, starch, glucose, and fat. In hepatic disorders, such as neonatal hepatitis or other obstructive cholangiopathies, in which there is a deficiency of bile flow, fat malabsorption is most prominent. Fat soluble vitamin malabsorption is an associated feature of fat malabsorption.

Just as specific intestinal diseases may result in either a generalized malabsorption of nutrients or the malabsorption of a specific nutrient, the same is true for pancreatic diseases. In generalized pancreatic insufficiency states such as cystic fibrosis, a deficiency of all exocrine pancreatic enzymes results in a generalized malabsorption of carbohydrates, fats, and proteins. In contrast, a single pancreatic enzyme deficiency, such as congenital lipase deficiency, results in malabsorption of fat. Secondary adverse effects on pancreatic function occur when malnutrition becomes severe. Generalized malabsorption occurs (secondary to pancreatic dysfunction) and further accentuates the malabsorptive state induced by intestinal malfunction. Impaired secretion of secretogogues, at rest and after stimulation, occurs. Trypsin activity seems to be preserved, whereas amylase and lipase activities are severely depressed in response to the stress of malnutrition (Rossi, Lee, & Lebenthal, 1987).

In contrast to losses of nutrients into the GI tract that occur from malabsorption, systemic infections impose nutritional burdens by a different mechanism. During periods of infection, there is usually a marked reduction in appetite, a tendency for solid foods to be withdrawn, an increase in caloric need, and a decrease in utilization of nutrients. Nitrogen is lost into the urine, and amino acids are shunted from peripheral muscle to alternative metabolic pathways involved in gluconeogenesis. In addition, synthesis of acute phase reactants (such as haptoglobin, C-reactive protein, and alpha-1-antitrypsin) may also take place. When infection occurs within the GI tract, a synergism occurs between these systemic metabolic effects and the specific effects induced in the intestine (Scrimshaw, 1981). Villus atrophy, which results in malabsorption of nutrients, exerts a summative deleterious effect on nutritional status and further compromises nutritional status (Rossi & Lebenthal, 1983).

Effects on Immune System

The adverse effects that malnutrition exerts on the immune system are emphasized by the fact that infection is the most frequent cause of death in malnourished individuals. As stated above, infection is often a major factor in precipitating acute nutritional deficiencies. Nutritional deficiencies, in turn, commonly impair immune responses, often before the development of any clinical signs or symptoms. Indeed, malnutrition is the most common cause of secondary immunodeficiency. Immunologic deficiencies have been well documented in patients with malnutrition. As malnutrition progresses, reduction occurs in the total lymphocyte count; lymphocyte response to phytohemagglutinins; neutrophil chemotaxis; immunoglobulin G levels; and skin test reactivity to mumps, Candida, streptokinase-streptodornase, and tuberculin antigens. Serum complement is also responsive to nutritional changes. Markedly depressed levels occur in severe protein energy malnutrition and may be an additional factor in the susceptibility to bacterial infections (Chandra, 1982; Meakins, Pietsch, & Bubernick, 1977).

■ METHODS OF DELIVERY OF FEEDINGS

Infants and children with swallowing and feeding problems often require alternative methods of feeding to obtain adequate nutrients and fluids for normal growth and development. If adjustments in breast- or bottle-feeding practices do not result in improved oral intake, other options must be considered (Chapters 6 and 9). The options available are enteral feedings, which utilize the GI tract, and parenteral feedings, which provide nutrients directly into the bloodstream and bypass the GI tract. Enteral feedings, when feasible and effective, are always preferred. The types of enteral and parenteral feeds, with their advantages and disadvantages, are found in Table 5–1.

Table 5–1. Advantages and Disadvantages of Alternate Routes for Feeding

Route	Advantages	Disadvantages
Orogastric	• Uses mouth • Good for neonates and infants • Preserves GI tract function	• Interferes with sucking • Not well tolerated in older children • Obstruction and dislodgement
Nasogastric	• Better for older infants and children • Preserves GI tract function	• Interferes with infant's nose breathing • Uncomfortable • Obstruction and dislodgement
Gastrostomy tube (PEG or surgical)	• Comfortable • Hidden • Preserves GI tract function	• Requires a surgical procedure • Obstruction and dislodgement • Complications (see text)
Parenteral	• Lifesaving when GI tract is not functioning • High energy, concentrated solutions available • Directed nutrient therapy possible	• Surgical procedure for long-term catheter • Metabolic and catheter complications are significant (see text)

Note. GI = gastrointestinal; PEG = percutaneous endoscopic gastrostomy.

Tube Feeding

Naso/Orogastric Tube Feeding

Enteral feedings by tube are usually the initial approach in infants and children who have either an inability to coordinate the suck and swallow sequence and feed orally or who have excessive or unusual nutrient requirements that preclude the use of oral feedings alone. The most direct and simple way to provide enteral feedings is by an orogastric (OG) or nasogastric (NG) tube. OG feedings are preferred by some clinicians for young infants. Young infants are primarily nose breathers and care must be taken to prevent even partial obstruction of the nasal airway. OG or NG feedings can be provided by continuous infusion or intermittent bolus feeds. Although intermittent bolus feeds more nearly simulate a normal feeding pattern, continuous infusion feedings may be better tolerated in some infants with gastroesophageal reflux or delayed gastric emptying.

If gastric feedings are poorly tolerated, it is possible to feed directly into the duodenum or jejunum. While lowering the risk of reflux, aspiration, and distension, tube placement under fluoroscopy is needed to assure proper placement. Duodenal and jejunal tube feedings must be given as a slow continuous infusion to avoid a rapid infusion of a high glucose and solute load into the small intestine, resulting in the dumping syndrome.

Gastrostomy Tube Feeding

If long-term (greater than 1–3 months) enteral feedings are required, a gastrostomy tube (GT) should be considered. The development and widespread use of gastrostomy tubes has made long-term delivery of enteral feedings a feasible alternative for children who cannot or will not meet nutritional needs orally. They are particularly useful when anatomic restrictions, e.g., tracheoesophageal fistula, short bowel syndrome; developmental delay, e.g., cerebral palsy, mental retardation; or increased needs, e.g., postoperative trauma, preclude full oral feeds. In infants and children with severe developmental delay or inadequate suck and swallow due to a chronic condition, particularly aspiration, gastrostomy tube placement early in the medical course is generally recommended. Each case must be decided on an individual basis, but most caregivers find gastrostomy tube feedings much preferable to nasogastric feedings for home use because of ease of care, patient comfort, and elimination of frequent tube changes. Gastrostomy tubes can be hidden under clothing, are not uncomfortable, and require less skill in care. In select cases, a gastrostomy can be placed via endoscopy (percutaneous endoscopic gastrostomy, PEG), thereby eliminating the need for general anesthesia (Figure 5–1).

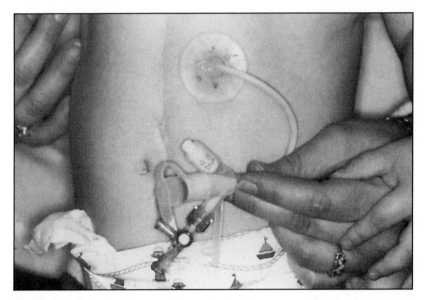

Figure 5–1. Patient with gastrostomy tube in place.

The percutaneous endoscopic approach to gastrostomy (PEG) place-ment offers an attractive alternative to the open intra-abdominal technique. PEG does not usually require general anesthesia and therefore can be safely performed in the endoscopy suite in most children. In children, both adequate sedation and control of the airway are important during the pro-cedure. The patient must lie still for PEG to be performed safely. The endo-scopist must be familiar with the child and judge whether the procedure can be performed safely with intravenous sedation. If there are any questions related to achieving proper sedation or adequate airway support, the pro-cedure should be performed in the operating room or intensive care unit, where adequate personnel, monitoring, and equipment are available. Some procedures may need to be terminated even after the administration of intravenous sedation if an inadequate response to sedation or interference with adequate oxygenation occur. Although the use of the operating room imposes additional costs to the procedure, safety certainly outweighs cost. Figures 5–2 A and B highlight the endoscopic features of PEG placement.

Complications of Tube Feedings

Potential complications of tube feedings can be divided into gastrointesti-nal, metabolic, or mechanical. The most common gastrointestinal compli-cations are vomiting, abdominal distention, diarrhea, and induction or worsening of GERD/EERD by tube placement, although this last situation

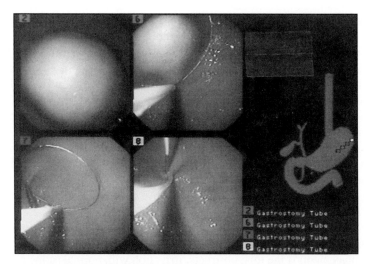

Figure 5–2A. Photographs taken during percutaneous endoscopic gastrostomy placement. Frame 2 illustrates a bulge in the stomach wall made by the endoscopy assistant's finger pressure on the abdomen during attempts to identify a proper location for tube placement. Frames 6 and 7 show the placement of a snare by the endoscopist at the site selected for tube placement. Frame 8 depicts the closure of the snare on the needle introduced from the anterior abdominal wall into the stomach. The guidewire coming through the needle is also identified.

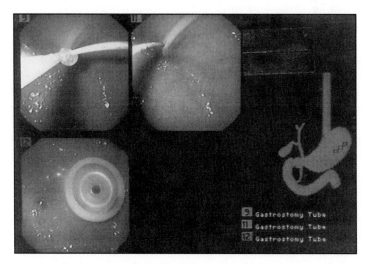

Figure 5–2B. Photographs taken during percutaneous endoscopic gastrostomy placement. Frames 9 and 11 demonstrate the guidewire over which the gastrostomy tube is placed. Frame 12 demonstrates the endoscopic appearance of the gastrostomy tube in place.

continues to be debated (Heine, Reddihough, & Catto-Smith, 1995; Jolley, Smith, & Tunell, 1985; Langer et al., 1988; Launay et al., 1996). If vomiting or distention is a consistent problem, investigation for GERD/EERD or delayed gastric emptying should be performed. GI disorders, GI infection, and immune deficiency diseases, which should be identified and treated, are not uncommon causes of vomiting and distension. A non-milk-based formula of relatively low osmolality should be used, with change to a more elemental formula considered if diarrhea does not resolve. In general, continuous feedings will be better tolerated than bolus feeds in infants and children with any GI complication. Metabolic complications of tube feedings are less common than GI complications. In sensitive premature infants or sick full-term infants, care must be taken to avoid sodium, protein, or fluid overload.

Mechanical complications of enteral feedings vary, depending on the method of delivery. NG or OG tubes must be checked carefully for proper tube placement. If the tube obstructs, irrigation with normal saline or proteolytic agents may be helpful; otherwise, the tube should be replaced. Reported complication rates from surgical gastrostomy tube placement range from 2 to 75%, with the higher incidence being attributed to the debilitated state of some of the patients. The risk of general anesthesia is great in these high-risk patients. Most patients reported in these series are elderly individuals with cancer or neurologic disorders (stroke), who are malnourished and have poor wound healing (Mequid & Williams, 1979).

Cited advantages of PEG include decreased procedure time, local anesthesia, and decreased likelihood for complications (Gauderer, 1991; Kirby, Craig, Tsang, & Plotnick, 1986). With increased use, however, complications are more often reported. These include GI bleeding, leakage of gastric contents, esophageal laceration, colonic perforation, gastrocolonic fistula, peritonitis, subcutaneous emphysema, external migration of the inner phalange, wound infections, peristomal excoriations, and symptomatic GERD/EERD (Kimber & Beasley, 1999; Ponsky, Gauderer, Stellato, & Aszodi, 1985). Up to 17% may need another procedure directly related to the PEG (Mehta & Schou, 1988).

Parenteral Nutrition

In the past, parenteral nutrition was reserved primarily for infants or children with severe GI disorders that prevented the use of the GI tract. Recently, however, parenteral nutrition has become a standard mode of feeding for very small premature infants and for infants or children in need of short-term intensive nutritional rehabilitation. The parenteral route offers the advantage of nutritional supplement in GI tract malfunction (Case Study 1).

If parenteral nutrition is needed for a relatively short period of time (1–2 weeks), peripheral vein access may be preferable to the use of a central venous catheter. Placement of a peripheral access catheter can be done at the bedside. Patients with higher than normal calorie requirements, fluid restriction (requiring highly concentrated formulations), or those requiring long-term parenteral nutrition require central venous access (e.g., Broviac or Hickman catheter). The recent development of a central percutaneous intravascular catheter (PIC line), which is placed via a peripheral vein but fed through to a central venous location, has improved access for central parenteral nutrition.

Complications of parenteral nutrition can be categorized as metabolic or technical. Metabolic complications remain a particular concern for patients receiving long-term parenteral nutrition. Close monitoring of laboratory values, including glucose, serum protein, liver function tests, and electrolytes, can be used to assess tolerance to the therapy. Alterations can thus be made rapidly if metabolic intolerance is observed.

Technical problems are associated primarily with the use of central venous catheters for access. Problems include those that arise at the time of insertion of the catheter and problems with the long-term use of catheters. Problems encountered at the time of insertion of a central venous catheter include pneumothorax, injury to the vein or artery, and air embolism. Technical complications that may arise with use of the catheter include venous thrombosis, sepsis, catheter dislodgement, perforation or leakage, sometimes with skin slough when a peripheral vein is used. Heparin is usually added to parenteral nutrition solutions to prevent thrombosis. Strict aseptic technique must be used in caring for the catheter site and during infusion of the parenteral nutrition solutions. Although parenteral nutrition can be lifesaving for some infants, disuse atrophy of the GI tract and cholestasis, leading to irreversible liver damage, can and should be avoided by the introduction of enteral feeds as soon as possible. A more complete discussion of parenteral nutrition in the pediatric population is found in Baker and Baker, 1997.

■ DYSPHAGIA SECONDARY TO GI DISEASE

GI problems that can present with swallowing and feeding problems include structural abnormalities of the esophagus and stomach, dysmotility disorders, inflammatory diseases (discussed under the differential diagnosis section of GERD below), and constipation (Table 5–2).

Table 5–2. Gastrointestinal Problems Causing Dysphagia

Structural Abnormalities
Esophagus
  • Tracheoesophageal fistula
  • Esophageal atresia
  • Esophageal webs/strictures
Stomach
  • Pyloric stenosis

Dysmotility Disorders
  • Esophageal or cricopharyngeal achalasia
  • Esophageal dysmotility (nonspecific)
  • Esophageal spasm

Inflammatory Diseases
Esophagitis
  • Eosinophilic esophagitis
  • Barrett's esophagus
  • Secondary to gastroesophageal reflux disorder
Eosinophilic gastroenteropathy

Miscellaneous
  • Esophageal compression (intrinsic/extrinsic lesions)
  • Constipation

Tracheoesophageal Fistula and Esophageal Atresia

Abnormal development of a separate and fully patent trachea and esophagus is not uncommon, occurring in about 1 in every 3,000 to 5,000 births. The embryologic relationships and clinical implications that result in such anomalies are discussed in Chapters 2 and 4.

About 87% of tracheoesophageal fistulae (TEF) with esophageal atresia present with a proximal esophageal atresia (EA) and a distal TEF (Figure 4–11). These are usually readily recognized soon after birth when the infant is unable to swallow. Passage of NG tube results in coiling in the proximal esophageal segment; a chest and abdominal X-ray shows large amounts of air in the stomach. Isolated esophageal atresia occurs in about 8% of cases. An H-type fistula, which can be difficult to recognize until the child becomes seriously ill with recurrent pneumonia during the first 2 years of life, occurs in 4% of cases (Chapter 4) (Adkins, 1990).

TEF and EA often present with other congenital anomalies, therefore a careful search for associated problems is necessary. The most common are congenital cardiac disease, other GI abnormalities (e.g., malrotation, intes-

tinal atresia, imperforate anus), genitourinary abnormalities, musculoskeletal abnormalities, and cleft lip or palate (Adkins, 1990). Until the
1940s, TEF and EA were uniformly fatal. Modern surgical techniques have
allowed repair to occur with a fairly high success rate, although habilitation
to normal feeding and swallowing remains challenging in some children.
Preoperative radiographic imaging should be performed in the institution
at which the surgical repair will take place. Experienced pediatric surgeons
and pediatric intensivists, with a dedicated pediatric intensive care unit, are
mandatory for the optimal outcomes.

Reanastamosis of the esophagus can be quite challenging, and stricture
at the anastomosic site is reported in 40% of cases. Almost all children have
some degree of GERD after surgery, which can aggravate the potential for
stricture. Esophageal motility also may be compromised, especially when
colon interposition is needed to reconstruct the esophagus. Feeding gastrostomy is always needed when EA is present.

The segment of trachea at the site of the TEF usually has a fair amount
of tracheomalacia due to tracheal ring abnormalities that compromise the
stiffness of the trachea. Airway problems from correction of this anomaly are
discussed in Chapter 4 (and highlighted by Case Study 2 in that chapter).

The complications of stricture formation and GERD/EERD often
result in prolonged periods during which the infant or child is unable to eat
orally, even though their oral sensorimotor function may be quite good.
Multiple procedures to dilate the esophagus or remove impacted foreign
bodies, as well as early alterations in feeding and eating patterns, dysphagia from GERD/EERD, and airway compromise are a few of the reasons
these children experience significant management challenges through most
of their early childhood.

Pyloric Stenosis

Pyloric stenosis is a narrowing of the muscle sphincter between the stomach and the duodenum. It occurs secondary to thickening of the muscles
that make up the pyloric valve. As one of the most common congenital GI
anomalies, recurrent projectile vomiting, present soon after birth, is its
hallmark. Surgical repair is warranted and highly successful.

Dysmotility Disorders

Esophageal motility may be impaired by four mechanisms: (a) lack of contractions, (b) absent relaxations (achalasia), (c) excessive contractions
(spasms), and (d) uncoordinated contractions. Neurologic impairment,
abnormal muscle function, and mucosal/muscle replacement, usually by
cicatrix, are the most common reasons for these motility problems to occur
in the esophagus.

The most common reason for abnormal esophageal motility in children is GERD/EERD (Fouad, Hatlebakk, & Castell, 1999), especially when airway symptoms are present. This is particularly true in the neurologically impaired child in whom generalized GI dysmotility may be present (Sullivan, 1997) and for whom GERD/EERD is a common and often vexing condition (Fouad, Hatlebakk, & Castell, 1999; Rosario et al., 1999; Sullivan).

The effects of GERD/EERD on motility are discussed in detail in the next section. Rarely, other disorders of motility, more common in adults, will present in a normal child without neurologic impairment or GERD/EERD. Esophageal achalasia, cricopharyngeal achalasia, esophageal spasm, and nonspecific esophageal motility disorders are included in this group of poorly understood disorders (Rosario et al., 1999; Sieber, 1990).

Esophageal achalasia is characterized by abnormal esophageal motility and relaxation failure of the lower esophageal sphincter. Cricopharyngeal achalasia is a relaxation failure of the upper esophageal sphincter, the cricopharyngeus muscle. Both forms of achalasia are rare in children. Radiologic and manometric studies are helpful in diagnosis. Surgical myotomy of the affected segment(s) is usually worthwhile and is performed with few complications. The laparoscopic approach has proven to be both feasible and effective (Esposito et al., 2000).

Esophageal spasm is rarely a problem in infants and children. A disorder of hypermotility, it can be intermittent and cause chest pain and dysphagia. Esophagram shows the typical "corkscrew" esophagus, indicating localized areas of contraction (Sieber, 1990).

Dysmotility of the stomach and intestines may also have untoward effects on swallowing and feeding. Especially in children with GERD/EERD, a high index of suspicion should be raised for this problem. Evaluation is difficult in that many centers do not have the expensive equipment or expertise to study such problems thoroughly. When gastric emptying is a problem, pylorotomy is sometimes recommended. Fundoplication in these instances may be detrimental to motility.

Miscellaneous

Compressive Lesions

Masses, cysts, and major blood vessels intrinsic and extrinsic to the esophagus can all cause compressive symptoms and dysphagia (Kosko, Moser, Erhart, & Tunkel, 1998; Sieber, 1990). Radiologic evaluation consists of a barium esophagram, computerized tomographic (CT) scan of the chest, and often magnetic resonance imaging (MRI) of the chest. Treatment will depend on the underlying problem.

Nonspecific motility disorders of the esophagus have been reported in approximately 8% of neurologically normal children who have upper GI symptoms and no GERD (Rosario et al., 1999). These symptoms include vomiting (62%), dysphagia (46%), chest pain (31%), food impaction (31%), and epigastric pain (23%). Boys are affected more often than girls. Manometric study reveals a wide range of esophageal malfunction including simultaneous contractions, delayed contractions, prolonged contractions, low-amplitude contractions, retrograde contractions, and aperistalsis. Treatment is unpredictable with improvement seen in about 50% of cases. Prokinetic agents and antacids are tried empirically. Food impaction in the mid-esophagus is problematic for these children. Long-term outlook is not well defined (Rosario et al., 1999).

Constipation

Chronic constipation is a common and aggravating problem for neurologically impaired children with swallowing and feeding problems, occurring in 74% of children with cerebral palsy (Del Giudice et al., 1999). Multifactorial in origin, constipation occurs because of faulty innervation of the entire GI tract, decreased intake of fluids, patient immobility, and inappropriate feeding regimens (Del Giudice et al.; Sullivan, 1997). Children with dysphagia are particularly susceptible because the decreased oral intake may be fluid poor. Careful attention to diet is important and should consist of enough fluid and fiber to enable easy, pain-free defecation. Maintenance laxative therapy is very helpful. In severe cases of stool impaction, manual removal of the stool is necessary (Sullivan).

■ REFLUX DISEASE—GERD/EERD

Definitions

Gastroesophageal reflux (GER) is defined as the return of stomach contents into the esophagus caused by a dysfunction of the lower esophagus. The lower esophageal sphincter[2] (LES) at the distal end of the esophagus

---

[2]Terminology in this field is evolving. The lower esophageal sphincter (LES) is alternatively called the gastroesophageal sphincter (GES). The upper esophageal sphincter (UES) more recently has been called the pharyngoesophageal sphincter (PES), referring primarily to the cricopharyngeus muscle. For purposes of this book, the still-familiar terms UES and LES will be used.

normally prevents free reflux of gastric contents into the esophagus. When symptoms result, then GERD is present and warrants evaluation and treatment. Physiologic GER is reflux that occurs in the absence of clinical signs or symptoms.

The term extraesophageal reflux is used to denote regurgitation of stomach contents through the upper esophageal sphincter (UES) into the pharynx, larynx, mouth, nose/paranasal sinuses, and tracheobronchial tree and lungs. When symptoms result, then EERD is present and warrants evaluation and treatment. Although it may seem intuitive that GERD always exists when EERD is present, this may not be the case. It is possible that a very small amount of refluxate in the hypopharynx, for example, may be life threatening without any ill effects being experienced in the esophagus. The recognition of EERD is a relatively recent development, and a high index of suspicion must be maintained to diagnose these individuals accurately. For further discussion of EERD, see Chapter 4.

Duodenogastric reflux (DGR) is retrograde flow of bile acids and pancreatic enzymes from the duodenum into the stomach. If the LES and UES are incompetent, then the refluxate can enter the esophagus and upper aerodigestive tract. The contents of the refluxate have been shown to have noxious effects on the esophagus (Tovar, Wang, & Eizaguirre, 1993). The incidence and implications of DGR are better understood in adults than in children (Iftikhar et al., 1995). When the clinician is faced with a difficult diagnostic situation, consideration of this diagnosis should occur. Treatment will vary from that of GERD/EERD (see below).

This section will emphasize the information known about GERD/EERD. A brief description of DGR will be provided in the next section about reflux disease.

Epidemiology

The incidence of GERD/EERD is not known. It has long been taught that GER in infants is normal and will resolve over time. It is estimated that about half (55%) of infants with reflux will resolve by 9 months of age (Shepherd & Wren, 1987). Many are actually symptomatic, however, although not recognized as such. These infants and children would therefore benefit from identification and treatment. A number of neonatal respiratory disorders are caused by reflux (Chapter 4). The irritable baby who refuses food, fails to sleep, and is generally regarded to have colic, may indeed be experiencing GERD/EERD.

The number of older children with GERD/EERD is difficult to estimate; the natural history of the disease is essentially unknown but appears to be increasing in today's fast-paced world (see below). In previous centuries, up to 10% of children with untreated reflux developed significant complications (Carre, 1959). The increased incidence of GERD/EERD is found in neurologically impaired infants and children (Del Giudice et al., 1999; Heine et al., 1995; Sullivan, 1997). The cause and effect of feeding and swallowing problems in this particular group of children will be discussed below.

Pathophysiology

The anatomy and physiology of the esophagus is presented in Chapter 2. Pathophysiology of GERD/EERD is summarized in Table 5–3 and described in further detail in this section. All of these factors appear to be interrelated and their relative importance is unknown at this time. The poor correlation between esophageal histology and reflux exposure implies that multiple factors must play a role.

Role of LES Pressure Gradient in GER

Several investigators have studied the role of the pressure gradient at the LES. In a group of pediatric patients suspected of reflux, only 12% of reflux episodes occurred while there was a *continuous* reduction in resting LES pressure (Werlin, Dodds, Hogan, & Arndorfer, 1980). The majority of reflux episodes (54%) occurred during *transient* increases in intra-abdominal pressure above the level of the resting LES pressure. These transient increases, occurring mainly while awake, were a result of normal activities such as crying, coughing, moving about, and defecating. The remainder of reflux episodes (34%) occurred during transient, spontaneous, and complete relaxations of the LES (TLESRs). A common cavity phenomenon between stomach and esophagus was thus produced. Transient lower esophageal sphincter relaxations (TLESRs) were brief and were neither associated with esophageal peristalsis nor as the result of a swallow. Spontaneous TLESRs have been observed in normal individuals as well as those with GERD/EERD (Dent et al., 1980; Orenstein, 1992). In comparison to normal individuals, however, patients with GERD have more frequent and more complete spontaneous relaxations, and TLESRs are thus more often associated with reflux in these individuals (Eastwood, Castell, & Higgs, 1975). It has been suggested that TLESRs are responsible for up to 94% of reflux episodes (Taminiau, 1997).

Reflux of gastric contents into the esophagus occurs during transient increases in intra-abdominal pressure. Intra-abdominal pressure elevations are also more frequent in GERD/EERD patients. The underlying etiology and reason for these differences between normal individuals and those with reflux is unclear.

Table 5–3. Pathophysiologic Mechanisms of Reflux Disease

Gastroesophageal Reflux Disease(GERD):

1. Anatomic/mechanical
   - Intrathoracic esophagus
   - Surgical alterations (TEF repair, GT placement)
   - Neurologic reflex hyper- or hyporeactivity

2. Physiologic
   - Increased frequency of reflux episodes
     Transient lower esophageal sphincter relaxations
     Increased abdominal pressure
     Decreased thoracic pressure
     Decreased tone in lower esophageal sphincter
     Gastric distention (increased volume)
     Gastric dysmotility (incoordination or delayed gastric emptying)
     Increased gastric secretion
   - Increased duration of reflux episodes
     Posture, position
     Deficiency of saliva
     Dysmotility of esophagus or stomach
   - Content of refluxate
     Acid
     Gastric enzymes
     Bacteria
     Undigested food

Extra-Esophageal Reflux Disease (EERD):[a]

1. Anatomic/mechanical:
   - Surgical (TEF, colonic interposition)
   - Upper airway obstructive lesions

2. Physiologic
   - Decreased upper esophageal sphincter tone (especially at night)
   - Impaired reflexes (e.g., esophagolaryngeal, esophagopulmonary)
   - Esophagitis
   - Refluxate contents (same as for GERD, but effect on respiratory mucosa may be much greater than on squamous epithelium of esophagus)

Duodenal Gastric Reflux:[a]

1. Anatomic
   - Pyloric incompetence

2. Physiologic
   - Bile salts
   - Pancreatic enzymes

[a]Most, if not all, of the pathophysiologic mechanisms for GERD are operant with EERD and DGR. The list here includes additional effects.

Gastric Emptying and Dysmotility

The rate of gastric emptying is one of the factors associated with GERD/EERD. Delay in gastric emptying of a liquid meal occurs commonly in both pediatric and adult patients who manifest GERD/EERD (Hillemeier, Grill, McCallum, & Gryboski, 1983; McCallum, Berkowitz, & Lerner, 1981; Papamihalis, Wilpizeski, & Grosfeld, 1989). Delay in gastric emptying may be one factor that increases the likelihood of GERD/EERD by increasing the time available for reflux to occur. Gastric distention has also been demonstrated to increase the number of spontaneous TLESRs but does not appear to increase intragastric pressure significantly (Holloway, Hongo, Berger, & McCallum, 1985; Martin, Patrinos, & Dent, 1986); however, the fact that delayed gastric emptying results in a full stomach for longer periods of time may result in greater ease of acid reflux during periods of increased intra-abdominal pressure (Sondheimer, 1988). The presence of delayed gastric emptying should raise the consideration that an underlying motility disorder is present.

Acid Clearance

Abnormalities of acid clearance may be primary to the development of GERD/EERD. Interruption of the normal mechanisms for acid clearance (Chapter 2) predisposes to the creation of a cycle of esophagitis–reflux. Patients with oral sensorimotor problems may be particularly prone to the development of esophagitis because they have decreased abilities for acid clearance. Difficulty handling oral secretions (drooling), prolonged recumbency, and less frequent swallows all play a role. In adults, hyperacidity also seems to play a role (Singh et al., 1993).

Some investigators have postulated that the cause of reflux is acid induced change in LES pressure. In animal studies, reduction of LES pressure follows perfusion of the distal esophagus with 0.1N hydrochloric acid. Esophagitis then results. With resolution of the esophagitis, however, LES pressure returns to normal (Eastwood et al., 1975). As local mediators of inflammation (such as prostaglandins) are released, the duration of both the reflux episodes and acid clearance time is longer for patients with GERD/EERD than for control subjects. This indicates that the ability of patients to clear refluxate from the esophagus and to restore a normal pH is impaired (Stanciu & Bennett, 1974). Exposing the esophageal mucosa to acid can alter LES function and esophageal peristalsis. Thus, reflux continues based on defective acid clearance.

Clinical Presentation

Vomiting is classically thought of as the hallmark of GERD; however, it has become increasingly apparent that reflux of gastric contents to any level of the esophagus, pharynx, larynx, and oral cavity is not always accompanied by clinically apparent emesis. The clinician must keep in mind the large number and type of symptoms associated with GERD/EERD when evaluating a child for reflux. No further evaluation is indicated when a healthy, thriving infant intermittently regurgitates small amounts of formula after feedings. In severe cases or those with unusual symptoms, documentation of GER is advisable. This is particularly true for patients who first manifest symptoms after infancy. However, when vomiting is present, it can be so severe that calorie loss results in rapid weight loss and undernutrition. The common clinical manifestations of GERD/EERD are listed in Table 4–2. Another way to look at clinical classification is based on major symptom complexes, that is, regurgitation, respiratory, neurobehavioral, and those due to esophagitis (Table 5–4) (Orenstein, 1992; Putnam, 1998).

It is important to identify the common daily activities and behaviors that can lead to or worsen GERD/EERD. These include use of certain medications, dietary habits, lifestyle habits, and exposure to environmental allergens. Tobacco (passive smoke), alcohol, and caffeine all increase the potential for reflux because of their adverse effects on LES pressure and GI peristalsis. An abundance of poor dietary choices may contribute. Foods associated with GERD/EERD include carbonated beverages; chocolate; caffeinated beverages; citrus fruits and juices; fried, greasy, or spicy foods; and tomato-based products. Overeating, late-night eating, excessive exercise after eating, or assuming a recumbent position immediately after eating are commonly found in older children with GERD/EERD. Environmental allergens, particularly milk, may be the cause of up to 42% of GERD/EERD (Iacono et al., 1996).

Complications of GERD/EERD

Esophagitis is the histopathologic marker for GERD. Acid contact with the stratified squamous epithelium lining the esophagus is the inciting incident. It is apparent, however, that more than 50% of children who have clinically significant GERD and EERD in particular can manifest without the presence of esophagitis (Fouad et al., 1999; Stroh, Faust, & Rimell, 1998).

Complications of esophagitis include bleeding from the inflamed tissue, which can result in iron deficiency anemia, melena, or hematemesis. Long-standing esophagitis manifests as mucosal ulcerations, erosions, granulation tissue, and esophageal stricture formation. Esophagitis has been reported in 60 to 80% of infants and children with signs and symptoms of GERD (Baer et al., 1986; Biller, Winter, Grand, & Allerd, 1983).

Endoscopic evidence of esophagitis includes mucosal erosions, exudate, and ulcers (Figure 5–3). Barrett's esophagus, strictures, and adenocarcinoma are other concerns, albeit rare (Orenstein et al., 1999). In infants and

Table 5–4. System-Oriented Classification for Signs and Symptoms of GERD/EERD

Signs and Symptoms From Regurgitation
- Emesis (with malnutrition)
- Gagging
- Choking
- Cough
- Apnea
- Halitosis
- Frequent swallowing
- Burping

Respiratory Symptoms and Signs
- Recurrent pneumonia
- Apnea (central and obstructive)
- Blue spells
- Recurrent croup
- Stridor
- Chronic cough
- Asthma
- Hiccups
- Acute Life-Threatening Events
- Gurgly respirations

Signs and Symptoms From Acid-Related Inflammation
- Heartburn
- Irritability
- Food refusal
- Swallowing problems (dysphagia)
- Opisthotonus (back arching)
- Otalgia
- Torticollis (Sandifer's syndrome)
- Chest/abdominal pain
- Hematemesis (with anemia)
- Esophageal obstruction (secondary to stricture from esophagitis)
- Chronic laryngitis
- Chronic rhinosinusitis
- Bronchospasm/laryngospasm

Neurobehavioral Signs and Symptoms
- Infant "reflux" spells (seizure-like with posturing, apnea, cyanosis)
- Severe sleep disturbances
- Irritability
- Food refusal

Note. EERD = extra-esophageal reflux disease; GERD = gastroesophageal reflux disease

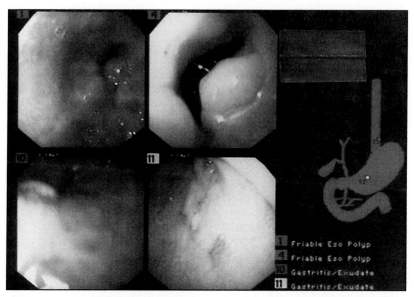

Figure 5–3. Severe esophagitis with polyp formation as a result of chronic inflammation of the lower esophagus is demonstrated in frames 1 and 4. Frames 10 and 11 show gastric inflammation.

young children, the diagnosis of esophagitis relies upon histologic criteria (Heikenen & Werlin, 2000; Stroh et al., 1998). Three criteria generally used are the presence of intraepithelial inflammatory cells (eosinophils, lymphocytes, or neutrophils), basal cell hyperplasia (greater than 25% of the thickness of the epithelium), and papillary elongation (greater than 50% of the thickness of the epithelium).

Barrett's Esophagus

With progressive injury to the mucosa of the esophagus, undifferentiated basal stem cells reepithelialize the mucosal defect. In the presence of as-yet-unspecified growth factors in the refluxate, these pluripotential cells differentiate into more acid-resistant columnar epithelium. The presence of the columnar epithelium is a condition termed Barrett's esophagus. This is rare in childhood but is more likely to occur in neurologically impaired children in whom the reflux is chronic (Hassal, Weinstein, & Ament, 1985). Barrett's esophagus has been reported in 5 to 15% of patients with chronic GER. Progression to adenocarcinoma is reported in 10% of untreated cases (Naef, Savary, & Ozzello, 1975). Endoscopically one sees an irregular, sharply demarcated change from the pale color of squamous mucosa to a velvety, erythematous mucosa typical of columnar epithelium as is present in the stomach.

Differential Diagnosis

Recurrent vomiting and malnutrition may be caused by other medical conditions other than GERD/EERD. These include urinary tract obstruction and recurrent infections, pyloric stenosis, increased intracranial pressure from a central nervous system (CNS) disorder (most often brain tumor), milk protein intolerance, cyclic vomiting, and eosinophilic gastroenteropathy. Cyclic vomiting is a poorly understood disorder in which vomiting lasting hours to days continues unabated. It has been mistaken for or may masquerade as GERD/EERD or any of these other problems. Therefore, a careful clinical examination, supplemented by appropriate diagnostic studies, is critical in the infant or child who has symptoms of regurgitation and vomiting (Catto-Smith, 1998).

Eosinophilic Gastroenteropathy and Milk Protein Allergy

The presence of eosinophils in esophageal mucosa has been regarded as pathognomonic for reflux esophagitis. Recently this has been challenged. Both esosinophilic gastroenteropathy and milk protein allergy may also manifest with similar symptoms to GERD/EERD, but the histology is different. In eosinophilic gastroenteropathy, peripapillary, or juxtaluminal eosinophil clustering is seen. Eoinophils in the mucosa of the stomach, small intestine, and colon are not uncommon (Orenstein et al., 2000).

Eosinophilic gastroenteropathy is a chronic relapsing disorder in which the eosinophil constitutes the major cell type of the inflammatory infiltrate in the GI tract. Clinical presentation correlates with the extent of eosinophilic infiltration (diffuse vs. circumscribed) and the depth of eosinophilic reaction (mucosal, muscularis, and serosal). It may involve the entire GI tract, but the stomach and small intestine are more commonly involved. Mucosal involvement is most common and produces either bleeding or protein loss. Muscularis infiltration produces stricture and obstruction, and serosal activity leads to eosinophilic ascites. Because of the diversity of presentation, it may be that several distinct, as-yet-unrecognized diseases have eosinophilic infiltration as the unifying feature.

A family or personal history of allergy is quite common. Food sensitivity may play a role, but the exact etiologic basis of this condition is unknown. Immunoglobulin E (IgE)-mediated and IgE-independent hypersensitivities are possibilities. Manifestation of this entity may include vomiting, abdominal pain, growth failure, diarrhea with or without rectal bleeding, peripheral edema, anemia, and hypoproteinemia.

Radiographic studies may demonstrate narrowing and nodularity of the gastric antrum and/or duodenum or thickened mucosal folds in the intestine. Endoscopy is often contributory, because it may show erythema, nodularity, friability erosions, and ulcerations in the affected areas, and it affords the ability to perform mucosal biopsies.

When food provokes characteristic symptoms, dietary elimination circumvents the problem. When symptoms persist, corticosteroids (1–2 mg/kg/day) and oral disodium cromoglycate (50–200 mg per dose given 4 times per day) may help control the symptoms. Surgery is usually not required except in cases of intractable strictures (Case Study 2).

When milk protein allergy is present, peripheral blood eosinophilia may also be present in this condition. An elevated eosinophil cationic protein or alpha-1-antitrypsin activity in the feces also supports the diagnosis.

Manifestations should resolve completely once cow's milk is stopped. Breast-feeding mothers should eliminate milk from their diet. With continuation of symptoms, proctosigmoidoscopy or endoscopy with biopsy should be considered, as well as a therapeutic and diagnostic trial first of hydrolysable formulas; amino acid formula may be tried as well. Oral cromolyn may be beneficial in those with persistent symptoms.

Swallowing and Feeding Problems and GERD/EERD

In adults, heartburn is an extremely common symptom. It may or may not be associated with visible esophagitis. It is often encountered in older children who are able to describe their symptoms. Infants, on the other hand, exhibit a wide variety of often nonspecific symptoms. Extreme irritability, sometimes difficult to differentiate from colic, is thought to be indicative of an infantile form of heartburn. With long-standing inflammation from reflux, stricture formation and associated dysphagia may also develop. Esophageal spasm leading to pain on swallowing food (odynophagia) can occur in the presence of esophagitis. Especially in the absence of regurgitation or vomiting, it may be assumed that this food "sticking" represents an anatomic obstruction or is secondary to a primary motility disorder (Case Study 3).

Patients with tracheoesophageal fistula (TEF) repair have abnormal esophageal motility, which leads to GERD/EERD in most, if not all, patients. These children are particularly susceptible to strictures, both at the anastomotic site and as a result of reflux. Dysphagia can result from the structural esophageal obstruction or a reflux induced esophageal stricture. Furthermore, esophagitis can cause secondary esophageal motor abnormalities, "food sticking," and dysphagia (Hillemeier et al., 1983). Peristaltic dysfunction increases with increasing severity of peptic esophagitis (Kahrilas et al., 1986). Indeed, either dysphagia or "food sticking" may be a presenting symptom of reflux esophagitis in childhood in the absence of the more common history suggestive of GER and without evidence of a peptic stricture (Catto-Smith, Machida, Butzner, Gall, & Scott, 1991). Determining the primary pathogenic process is often impossible.

In individuals with handicaps, many of whom have little to no functional communication skills, dysphagia also can lead to food aversion, a significant factor in the development of primary malnutrition. Similarly, arching of the spine, opisthotonic posture, and neck rubbing may indicate unrecognized GERD/EERD in these individuals.

Respiratory Distress and GERD/EERD

Respiratory symptoms are less obvious manifestations of GERD/EERD (Table 4–2). These are well described in Chapter 4.

Diagnostic Evaluation

The diagnosis of GERD/EERD, suspected after the clinical history and physical examination are completed, is made using either diagnostic tests or a therapeutic trial. Many children can be given a therapeutic trial of antacids, dietary control, and positional therapy (Orenstein, 1992; Putnam, 1998; Tsou & Bishop, 1998). A complete response is evidence enough to diagnose GERD/EERD as the cause of the symptoms. The relative usefulness of commonly used diagnostic studies is outlined in Table 5–5. Although no one test is considered diagnostic, there is some evidence that two positive tests are highly predictive of reflux (Meyers, Roberts, Johnson, & Herbst, 1985).

Barium Esophagram

The barium esophagram is a radiographic study in which the child swallows a liquid mixed with barium, that is a radiopaque, inert element. Although the barium esophagram has a low sensitivity for reflux, in part because of the short duration of the study, it is a good contrast radiographic study to delineate the structure of the esophagus and stomach. Pyloric stenosis, esophageal webs, strictures, TEF, esophageal compression from vascular anomalies, intrinsic masses, achalasia, and malrotation of the gut may be demonstrated. Aspiration may be seen; however, the esophagram has low sensitivity for this condition (see Chapters 8 and 10) (Putnam, 1998; Sondheimer, 1988).

Scintigram

A gastric scintiscan uses a substance labeled with radioactive technecium 99m added to commonly eaten foods. The course of a meal, after it is

Table 5–5. The Advantages and Disadvantages of Commonly Used Diagnostic Modalities for GERD/EERD in Children

Test	Advantages	Disadvantages
Barium esophagram	• Readily available • Shows anatomic abnormalities	• Shows only obvious reflux • Short test • Artificial food • Radiation exposure • Low sensitivity
Gastric scintiscan w/gastric emptying	• Uses regular food • Longer test time (1 hour) • Estimates gastric emptying (a measure of motility) • May show aspiration • High specificity • Shows any reflux (acid and alkaline)	• Does not quantitate reflux • Limited time for test • Low sensitivity • Postprandial only
Direct rigid laryngosocpy or FFNL	• Readily available • Shows airway structure	• Minimally invasive • Requires otolaryngologist
Bronchoscopy w/ bronchial washings[a]	• Shows airway structure • Helps diagnose aspiration	• Invasive
Esophagoscopy	• Can evaluate other conditions w/biopsy • Can treat strictures	• Invasive • Low sensitivity for EERD
Suction catheter esophageal biopsy	• Diagnostic if present • Minimally invasive	• Low sensitivity
24-hour dual-channel pH probe	• High sensitivity • Quantitates acid insult • May be used for alkaline reflux	• Invasive • Does not always evaluate for non-acid reflux unless calibrated and requested

Note: EERD = extra-esophageal reflux disorder; FFNL = flexible fiberoptic nasopharyngo-laryngoscopy; GERD = gastroesophageal reflux disorder.
[a]Bronchial washings for lipid laden macrophages and amylase are indirect indicators for aspiration, often secondary to GERD/EERD.

ingested, is followed through the upper aerodigestive tract for 1 complete hour. Typically done in the supine position, the scintiscan evaluates for both reflux and gastric emptying. It is a good screening test although the sensitivity is quite low. Limited anatomic information is gained, but the food used is that of the normal diet of the child. Observation time is increased over that allowed by barium esophagram; however, standardization of this test is lacking (Putnam, 1998; Tsou & Bishop, 1998). The presence of low gastric emptying is important because it will usually herald a positive pH probe. Low gastric emptying is used by some to indicate reflux (Papamihalis et al., 1989) (Figure 5–4A, B).

24-Hour Multi-Channel pH Probe Monitoring

Prolonged pH probe monitoring using upper esophageal and lower esophageal channels is considered, at the time of this writing, the most sensitive indicator of GERD/EERD. Its greatest usefulness is in establishing the diagnosis of silent or difficult-to-diagnose reflux. In children with respiratory symptoms, such as apnea, acute life-threatening events, or sleep disturbances, pH monitoring may establish a temporal relationship between the reflux and these less common presentations (Case Study 4). The test is also

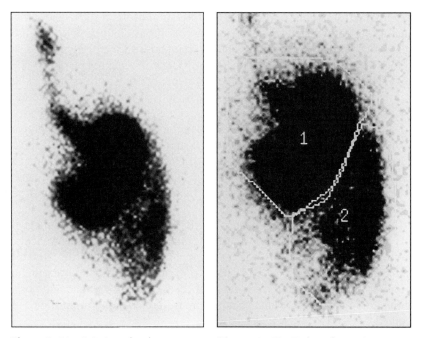

Figure 5–4A. Scintigraphy demonstrating reflux to upper esophagus.

Figure 5–4B. Delayed gastric emptying as evidenced by only 10% of the stomach emptied at 1 hour as depicted by the large amount of isotope still in the stomach (labelled #1).

useful to document effectiveness of medical or surgical therapy in difficult cases. Use of the probe to diagnose alkaline or acidoalkaline reflux is not yet in widespread use in children.

Most clinicians place the probe 2 to 5 cm above the LES. Specially sized probe tips are necessary for neonates, infants, and small children (DiLorenzo & Hyman, 1997). Using various length probe catheters with varying interprobe distances, the proximal probe placement can be determined by the probe tip length (Postma, 2000). The sensors are set to capture events when acidification of the esophagus drops below a pH of 4.0. Data are obtained regarding the time and number of reflux episodes, the number of episodes lasting more than 5 min, number of episodes in either the supine or upright position, and the total percentage of time when reflux is present. Different methodologies for quantification and definition of pathologic GERD are reported (Andze, Brandt, St. Vil, Bensoussan, & Blanchard, 1991; Contencin & Narcy, 1991; Contencin & Philippe, 1992; Little et al., 1997; Postma). The presence of an NG or OG tube, dietary frequency and composition, the position of the patient, and the simultaneous use of medical therapy during the study are factors that must be considered before the test is done and during interpretation of the results. The information sought will determine the testing conditions. For example, because gastric acid production may be deficient in infants less than 1 month of age, it may be difficult to diagnose GERD/EERD in this age group by pH probe testing (Euler, Byrne, Meis, Leake, & Ament, 1979). Gastric contents that reflux into the lower esophagus may not be sufficiently acidic for detection by esophageal pH probe. In these cases, stomach pH must be tested prior to a pH probe study. A gastric pH of 1–2 indicates that the test should give valid results. In cases where gastric pH is high, the infant may be fed apple juice, which has a pH slightly less than 4. This will acidify gastric contents and thus overcome the problem in the patient with hyposecretion of acid. The use of dual channel pH probe in the diagnosis of duodenal gastric reflux (DGR) will be discussed below.

The criteria for the diagnosis of GERD by prolonged intraesophageal pH monitoring are controversial. Despite attempts to standardize protocols, normal scoring values for prolonged esophageal pH monitoring are still subjective, and pH probe studies reported in the literature may vary in the monitoring time, feeding time, types of feeds, feeding volume, and positioning (Boyle, 1989). Thus, results from different studies are difficult to compare.

Age is also an important factor affecting pH probe results. Infants have more frequent reflux episodes than older children. One study in children over 1 year of age indicated that normal children may exhibit a distal esophageal pH <4.0 for a mean of 3.2 ± 1.9% of the total monitored time and that reflux episodes occur 0.84 ± 0.36 times per hour (Sondheimer, 1988).

Boyle (1989) proposed that two or more of the following indicate abnormal reflux:

1. greater than 1.5 episodes per hour,
2. more than 0.3 episodes per hour that exceed 5 min,
3. more than 6% of time when esophageal pH is less than 4.0,
4. more than 12% of episodes exceed 5 min duration,
5. mean acid clearance of more than 4 min, and
6. duration of the longest episode greater than 20 min.

These criteria are useful in the prediction of the development of esophagitis; however, the vagally mediated responses of GERD/EERD may be caused by much less acid exposure and are not taken into account by these criteria.

Although the dual channel 24-hour pH probe is regarded as the gold standard in the diagnosis of GERD, it has some limitations. Intertest reliability is only fair, with 25 to 30% of probes missing GERD (Mahajan et al., 1998; Vaezi, Schroeder, & Richter, 1997). The correlation to symptoms or to the presence of esophagitis is unreliable (Bollschweiler, Feussner, Holscher, & Siewert, 1993; Ferreira et al., 1993). The pH probe only tests for the presence of acid, pH less than 4, unless the study is calibrated to evaluate for alkaline reflux (Igarashi, Lee, Evans, Yusuf, Steele, & Atkinson, 1995; Tovar et al., 1993). The time commitment need for skilled nursing for insertion, patient discomfort, and cost are other concerns that limit the use of the pH probe. Four-channel esophageal pH monitoring may be more sensitive, particularly in young patients (Haase, Ross, Gance-Cleveland, & Kolack, 1988). The negative predictive value for the distal pH probe, especially when airway symptoms are present, continues to be of concern (Bauman, Sandler, Bishop, & Smith, 2000; Bollschweiler et al., 1993; Vaezi et al., 1997).

The usefulness of the pH probe for evaluation of respiratory symptoms and atypical symptoms of GERD/EERD is highlighted by several reports (Andze et al., 1991; Bauman et al., 2000; Little et al., 1997; Matthews, Little, McGuirt Jr., & Koufman, 1999; Vaezi et al., 1997). There continues to be a lack of normative data regarding acid reflux to the upper probe. In a recent report claiming normative data, the authors do not meticulously exclude airway and other atypical presentations from their "normal" group (Bagucka, Badriul, Vandemaele, Troch, & Vandenplas, 2000). Nasopharyngeal monitoring has been reported; however, the technical difficulties of keeping the probe tip moist and accurately assessing the origin of the secretions causing the pH change are significant limitations of this technique (Contencin & Narcy, 1991). Thus, although pH probe assessment is highly useful, its limitations require clinicians to seek better diagnostic tools for the difficult to diagnose patient (Cucchiara et al., 1995).

Endoscopy

Both flexible fiberoptic and rigid esophagogastroscopy are useful in determining the presence of esophagitis and other esophageal mucosal manifestations of GERD/EERD. Direct visualization of the esophagus with histopathology for evidence of esophagitis is discussed above under differential diagnosis. The use of esophageal suction biopsy is performed without direct visualization. This technique is also useful, less invasive, and, if positive, provides enough information to justify treatment (Orenstein, 1992). The endoscopic diagnosis of EERD is discussed in Chapter 4.

Treatment of GERD/EERD

The treatment of pathologic GERD/EERD is multifaceted and depends on the age of the patient, the severity of symptoms, underlying medical conditions, and contributing environmental factors. Empiric therapy, for those in whom the diagnosis is suspected, but in whom diagnostic tests are unavailable or unwanted, is a reasonable alternative (Schindlbeck, Klauser, Voderholzer, & Muller-Lissner, 1995). A summary of treatment modalities used is found in Table 5–6.

Medical, Non-Pharmacologic Therapy

In smaller infants, the "time honored" recommendations have been elevation of the head of bed, change to a non-cow's-milk formula, thickened feedings, and small frequent feedings (Orenstein, 1992; Putnam, 1998; Tsou & Bishop, 1998). Positional treatment is the mode of therapy used most

Table 5–6. Treatment Modalities for GERD/EERD

Non-medical, Non-surgical
- Dietary
- Position
- Activity

Pharmacologic
- Antacids
- Prokinetics

Surgical
- Jejunostomy feeding
- Fundoplication
- Gastroesophageal separation

Note: EERD = extra-esophageal reflux disorder; GERD = gastroesophageal reflux disorder.

frequently. In light of new information regarding sudden infant death syndrome, having the infant suspected of GERD/EERD sleep on one side is probably most beneficial and safe. Although recent reports have questioned the benefit of positional therapy in infants (Orenstein), older children often will state that they sleep more comfortably in an upright position, often with multiple pillows. Other activities that might impair gastric emptying are hurried meals, immediately assuming a recumbent position after meals, and excessive exercise immediately after eating. Adolescents in particular are prone to these situations.

Thickened feedings of 1–2 teaspoons of rice cereal per ounce of formula are often recommended for the treatment of infant GERD/EERD. This therapy may actually worsen the problem if gastric emptying is slow. The use of non-cow's-milk formulas is discussed above. A diet free of reflux inducing foods is also helpful.

Pharmacologic Therapy

Pharmacologic therapy is the mainstay for GERD/EERD. Prokinetic agents include metoclopramide and bethanecol. H-2 receptor antagonists such as cimetidine or ranitidine are designed to lower gastric acid production and are therefore useful in preventing or treating esophagitis as a result of GER. Proton pump inhibitors, such as omeprazole, are extremely effective in reducing acid production. The antacid Gaviscon, a formulation of alginaic acid, is stated to form a "floating barrier" of viscous, foamy material to provide a mechanical barrier to reflux. Table 5–7 lists the most commonly used pharmacologic agents, their mechanism of action and dose, and their side effects.

Surgical Therapy

Surgical therapy is reserved for those patients who have severe reflux that is unresponsive to medical therapy. Watchful waiting, if at all possible, is especially recommended for those patients who are less than 18 months of age. Older children are less likely to have spontaneous resolution of their symptoms. Patients with neurologic disease or those with life-threatening complications that can be directly related to GERD/EERD are prime candidates for surgical intervention. Patients with choking, aspiration, recurrent apnea, chronic pulmonary disease, Barrett's esophagus, esophageal strictures, large fixed hiatal hernias, bleeding, and malnutrition unresponsive to medical therapy all have reason to undergo surgery.

The procedure of choice is fundoplication. In this procedure the fundus of the stomach is wrapped around the distal esophagus. Jolley et al. (1980) reported 96% control of vomiting in 135 infants and improvement in respiratory symptoms in 56 of 61 children. There is general agreement

Table 5–7. Commonly Used Pharmacologic Agents in Infants and Children with GERD/EERD

Drug	Mechanism of Action	Dosage	Side Effects
Metoclopramide (Reglan)	Inhibits dopamine Increases acetylcholine release	0.1–0.2 mg/ kg/dose q.i.d.	Insomnia Restlessssness Diarrhea
Bethanecol (Urecholine)	Cholinergic stimulator	0.1 mg/ kg/dose t.i.d.	Cramps Fatigue Increased urination and salivation
Cimetidine (Tagamet)	H-2 receptor antagonist	10–15 mg/ kg/dose b.i.d.	Headache, confusion Pancytopenia Gynecomastia
Ranitidine (Zantac)	H-2 receptor antagonist	2–4 mg/ kg/dose b.i.d.	Headache, malaise Thrombo- cytopenia Hepatotoxicity
Omeprazole (Prilosec)	Proton pump inhibitor	1.0 mg/ kg/day q.h.s.	Headache, rash Hypergastrinemia Diarrhea
TUMS	Antacid	prn	Constipation
Alginate-antacid (Gaviscon)	Mucosal protection, acid neutralizer	5–15 ml/dose after meals	Diarrhea
Aluminum/ Magnesium Hydroxide (Mylanta/Maalox)	Mucosal protection, acid neutralizer	0.5–1.0 mg/ kg/dose t.i.d. or q.i.d.	Diarrhea
Carafate (Sucralfate)	Mucosal protection	20 mg/kg/ dose q.i.d.	Constipation

Note: EERD = estraesophageal reflux disorder; GERD = gastroesophageal reflux disorder.

that the operative mortality is less than 1%. Gas bloat may occur with the inability to belch or vomit. Nausea, retching, gagging, and abdominal full-ness also may be symptoms of gas bloat. Dysphagia from too tight a wrap of the stomach can occur. "Dumping," defined as the occurrence of diar-rhea, nausea, diaphoresis, or retching within 30 min following feedings, is another potential problem. This results from rapid gastric emptying of hyperosmolar gastric contents into the duodenum. Gastrointestinal obstruction is also a rare complication, as is new onset oral dysfunction (Borowitz & Borowitz, 1992).

Contraindication to fundoplication includes chronic intestinal pseudo-obstruction syndrome, which describes a heterogeneous group of enteric neuromuscular disorders that vary widely in their symptoms. The most common symptoms are abdominal pain, vomiting, distention, constipation, or diarrhea. Abnormal motility may be anatomically limited or diffuse throughout the entire GI tract. When present, fundoplication is rarely, if ever, indicated. If, however, fundoplication is performed, symptoms may change from vomiting to repeated retching due to abnormal esophageal and gastric peristalsis. Pyloroplasty has not proven effective in treating this problem because of the overall motility problem and delay in gastric emptying.

Treatment of Patients With Neurologic Impairment and GERD/EERD

Patients who have neurologic impairment from mental or motor retardation pose special problems in regard to nutritional support and control of GERD/EERD. The use of gastrostomy tubes has been well received by caregivers (Tawfik, Dickson, Clarke, & Thomas, 1997) and has enabled the reversal of nutritional deficiencies in many of these patients with oral–motor problems. This has been an important advancement in their therapy. Improvement in overall nutrition (Gerber, Gaugler, Myer, & Cotton, 1996) and the use of antireflux medications are often enough to keep the GERD/EERD under control. Because up to 70 or 80% of patients with mental or motor retardation also suffer from GERD/EERD, some clinicians advise that antireflux surgery should be performed at the time of gastrostomy tube placement (Fonkalsrud, Ashcraft, Coran, et al., 1998; Heine et al., 1995; Jolley et al., 1985). This has been recommended because surgical gastrostomy placement itself has been reported to induce or contribute to GER by altering the angle at the gastroesophageal junction and also by lowering LES pressure (Canal, Vane, Goto, Gardner, & Grosfeld, 1987). In patients who do not have pathologic GER and who do not suffer from the complications of GER listed above, it is difficult to make a definitive statement that antireflux surgery is necessary at the time of feeding gastrostomy (Orenstein, 1992). Each case must be assessed individually. One investigator indicates that if nasogastric feedings are well tolerated preoperatively, the patient probably will do well with only gastrostomy tube placement (Boyle, 1989).

Gastrostomy tube placement in this situation can be performed using the percutaneous endoscopic technique. If significant GER subsequently develops, antireflux surgery may then be performed. The fundoplication can be done with open or laparoscopic techniques (Ritter, Vanderpool, & Westmoreland, 1997; Rothenberg et al., 1997). This approach seems rational, and with it, major intra-abdominal surgery will be avoided in some patients. Unfortunately, there is a not-insignificant failure rate for fundoplication (Kimber et al., 2000; Martinez, Ginn-Pease, & Caniano, 1992). A high index of suspicion and repeated testing may be necessary to make the diagnosis of recurrent reflux. The complications in this group of children are similar to those in children who are neurologically normal.

Esophagogastric dissociation is the complete separation of the esophagus from the stomach (Bianchi, 1997; Danielson & Emmens, 1999). This procedure entails a feeding gastrostomy and an anastomosis between the esophagus and jejunum (Bianchi). Although reserved for failures of fundoplication, some have recommended this as a first-line treatment for children with severe neurologic impairment in whom GERD/EERD is highly probable and feeding by mouth is impossible (Bianchi; Danielson & Emmens).

■ DUODENOGASTRIC REFLUX (DGR)

The incidence of duodenogastric reflux (DGR) was found to be high in a group of 109 children studied by 24-hour dual-channel pH probe, using both gastric and esophageal monitors. Of the total group, 69 were considered clinically to be refluxers, and 40 were nonrefluxers. Of the total group, 11% were found to have alkaline reflux and 22% acidalkaline reflux (Tovar et al., 1993). Alkaline reflux (above pH 7.0) may have deleterious effects on the mucosa of the stomach and upper aerodigestive tract (Tovar et al.). The refluxate consists of gastric enzymes, bile salts, and pancreatic enzymes. Their effects are better understood in adults than in children at this time. It is suggested that DGR be considered in difficult cases in which GERD/EERD signs and symptoms are apparent but no evidence confirms the diagnosis. Treatment options for this disorder are not yet well developed.

■ CASE STUDIES

Case Study 1

"Peter" is a 26-month-old boy with severe short bowel syndrome, secondary to necrotizing enterocolitis; he has been nourished by parenteral nutrition since birth. Peter is averse to oral feedings and tolerates only tiny quantities of tube feedings (5 cc/hour for 12 hours overnight via gastrostomy). He has a central catheter placed for parenteral nutrition. He weighs 11 kg and is 88 cm in length. He exhibits normal development and activity for age. The feeding team was consulted to assess nutrient needs and to help arrange home nutrition support.

Assessment

Weight is at the 5th percentile for age. Length is at the 50th percentile for age. Weight for length is at the 5th percentile. His appropriate weight for his length is 12.5 kg.

Energy needs are estimated based on ideal weight (12.5 kg) for length to allow for catch up growth; according to estimated requirements from total parenteral nutrition (TPN), he needs approximately 102 calories/kg, or 1,275 calories/day. Protein requirements are 1.5 to 2 g/kg/day or 16 to 22 g/day. Fluid needs are 100 cc/kg/day or 1,100 cc/day (Baker & Baker, 1997).

Recommendation

An appropriate TPN solution for Peter was determined to be 1,100 cc of fluid containing 800 cc of 20% dextrose (544 calories); 16 g of protein (64 calories) and 300 cc of fat (60 g) provided as a 20% lipid emulsion (600 calories). The parenteral nutrition was initiated at full volume (1,100 cc) provided over 24 hours. Concentrations of dextrose, protein, and fat were increased gradually to reach goal caloric and protein intake. Once full nutrient levels were obtained, the hours of infusion were gradually reduced, with the volume infused per hour gradually increased. Most children can tolerate infusion over 10 to12 hours so that the infusion can be provided at night only. Serum glucose, triglycerides, proteins, and liver function were monitored weekly throughout the course of TPN infusion. It was found that when the hours of infusion were decreased to under 16 hours per day (approximately 68 cc/hr), hyperglycemia became a problem. Although insulin could have been provided in the TPN solution, the parents preferred to maintain the infusion at 16 hours/day.

Portable infusion pumps and overnight infusions have made home delivery of parenteral nutrition a viable option. Peter's parents were trained to provide TPN at home so he could be discharged from the hospital. Enteral feedings continued to be encouraged throughout the course of TPN therapy. Once he was at home, Peter began to eat more by mouth. The dietitian evaluated his caloric intake on a monthly basis and adjusted his TPN infusion to maintain a constant calorie, protein, and fluid intake.

Comment

This case illustrates the need for detailed evaluation of the nutritional needs of patients requiring parenteral nutrition. A coordinated approach allowed this child to be discharged to his home despite his need for complex nutritional support.

Case Study 2

"Catherine" is a 15-year-old young woman who complained of "very bad heartburn" for 6 months with fluid "shooting up her chest and acid taste in her mouth." She also had intermittent episodes of difficulty swallowing with "food sticking" in her chest. Symptoms were aggravated by stress and foods such as chocolate, acidic foods, and carbonated beverages. She avoided these substances but continued with symptoms.

A 3-month trial of antacids (ranitidine 150 mg p.o. b.i.d.) did not help, but Prevacid (30 mg p.o. q.d.) ameliorated her symptoms. An upper GI series was normal with no evidence of hiatal hernia or gastroesophageal stricture. The persistent symptoms led to an upper intestinal endoscopy that revealed cicatricial granular mucosa of the esophagus. Biopsies demonstrated greater than 40 eosinophils per high powered field. A 24-hour dual-channel pH probe did not reveal acid reflux. The young woman was treated with diet restriction for milk products, continuation of Prevacid, and the addition of oral Flovent (fluticasone) 220 mg sprayed orally and swallowed 3 times daily led to amelioration of symptoms. Symptoms abated, and Catherine is doing well.

Comment

Catherine had many of the symptoms of GERD/EERD. When a therapeutic trial is undertaken, close follow-up is essential. When medical therapy failed, however, investigation for an alternative diagnosis was undertaken successfully. This case highlights the need to be vigilant about diagnostic accuracy.

Case Study 3

"Phyllis" is an 11-year-old girl who presented with an acute onset of dysphagia after eating shrimp with cocktail sauce. She described a burning sensation in the back of her throat. From that time she had taken only liquids and had lost 5 pounds. This was very distressing to her mother, who described Phyllis' life as stressful, particularly at the time of onset because of church readings that she was preparing. She participates in competitive gymnastics and maintains an A average. Dietary history revealed almost daily consumption of carbonated beverages, citrus juice, tomato-based sauces, hot sauce, chocolate, and processed lunch meats. Many meals were eaten on the run either to or from a competition. Her last meal is usually eaten at 10 p.m. before going to sleep. No smoke exposure was noted.

Review of systems revealed occasional chest pain, throat clearing, and stomach aches.

Physical examination revealed an anxious, very thin girl in no acute distress. The remainder of the physical examination was normal. Video flouroscopic swallow study revealed no abnormalities and barium esophagram was also normal. Flexible fiberoptic nasopharyngolaryngoscopy revealed severe hypopharyngeal erythema, edema, lingual tonsillar hyperplasia, posterior glottic swelling, vocal fold edema, and loss of arytenoid architecture.

A diagnosis of severe hypopharyngeal EERD was made. The family and child were counseled about dietary control. Elevation of the head of the bed was recommended. Gymnastic competitions continued at the same pace, although Phyllis did not eat directly before a competition or late at night. Ranitidine (50 mg p.o. b.i.d.) was begun.

One month later, Phyllis returned with her mother and reported that her symptoms were much better. She was beginning to tolerate solids. When she ate foods off her diet, she reported an increased incidence of heartburn. Metoclopramide (8 mg p.o. b.i.d.) was added to the regimen, and ranitidine was replaced with omeprazole (20 mg p.o. q.d.). Stress reduction counseling was suggested, and she was referred to a psychologist.

One month follow-up revealed that the metoclopramide had to be discontinued because of excessive sleepiness, even at a very low dose. She was doing well and had begun to gain some weight. The stress reduction was quite helpful.

Phyllis was seen 3 months later. She was eating normally, had gained 7 pounds, and was able to continue her gymnastics. Omeprazole was discontinued and the diet liberalized.

Comment

This case study demonstrates the need to keep in mind the atypical presentations of GERD/EERD. A wholistic approach to the patient's diet and lifestyle was necessary to effect a cure in this preadolescent

Case Study 4

"Tony" is a 4-month-old infant who successfully underwent correction of transposition of the great vessels on the 3rd day of life. On three separate occasions following discharge, he suffered cessation of breathing, cyanosis, and loss of muscle tone requiring cardiopulmonary resuscitation. These acute life threatening events (ALTEs) occurred within 1 hour of feeding; on one occasion he had regurgitation at the onset of feeding. Upper GI, scintiscan, endoscopy, and two pH probe examinations were read as normal. One ALTE occurred while the infant was receiving medical treatment, which included metoclopramide and omeprazole. The severe nature of these symptoms led to the recommendation for fundoplication. Since the surgery, no further acute life-threatening events have occurred.

Comment

This case emphasizes that one needs to consider GERD/EERD on clinical grounds alone, even when the diagnostic tests are not helpful in establishing the diagnosis. Although the pH probe was technically normal, some reflux did occur although not meeting criteria for pathologic reflux. This infant may have been particularly susceptible to reflex induced laryngospasm from lower esophageal reflux or direct acid contact laryngospasm, or both. In this case, the consequences of not effectively treating reflux could possibly have been fatal.

■ REFERENCES

Adkins, J. C. (1990). Congenital malformations of the esophagus. In C. Bluestone and S. Stool (Eds.), *Pediatric Otolaryngology* (2nd ed) (973–984). Philadelphia: Saunders.

Amundson, J. A., Sherbondy, A., Van Dyke, D. C., & Alexander, R. (1994). Early identification and treatment necessary to prevent malnutrition in children and adolescents with severe disabilities. *Journal of American Dietetic Association, 94,* 880–883.

Andze, G. O., Brandt, M. L., St. Vil, D., Bensoussan, A. L., & Blanchard, H. (1991). Diagnosis and treatment of gastroesophageal reflux in 500 children with respiratory symptoms: The value of pH monitoring. *Journal of Pediatric Surgery, 26,* 295–299.

Baer, M., Maki, M., Nurminen, J., Turjanmaa, V., Pukander, J., & Vesikari, T. (1986). Esophagitis and findings of long-term esophageal pH recording in children with repeated lower respiratory tract symptoms. *Journal of Pediatric Gastroenterology and Nutrition, 5,* 187–190.

Bagucka, B., Badriul, H., Vandemaele, K., Troch, E., & Vandenplas, Y. (2000). Normal ranges of continuous pH monitoring in the proximal esophagus. *Journal of Pediatric Gastroenterology & Nutrition, 31,* 244–247.

Baker, R., & Baker, S. (1997). *Pediatric Parenteral Nutrition.* New York: Chapman and Hall.

Bauman, N., Sandler, A., Bishop, W., & Smith, R. (2000). Value of pH probe testing in pediatric patients with extraesophageal manifestations of gastroesophageal reflux disease: A retrospective review. *Annals of Otorhinology and Laryngology, 109,* 18–24.

Beghin, I. D., & Viteri, F. E. (1973) Nutritional rehabilitation centers: an evaluation of their performance. *Journal of Tropical Medicine and Environmental Health. 19,* 403–416.

Bianchi, A. (1997). Total esophagogastric dissociation: An alternative approach. *Journal of Pediatric Surgery, 32,* 1291–1294.

Biller, J. A., Winter, H. S., Grand, R. J., & Allerd, E. (1983). Are endoscopic changes predictive of histologic esophagitis in children? *Journal of Pediatrics, 103,* 215–218.

Bollschweiler, E., Feussner, H., Holscher, A. H., & Siewert, J. R. (1993). pH monitoring: The gold standard in detection of gastrointestinal reflux disease? *Dysphagia, 8,* 118–121.

Borowitz, S. M., & Borowitz, K. C. (1992). Oral dysfunction following Nissen fundoplication. *Dysphagia, 7,* 234–237.

Boyle, J. T. (1989). Gastroesophageal reflux in the pediatric patient. *Gastroenterology Clinics of North America, 18,* 315-337.

Canal, D. F., Vane, D. W., Goto, S., Gardner, G. P., & Grosfeld, J. L. (1987). Changes in lower esophageal sphincter pressure (LES) after Stamm gastrostomy. *Journal of Surgical Research, 42,* 570–574.

Carre, I. J. (1959). The natural history of the partial thoracic stomach (hiatal hernia) in children. *Archives in Childhood Diseases, 34,* 344–353.

Catto-Smith, A. G. (1998). Gastroesophageal reflux in children. *Australian Family Physician, 27,* 465–469, 472–473.

Catto-Smith, A. G., Machida, H., Butzner, J. D., Gall, D. G., & Scott, R. B. (1991). The role of gastroenterology reflux in pedactric dysphasia. *Journal of Gastroenterology and Nutrition, 12,* 155–165.

Chandra, R. K. (1982). Immunocompetence testing and nutritional status. *Diagnostic Medicine, 5,* 53–57.

Cloud, H. H., & Bergman, J. (1991). Eating/feeding problems of children: The team approach. *Nutrition Focus, 6,* 1–8.

Contencin, P., & Narcy, P. (1991). Nasopharyngeal pH monitoring in infants and children with rhinopharyngitis. *International Journal of Pediatric Otorhinolaryngology, 22,* 249–256.

Contencin, P., & Philippe, N. (1992). Gastropharyngeal reflux in infants and children: A pharyngeal pH monitoring study. *Archives of Otolaryngology and Head and Neck Surgery, 118,* 1028–1030.

Cucchiara, S., Santamaria, F., Minella, R., Alfieri, E., Scoppa, A., Calabrese, F. F. M., Rea, B., & Salvia, G. (1995). Simultaneous prolonged recordings of proximal and distal intraesophageal pH in children with gastroesophageal reflux disease and respiratory symptoms. *American Journal of Gastroenterology, 90,* 1791–1796.

Danielson, P., & Emmens R. W. (1999). Esophagogastric disconnection for gastroesophageal reflux in children with severe neurological impairment. *Journal of Pediatric Surgery, 34,* 84–87.

Del Giudice, E., Staiano, A., Capano, G., Romano, A., Florimonte, L., Miele, E., Ciarla, C., Campanozzi, A., & Crisanti, A. F. (1999). Gastrointestinal manifestations in children with cerebral palsy. *Brain & Development, 21,* 307–311.

Dent, J., Dodds, W. J., Friedman, R. H., Sekiguchi, T., Hogan, W. J., Arndorfer, R. C., & Petrie, D. J. (1980). Mechanism of gastroesophageal reflux in recumbent asymptomatic human subjects. *Journal of Clinical Investigation, 65,* 256–267.

DiLorenzo, C. & Hyman, P. E. Pediatric applications of pH monitoring. In *Ambulatory Esophageal pH Monitoring.* J. E.Richter, (Ed.). Baltimore: Williams and Wilkins.

Eastwood, G. L., Castell, D. O., & Higgs, R. H. (1975). Experimental esophagitis in cats impairs lower esophageal sphincter pressure. *Gastroenterology, 69,* 146–153.

Esposito, C., Mendoza-Sagaon, M., Roblot-Maigret, B., Amici, G., Desruelle, P., & Montupet, P. (2000). Complications of laparoscopic treatment of esophageal achalasia in children. *Journal of Pediatric Surgery, 35,* 680–683.

Euler, A. R., Byrne, W. J., Meis, P. J., Leake, R. D., & Ament, M. E. (1979). Basal and pentagastrin stimulated acid secretion in newborn human infants. *Pediatric Research, 13,* 36–37.

Ferreira, C., Lohoues, M. J., Bensoussan, A., Yazbeck, S., Brouchu, P., & Roy, C. (1993). Prolonged pH monitoring is of limited usefulness for gastroesophageal reflux. *American Journal Diseases Children, 147,* 662–664.

Fonkalsrud, E., Ashcraft, K., Coran, A., Ellis, D., Grosfeld, J., Tunell, W., & Weber, T. (1998). Surgical treatment of gastroesophageal reflux in children: A combined hospital study of 7467 patients. *Pediatrics, 101,* 419–422.

Fouad, Y. M. K. P. O., Hatlebakk, J. G., & Castell, D. O. (1999). Ineffective esophageal motility: The most common motility abnormality in patients with GERD-associated respiratory symptoms. *American Journal of Gastroenterology, 94,* 1464–1467.

Gauderer, M. W. L. (1991). Percutaneous endoscopic gastrostomy: A 10-year experience with 220 children. *Journal of Pediatric Surgery, 26,* 288–294.

Gerber, M. E., Gaugler, M. D., Myer C. M. III, & Cotton, R. T. (1996). Chronic aspiration in children. When are bilateral submandibular gland excision and parotid duct ligation indicated? *Archives of Otolaryngology Head and Neck Surgery, 122,* 1368–1371.

Haase, G., Ross, M., Gance-Cleveland, B., & Kolack, K. (1988). Extended four-channel esophageal pH monitoring: The importance of acid reflux patterns at the middle and proximal levels. *Journal of Pediatric Surgery, 23,* 32–37.

Hassal, E., Weinstein, W. M., & Ament, M. E. (1985). Barrett's esophagus in childhood. *Gastroenterology, 89,* 1331–1337.

Heikenen, J., & Werlin, S. L. (2000). Esophageal biopsy does not predict clinical outcome after percutaneous endoscopic gastrostomy in children. *Dysphagia, 15,* 167–169.

Heine, R. G., Reddihough, D. S., & Catto-Smith, A. G. (1995). Gastroesophageal reflux and feeding problems after gastrostomy in children with severe neurological impairment. *Developmental Medicine and Child Neurology, 37,* 320–329.

Hillemeier, A. C., Grill, B. B., McCallum, R., & Gryboski, J. (1983). Esophageal and gastric motor abnormalities in gastroesophageal reflux during infancy. *Gastroenterology, 84,* 741–746.

Holloway, R. H., Hongo, M., Berger, K., & McCallum, R. W. (1985). Gastric distention: A mechanism for postprandial gastroesophageal reflux. *Gastroenterology, 89,* 779–784.

Iacono, G., Carroccio, A. C. F., Montalto, G., Kazmierska, I., Lorello, D., Soresi, M., & Notarbartolo, A. (1996). Gastroesophageal reflux and cow's milk allergy in infants: A prospective study. *Journal Allergy Clinics Immunology, 97,* 822–827.

Iftikhar, S., Ledingham, S. S. E., Yusuf, S., Steele, R., Atkinson, M., & Hardcastle, J. (1995). Alkaline gastro-esophageal reflux: Dual probe pH monitoring. *Gut, 37,* 465-470.

Igarashi, S., Lee, A.W., Evans, D., Yusuf, S., Steele, R., & Atkinson J. D. (1995). Alkaline gastro-esophageal reflux: Dual probe pH monitoring. *Gut, 37,* 465–470.

Jolley, S. G., Herlost, J. J., Johnson, D. G., Matlak, M. E., Boote, L. S., (1980). Surgery in children with gastroesophageal reflux and respiratory symptoms. *Journal of Pediatrics, 9,* 194–198.

Jolley, S., Smith, E., & Tunell, W. P. (1985). Protective anti-reflux operation with feeding gastrostomy: Experience with children. *Annals of Surgery, 201,* 736–740.

Kahrilas, P. J., Dodds, W. J., Hogan, W. J., Kern, M., Arndorfer, R. C., & Reece, A. (1986). Esophageal peristaltic dysfunction in peptic esophagitis. *Gastroenterology, 91,* 897–904.

Kimber, C., Kiely, E., & Spitz, L. (2000). The failure rate of surgery for gastro-esophageal reflux. *Journal of Pediatric Surgery, 33,* 64–66.

Kimber, C., & Beasley, S. (1999). Limitations of percutaneous endoscopic gastrostomy in facilitating enteral nutrition in children: Review of the shortcomings of a new technique. *Journal of Pediatrics & Child Health, 35,* 427–431.

Kirby, D. F., Craig, R. M., Tsang, T. K., & Plotnick, B. H. (1986). Percutaneous endoscopic gastrostomies: A prospective evaluation and review of the literature. *Journal of Parenteral & Enteral Nutrition, 10,* 155–159.

Kosko, J., Moser, D., Erhart, N., & Tunkel, D. (1998). Differential diagnosis of dysphagia in children. *Otolaryngologic Clinics of North America, 31,* 435–451.

Langer, J. C., Wesson, D. E., Ein, S. H., Filler, R. M., Shandling, B., Superina, R. A., & Papa, M. (1988). Feeding gastrostomy in neurologically impaired children: Is an antireflux procedure necessary? *Journal of Pediatric Gastroenterology and Nutrition, 7,* 837–841.

Launay, V., Gottrand, F., Turck, D., Michaud, L., Ategbo, S., & Farriaux, J. P. (1996). Percutaneous endoscopic gastrostomy in children: Influence on gastroesophageal reflux. *Pediatrics, 97,* 726–728.

Little, J. P., Matthews, B. L., Glock, M. S., Koufman, J. A., Reboussin, D. M., Loughlin, C. J., & McGuirt, W. F., Jr. (1997). Extraesophageal pediatric reflux: 24-hour double-probe pH monitoring of 222 children. *Annals of Otorhinology and Laryngology, 106 (Suppl. 169),* 1–16.

Mahajan, L., Wyllie, R., Oliva, L., Balsells, F., Steffen, R., & Kay, M. (1998). Reproducibility of 24-hour intraesophageal pH monitoring in pediatric patients. *Pediactrics, 101,* 260–263.

Marino, A. J., Assing, E., Carbone, M. T., Hiatt, I. M., Hegyi, T., & Graff, M. (1995). The incidence of gastroesophageal reflux in preterm infants. *Journal of Perinatology, 15,* 369–371.

Martin, C. J., Patrinos, J., & Dent, J. (1986). Abolition of gas reflux and transient lower esophageal sphincter relaxation by vagal blockade in the dog. *Gastroenterology, 91,* 890–896.

Martinez, D. A., Ginn-Pease, M. E., & Caniano, D. A. (1992). Recognition of recurrent gastroesophageal reflux following antireflux surgery in the neurologically disabled child: High index of suspicion and definitive evaluation. *Journal of Pediatric Surgery, 27,* 983–990.

Matthews, B. L., Little, J. P., McGuirt, W. F., Jr., & Koufman, J. A. (1999). Reflux in infants with laryngomalacia: Results of 24-hour double-probe pH monitoring. *Otolaryngology Head Neck Surgery, 120,* 860–864.

McCallum, R. W., Berkowitz, D. M., & Lerner, E. (1981). Gastric emptying in patients with gastroesophageal reflux. *Gastroenterology, 80,* 285–291.

Meakins, J. L., Pietsch, J. B., & Bubernick, D. (1977). Delayed hypersensitivity: An indicator of acquired failure of host defenses in sepsis and trauma. *Annals of Surgery, 186,* 241–250.

Mehta, Y., & Schou, H. (1988). The anaesthetic management of an infant with frontometaphyseal dysplasia (Gorlin-Cohen syndrome). *Acta Anaesthesia Scandinavia, 32,* 505–507.

Mequid, M. M., & Williams, L. F. (1979). The use of gastrostomy to correct malnutrition. *Surgery, Gynecology & Obstetrics, 149,* 27–32.

Meyers, W., Roberts, C., Johnson, D. G., & Herbst, J. (1985). Value of test for evaluation of gastroesophageal reflux in children. *Journal of Pediatric Surgery, 20,* 515–520.

Naef, A. P., Savary, M., & Ozzello, L. (1975). Columnar-lined lower esophagus: An acquired lesion with malignant predisposition. Report on 140 cases of Barrett's esophagus with 12 adenocarcinomas. *Journal of Thoracic & Cardiovascular Surgery, 70,* 826–835.

Orenstein, S. R. (1992). Controversies in pediatric gastroesophageal reflux. *Journal of Pediatric Gastroenterology and Nutrition, 14,* 338–348.

Orenstein, S. R., Izadnia, F., & Khan, S. (1999). Gastroesophageal reflux disease in children. *Gastroenterology Clinics of North America, 28,* 947–969.

Orenstein, S. R., Shalaby, T. M., DiLorenzo, C., Putnam, P. E., Sigurdsson, L., & Kocoshis, S. A. (2000). The spectrum of pediatric eosinophilic esophagitis beyond infancy: A clinical series of 30 children. *American Journal of Gastroenterology, 95,* 1422–1430.

Papamihalis, T., Wilpizeski, C., & Grosfeld, J. (1989). Increased incidence of delayed gastric emptying in children with gastroesophageal reflux. *Archives of Surgery, 124,* 933–936.

Patrick, J., Boland, M., Stoski, D., & Murray, G. E. (1986). Rapid correction of wasting in children with cerebral palsy. *Developmental Medicine and Child Neurology, 28,* 734–739.

Ponsky, J. L., Gauderer, M. L., Stellato, T. A., & Aszodi, A. (1985). Percutaneous approaches to enteral alimentation. *American Journal of Surgery, 149,* 102–105.

Postma, G. (2000). Ambulatory pH monitoring methodology. *Annals of Otorhinology and Laryngology, 109,* 10–14.

Putnam, P. E. (1998). Gastroesophageal reflux. In *Head & Neck Surgery* (1144–1156). Philadelphia: Lippincott.

Ritter, D., Vanderpool, D., & Westmoreland, M. (1997). Laparoscopic Nissen fundoplication for gastroesophageal reflux disease. *American Journal of Surgery, 174,* 715–718.

Rosario, J., Medow, M., Halata, M., Bostwick, H., Newman, L., Schwarz, S., & Berezin, S. (1999). Nonspecific esophageal motility disorders in children without gastroesophageal reflux. *Journal of Pediatric Gastroenterology and Nutrition, 28,* 480–485.

Rossi, T. M. (1986). Effects of total parenteral nutrition on the digestive organs. In E. Lebenthal (Ed.), *Total parenteral nutrition* (173–184). New York: Raven Press.

Rossi, T. M., & Lebenthal, E. (1983). Pathogenic mechanisms of protracted diarrhea. In L. Barness (Ed.), *Advances in pediatrics* (595–633). Chicago: Year Book Medical Publishers.

Rossi, T. M., Lee, P. C., & Lebenthal, E. (1987). Nutrition and exocrine pancreatic function in infancy: Effects of total parental nutrition and first degree malnutrition. *Pancreas, 2,* 463-469.

Rothenberg, S. S., Bratton, D., Larsen, G., Deterding, R., Milgrom, H., Brugman, S., Boguniewicz, M., Copenhaver, S., White, C., Wagener, J., Fan, L., Chang, J., & Stathos, T. (1997). Laparoscopic fundoplication to enhance pulmonary function in children with severe reactive airway disease and gastroesopheagal reflux disease. *Surgical Endoscopy, 11,* 1088–1099.

Sanders, K. D., Cox, K., Cannon, R., Blanchard, D., Pitcher, J., Papathakis, P., Varella, L., & Maughan, R. (1990). Growth response to enteral feeding by children with cerebral palsy. *Journal of Parenteral & Enteral Nutrition, 14,* 23–26.

Sasaki, C. T., & Toohill, R. J. (2000). Ambulatory pH monitoring for extraesophageal reflux—Introduction. *Annals of Otology, Rhinology, & Laryngology, 109 (Suppl.),* 2–3.

Schindlbeck, N. E., Klauser, A. G., Voderholzer, W. A., & Muller-Lissner, S. A. (1995). Empiric therapy for gastroesophageal reflux disease. *Archives of Internal Medicine, 155,* 1808–1812.

Scrimshaw, N. S. (1981). Significance of the interaction of nutrition and infection in children. In R. Suskind (Ed.), *Textbook of pediatric nutrition* (229–240). New York: Raven Press.

Shapiro, B. K., Green, P., Krick, J., Allen, D., & Capute, A. J. (1986). Growth of severely impaired children: Neurological versus nutritional factors. *Developmental Medicine & Child Neurology, 89,* 729–733.

Shepherd, R., & Wren, J. E. S. (1987). Gastroesophageal reflux in children. *Clinical Pediatrics, 26,* 55

Sieber, W. K. (1990). Functional abnormalities of the esophagus. In C. Bluestone and S. Stool (Eds.), *Pediatric Otolaryngology* (2nd ed) (985–997). Philadelphia: Saunders.

Singh, S., Hinder, R., Naspetti, R., Jamieson, J., Polishuk, P., & DeMeester, T. (1993). Cervical dysphagia is associated with gastric hyperacidity. *Journal of Clinical Gastroenterology, 16,* 98–102.

Sondheimer, J. M. (1988). Gastroesophageal reflux: Update on pathogenesis and diagnosis. *Pediatric Clinics of North America, 35(1),* 103–116.

Stanciu, C., & Bennett, J. R. (1974). Oesophageal acid clearing: One factor in the production of reflux esophagitis. *Gut, 15,* 852–857.

Stallings, V. A., Charney, E. B., Davies, J. C., Cronk, C. E. (1993). Nutritional status and growth of children with diplegic or hemiplegic cerebral palsy. *Developmental Medicine and Child Neurology, 35,* 997–1006.

Stroh, B., Faust, R., & Rimell, F. (1998). Results of esophageal biopsies performed during triple endoscopy in the pediatric patient. *Arch Otolaryngol Head Neck Surg, 124,* 545–549.

Sullivan, P. B. (1997). Gastrointestinal problems in the neurologically impaired child. *Bailliere's Clinical Gastroenterology, 11,* 529–546.

Taminiau, J. A. (1997). Gastro-esophageal reflux in children. *Scandinavian Journal of Gastroenterology, 332(suppl. 223),* 18–20.

Tawfik, R., Dickson, A., Clarke, M., & Thomas, A. G. (1997). Caregivers' perceptions following gastrostomy in severely disabled children with feeding problems. *Developmental Medicine & Child Neurology, 39,* 746–751.

Tovar, J., Wang, W., & Eizaguirre, I. (1993). Simultaneous gastro-esophageal pH monitoring and the diagnosis of alkaline reflux. *Journal of Pediatric Surgery, 28,* 1386–1392.

Tsou, Y. K., & Bishop, P. R. (1998). Gastroesophageal reflux in children. *Otolaryngologic Clinics of North America, 31,* 419–434.

Vaezi, M., Schroeder, P., & Richter, J. (1997). Reproducibility of proximal probe pH parameters in 24-hour ambulatory esophageal pH monitoring. *American Journal of Gastroenterology, 92,* 825–829.

Viteri, F. E. (1981). Primary protien-energy malnutrition: Clinical biochemical and metabolic changes. In R. Suskind (Ed.), *Textbook of pediatric nutrition* (189–215). New York: Raven Press.

Viteri, F. E., & Alvarado, J. (1970). The creatine height index: Its use in the estimation of the degree of protein depletion and repletion in protein calorie malnourished children. *Pediatrics, 46,* 696–706.

Waterlow, J. C. (1973). Note on the assessment and classification of protein-energy malnutrition in children. *The Lancet, 2,* 87–89.

Werlin, S. L., Dodds, W. J., Hogan, W. J., & Arndorfer, R. C. (1980). Mechanisms of gastroesophageal reflux in children. *The Journal of Pediatrics, 97,* 244–249.

■ CHAPTER 6

Pediatric Nutrition

Joan Arvedson, Linda Brodsky, and Nancy Claxton

■ SUMMARY

All children need and are entitled to adequate nutrition. Children with special health needs include those who have congenital or acquired conditions that affect physical or cognitive growth and development. They may have or be at risk for developmental disabilities and chronic, often debilitating health-related problems (Ireys & Nelson, 1992). Increased utilization of medical care, educational services, and nutritional guidance is frequent and should be be provided within a system of coordinated interdisciplinary services in a manner that is preventive, family centered, community based, and culturally competent (American Dietetic Association [ADA], 1995, p. 809). Specifically for children with feeding and swallowing problems, the ADA states that nutrition services, in particular, are an essential component of comprehensive care for children with special health needs (CSHN; ADA, 1995).

Early recognition of feeding problems is essential to avoid growth failure in those infants and children who often have little nutritional reserve. The term "failure to thrive" (FTT) describes infants and young children who fail to grow as expected on the basis of established growth standards for age and gender. FTT is a multifactorial induced problem, is descriptive, and is not a diagnosis per se. Favored terminology today is "pediatric undernutrition"(PUN) which refers more specifically to growth impairment (Kessler, 1999).

The role of the nutritionist or dietitian in the interdisciplinary team caring for undernourished CSHN cannot be overemphasized. The nutritional needs of such children, assessment, and management strategies are all described in this chapter.

■ INTRODUCTION

Estimate of risk for nutrition problems in CSHN ranges from 40% (Lichtenwalter, Freeman, Lee, & Cialone, 1993) to 92% (Bayerl, Ries, Bettencourt, & Fisher, 1993). The need for nutrition intervention is related to the feeding process (mechanical and behavioral), underlying medical problems, and the amount and route of nutritional intake. Although improved nutrition can be the most critical factor for survival in some children, for others it can markedly reduce the potentially debilitating effects of their chronic conditions (ADA, 1995). Improved nutrition and normalized feeding patterns have the potential to increase the child's level of independence and provide a positive perception of self. It can also increase the caregiver's satisfaction in meeting a fundamental need of the child. Nutrition status has direct implications for the child's level of impairment, activities, and participation with family and society.

Nutrition support must be integrated with other health, education, and social services. Professionals work in partnership with families and other caregivers to achieve agreed-upon goals. As the demands increase for continuous care for increasingly complex CSHN, the challenges become enormous. Some children encounter multiple caregivers every day as they move from child-care settings to schools and then home. Others are challenged by lack of access to specialized services and particularly by the dearth of trained practitioners who are able to respond to unfamiliar racial, ethnic, and socioeconomic conditions that have become more characteristic of our rapidly changing society. By 2020, it is predicted that one in three Americans will be of African, Asian, Hispanic, or Native American ancestry (Day, 1993). Strategies are needed for effective communication and follow-up within these communities to make nutrition services culturally sensitive and competent for CSHN from these populations (ADA, 1995). Despite 1987 legislation that mandated care of children with special needs, governmental initiatives continue to call for statewide networks of comprehensive, community-based, health care systems for CSHN that also ensure family-centered, culturally competent, coordinated services (U.S. Department of Health and Human Services, 1990). Nutritionists are identified as qualified personnel who provide developmental services that include "health services necessary to enable the infant or toddler to benefit from the other early intervention services" (Education of the Handicapped Act Amendments of 1986).

Failure to thrive (FTT) refers to infants and children who fail to grow as expected based on normal growth patterns. FTT was often differentiated as organic (OFTT from organ illness or dysfunction) or nonorganic (NOFTT when no organic reason is found). This dichotomy appears overly simplistic and time-consuming (Skuse, 1993). The degree of weight deficit that is labeled FTT in the United States and other Western nations is identical to the degree of deficit that is endemic in developing countries. Thus, some recommend that the term "undernutrition" be applied to children in industrialized ("First World") countries (Ward, Brazelton, & Wust, 1999). FTT is not an accepted medical terminology diagnosis. Undernutrition will be used throughout this chapter to encompass both FTT and malnutrition.

Undernutrition is of particular concern in the first 2 years of life. During this time, rapid development of the central nervous system (CNS) occurs, especially myelination of central and peripheral nerves (Chapters 2 and 3) (DeLong, 1993). Children under the age of 2 years who do not get adequate nutrition may never recover from the effects on the developing CNS (Bithoney & Dubowitz, 1985). Growth impairment can often be accompanied by developmental delays, cognitive disabilities, and behavior problems (e.g., Drotar & Sturm, 1992; Heffer & Kelley, 1994). The infants at highest risk for cognitive retardation can be identified in the neonatal period using social risk assessments, which are particularly important for infants who have medical or neurologic problems (Engelke, Engelke, Helm, & Holbert, 1995). In addition to inadequate intake, undernutrition may result from primary gastrointestinal disease, cardiopulmonary disease, and neurologic problems, especially those associated with difficulty in swallowing and feeding.

This chapter first describes the etiology of undernutrition. Understanding this complex, multifactorial process will serve as a foundation for the discussion of the assessment and management of nutritional status in normal infants and children and CSHN. Special topics include advancing feeds, alternative methods for feeding, and approaches to children who have significant acute nutritional needs due to medical illness. Finally, case studies are used to illustrate pertinent points.

■ ETIOLOGY OF UNDERNUTRITION

The prevalence of inadequate growth both for low height for age and low weight for height is about 5% among 2- to 5-year-olds. These rates have remained stable with no major changes in the past 20 to 25 years (Federation of American Societies for Experimental Biology, Life Sciences Research Office, 1995). In 1996, the Pediatric Nutrition Surveillance System data documented that infants from birth to age 2 months had the highest prevalence by age group for both indicators—12.0% for low height for age and 4.1% for low weight for height (Centers for Disease Control and Prevention, 1997).

Undernutrition in CSHN can result from an increased caloric need because of abnormalities in tone and posture that increase work efforts, insufficient caloric intake for a variety of reasons, altered absorption, behavior disturbances, and early satiety along with other factors (Table 6–1); however, decreased oral intake is a prominent factor in the etiology of

Table 6–1. Contributing Factors to Undernutrition in Children with Special Needs

- Inadequate nutrient/caloric intake
- Increased caloric needs due to increased work to maintain normal tone and posture
- Altered absorption
- Behavior disturbances
- Early satiety
- Poor dentition
- Genetically programmed growth failure
- Limited communication abilities
- Associated medical conditions
  - Respiratory failure
  - Complex cardiac disease
  - Airway obstruction
  - Scoliosis

growth deficiency of these children. Gastrostomy feedings reverse weight-for-length ratios and result in the development of improved proportionality. This is in contrast to intensive nutritional support via oral feedings, which resulted in only minimal growth (Shapiro et al., 1986). The earlier an adequate nutritional management plan is initiated, the more readily the nutritional deficiencies can be reversed. For example, children with severe cerebral palsy given enteral tube feedings within 1 year of the CNS damage normalized weight within 6 months of therapy (Sanders et al., 1990). Those treated within 8 years of their CNS damage exhibited improvements in their weight-for-length ratio, but gains in length reached a plateau at 90% of ideal length for age. The third group of children, however, who were treated after 8 years of their CNS damage and were markedly malnourished, exhibited only a slight improvement in weight and no significant improvement in length for age. Growth disturbances do appear to be reversible with early aggressive nutritional intervention.

Decreased caloric intake is thus believed to explain the chronic undernutrition of handicapped individuals, especially when oral sensorimotor problems are present. The feeding of these children may be further compromised by an element of food aversion related to gastrointestinal problems (e.g., gastroesophageal reflux disease and extra-esophageal reflux disease [GERD/EERD]), airway compromise, or behavioral and psychosocial factors. Interactions between caregiver and child also must be considered. Development of an appropriate nutritional plan at the outset may prevent more severe nutritional problems from arising later (Cloud & Bergman, 1991).

Undernutrition can be differentiated into two categories: primary and secondary. Primary undernutrition occurs when there are inadequacies and imbalances in the quantity or quality of foods consumed (Ekvall, 1993). Persons in economically, socially, and educationally deprived populations are at risk for primary undernutrition. Secondary undernutrition is produced by disease and disability. Three states of primary undernutrition are described (Table 6–2) (Ekvall):

1. A visceral attrition state of kwashiorkor-like syndrome resulting primarily from a diet with a low protein/energy ratio,
2. marasmus-like syndrome, and
3. acute state combining both kwashiorkor and marasmus.

Table 6–2. Three States of Primary Undernutrition Described With Their International Classification of Disease (ICD) Codes

State of Undernutrition	Appearance	Problems and Needs
A visceral attrition state of Kwashiorkor-like syndrome (ICD 267)	Well-nourished; Anthropometric measures are maintained	Depressed serum levels of albumin, transferrin, and other circulating proteins; Cellular immunity compromised; Requires protein, fluid, electrolytes, extra calories, vitamins, and minerals.
Marasmus-like syndrome (ICD 268)	Visibly underweight; Serum proteins maintained until late in course	Depleted muscle and fat stores; Requires high-calorie, high-protein food, often augmented by oral supplements.
Acute state combining kwashiorkor and marasmus (ICD 269.9)	Mildly under-nourished; Shows signs of both visceral attrition and cachexia	Severe trauma and stress are often the cause; Needs vigorous nutritional support; Oral feeding of high nutrient and caloric density; May need peripheral or total parenteral nutrition.

Secondary undernutrition may be produced by diseases such as diabetes mellitus, cystic fibrosis, muscular dystrophy, cardiovascular anomalies, and cerebral palsy. Other disease-related problems are malabsorption, anorexia, hypermetabolic and metabolic dysfunction, organ failure, and iatrogenic problems (Gilbride, Cowell, & Simko, 1989). Obesity, considered by some to be a form of undernutrition, is found especially in children who are not mobile. Although treatment of obesity is important for CSHN, its assessment and management will not be a focus of this chapter.

■ NUTRITIONAL STATUS ASSESSMENT

Nutrition Screening

Nutrition screening can identify children at risk for nutritional problems. On the basis of the screening, children with more severe problems can be referred for further investigation and treatment. Given some basic knowledge of nutrition and growth, public health nurses, as well as teachers, therapists, and social workers, should be able to perform a basic nutrition screen. Weight, height, and head circumference measures can be plotted on the appropriate National Center for Health Statistics (NCHS) growth chart (Hamill, Drizd, & Johnson, 1979) and revised growth charts (Centers for Disease Control and Prevention, 2000). These growth charts should be used for charting weight, length, weight-for-length ratio, and head circumference at regular intervals (Figure 6–1). Weight-for-length is an important indicator of proportionality and can be used to assess appropriate weight for an individual, particularly if growth is delayed. Growth charts are available for some specific populations (e.g., premature infants and Down syndrome) (Cronk, 1983). In addition, growth charts are available for children with myelomeningocele, Prader-Willi, sickle cell anemia, and Turner syndrome. It is likely that growth charts for other groups will be developed, or may be in process. Nutrition screening programs can provide anticipatory guidance and educational materials to families with a goal for prevention of nutritional problems.

Nutritional Assessment

A nutritional assessment consists of anthropometric measurements, dietary history, clinical findings, biochemical profile, feeding skills development, and observations of behavioral interactions with caregivers. A diet history is an essential part of the assessment. Typically a 3-day diary of all food and liquid consumed, timing and duration of feedings, and problems associated with eating and feeding are recorded. Information about the physical activity is also

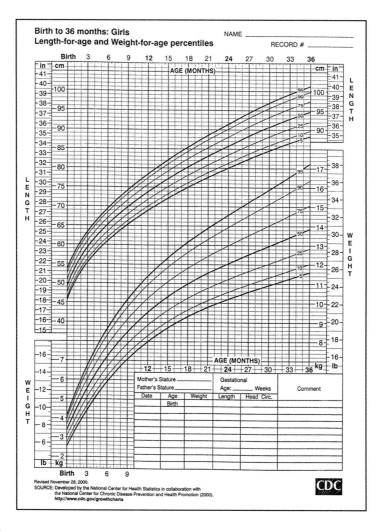

Birth to 36 months: Girls
Length-for-age and Weight-for-age percentiles

NAME _____

RECORD # _____

Revised November 28, 2000.
SOURCE: Developed by the National Center for Health Statistics in collaboration with
the National Center for Chronic Disease Prevention and Health Promotion (2000).
http://www.cdc.gov/growthcharts

A

Figure 6–1A. Physical growth chart (revised, 2000). National Center for Health Statistics Percentiles. Girls Birth to 36 months. Weight for age, length for age.

recorded so that both caloric intake and energy expenditure can be calculated. The Food Guide Pyramid accepted by the U.S. Department of Agriculture has recently emphasized an increase in grains, fruits, and vegetables. Figure 6–2 has a guide in English for Children 1 to 3 years. Figure 6–3 has the figure in Spanish. Figure 6–4 has a food guide pyramid with popular Chinese fare.

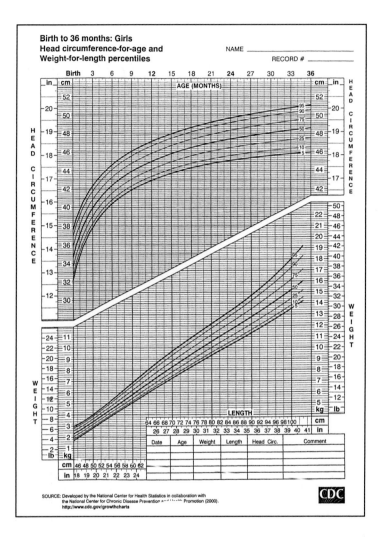

B

Figure 6–1B. Physical growth chart (revised, 2000). Head circumference, weight-for-length.

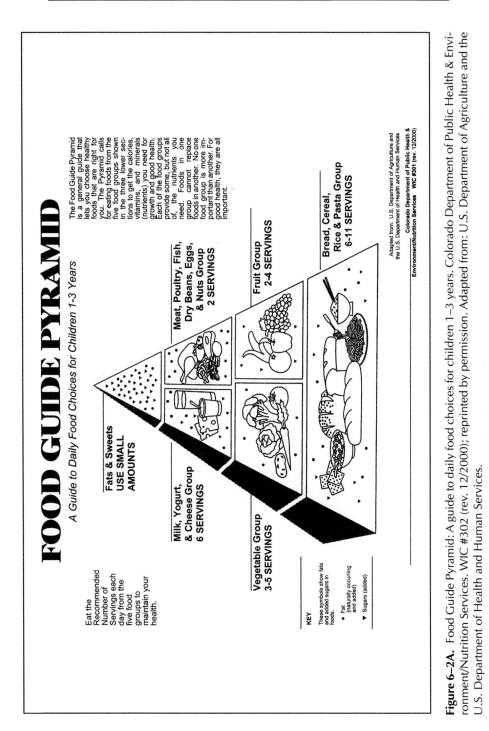

Figure 6–2A. Food Guide Pyramid: A guide to daily food choices for children 1–3 years. Colorado Department of Public Health & Environment/Nutrition Services. WIC #302 (rev. 12/2000); reprinted by permission. Adapted from: U.S. Department of Agriculture and the U.S. Department of Health and Human Services.

What Counts as 1 Serving?

▲ Children's serving sizes are smaller than adults'. The amount your child eats may be more than one serving. For example, a dinner portion of spaghetti would count as 2 or 3 servings.

Bread, Cereal, Rice, & Pasta Group
½ slice of bread
¼ cup of cooked rice or pasta
¼ cup of cooked cereal
½ cup of ready-to-eat cereal
crackers (1 large rectangle graham or 5 animal or wheat
½ tortilla (6")
¾ cups popped corn
¼ English muffin or bagel
½ roll/muffin
¼ hamburger/hot dog bun
½ pancake or waffle (5")

Vegetable Group
¼ cup of chopped raw or cooked vegetables
½ cup of leafy raw vegetables

Fruit Group
½ piece of fruit or melon wedge
½ cup of juice
¼ cup of canned fruit
⅙ cup of dried fruit

Milk, Yogurt, & Cheese Group
½ cup of milk or yogurt
¾ ounces of natural cheese
1 ounce of processed cheese
¾ cup of ice cream or frozen yogurt
¾ cup cottage cheese

Meat, Poultry, Fish, Dry Beans, Eggs, & Nuts Group
1 ounce of cooked lean meat, poultry, or fish
½ cup of cooked beans
1 egg
2 tablespoons of peanut butter
¼ cup tuna salad
½ cup tofu

Fats & Sweets
Eat in moderation

A Closer Look at Fat and Sugar

The tip of the Food Guide Pyramid contains the fats and sweets. These foods include salad dressing, cream, butter, margarine, sugar, candy, soda pop, sweet desserts, and some snack and fast foods. These foods provide calories but not many vitamins and minerals. They can be used in moderation to add variety to your child's diet once he or she has eaten foods from the other food groups.

When choosing foods for a healthful diet, consider the fat and sugar that might be in foods in the other food groups--for example, French fried potatoes. Fat and sugar is not just in the tip of the Pyramid, but it is also hidden in many of the fast and convenience foods we eat. The best idea is to choose foods from the five groups of the Pyramid that are as close to natural as possible--not precooked, boxed, or bagged. That way it is easiest to choose a healthful diet without a lot of added fat, sugar, and salt. Foods already processed are often more expensive than those you fix yourself.

Some children may need foods that are high in fat or calories to improve their growth. The WIC staff will let you know if this applies to your child.

Figure 6–2B. What counts as 1 serving?

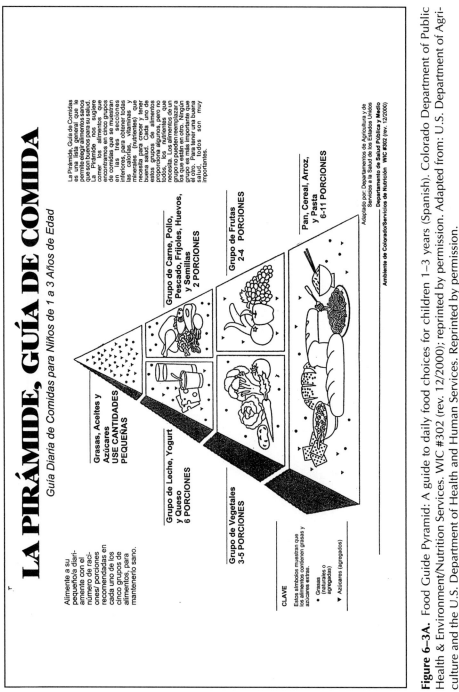

Figure 6–3A. Food Guide Pyramid: A guide to daily food choices for children 1–3 years (Spanish). WIC #302 (rev. 12/2000); reprinted by permission. Colorado Department of Public Health & Environment/Nutrition Services. WIC #302 (rev. 12/2000); reprinted by permission. Adapted from: U.S. Department of Agriculture and the U.S. Department of Health and Human Services. Reprinted by permission.

¿Qué es Una Ración/Porción?

▲ Las porciones/raciones para niños son más pequeñas que las de los adultos. Su niño/a podría comer más que una ración/porción. Por ejemplo, un plato de fideos a la hora de la comida podría ser igual a 2 ó 3 raciones/porciones.

Pan, Cereal, Arroz, y Pasta Grupo
½ rebanada de pan
¼ de taza de arroz o pasta
¼ de taza de cereal cocido
½ taza de cereal preparado
galletitas (1 rectángulo de graham
5 de animalitos o de trigo)
½ tortilla (6 pulgadas)
¾ de taza de palomitas de maíz
¼ de English muffin, rosquilla, o bagel
½ panecito, rol, bollo, o "muffin"
¼ pan para hamburguesa o hot dog
½ panqueque/waffle (5")

Grupo de Vegetales
¼ de taza de trozos de vegetales, cocidos o crudos
½ taza de vegetales de hojas, crudos

Grupo de Frutas
½ fruta o una tajada, rebanada de melón
½ taza de jugo
¼ de taza de fruta de lata
⅛ de taza de fruta seca

Grupo de Leche, Yogurt, y Queso
½ taza de leche o yogurt
¾ de onza de queso natural (fresco)
1 onza de queso procesado
¾ de taza de helado o helado de yogurt
¾ de taza de requesón, "cottage cheese"

Carne, Pollo, Pescado, Frijoles, Huevos, y Semillas
1 onza de carne sin grasa, pollo, o pescado cocido
½ taza de frijoles, habichuelas, lentejas, etc. cocidos
1 huevo
2 cucharadas de mantequilla de cacahuate o maní
¼ de taza de ensalada de atún
½ taza de tofu

Grasas, Aceites, y Azúcares
Cómalos con moderación (no mucho)

Figure 6–3B. What counts as 1 serving? (Spanish)

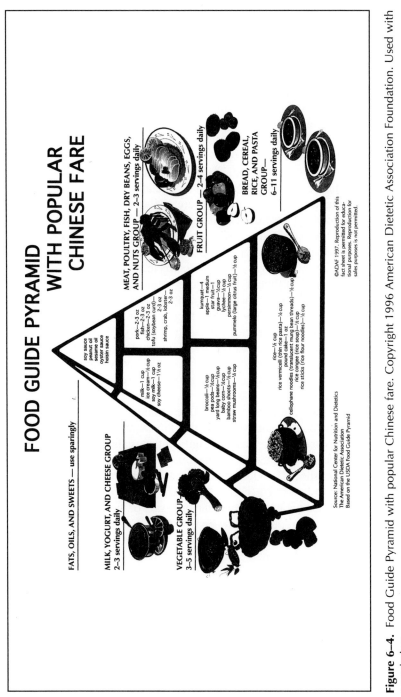

FOOD GUIDE PYRAMID WITH POPULAR CHINESE FARE

FATS, OILS, AND SWEETS — use sparingly

MILK, YOGURT, AND CHEESE GROUP
2–3 servings daily

milk—1 cup
ice cream—½ cup
soy milk—1 cup
soy cheese—1½ oz

VEGETABLE GROUP
3–5 servings daily

broccoli—½ cup
pea pods—½ cup
yard long beans—½ cup
baby corn—½ cup
bamboo shoots—½ cup
straw mushrooms—½ cup

MEAT, POULTRY, FISH, DRY BEANS, EGGS, AND NUTS GROUP — 2–3 servings daily

pork—2–3 oz
fish—2–3 oz
chicken—2–3 oz
tofu (soybean curd)—
2–3 oz
shrimp, crab, lobster—
2–3 oz

soy sauce
peanut oil
sesame oil
oyster sauce
hoisin sauce

FRUIT GROUP —2–4 servings daily

kumquat—4
apple—1 medium
star fruit—1
guava—½ cup
lychee—½ cup
persimmon—½ cup
pummelo (large citrus fruit)—½ cup

BREAD, CEREAL, RICE, AND PASTA GROUP—
6–11 servings daily

rice—½ cup
rice vermicelli (thin rice pasta)—½ cup
pound cake—1 oz
cellophane noodles (translucent mung bean threads)—½ cup
rice congee (rice soup)—½ cup
rice sticks (rice flour noodles)—½ cup

Source: National Center for Nutrition and Dietetics
The American Dietetic Association
Based on the USDA Food Guide Pyramid

©ADAF 1997. Reproduction of this fact sheet is permitted for educational purposes. Reproduction for sales purposes is not permitted.

Figure 6–4. Food Guide Pyramid with popular Chinese fare. Copyright 1996 American Dietetic Association Foundation. Used with permission.

Anthropometric Measurement in Premature and Term Infants and Children

Anthropometric measurement refers to the measures of body dimensions and relative fat and muscle composition of a child. Rapid, easily accessible, and inexpensive, anthropometric measurements are useful in helping to determine acute and chronic nutritional status. No single measure is sufficient to characterize nutritional status, however. Furthermore, it is important to compare the various measurements over time. As mentioned above, growth charts are used to track weight, height (length), weight–height ratios, and head circumference. These charts are available for typically developing children and for some special populations.

Growth charts based on fetal growth are available to provide a "standard" from which growth of premature infants can be assessed (Dancis, O'Connell, & Holt, 1948; Naeye & Dixon, 1978). These curves are useful until 40 weeks gestation, at which time the NCHS growth curves should be used. When standard NCHS growth curves are used, a corrected age (chronologic age corrected for prematurity) should be used for plotting weight, length, and head circumference until a child reaches 24 months chronologic age.

In sick premature infants, weight measures are recommended daily. Length and head circumference are measured weekly. Changes in fluid balance occur rapidly in these premature infants and can greatly alter body weight (Marks, 1986), so trends in growth over time are important. Appropriate growth is measured by an increase in all body compartments. Unfortunately, standards are not available for triceps skin fold or midarm circumference measurements in premature infants.

Full-term infants should be weighed to the nearest 0.01 kg with no diaper or a dry diaper on a table beam or digital infant scale (Figure 6–5). Older children should be weighed to the nearest 0.1 kg with little or no outer clothing and no shoes. In addition to standard scales, there are scales that allow children to be seated (Figure 6–6). The same trained observer who uses the same scale greatly increases the precision of measurement for more meaningful interpretation of follow-up over time (Grant & DeHoog, 1991).

Length is measured to the nearest 0.1 cm. Children less than 2 to 3 years of age are measured in supine position (Figure 6–7). Lengths should be obtained with the infant in supine position on a measuring board, with the head held securely against the stationary headboard, the legs in full extension and the slide moved to press firmly against the bottom of the feet. Children over the age of 2 to 3 years who are able to stand are measured in standing position. A height–weight percentile is then plotted on the growth chart. The nutritional assessment is made on the basis of weight in relation to current height. This height–weight percentile is more meaningful than weight for age, particularly when a limited number of measurements is available.

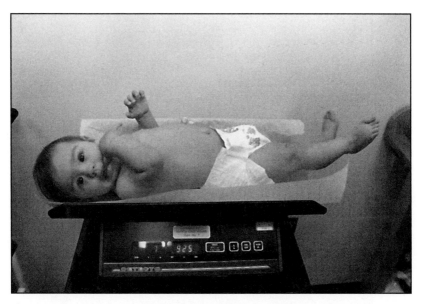

Figure 6–5. Infant in a dry diaper being weighed on a digital infant scale.

Acute versus chronic undernutrition needs to be defined to determine cause(s). In acute undernutrition, a low weight for height or length is the first noticeable sign, usually being less than the 5th percentile. This reflects the relatively short-term onset of slowed weight gain with length growth maintained in the normal range. This finding may be caused by a recent onset of a medical illness, by a change in nutritional needs, or by alterations in nutritional intake. In chronic undernutrition, low weight and low height/length are seen. Weight tends to remain proportional to length, so that weight-for-length ratio will be within the normal range (10th–90th percentile on the growth curve). In these cases, chronic undernutrition from slow growth must be distinguished from that due to genetic factors, such as constitutional short stature.

Head circumference should be measured routinely with a flexible metal or non-stretchable plastic coated tape. This measurement is especially important during the first 2 to 3 years of life because of the rapid brain growth occurring during that time. Head circumference is usually maintained in the face of mild to moderate undernutrition. Only in the case of chronic severe undernutrition does the head circumference fall off the growth curve. A small head circumference should be investigated because it may be due to other medical conditions, such as microcephaly, from a variety of etiologies.

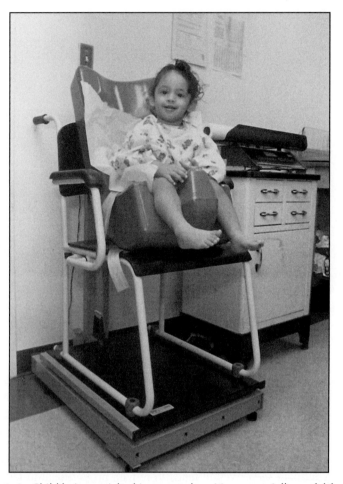

Figure 6–6. Child being weighed in a seated position, especially useful for children who cannot stand on a regular scale.

Continued growth of an infant in terms of weight, length, and head circumference along any given percentile of the growth curve over time is termed *channeling* and is usually a good indicator that nutrient needs are being met. For example, if an infant's length consistently plots along the 50th percentile on the length curve, but weight "crosses channels" on the weight curve from the 50th percentile at birth to the 5th percentile at 6 months, there should be investigation of the nutritional adequacy of the diet. Whenever there is a concern about change in nutritional status, underlying medical conditions, such as endocrine abnormalities and digestive malfunction, must be considered.

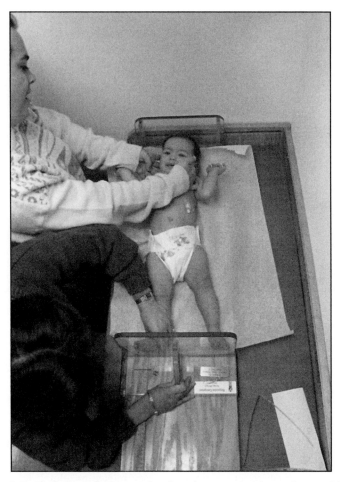

Figure 6–7. Technique for measuring length or stature in supine position for infants and young children < 2–3 years of age.

Anthropometric Measurements in Children With Physical Disabilities

Standard measures are sometimes difficult to obtain with children who have physical disabilities (e.g., scoliosis or joint contractures). Other measures for these children with physical disabilities include triceps skinfold thickness (TSF; Figure 6–8) and subscapular skinfold thickness (SSF) (van den Berg-Emons, van Baak, & Westerterp, 1998). The TSF is particularly useful as a measure of nutritional status. It is a good indicator of energy reserves because it correlates well with total body fat stores. Midarm

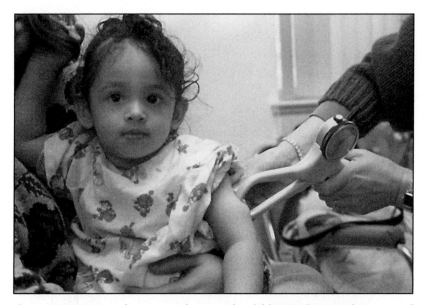

Figure 6–8. Segmental measure of triceps skin fold (TSF) that correlates to total body fat stores.

circumference can estimate muscle mass (Frisancho, 1974). These measures are most useful for longitudinal assessment of changes in body fat and muscle stores (Grant & DeHoog, 1991).

Alternative measures of length for children with disabilities include upper arm and lower leg length, or knee height (Figure 6–9) for children with spinal curvature, contractures, or any musculoskeletal deformities. Standards for upper arm and lower leg lengths of normal children are based on the work of Snyder et al. (1977). These standards are compared with the upper arm and lower leg lengths of 110 children with cerebral palsy (CP) (Spender, Cronk, Charney, & Stallings, 1989). Approximately one-third of patients with CP fell below the 5th percentile for upper arm and lower leg length. Patients with quadriplegia were most likely to be below the 5th percentile for either measure. These measurements performed by a trained technician can provide additional information in patients with disabilities when standard height measurements are not available or not helpful. Monitoring of linear growth by leg or arm measurement can also be useful in determining response to nutritional rehabilitation. If increased caloric intake and weight gain are not accompanied by linear growth, calorie needs can be reassessed to prevent obesity.

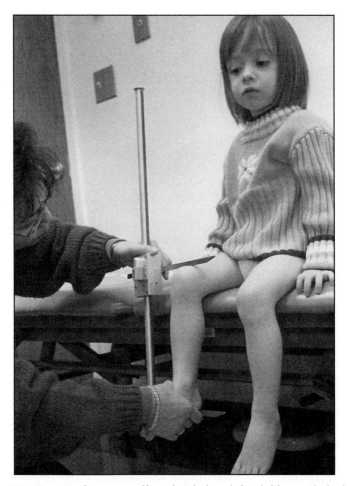

Figure 6–9. Segmental measure of knee height length for children with disabilities

.

Clinical Assessment

Review of history of present illness, past medical problems, surgical history, and systems is another tool to help determine etiologies of poor nutritional status. When specific nutritional disorders or inheritable metabolic disease are found, referral is made to the appropriate specialist. Children with phenylketonuria (PKU), maple syrup urine disease, cystic fibrosis, and sickle cell anemia are all at risk. Furthermore, dietitians should routinely screen for dysphagia as part of the standard nutrition assessment. This practice may aid in decreasing dysphagia-related complications (Brody et al., 2000).

Biochemical Profile

In some children, biochemical information is helpful in determining present nutritional status or current dietary intake. Those biochemical measures that are most readily available and supply a fair amount of information include complete blood counts, urine analysis, total serum protein, albumin levels, transferrin saturation, blood urea nitrogen, and creatinine. Low levels of serum protein and albumin are indicative of chronic undernutrition.

Dietary Intake History

This part of the nutrition assessment helps to determine a usual dietary pattern or nutrient intake. A diet history or log is maintained by the caregivers for 3 days, 2 weekdays and 1 weekend day. They are asked to record portion size consumed, time and duration of meals, and bowel movements. These data are used along with pertinent history information related to feeding that might influence dietary intake.

Behavioral and Feeding Skills

The influence of level of feeding development and behavior on nutritional status cannot be underestimated. This is so important that these skills often are evaluated by a feeding specialist (e.g., speech–language pathologist or occupational therapist) or a child psychologist.

When the evaluation of all the above areas is completed, the dietitian summarizes the findings with caregivers and other professionals. A plan is recommended that takes into account the oral sensorimotor feeding skills, health issues, family food habits, and the child's preferences where applicable. Figure 6–10 shows a decision process when children demonstrate poor growth and undernutrition.

■ MEETING NUTRITIONAL NEEDS

Full Term Infants

Breast milk is the optimal sole source of nutrition for healthy infants for the first 6 months of life. Its continuation is encouraged through the first 12 months of life or longer, when possible (American Academy of Pediatrics [AAP], 2000). Breast-feeding exclusively for at least 6 months appears to reduce the risk of later respiratory ailments, allergic symptoms, and eczema (Lucas, Brooke, Morley, Cole, & Bamford, 1990; Saarinen & Kajosaari,

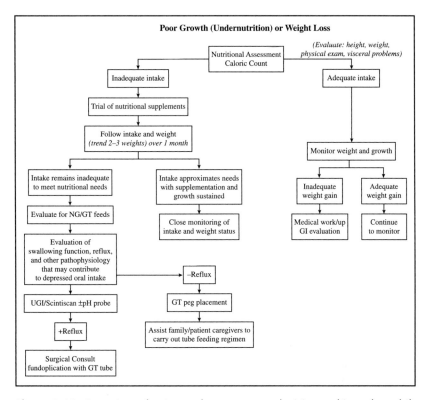

Figure 6–10. Steps in evaluation and management decision making when children demonstrate poor growth/undernutrition.

1995). In those infants who are formula-fed and develop symptoms of food allergy, a hypoallergenic formula is suggested as an alternative to breast-feeding (e.g., Nutramigen, Neocate). Hypoallergenic formulas must demonstrate nutritional suitability to support infant growth and development.

Nutrient, energy, and fluid needs (on a per-kilogram basis) tend to be quite standard in normal healthy infants (Fomon, Filer, Anderson, & Ziegler, 1979). The recommended dietary allowances (RDA) are the levels of intake of nutrients considered to be adequate to meet the known nutritional needs of all healthy people. The RDAs provide a margin of safety for all nutrients, and although the allowances are designed for assessing the diet of a population, they provide the best available guidelines for assessing the adequacy of an individual's diet as well, except for energy, which can vary markedly as described below. The RDAs are available through the National Academy of Sciences—National Research Council (1989).

Energy Requirements

Energy requirements are determined by body size, age, gender, physical activity, and rate of growth. Term infants have caloric requirements 2 to 3 times greater than adults on the basis of body weight; for example the RDA for an infant from birth to 6 months of age is 108 kcal/kg/day and from 6 to 12 months the requirement is 98 kcal/kg/day, whereas for a 70-kg adult, it is only 35 to 40 kcal/kg/day. The RDAs assume that 50% of calories will be expended for maintenance, 25% for activity, and 25% for growth during infancy. Alterations in any of these components will affect caloric requirements. Immediate energy needs are met though carbohydrates and fat, with each contributing approximately 50% of calories. Protein will also be broken down for energy, when calorie intake is insufficient.

Protein Requirements

Protein requirements are relatively high at birth because of the very rapid rate of somatic growth occuring in young infants. Protein requirements begin to decline late in the 1st year of life, as somatic growth slows and activity requiring immediate energy sources increases. These protein requirements assume adequate caloric intake so that protein is not broken down to supply energy. The recommended allowance for protein for an infant from birth to 6 months is 2.2 gm/kg per day and for an infant from 6 to 12 months 1.6 gm/kg/day (AAP, 1998). This recommendation assumes a protein quality equal to that of cow's-milk protein, casein, or whey. Soy protein is not considered a complete protein providing all essential amino acids. Therefore, soy-based formulas are supplemented with methionine to compensate for the low concentration of this amino acid. Examples of soy-based formulas include ProSobee (Mead-Johnson), Isomil (Ross), Nursoy (Wyeth), Alsoy (Carnation), and I-Soyalac (Loma-Linda). Soy formulas in the United States are free of lactose and used for infants with lactase deficiency or galactosemia.

Fluid Requirements

Standard infant formulas are prescribed with a caloric density of 67 to 70 kcal/dl (20 kcal/oz), similar to human milk, and should be offered ad libitum (AAP, 1998). The usual intake will be 150 to 200 ml/kg/day. This provides 100 to 135 kcal/kg/day and should result in an initial weight gain of 20 to 30 g/day, gradually decreasing to 15 to 25 g/day. Newborn infants have a relatively inefficient concentrating mechanism in the kidneys, and therefore, obligatory water loss may be high, and dehydration can occur quite rapidly. In general, infants receiving standard infant formulas providing 67 to 70 kcal/dl (20 kcal/oz) or breast milk alone get adequate fluid if calorie needs are being met. Healthy infants usually require little or no supplemental water. However, infants with high fluid losses in hot weather or during an illness should be monitored closely and supplemented when necessary.

Vitamin and Mineral Requirements

Supplementation with vitamin D (400 IU/day) is recommended for breast-feeding infants. Fluoride (0.25 mg/day) is recommended if the mother's drinking water is not fortified with fluoride (AAP, 1998). Although the need for iron supplements is not clearly demonstrated in well-controlled studies, the AAP (1998) recommended that all formulas should be fortified with iron. Breast-feeding infants should receive 7 mg of iron/day (Fomon et al., 1979).

Premature Infants

Specialized nutritional intervention plays a major role in making survival possible for very-low-birth-weight (VLBW) infants (e.g., 23–24 weeks gestation with birth weight at 500–650 g). Infants at 22–24 weeks gestation are entering what would be a period of very rapid weight gain in utero; a 22-week gestation fetus doubles weight twice in the next 2 months (Marks, 1986). This rate of weight gain is difficult to achieve after birth because of the limitations of intravascular and gastric fluid capacity. The incomplete development of the gastrointestinal tract and renal system is another factor (Neu, Valentine, & Meetze, 1990). Problems of delayed gastric emptying and abnormal motility, often accompanied by GERD/EERD, also complicate the provision of adequate nutrition in some premature infants (Lebenthal, 1989; Siegel & Lebenthal, 1989) (Chapter 5).

Provision of adequate nutrition is also complicated by the fact that premature infants have very low fat stores (1% of body weight vs. 16% in term infants) (Marks, 1986). Under conditions of total starvation, this energy reserve would allow survival for 1 month in a term infant, 12 days in a 2,000 g infant, and only 4.5 days for a 1,000 g infant (Kerner, 1983). Thus, provision of maintenance calories to prevent loss of fat stores is a high priority in the initial treatment of VLBW infants. Low fat stores greatly increase their surface-area–to–weight ratio, thereby increasing their potential for energy loss through heat (Field et al., 1982). Adequate temperature control can help decrease energy requirements and thereby improve growth. Formulas for low-birth-weight and premature infants include Enfamil Premature 24 (Mead Johnson) and Similac Special Care 24 (Ross).

Energy Requirements

Energy needs are estimated at 125 to 140 kcal/kg/day. This estimate allows for growth rates comparable to intrauterine growth rates at similar gestational ages, at least 15 g/kg/day (AAP, 1993). Energy needs are partitioned among basal metabolic rate, growth, physical activity, protein synthesis, fecal and urinary losses, and cold stress. Energy expenditure may be increased with chronic lung disease or congestive heart failure. Small-for-gestational-age neonates also frequently expend more energy because of increased metabolic needs and higher energy costs for synthesis of new tissue. If caloric intake is inadequate, dietary and somatic protein will be broken down to supply energy for life-sustaining activities, reducing the protein available for anabolic processes such as brain growth and development (Marks, 1986).

Protein Requirements

Recommended allowance for protein in VLBW infants is 3.0 to 3.6 g/kg per day and may be up to 3.8 g/kg per day (Ziegler, 1991). The poorly developed kidneys in the premature infant may make excretion of excess protein difficult, resulting in an elevated blood urea nitrogen level. Excessive protein intake may occur easily if infant formulas are concentrated to provide increased caloric density or if nutrition is being provided by combining the enteral and parenteral routes (Ostertag & Frayer, 1983). Total protein intake from all sources should be calculated on a regular basis, with close monitoring of tolerance.

Fluid Requirements

Fluid needs of premature infants are highly variable and must be assessed on a daily basis, even in relatively healthy premature infants. A minimum of 130 to 150 cc/kg/day is usually required to meet fluid needs (Neu et al., 1990). During the 1st week of life, fluid intake of up to 200 cc/kg/day may be required because of increased water loss. Fluid restrictions with increased caloric density of feedings may be necessary for infants with respiratory distress syndrome, chronic lung disease, congestive heart failure, patent ductus arteriosis, and renal insufficiency (Sun et al., 1998).

Mineral Requirements

Minerals of special concern in premature infants include calcium, phosphorus, and iron (Neu et al., 1990). Third-trimester calcium accumulation is greater than the amount of calcium a preterm infant can ingest from human milk. Human milk fortifier that contains calcium and phosphorus must be added to support bone mineralization in breast-fed infants. Premature infant formulas must meet the recommendations for calcium and phosphorus. It is important to prevent osteopenia and rickets that may be complications of severe prematurity.

Iron stores accrued during the last trimester are generally adequate for term infants up to 4 months of age. Preterm neonates have diminished stores, and iron supplementation is started once tolerance of full feeds is achieved (Sun et al., 1998). Iron supplementation will not prevent the physiologic anemia of prematurity. Vitamin supplementation is also recommended (AAP, 1985). Iron supplementation is recommended until at least 1 year of age in this population (Neu et al., 1990; Ostertag & Frayer, 1983).

■ CHILDREN IN TRANSITION FEEDING

By 6 months of age, infants are usually ready for adding cereal by spoon even though nutritional needs are met with breast milk or standard infant formulas up to 12 months of age. Fortified infant cereal is an optimal first food for infants because it is an excellent source of iron. The texture may be altered to suit the infant's needs and abilities as oral sensorimotor and swallowing abilities become more fully developed. Small amounts of new foods should be introduced, and single-ingredient foods should be introduced one at a time for 4 to 5 days' use before introducing another new food (Finney, 1986; Satter, 1990). Table 6–3 provides general guidelines for types and volumes of foods appropriate for infants up to 12 months of age.

As children in the 2nd year of life transition to a modified adult-style diet, intake of some key nutrients appears to be low. The intake of some nutrients actually decreases despite increases in energy intake. A considerable portion of children studied (55 children from 12 to 18 months of age with their parents) consumed low-fat diets. These findings argue for development of dietary guidance to assist parents in selecting more appropriate diets that support optimum growth and development in young children (Picciano, et al., 2000; Tamborlane, 1997).

■ CHILDREN WITH MULTIPLE DISABILITIES

Infants With Special Needs

Young infants with developmental delay or multiple handicaps usually have nutrient needs similar to those of typically developing infants. These infants can meet their nutritional needs through oral feeding with standard infant formulas. The RDAs can be used to set feeding goals. Some infants with oral sensorimotor dysfunction exhibit problems in the neonatal period, whereas others may have functional suck/swallow/breathe pattern for the first few months. Problems may become evident when children with oral sensorimotor dysfunction start on solid foods.

Table 6–3. Recommended Feeding Schedule—Birth to 12 Months[a]

Food Group	Birth–4 months	4–6 months	6–8 months	8–10 months	10–12 months
Milk	Breast milk or formula	Breast milk or formula	Breast milk or formula	Breast milk or formula	Breast milk or formula; whole milk after 12 months
Cereal and bread group	None	Begin iron-fortified rice cereal, mixed with formula or pumped breast milk	Begin 1 new grain at a time	Good finger foods to try include crackers, bread, pasta, regular cereals	Grains provide B vitamins and iron: try to include 4 servings/day
Fruit and vegetable group	None	None	Commercial baby food or mashed table food; no added sugar or salt	Juices may be introduced one at a time, preferably from a cup. Use real juice, not fruit drinks	Include 1 good vitamin A source 3 times/ week, 1 vitamin C source daily
Meat and other protein sources	None	None	None	Commercial baby food or finely ground meat; casseroles, eggs, fish, poultry, legumes, and cheese are all good protein sources	Aim for 1–2 oz/day

Source: Based on the recommendations of the Committee on Nutrition of the American Academy of Pediatrics. (1998). *Pediatric Nutrition Handbook.* Elk Grove Village, IL: American Academy of Pediatrics; and adapted from W. A. Walker & K. M. Hendricks. (1985). *Manual of Pediatric Nutrition* (p. 46). Philadelphia: W. B. Saunders, with permission.

[a]This is an approximate schedule as each infant will progress at his or her own rate. In all instances: (1) start with small serving sizes of 1–2 tsp and increase gradually to 3–4 tbs/feeding; (2) introduce single-ingredient foods one at a time and continue for 4 to 5 days before introducing another food.

Premature or full-term infants who are small for gestational age have increased energy needs to achieve catch-up growth. It is common for sick infants to have periods of slow weight gain or even weight loss due to other medical complications (Schanler, 1988). Once adequate nutrition is resumed, a need for catch-up growth means increased energy requirements. Infants with severe undernutrition may need an additional 30 to 50% increase in caloric intake beyond standard needs for age and weight to catch up to their appropriate weight (Marks, 1986; Pridham, Martin, Sondel, & Tluczek, 1989). Caloric requirements are estimated on the basis of ideal weight for length to determine the calories required for catch-up weight gain (Walker & Hendricks, 1985).

Infants need alternative modes for nutrition when suck/swallow/ breathe sequencing is not functional or when other situations preclude oral feeding. Nonnutritive sucking should be encouraged for infants who are unable to eat because of a structural or digestive constraint, e.g., children with short bowel syndrome or esophageal atresia (Chapters 5 and 9) (Field et al., 1982; Zisserman, 1986). Many of these children lose interest and skills for oral feeding if oral stimulation is not provided consistently. This interest may be difficult to reestablish, so that even when children are medically able to eat, they may have severe feeding problems in later months or years (Geertsma, Hyams, Pelletier, & Reiter, 1985; Handen, Mandell, & Russo, 1986; Thommessen, Heiberg, Kase, & Riis, 1991). Close evaluation and guidance by oral–motor/swallow specialists can help diminish the consequences of prolonged nonoral feeding.

As the infant grows, oral sensorimotor incoordination of suck and swallow may become exaggerated because of behavioral factors or other developmental delays. Optimal methods of feeding children with poor or delayed ability to suck and swallow should be determined by a team effort that includes medical personnel and family or other caregivers (Humphrey, 1991; Hynak-Hankinson et al., 1984).

Children With Special Needs

Calorie requirements for children with special needs and multiple handicaps cannot be estimated accurately from the RDAs because the RDAs assume normal activity levels. One good estimate can be obtained from determination of the basal metabolic rate (Table 6–4) adjusted for activity level (Table 6–5). Severely malnourished children may gain weight initially with very low caloric intake because of their low body weight and reduced basal metabolic rate. Once the episode of acute undernutrition has been treated, caloric requirements are higher for children to achieve "catch-up" growth. Individual variation in caloric requirements is so great that general guidelines for assessing calorie requirements are insufficient, and close monitoring of weight gain in each individual is essential.

Table 6–4. Metabolic Rates (BMR) for Children

Age 1 week–10 months		Age 11–36 months			Age 3–16 years		
Weight (kg)	**Metabolic Rate (Kcal/hr)** Male or Female	**Weight (kg)**	**Metabolic Rate (Kcal/hr)** Male	Female	**Weight (kg)**	**Metabolic Rate (Kcal/hr)** Male	Female
3.5	8.4	9.0	22.0	21.2	15	35.8	33.3
4.0	9.5	9.5	22.8	22.0	20	39.7	37.4
4.5	10.5	10.0	23.6	22.8	25	43.6	41.5
5.0	11.6	10.5	24.4	23.6	30	47.5	45.5
5.5	12.7	11.0	25.2	24.4	35	51.3	49.6
6.0	13.8	11.5	26.0	25.2	40	55.2	53.7
6.5	14.9	12.0	26.8	26.0	45	59.1	57.8
7.0	16.0	12.5	27.6	26.9	50	63.0	61.9
7.5	17.1	13.0	28.4	27.7	55	66.9	66.0
8.0	18.2	13.5	29.2	28.4	60	70.8	70.0
8.5	19.3	14.0	30.0	29.3	65	74.7	74.0
9.0	20.4	14.5	30.8	30.1	70	78.6	78.1
9.5	21.4	15.0	31.6	30.9	75	82.5	82.2
10.0	22.5	15.5	32.4	31.7			
10.5	23.6	16.0	33.2	32.6			
11.0	24.7	16.5	34.0	33.4			

Source: From Altman, P. L., & Dittmer, D. S. (Eds.). (1968). *Metabolism.* Bethesda, MD: Federation of Societies for Experimental Biology, with permission. (p. 344)

Note: To calculate BMR: (a) determine age of patient and locate appropriate column on table, (b) find weight in kg of child and read across to appropriate gender, (c) read kcal/hr and multiply by 24 to determine daily BMR. There is only one BMR for children of either gender at ages 1 week to 10 months.

Table 6–5. Adjustments of Basal Metabolic Rate for Activity in Children[a]

Activity	Increase
Bed rest	+10%
Light activity	+30% (out of bed, quiet play)
Moderate activity	+50% (standing, playing)
Heavy activity	+75% or greater (vigorous play or work)

Source: Adapted from Walker, W. A., & Hendricks, K. M. (1985). *Manual of Pediatric Nutrition* (p. 60). Philadelphia: W. B. Saunders.

[a]Medical conditions may increase caloric needs further.

■ FEEDING TO MEET NUTRITION NEEDS

Feeding for Term Infants

It is recommended that infants receive breast milk or infant formula as their only source of nutrition for the first 4 to 6 months of life (Table 6–3) (AAP, 1998). Infants younger than 4 to 6 months tend to produce a tongue thrust in response to solid foods in the mouth. During these first few months, the infant's pattern for nipple-feeding is the most efficient means of obtaining adequate nutrition (Chapters 2 and 3).

Breast-feeding

Breast milk is almost perfectly formulated to meet the needs of healthy infants, particularly because of its immunochemical and cellular components. Breast-feeding should be encouraged whenever possible for reasons beyond meeting nutrition requirements. Other reasons include bonding between mother and infant, economics, and convenience. Infants with oral sensorimotor difficulties may require special assistance with breast-feeding. These difficulties should not automatically preclude breast-feeding, because in many instances adaptations can be made (Lawrence, 1980). Frequent assessment of weight and growth by a professional can allay concern for adequate intake in a breast-fed infant. The volume of milk consumed can be determined indirectly by "before-and-after" weights in breast-fed infants, and this method is useful when accurate estimates of intake are required.

Infant Feeding with Commercial Formulas

Commercial infant formulas are the best substitute for breast milk. Mothers who cannot or choose not to breast-feed should be reassured that they are providing an extremely satisfactory alternative to their infant if they use an appropriate commercial infant formula (Greer, 1995). Standard formulas in the United States provide 20 calories per 30 cc when prepared according to standard directions and are available in powder, liquid concentrate, and ready-to-feed formulations. They are fortified with all essential vitamins and minerals to meet the RDAs for normal infants when consumed in volumes adequate for normal growth.

A cow's-milk–based formula at 20 or 24 cal/oz should be used (e.g., Similac, Ross; Enfamil, Mead-Johnson; Good Start, Carnation; Gerber) unless there is a known or suspected allergy to cow's milk. Enfamil AR (Mead-Johnson, 1998) is a thickened infant formula with added rice (AR) starch that has a viscosity 10 times that of routine formula. It is designed to allow free flow of formula through a standard nipple in a more reliable preparation with fewer steps than adding rice cereal to formula. Soy-based formulas (see "Protein Requirements" section in this chapter) should be used only when poor tolerance to cow's milk or cow's-milk protein allergy is known or suspected because the quality of soy protein is not as high as that of milk protein. Infants with lactase deficiency may do well with Lactofree (Mead-Johnson).

Specialized formulas are designed for a variety of congenital and neonatal disorders, including allergy, malabsorption syndromes, and several inborn errors of amino acid, organic acid, urea, or carbohydrate metabolism (Sun et al., 1998) (Table 6–6). They are complete formulas and may be used throughout life for some genetic disorders.

Children with cow's-milk protein allergy have increased incidence of soy protein allergy. Specialized infant formulas that provide protein in hydrolysate form or that use sodium caseinate may be helpful. An overview of problems in infancy, suggested formulas and rationale for use is shown in Table 6–7.

Feeding for Preterm Infants

Breast-feeding

Determination of optimal feeding strategies for premature infants involves many factors. Human breast milk is the ideal food for healthy full-term infants and has advantages for premature infants because of its low renal solute load, protective immunologic function, and easy digestibility (Fomon et al., 1977). Nonetheless, the protein and calcium content may not be optimal for small premature infants with very high requirements. Schanlcr (1988) recommended the use of human milk for any healthy infant over 1,250 g, but lower birth weight infants may require specialized premature formulas. The mother can express milk by pump or manually to maintain lactation (Lawrence, 1980) until appropriate weight gain occurs when she can initiate or resume human milk feedings. A human milk fortifier that provides calcium and phosphorus can be added to human breast milk to increase mineral content to a more appropriate range.

Formulas for Premature Infants

Formulas designed for premature infants generally provide 24 calories per ounce (e.g., Similac Special Care 24 (Ross) and Enfamil Premature 24 (Mead Johnson)) compared with 20 calories per ounce for human milk and standard infant formulas. The higher density formula helps the infant meet calorie requirements without fluid overload. The common features of these commercial infant formulas are (a) use of whey-predominant proteins, (b) carbohydrate mixtures of lactose and glucose polymers, and (c) fat mixtures

Table 6–6. Specialized Formulas and their Composition for Full-Term Infants With Selected Problems

Formula	Problem	Composition
Protein Hydrolysate-based Formulas		
Pregestimil	Malabsorption (e.g., CF), short bowel syndrome, or impaired intestinal function	Casein protein, fat 50% MCT, high in fat-soluble vitamins, carbohydrate is glucose polymers
Alimentum	Similar malabsorption problems (see Pregestimil)	Carbohydrate is sucrose; ready-to-feed liquid, cannot be concentrated
Nutramigen	Protein allergies or lactose intolerance	Hypoallergenic formula, same protein hydrolysates as Pregestimil; fat source is safflower, coconut, and soy oils; lactose and sucrose free
Neocate	Severe cow's-milk protein allergy	100% free amino acids as protein source, no hydrolyzed casein
Milk based with special components		
Portagen	Fat malabsorption (e.g., chronic liver disease or pancreatic insufficiency)	Carbohydrate: 75% glucose polymers, 25% sucrose; protein is casein; fat slightly less than standard formulas
PM60/40	Hypocalcemia and hyperphosphatemia	Cow's-milk–based, whey predominant; low sodium & phosphate, high calcium-phosphate ratio (2:1); has lactose
Lacto-Free	Lactose intolerance	Milk protein isolate; carbohydrate by corn syrup solids; fat source palm olein, soy, coconut, and sunflower oils
Milk based and concentrated		
Similac 27	Fluid restrictions (CHF & BPD)	High energy with lactose, protein (whey-predominant), and fat composition similar to full-term formulas; higher in protein, calcium, phosphorus, and electrolytes

Note: CF: cystic fibrosis; CHF: congestive heart failure; BPD: bronchopulmonary dysplasia; MCT: medium chain triglyceride

Table 6–7. Indications for Use of Infant Formulas

Problem in Infancy	Suggested Formula	Rationale
Allergy to cow's-milk protein or soy protein	Protein hydrolysate (Nutramigen, Pregestimil, Alimentum, or Neocate)	Protein sensitivity
Biliary atresia	Portagen Pregestimil	Impaired intraluminal digestion and absorption of long-chain fats
Cardiac disease	Enfamil	Low electrolyte content
Celiac disease	Pregestimil or Alimentum followed by soy-based formula followed by cow's-milk formula	Advance to more complete formula as intestinal epithelium becomes normal
Constipation	Routine formula, increase sugar	Mild laxative effect
Cystic fibrosis	Regular infant formula unless short bowel	Impaired intraluminal digestion and absorption of long-chain fats
	Pregestimil, Alimentum	Whey protein and disaccharide digestion and absorption impaired, indicated for short bowel
Diarrhea: chronic, nonspecific	Isomil D&F (dietary fiber); Pedialyte	
Diarrhea: intractable	Pregestimil, Alimentum, Neocate, Nutramigen	Impaired digestion of intact protein, long-chain fats, and disaccharides
Failure to thrive (when damage is suspected)	Pregestimil, Alimentum, Neocate, Nutramigen	Advance to more complete formula as intestinal epithelium returns to normal

continues

Table 6–7. *(continued)* Indications for Use of Infant Formulas

Problem in Infancy	Suggested Formula	Rationale
Gastroesophageal reflux (consider allergy)	Routine formula	Thicken with 2 to 3 tsp cereal/oz; small frequent feeds
	Enfamil/AR	Added rice, thickens when reaches stomach acids
Gastrointestinal bleeding (consider allergy)	Consider formula free of soy or cow's milk; Nutramigen, Alimentum, Pregestimil, Neocate	Milk toxicity in infants
Hepatic dysfunction (major complication of parenteral nutrition)	Portagen	Impaired intraluminal digestion and absorption of long-chain fats; 80% medium chain triglyceride
Lactose intolerance	Soy-based formula (e.g., Isomil, Prosobee)	Impaired digestion or utilization of lactose
Necrotizing enterocolitis (after resection)	Pregestimil, Alimentum (when feeding is resumed)	Impaired digestion
Renal insufficiency	PM 60/40	Low phosphate content, low renal solute load

Source: Modified from Grybowsky, J., & Walker, W. A. (1993). *Gastrointestinal Problems in the Infant* (2nd ed.). Philadelphia: W. B. Saunders; and Walker, W. A., & Hendricks, K. A., (1985). *Manual of Pediatric Nutrition.* Philadelphia: W. B. Saunders.

that are combinations of medium-chain triglycerides (MCT) and relatively unsaturated long-chain triglycerides (LCT). Carbohydrate mixtures of 40 to 50% lactose and 50 to 60% glucose polymers are used to compensate for infants' relative lactase deficiency (Sun et al., 1998). Semielemental formulas are used with some infants who have very low birth weights.

Concentration of standard infant formulas to increase caloric density will increase osmolarity and renal solute load and may not be as well tolerated as premature formulas, which are iso-osmolar and have a relatively low renal solute load.

Formulas for premature infants contain a portion of their fat as MCT oil. These do not require bile salts for digestion and are emptied more rapidly from the stomach than are LCT. MCT oil does not contain essential fatty acids, however. A small amount of long-chain fatty acids (approximately 1 cc of vegetable oil per kg body weight per day) is necessary to prevent essential fatty acid deficiency. Most infant formulas, even those high in MCT oil, provide adequate quantities of long-chain fat. Portagen does not contain adequate long-chain fatty acids and should not be used for the long term. Vegetable oil is used as the source of long-chain fat in premature formulas because of its easy digestibility. Although animal fat is, in general, not as easily digested, human milk contains a bile-salt-activated lipase that may help explain the excellent absorption of human milk fat by premature and term infants (AAP, 1985).

Most premature infant formulas provide protein as a mixture of 60% whey and 40% casein, similar to the mixture found in human milk. Most cow's-milk–based standard infant formulas have a greater quantity of casein (80% casein, 20% whey). Whey protein forms a smaller, softer curd in the stomach than does casein and is therefore more easily digested (Fried et al., 1992; Suchow, 1983). Low-birth-weight infants who receive formulas with a high percentage of protein from whey also tend to have lower serum ammonia and blood urea nitrogen levels, indicating more efficient protein metabolism (Menenstein & Gardner, 1985; Steichen, Krug-Wispe, & Tsang, 1987). When protein hypersensitivity (protein allergy) is related to intolerance of formulas, hypoallergenic formulas may be considered (AAP, 2000). The diet of premature infants does appear to influence later outcomes and thus demands caregiver attention to make sure the diet is adequate (Morley & Lucas, 1994).

■ FEEDING FOR CHILDREN WITH SPECIAL HEALTH NEEDS (CSHN)

The very-low-birth-weight or multiply handicapped infant is at high risk to develop feeding problems within the 1st year of life. These problems may be from incoordination of suck/swallow/breathe sequencing, developmental delay, anatomic abnormalities, or misconceptions on the part of caregivers as to appropriate feeding for age and developmental stage, among other contributing factors (Table 6–1). The initiation of solid food and cow's milk tends to be based on the infant's chronologic rather than corrected age according to a study of very-low-birth-weight infants during the first year of life (Ernst, Bull, Rickard, Brady & Lemons, 1990). A majority of these infants were receiving infant cereal by 2 months corrected age via bottle or infant feeder, because the tongue protrusion response to the spoon was strong. When such foods are introduced inappropriately, the child may find it detrimental to the development of normal feeding patterns.

Addition of cow's milk before 6 months corrected age was observed in 20% of infants and before 12 months corrected age in 90% of infants. Fifty percent of these were receiving low-fat cow's milk.

Introduction of cow's milk is not usually recommended until 12 months of age, unless the diet contains a wide variety of nutrients from solid foods and appropriate supplements to meet iron, zinc, and copper needs. Low-fat cow's milk is not recommended for any child before 2 years of age, because its use has been found to be associated with slowed growth and decreased fat stores. These findings indicate the need for improved parent/caregiver counseling. Also, consistent monitoring of premature, low-birth-weight, and multiply handicapped infants is necessary to insure that nutritional needs are met and the diet is advanced in stages appropriate to the infant's developmental abilities (Chapter 2). In children with oral sensorimotor delay or incoordination, the advancement of textures may be a slow process (Blackman & Nelson, 1985).

Nutritional needs can be met with many types of food textures. As textures are changed, the total composition of the diet must be monitored to assure nutritional adequacy. For example, reducing formula intake for prolonged periods as a means to increase "hunger" for solids may be counterproductive, because the child's lack of hunger may actually be a lack of skill in dealing with the texture of the food (Gisel, 1991). The reduction will result in hunger and frustration for the child, and undernutrition and dehydration may develop. Thus, if a child is not progressing as expected in consuming solid foods, it is important to investigate the child's ability to handle various textures using a detailed clinical evaluation and appropriate instrumental studies (Chapters 7 and 8). Total calories and protein are more important than variety for children in this stage of development. Caregivers and school staff members need to work closely together to assure adequate nutrition for CSHN (Cloud, 1994)

Children over 12 months of age who require liquid feedings, orally or by tube, to meet nutritional needs should be taken off infant formulas and placed on other special formulas. These formulas are nutritionally complete, balanced, isotonic enteral formulas especially designed for tube or oral feeding of children 1 to 10 years of age (e.g., Pediasure and Kindercal). They may be used as the sole source of nutrition or as a supplement. Patients with severe motor delays that alter caloric requirements may need to have formulas changed by dilution or addition of supplemental nutrients (protein, vitamins, and minerals) to meet fluid and nutrition needs without excessive calories. There are many special formulas available, and more become available regularly.

Likewise, special diets have been developed for children with specific metabolic deficits and CNS disorders. For example, the ketogenic diet is used with some children who have intractable seizures and as a diagnostic test for ketotic hypoglycemia (AAP, 1998). The ketogenic diet is a non-pharmacologic therapy based on maintaining ketosis used to treat intractable pediatric epilepsy. This diet that is low-carbohydrate and high-fat was first made known to the American public on a 1994 NBC television special. Fat (ketogenic) makes up 90% of calories, with the other 10% from protein (neutral) and CHO (antiketogenic). This diet restricts total fluid intake and requires vitamin and mineral supplements. Calories are about 75% of the RDA level. Advantages and disadvantages are seen in Table 6–8. Preliminary results also indicate that this diet may be beneficial to some pediatric oncology patients (Nebeling, Miraldi, Shurin, & Lerner, 1995).

Children with cerebral palsy are known to be at risk for poor nutritional status and delayed growth (e.g., Suresh-Babu & Thomas, 1998). In a study with children who have diplegia or hemiplegia, it has been suggested that these children have significantly reduced linear growth compared with norms for healthy children. Children in the youngest age group are most at risk for undernutrition, whereas all have some degree of abnormalities of growth and nutritional status (Stallings, Charney, Davies, & Cronk, 1993a). Children with quadriplegia show significant reductions in growth and nutrition status indicators, even at 2 to 4 years. Linear growth measures are correlated significantly with measures of nutritional status. (Stallings, Charney, Davies, & Cronk, 1993b). Growth can be improved with gastrostomy feeds in some children with CP (Rempel, Colwell, & Nelson, 1988). It is also important to be aware that nonnutritional factors related to disease severity have an effect on growth of children with CP, even in the absence of undernutrition (Stevenson, Roberts, & Vogtle, 1995). Children with neuromuscular conditions need nutrition guidance, with special consideration paid to risks for pharyngeal phase swallow problems (Bartz & Deubler, 1990; Tilton, Miller, & Khoshoo, 1998).

Table 6–8. Advantages and Disadvantages of Ketogenic Diet for Intractable Pediatric Epilepsy

Advantages	Disadvantages	Side Effects
Improved seizure control (67% improved)	Strictly regulated medical diet (may require hospital admission to initiate)	Constipation
Reduction in antiepileptic drugs (64%)	Requires a team for success	Renal stones
Increased alertness (36%)	Rigorous work to initiate and maintain by parents and dietitian	
Improved behavior (23%)		

For children in whom fluid overload is of concern, additional nutritional needs can be met without fluid overload by use of protein powder, vitamin additives, and mineral supplements. Intake can be calculated and adjustments made to meet the RDAs. If needs are higher because of drug–nutrient interactions or other factors, adjustments should be made. Many single or multiple supplements are available and can be crushed or given in liquid form. The liquid forms can be taken orally or delivered through a feeding tube as needed. A dietitian should be consulted whenever there are concerns about adequacy of nutrient intake. A dietitian or pharmacist can make recommendations for appropriate supplements once needs are determined.

In children with motor delay, caloric requirements may begin to decrease markedly during the toddler years when a larger percentage of caloric requirements are normally used for activity. When caloric intake needs to be reduced to avoid obesity, proper attention must be paid to avoid fluid imbalance. Fluid intake in the range of 75 to 80% of maintenance needs is usually adequate if fluid losses are not high, but it is important to monitor children for signs of dehydration. Losses from drooling, mechanical ventilation, emesis, and diarrhea are considered in determining fluid needs.

Drug–nutrient interactions can lead to nutrient deficiencies in patients requiring long-term medications. The association between long-term use of anticonvulsants and the development of rickets is of particular concern for this population. As many as 25% of children requiring chronic anticonvulsant therapy may be affected (Deitz, 1987). Risk increases further in children who are nonambulatory. Prophylactic treatment with vitamin D should be considered in those children who require long-term anticonvulsant therapy. Other drug–nutrient interactions may be of significance in this population, because medication use tends to be high. A dietitian can assess whether micronutrient needs are being met for any child requiring long-term medications (Grant & DeHoog, 1991).

■ NONORAL FEEDING DELIVERY FOR INFANTS AND CHILDREN

Whenever children cannot meet nutrition needs orally, alternate methods of feeding are needed. The options include enteral feedings through the gastrointestinal tract (e.g., MacBurney, Russell, & Young, 1990) and parenteral feedings that provide nutrients directly into the bloodstream and bypass the gastrointestinal tract. Figure 6–11 shows factors in decision making regarding parenteral versus enteral feeding. Multiple options for both enteral and parenteral routes of feeding are now available. Enteral feedings can be given via nasogastric, orogastric, gastrostomy, and jejunostomy tubes (Minard, 1994). Parenteral nutrition (PN) may be delivered by

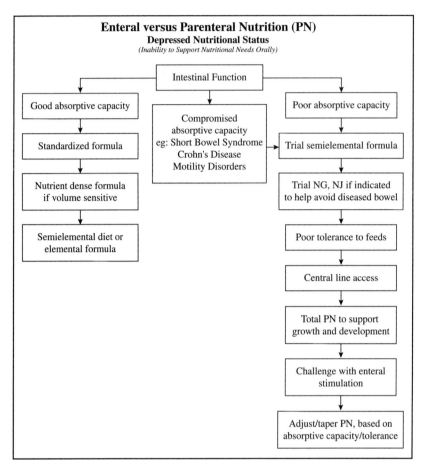

Figure 6–11. Decision making for determination of parenteral vs. enteral nutrition routes.

peripheral vein access (a percutaneous intravascular catheter that is guided into a central vein) or direct central venous access. These methods are described in detail in Chapter 5. Types of tubes and management decisions are described further in Chapter 9.

Enteral Tube Feeding

Formulas for Enteral Tube Feeding

The same considerations used when choosing a formula for oral feedings should be taken into account when choosing a formula for tube feeding.

Infant formulas available for oral intake are also appropriate for tube-fed infants. Pediasure and Kindercal are available for children from 1 to 10 years. These formulas meet the specific nutrient needs for this age group and are, in most cases, satisfactory tube feedings. If a specialized formula is required to treat an underlying condition, such as malabsorption, or if caloric requirements deviate from normal, modified formulas are available to meet individual needs.

Schedule of Enteral Tube Feedings

A feeding schedule is based on the underlying medical problem as well as on the type of tube and feeding used (Shauster & Dwyer, 1996). In general, continuous feeds are tolerated better than bolus feeds if vomiting, GERD/EERD, or delayed gastric emptying are concerns. Infants or children receiving some oral feeds supplemented with tube feeds may receive this supplemental bolus feed following each meal or as a continuous slow feeding overnight. Continuous feedings, whether 24 hours a day or overnight, should be delivered with an infusion pump to insure a constant flow. The rate and volume are calculated on the basis of what the child can tolerate and also what is needed to complete the requirements for total volume within each 24-hour period.

Children whose nutritional needs are met by tube feedings alone seem to have the best potential for progressing to oral feeding (providing they are safe oral feeders) when they can tolerate bolus feedings during family mealtimes. That schedule allows for the most physiologic feedings that are least upsetting to the normal family schedule and have the potential to promote hunger and appetite in children (Chapter 13). Bolus feedings may be provided by an infusion pump, which enables consistent regulation of flow. Patients without gastrointestinal problems typically tolerate gravity infusion of bolus feedings. If bolus feeds take longer than 30 to 45 minutes to infuse because of poor tolerance or the presence of high residuals, the feeding schedule may need to be altered, and continuous feeds may need to be instituted. Alternatively, small volumes of bolus feedings given during the day, with a continuous infusion given overnight, may be tolerated best by children and more convenient for families. A number of different feeding schedules may need to be tested by caregivers and professionals working as a team. Tolerance of bolus feedings is a positive indicator for oral feeding potential.

Complications of Enteral Tube Feedings

Potential complications of tube feedings can be divided into gastrointestinal, metabolic, or mechanical. The most common gastrointestinal complications are vomiting, abdominal distension, and diarrhea, which are likely related to GER (Chapter 5). Diarrhea is a frequent complication of tube feedings in children with gastrointestinal disorders or immune deficiency diseases. Initial treatment includes a non-cow's-milk–based formula of relatively low osmolality, with consideration for change to a more elemental formula if diarrhea does not resolve within a short time. Continuous feedings will, in general, be better tolerated than bolus feeds in infants and children with any gastrointestinal complications.

Metabolic complications of tube feedings are less common than gastrointestinal complications. Care must be taken to avoid sodium, protein, or fluid overload in sensitive premature infants or sick full-term infants.

Mechanical complications of enteral feedings vary, depending on the method of delivery. Nasogastric or orogastric tubes must be checked carefully for proper tube placement. If the tube obstructs, irrigation with water or proteolytic agents may be helpful; otherwise, the tube should be replaced.

Parenteral Nutrition

Parenteral nutrition (PN) is a standard mode of feeding for infants and children in whom the GI tract is nonfunctional or for those in need of short-term intensive nutritional rehabilitation. PN supports increased growth at slightly lower energy intakes than enteral feedings because energy is not lost in absorption and digestion. Venous access for PN is discussed in Chapter 5.

Composition of Parenteral Nutrition Fluid

Once an appropriate catheter is in place, concentration of nutrients can be increased gradually. Estimates are made for amino acid and energy requirements (Table 6–9). Distribution of calorics needs to be considered

Table 6–9. Amino Acid Energy Requirements of Infants and Children Receiving Parenteral Nutrition

Age Group	Amino Acids (gm/kg/d)	Energy (kcal/kg/d)
Premature neonates	3.0	90
Infants 0–1 year	2.5	80–95
Children, 2–9 years	1.5–2.0	60–75
10–13 years	1.5–2.0	50–60
Adolescents	1.0–1.5	40

Source: From Zlotkin, S. H., Stallings, V. A., & Rencharz, P. B. (1985). Total Parenteral Nutrition in Children. *Pediatric Clinics of North America, 32,* 381–400, with permission.

and may be provided by a combination of carbohydrate (dextrose) and fat emulsion. In general, an optimal distribution of calories is 50 to 60% of calories from carbohydrate and 40 to 50% of calories from fat.

Concentration of glucose is advanced in a methodical way to ensure tolerance. Protein (crystalline amino acids) should be provided at a rate of 1.5 to 3.0 g/kg/day (AAP, 1993). Infusion of intravenous lipid at 0.5 to 1.0 g/kg/day meets essential fatty acid requirements. Tolerance should be maximized by slow infusion of up to 3.0 g/kg/day. Parenteral solutions should contain vitamins, minerals, and trace elements.

Schedule and Advancement of Parenteral Nutrition Support

Dextrose concentration, lipids, and amino acids are given in small amounts initially and gradually advanced to meet nutritional needs. Transition to enteral nutrition should begin as soon as possible, with PN continued until full nutritional support is achieved via the gastrointestinal tract.

Cycling of PN is desirable to provide needed nutrients in shorter time periods than over 24 hours per day. This cycling helps to decrease the risk of metabolic complications, allows greater freedom of movement, and encourages oral intake when feasible. The total volume of solution should be held constant while the number of hours of infusion is gradually decreased. Then, during the last hour of the infusion, the rate should be decreased slowly to allow for normalization of insulin output and prevention of hypoglycemia (Rossi & Morrison-Willard, 1986).

Complications of Parenteral Nutrition Support

Complications of PN can be metabolic or technical. Patients receiving long-term PN are at some risk for metabolic complications. Tolerance to the therapy is monitored by regular laboratory values that include glucose, serum protein, liver function tests, and electrolytes. Alterations can be made immediately for metabolic intolerance.

Technical problems are associated primarily with the use of central venous catheters for access (Chapter 5). Complications with peripheral intravenous central catheter (PICC) lines are rare, but they include phlebitis and skin slough from extravasation of the PN solution into the interstitial space. Treatment for both these complications is removal of the catheter, warm soaks to the area, and close observation of the access site (Walker & Hendricks, 1985).

Small infusions of enteral feeds should be initiated as soon as possible to prevent gastrointestinal mucosal atrophy and cholestasis, which can lead to irreversible liver disease (AAP, 1998). Nutrition status must be monitored continuously to assure the adequacy of nutritional support. Evidence of benefit from minimal enteral nutrition (MEN) is not convincing in a review of clinical trials (Tyson & Kennedy, 2000). The reviewers concluded that particularly in relation to necrotizing enterocolitis (NEC) in infants during the neonatal period, it is unclear whether MEN should be used in lieu of an equal time without enteral feedings.

Transition From Parenteral to Enteral Feeds

Most children tolerate transition from total parenteral (TPN) to enteral nutrition when the transition is gradual. The rate of advancement from parenteral to enteral feedings in very-low-birth-weight infants with NEC is unclear because of multiple variables (Kennedy, Tyson, & Chamnanvanakij, 2000). In all circumstances, close monitoring is needed to assure that adequate nutrition is provided during the transition. In general, the concentration of enteral formulas should first be increased gradually to full strength, with volume kept low, so that PN fluid can continue to be provided in large volumes to meet calorie needs. Once enteral feeds are at full concentration, the enteral fluid volume is increased with an equivalent decrease in PN volume. If the increased enteral feeds are not well tolerated, volume should be decreased, and parenteral volume increased. When enteral feeds make up at least two thirds of necessary fluid, the PN usually may be discontinued.

Long Term Outcomes With Prolonged Parenteral Nutrition

Children who get prolonged PN in early life appear at risk for abnormalities in growth and nutritional status in later childhood (Leonberg et al., 1998). They require long-term dietary, growth, and nutritional monitoring.

The provision of adequate nutritional support for infants and CSHN is a challenge for the entire team caring for the child. The process involves assessment of nutritional status, choice of an appropriate feeding and method of delivery, and follow-up to assess tolerance and whether needs are being met. Nutritional therapy is not a static process, but one that requires continuous monitoring, reassessment, and alteration in the treatment plan as the infant or child grows and develops. The contribution of these ongoing evaluations cannot be overemphasized.

■ CASE STUDIES

Case Study 1

"Janice," a 20-week-old female infant, born at 24 weeks gestation, is now at a corrected age of 4 weeks. Weight is 3.5 kg, and length is 52 cm. Her weight and length should be plotted on the growth chart as a 4-week-old infant (40 weeks normal gestation minus 24 weeks actual gestation = 16 weeks premature; 20 weeks chronologic age minus 16 weeks premature =

4 weeks corrected age). On the NCHS growth chart as a 4-week-old infant, she is at nearly the 25th percentile for both weight and length, with weight-for-length at the 25th percentile. She is therefore growing quite well and is probably not malnourished. In contrast, if weight and length are plotted at her chronologic age of 20 weeks, she would be below the 5th percentile for both weight and length, which would lead to an erroneous interpretation that she is growing poorly. Weight is adjusted up to 24 months, height up to 40 months, and head circumference up to 36 months (Frank, Needlman, & Silva, 1993; Kraus & Mahank, 1984).

Comment

This case is an example of a preterm infant and how the corrected age is used to evaluate nutrition status.

Case Study 2

"Joseph" presented at 6 months of age. History revealed a term infant with normal prenatal and postnatal course. He weighs 6.6 kg (14.5 pounds) and is 67 cm (27.5 inches) in length. His head circumference is 44 cm (17.5 inches). He is at the 10th percentile for weight and the 50th percentile for length and head circumference on the growth curve. His weight-for-length is at the 5th percentile. He is acutely malnourished, noted by reduced weight, but length is maintained. His appropriate weight for his length can be determined by finding the weight for length that corresponds with the 50th percentile on the growth chart, which is approximately 7.5 kg.

Follow-up medical investigation revealed that this child has celiac disease, a reaction or intolerance to wheat, oats, rye, and barley that causes malabsorption and resultant undernutrition. This allergy did not become manifest until these grains were added to his diet at 4 months of age, and thus his undernutrition developed acutely in the 2 months following introduction of solid feedings. Removal of the offending agents from his diet resulted in rapid catch-up weight gain.

Comment

This case study reveals the critical need to determine the etiology for the undernutrition, and not simply to boost calories, without appropriate diagnostic work-up. This child would have been harmed further if he had continued with foods that he could not absorb adequately.

Case Study 3

"Paul," a 2-year-old with cerebral palsy, gets his nutritional needs met with a combination of oral feeding with pureed foods supplemented by formula via a gastrostomy tube (GT). He requires 1,200 calories per day. On a specific day he took in 800 calories by mouth from pureed foods. He thus requires an additional 400 calories that can be given as a continuous overnight tube feeding of a 1 calorie/cc formula, given as 40 cc/hour for 10 hours overnight.

Comment

This method insures a consistent daily intake despite inevitable variations in a child's oral intake. It also has the advantage of freeing the child from the tube during the more active daytime. Typical eating patterns throughout the day can be encouraged. Gradually the GT feeds should be shifted to bolus feeds if Paul can tolerate the increased volume in shorter time periods. As long as slow night feeds are needed, the prognosis for attainment of total oral feeding is guarded.

■ REFERENCES

American Academy of Pediatrics Committee on Nutrition. (1985). Nutritional needs of low-birth-weight infants. *Pediatrics, 75,* 976–986.

American Academy of Pediatrics Committee on Nutrition. (1998). *Pediatric nutrition handbook* (4th ed.). Elk Grove Village, IL: American Academy of Pediatrics.

American Academy of Pediatrics Committee on Nutrition. (2000). Hypoallergenic infant formulas. *Pediatrics, 106,* 346–349.

American Dietetic Association. (1995). Position of the American Dietetic Association: Nutrition services for children with special health needs. *Journal of the American Dietetic Association, 95,* 809–811.

Bartz, A. H., & Deubler, D. C. (1990). Identification of feeding and nutrition problems in young children with neuromotor involvement: A self-assessment. *Journal of Pediatric and Perinatal Nutrition, 2,* 1–13.

Bayerl, C. T., Ries, J. D., Bettencourt, M. F., & Fisher, P. (1993). Nutrition issues of children in early intervention programs: Primary care team approach. *Seminars in Pediatric Gastroenterology and Nutrition, 4,* 11–15.

Bithoney, W. G., & Dubowitz, H. (1985). Organic concomitants of nonorganic failure to thrive: Implications for research. In D. Drotar (Ed.), *New directions in failure to thrive: Implications for research and practice* (47–68). New York: Plenum Press.

Blackman, J. A., & Nelson, C. L. (1985). Reinstituting oral feedings in children fed by gastrostomy tube. *Clinical Pediatrics, 24,* 434–438.

Brody, R. A., Touger-Decker, R., VonHagen, S., & O'Sullivan Maillet, J. (2000). Role of registered dietitians in dysphagia screening. *Journal of the American Dietetic Association, 100,* 1029–1037.

Centers for Disease Control and Prevention, National Center for Health Statistics. CDC growth charts. United States. Retrieved from the World Wide Web May 30, 2000: http://www.cdc.gov/nchs/about/major/nhanes/growthcharts/charts.htm

Cloud, H. H. (1994). Role of school food service in providing nutrition to children with special needs. *Topics in Clinical Nutrition, 9*, 47–53.

Cloud, H. H., & Bergman, J. (1991). Eating/feeding problems of children: The team approach. *Nutrition Focus, 6*, 1–8.

Cronk, C. E. (1983). Growth of children with Down syndrome. *Pediatrics, 61*, 564–568.

Dancis, J., O'Connell, J. R., & Holt, L. E. (1948). A grid for recording the weight of premature infants. *Journal of Pediatrics, 33*, 570.

Day, J. C. (1993). *Population projections of the United States by age, race, and Hispanic origin: 1993-2050* (US Bureau of the Census, Current Population Reports P25–1104).Washington, DC: Government Printing Office.

Deitz, W. H. (1987). Nutritional requirements and feeding of the handicapped child. In R. Grand, J. Stephen, & W. H. Deitz (Eds.), *Pediatric nutrition* (387–392). Boston: Butterworth.

DeLong, G. R. (1993). Effects of nutrition on brain development in humans. *American Journal of Clinical Nutrition Supplement, 57*, 286S–290S.

Drotar, D., & Sturm, L. (1992). Personality development, personality solving and behavioral problems among preschool children with early histories of nonorganic failure to thrive: A controlled study. *Journal of Developmental and Behavioral Pediatarics, 13*, 266–273.

Education of the Handicapped Act Amendments of 1986. Pub L. No. 99-457, 100 Stat 1146.

Ekvall, S. W. (1993). Nutritional assessment and early intervention. In S. W. Ekvall, (Ed.), *Pediatric nutrition in chronic diseases and developmental disorders: Prevention, Assessment, and Treatment*. New York: Oxford University Press.

Engelke, S. C., Engelke, M. K., Helm, J. M., & Holbert, D. (1995). Cognitive failure to thrive in high-risk infants: The importance of the psychosocial environment. *Journal of Perinatology, 15*, 325–329.

Ernst, J. A., Bull, M. J., Rickard, K. A., Brady, M. S., & Lemons, J. A. (1990). Growth outcome and feeding practices of the very low birth weight infant (less than 1500 grams) within the first year of life. *The Journal of Pediatrics, 117*, 156–166.

Federation of American Societies for Experimental Biology, Life Sciences Research Office, (1995). *Third report on nutrition monitoring in the United States* (Vol. 2). Washington, DC: U.S. Government Printing Office. (Prepared for the Interagency Board for Nutrition Monitoring and Related Research.)

Field, T., Ignatoff, E., Stringer, S., Brennan, J., Greenberg, R., Widmayer, S., & Anderson, G.C. (1982). Nonnutritive sucking during tube feedings: Effects on preterm neonates in an intensive care unit. *Pediatrics, 70,* 381–384.

Finney, J. W. (1986). Preventing common feeding problems in infants and young children. *Pediatric Clinics of North America, 33,* 775–788.

Fomon, S. J., Filer, L. J., Anderson, T. A., & Ziegler, E. E. (1979). Recommendations for feeding normal infants. *Pediatrics, 63,* 52–59.

Fomon, S. J., Ziegler, E. E., & Vasquez, H. D. (1977). Human milk and the small premature infant. *American Journal of Diseases of Childhood, 131,* 463–467.

Frank, D., Needlman, R., & Silva, M. (1993). Failure to thrive: Mystery, myth, and method. *Contemporary Pediatrics,* 114–133.

Fried, M. D., Khoshoo, V., Secker, D. J., Gilday, D. L., Ash, J. M., & Pencharz, P. B. (1992). Decrease in gastric emptying time and episodes of regurgitation in children with spastic quadriplegia fed a whey-based formula. *The Journal of Pediatrics, 120,* 569–572.

Frisancho, A. (1974). Triceps skinfold and upper arm muscle size norms for assessment of nutritional status. *American Journal of Clinical Nutrition, 27,* 1052–1058.

Geertsma, M. A., Hyams, J. S., Pelletier, J. M., & Reiter, S. (1985). Feeding resistance after parenteral hyperalimentation. *American Journal of Diseases of Childhood, 139,* 255–256.

Gilbride, J. A., Cowell, C., & Simko, M. D. (1989). Overview of nutrition assessment: The process of nutrition assessment. In M. D. Simko, C. Cowell, & J. A. Gilbride, (Eds.), *Nutrition assessment: A comprehensive guide for planning intervention.* Rockville, MD: Aspen.

Gisel, E. G. (1991). Effect of food texture on the development of chewing of children between six months and two years of age. *Developmental Medicine and Child Neurology, 33,* 69–79.

Grant, A. & DeHoog, S. (1991). *Nutritional assessment and support.* Seattle: Grant and DeHoog Publishers.

Greer, F. R. (1995). Formulas for the healthy term infant. *Pediatrics in Review, 16,* 107.

Grybowsky, J., & Walker, W. A. (1993). *Gastrointestinal Problems in the Infant* (2nd ed.). Philadelphia: W. B. Saunders.

Hamill, P. V. V., Drizd, T. A., & Johnson, C. L. (1979). Physical growth: National Center for Health Statistics percentiles. *American Journal of Clinical Nutrition, 32,* 607–615.

Handen, B. L., Mandell, F., & Russo, D. C. (1986). Feeding induction in children who refuse to eat. *American Journal of Diseases of Childhood, 140,* 52–54.

Heffer, R. W., & Kelley, M. L. (1994). Nonorganic failure to thrive: Developmental outcomes and psychosocial assessment and intervention issues [Review]. *Research in Developmental Disabilities, 15*, 247–268.

Humphrey, R. (1991). Impact of feeding problems on the parent-infant relationship. *Infants and Young Children, 3*, 30–38.

Hynak-Hankinson, M. R., Agin, M., Gardner, C., Jones, P. L., Lichtenstein, S., Peiffer, S., & Rao, P. (1984). Dysphagia evaluation and treatment: The team approach, part II. *Nutrition Support Services, 4*, 30–33.

Ireys, H. T., & Nelson, R. P. (1992). New federal policy for children with special health care needs: Implications for pediatricians. *Pediatrics, 90*, 321–327.

Kennedy, K. A., Tyson, J. E., & Chamnanvanakij, S. (2000). Rapid versus slow rate of advancement of feedings for promoting growth and preventing necrotizing enterocolitis in parenterally fed low-birth-weight infants. *Cochrane Database System Review, 2* CD001241.

Kerner, J. A., (1983). *Manual of pediatric parenteral nutrition.* New York: John Wiley.

Kessler, D. B. (1999). Failure to thrive and pediatric undernutrition historical and theoretical context. In D. B. Kessler, & P. Dawson, (Eds.), *Failure to thrive and pediatric undernutrition: A transdisciplinary approach* (3–17). Baltimore: Paul H. Brookes.

Kraus, M., & Mahank, L. H. (1984). *Food nutrition and diet therapy.* Philadelphia: W. B. Saunders.

Lawrence, R. A. (1980). *Breastfeeding: A guide for the medical profession.* St. Louis: C.V. Mosby Co.

Lebenthal, E. (1989). Concepts in gastrointestinal development. In E. Lebenthal (Ed.), *Human gastrointestinal development* (3–18). New York: Raven Press.

Leonberg, B. L., Chuang, E., Eicher, P., Tershakovec, A. M., Leonard, L., & Stallings, V. A. (1998). Long-term growth and development in children after home parenteral nutrition. *The Journal of Pediatrics, 132*, 461–466.

Lichtenwalter, L., Freeman, R., Lee, M., & Cialone, J. (1993). Providing nutrition services to children with special needs in a community setting. *Topics in Clinical Nutrition, 8*, 75–78.

Lucas, A., Brooke, O. G., Morley, R., Cole, T. J., & Bamford, M. F. (1990). Early diet of pre-term infants and development of allergic or atopic disease: A randomized prospective study. *British Medical Journal, 300*, 837–840.

MacBurney, M. M., Russell, C., & Young, L. S. (1990). In J. L. Rambeau and M. D. Caldwell (Eds.), *Clinical nutrition: Enteral and tube feeding* (149–173). Philadelphia: W. B. Saunders.

Marks, K. H. (1986). Growth of sick premature infants. In S. A. Cohen (Ed.), *The underweight infant, child and adolescent* (56–65). Norwalk, CT: Appleton-Century-Crofts.

Menenstein, G., & Gardner, S. (1985). *Handbook of neonatal intensive care.* St. Louis: C.V. Mosby Co.

Minard, G. (1994). Enteral access. *Nutrition in Clinical Practice, 9,* 172–182.

Morley, R., & Lucas, A. (1994). Influence of early diet on outcome in preterm infants. *Acta Paediatrics Suppl. 405,* 123–126.

National Academy of Sciences. (1989). *Recommended dietary allowances* (9th ed.). Washington, DC: National Research Council, Food and Nutrition Board.

Naeye, R. L., & Dixon, J. B. (1978). Distortions in fetal growth standards. *Pediatric Research, 12,* 987–1003.

Nebeling, L. C., Miraldi, F., Shurin, S. B., & Lerner, E. (1995). Effects of a ketogenic diet on tumor metabolism and nutritional status in pediatric oncology patients: Two case reports. *Journal of the American College of Nutrition, 14,* 202–208.

Neu, J., Valentine, C., & Meetze, W. (1990). Scientifically-based strategies for nutrition of the high-risk low birth weight infant. *European Journal of Pediatrics, 150,* 2–13.

Ostertag, S. G., & Frayer, W. W. (1983). Feeding the premature infant—general principles. *Pediatric Annals, 12,* 46–54.

Picciano, M. F., Smiciklas-Wright, H., Birch, L. L., Mitchell, D. C., Murray-Kolb, L., & McConahy, D. L. (2000). Nutritional guidance is needed during dietary transition in early childhood. *Pediatrics, 106,* 109–114.

Pridham, K. F., Martin, R., Sondel, S., & Tluczek, A. (1989). Parental issues in feeding young children with bronchopulmonary dysplasia. *Journal of Pediatric Nursing, 4,* 177–185.

Rempel, G. R., Colwell, S. O., & Nelson, R. P. (1988). Growth in children with cerebral palsy fed via gastrostomy. *Pediatrics, 82,* 857–862.

Ross Laboratories. (1991). *Composition of feedings for infants and young children in the hospital.* Columbus, OH: Ross Laboratories.

Rossi, T. M., & Morrison-Willard, E. (1986). Home parenteral nutrition. In E. Lebenthal (Ed.), *Total parenteral nutrition* (253–276). New York: Raven Press.

Saarinen, U. M., & Kajosaari, M. (1995). Breast-feeding as prophylaxis against atopic disease: Prospective follow-up study until 17 years old. *Lancet, 346,* 1065–1069.

Sanders, K. D., Cox, K., Cannon, R., Blanchard, D., Pither, J., Papatakis, P., Varella, L., & Maughan, R. (1990). Growth response to enteral feeding by children with cerebral palsy. *Journal of Parenteral and Enteral Nutrition, 14,* 23–26.

Satter, E. (1990). The feeding relationship: Problems and interventions. *The Journal of Pediatrics, 117,* S181–189.

Schanler, R. J. (1988). Special methods in feeding the preterm infant. In R. C. Tsang & B. L. Nichols (Eds.), *Nutrition during infancy* (314–325). Philadelphia: Hanley and Belfus.

Shapiro, B. K., Green, P., Krick, J., Allen, D., & Capute, A. J. (1986). Growth of severely impaired children: Neurological versus nutritional factors. *Developmental Medicine and Child Neurology, 28,* 729–733.

Shauster, H., & Dwyer, J. (1996). Transition from tube feedings to feedings by mouth in children: Preventing eating dysfunction. *Journal of the American Dietetic Association, 96,* 277–281.

Siegel, M., & Lebenthal, E. (1989). Development of gastrointestinal motility and gastric emptying during the fetal and newborn periods. In E. Lebenthal (Ed.), *Human gastrointestinal development* (277–298). New York: Raven Press.

Skuse, D. (1993). Epidemiological and definitional issues in failure to thrive. *Child and Adolescent Psychiatric Clinics of North America, 2,* 37–59.

Snyder, R. G., Schneider, L. W., Owings, M. A., Reynolds, H. M., Golomb, D. H., & Schork, M. A. (1977). *Anthropometry of infants, children and youth to age 18 for product safety design* (Report No. UM-HSRI-77-17). Bethesda, MD: Consumer Product Safety Commission.

Spender, Q. W., Cronk, C. E., Charney, E. B., & Stallings, V. A. (1989). Assessment of linear growth of children with cerebral palsy: Use of alternative measures to height or length. *Developmental Medicine and Child Neurology, 31,* 206–214.

Stallings, V. A., Charney, E. B., Davies, J. C., & Cronk, C. E. (1993a). Nutritional status and growth of children with diplegic or hemiplegic cerbral palsy. *Developmental Medicine and Child Neurology, 35,* 997–1006.

Stallings, V. A., Charney, E. B., Davies, J. C., & Cronk, C. E. (1993b). Nutritional-related growth failure of children with quadriplegic cerebral palsy. *Dev Med and Child Neurology, 35,* 126–138.

Steichen, J. J., Krug-Wispe, S. K., & Tsang, R. C. (1987). Breastfeeding the low birth weight preterm infant. *Clinics in Perinatology, 14,* 131–171.

Stevenson, R. D., Roberts, C. D., & Vogtle, L. (1995). The effects of non-nutritional factors on growth in cerebral palsy. *Developmental Medicine and Child Neurology, 37,* 124–130.

Suchow, E. (1983). Feeding the premature infant. *Environmental Nutrition, 6,* 1–3.

Sun, Y., Awnetwant, E. L., Collier, S. B., Gallagher, L. M., Olsen, I. E., & Stewart, J.E. (1998). Nutrition. In J. P. Cloherty & A. R. Stark, (Eds.),

Manual of neonatal care (4th ed; 101–134). Philadelphia: Lippincott-Raven.

Suresh-Babu, M. V., & Thomas, A. G. (1998). Nutrition in children with cerebral palsy. *Journal of Pediatric Gastroenterology & Nutrition, 26,* 484–485.

Tamborlane, W. V. (Ed.) (1997). *The Yale guide to children's nutrition.* New Haven, CT: Yale Unversity Press.

Thommessen, M., Heiberg, A., Kase, B. F., & Riis, G. (1991). Feeding problems, height and weight in different groups of disabled children. *Acta Pediatrica Scandinavica, 80,* 527– 533.

Tilton, A. H., Miller, M. D., & Khoshoo, V. (1998). Nutrition and swallowing in pediatric neuromuscular patients. *Seminars in Pediatric Neurology, 5,* 106–115.

Tyson, J. E., & Kennedy, K. A. (2000). Minimal enteral nutrition for promoting feeding tolerance and preventing morbidity in parenterally fed infants. *Cochrane Database Systems Review, 2,* CD000504.

U.S. Dept of Health and Human Services. (1990). *Healthy People 2000: National Health Promotion and Disease Prevention Objectives* (DHHS (PHS) publication No. 50213). Washington, DC: Public Health Services.

van den Berg-Emons, R. J. F., van Baak, M. A., & Westerterp, K. R. (1998). Are skinfold measurements suitable to compare body fat between children with spastic cerebral palsy and healthy controls? *Developmental Medicine and Child Neurology, 40,* 335–339.

Walker, W. A., & Hendricks, K. M. (1985). *Manual of pediatric nutrition.* Philadelphia: W. B. Saunders Company.

Ward, M. J., Brazelton, T. B., & Wust, M. (1999). Toward understanding the role of attachment in malnutrition. In D. B. Kessler & P. Dawson, (Eds.), *Failure to thrive and pediatric undernutrition: A transdisciplinary approach* (411–423). Baltimore: Paul H. Brookes.

Ziegler, E. E., (1991). Malnutrition in the premature infant. *Acta Pediatrica Scandinavica (Suppl,) 374,* 58–66.

Zisserman, L. (1986). Feeding problems: Weaning an infant from a transpyloric tube. *Pediatric Nursing, 12,* 33–37.

Zlotkin, S. H., Stallings, V. A., & Rencharz, P. B. (1985). Total Parenteral Nutrition in Children. *Pediatric Clinics of North America, 32,* 381–400.

■ CHAPTER 7
Clinical Feeding and Swallowing Assessment

Joan Arvedson, Linda Brodsky, and Donna Reigstad

■ SUMMARY

The clinical evaluation for infants and children with feeding and swallowing problems is a basic part of the process to identify, as clearly as possible, the nature and extent of the problem. The importance of a professional's adequate knowledge base and experience cannot be overstated. Clinicians of all disciplines, especially non-physicians, should continually remind themselves that this area of practice is one of highest risk. Improper diagnoses or management recommendations place these children in jeopardy for poor nutrition and impaired health status, such as reduced energy and lower long-term cognitive, communication, and sensorimotor outcomes. On the other hand, well-thought-out and coordinated planning can enhance the lives of these children and their caregivers. Thus, no clinician should evaluate and treat these children with feeding and swallowing problems as a single discipline in isolation. An interdisciplinary team, whether in medical- or school-based settings, should compile findings from all evaluations or assessments for appropriate coordinated recommendations. Physician input is of utmost importance in developing and monitoring management plans for many children. Treatment options vary according to history, physical examination, and findings during the clinical feeding evaluation.

The clinical feeding and swallowing evaluation process is based on concepts from the International Classification of Impairment, Disability, and Handicap (ICIDH2) (World Health Organization, 1997). This classification system is used to describe levels of disablement to include impairments (body function level), activities (person level), and participation (society level). A comprehensive evaluation includes obtaining information on the social and physical mealtime environments in which the child participates (e.g., home, school, restaurants), the child's activity limitations during mealtime (e.g., self-feeding abilities, need for adaptive equipment), and specific observations regarding underlying impairment (e.g., motor skills, respiratory, neuromuscular conditions, orthopedic conditions). Using this approach, the clinician first considers the child's level of participation in various mealtime environments.

This information is generally obtained through interviews with caregivers and observations of the child. Specific information regarding a child's activity limitations in meal setup, food acceptance, and self-feeding is acquired through a mealtime observation and caregiver interview or a standardized functional assessment. Information regarding underlying impairments (neuromuscular status, respiratory status, etc.) may be obtained through history via chart reviews, caregiver interview, various medical and therapeutic assessments, and instrumental examinations. This holistic approach to evaluation and assessment assists the evaluator(s) in decision making during the treatment planning process because it focuses on the overall goal of promoting a meaningful and functional mealtime experience for children and their families.

■ INTRODUCTION

A comprehensive clinical evaluation typically includes: (a) a review of the family, medical, developmental, and feeding history; (b) a physical examination; and (c) an observation of a typical meal (Arvedson & Lefton-Greif, 1998). (See Figure 7–1 for steps in clinical or bedside feeding and swallowing evaluation for infants and children.) The clinical evaluation enables clinicians to:

- identify possible etiologies underlying the dysphagia,
- formulate a hypothesis about the nature and severity of the dysphagia,
- establish a baseline (e.g., oral sensorimotor skills and respiratory function),
- introduce therapeutic modifications,
- investigate feeding options that are safe for the child and sensitive to family and cultural differences,
- determine whether an instrumental assessment is warranted and identify appropriate instrumental assessment tools,
- assess the readiness or ability of a patient to participate in an instrumental procedure, and

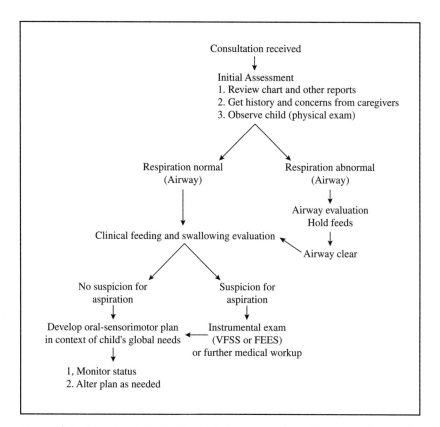

Figure 7–1. Steps in clinical or bedside feeding and swallowing evaluation for infants and children.

- develop and execute plans to modify specific instrumental procedures to address patient needs (e.g., Arvedson & Lefton-Greif, 1998; Case-Smith & Humphry, 2000; Groher, 1997; Langmore & Logemann, 1991; Logemann 1983, 1993, 1998).

The clinical evaluation provides an opportunity to appreciate multiple social, cultural, and environmental factors that interact with a child's unique developmental and medical/surgical profile. These environmental factors all influence the development of feeding. These factors include, but are not limited to, caregivers' responses to the child, family support systems, economic resources, cultural influences, and the iatrogenic effects of professional input. The clinician and team must consider any and all factors that can influence the development of deglutition before making decisions related to management, including possible referral for appropriate instrumental examination.

Setting the Stage for Clinical Evaluation

The earliest communication between parent and infant occurs through feeding. Thus, a feeding problem in the newborn period is usually perceived by parents as a significant concern. The ramifications of abnormal feeding permeate all aspects of their lives. Nonetheless, improvement can be anticipated as the central nervous system (CNS) matures, even in children with neurologic impairment. As infants develop increased muscle strength and learn to make compensatory movements, early feeding problems are likely to improve. On the other hand, feeding problems may become more prominent, or new problems may arise, as children get older.

The early promotion of optimal oral sensorimotor function in infants is a high priority. Unless effective changes are made early, oral sensorimotor and feeding problems in infancy frequently result in cycles of forced feeding and inadequate nutrition later in life. Delay in the development of sensorimotor skills can result in longer feeding times and also in increased tension in the caregiver, further exacerbating the feeding problems (Krick & Van Duyn, 1984; Ottenbacher, Bundy, & Short, 1983).

An oral sensorimotor and feeding assessment of infants and children takes many variables into account. Previous chapters have covered topics that are important to professionals who evaluate the oral sensorimotor functioning. Knowledge of anatomy, embryology, and physiology related to swallowing and feeding, as well as normal development and feeding, provides the basis for evaluation of swallowing and feeding problems. Professionals must keep in mind that the complexities of neurodevelopment, the airway, the gastrointestinal tract, nutrition, and tone and positioning have ramifications for the clinical oral sensorimotor and feeding evaluation. The clinical feeding evaluation focuses on a relatively narrow set of behaviors and skills potentially operant in the total feeding process.

Although assessment and treatment programs frequently have their major emphases on oral sensorimotor function and swallowing, the possible need for psychotherapeutic consultation and intervention also should be considered. Behavioral components related to feeding can be either primary or secondary complicating factors (Chapter 13). Children who are difficult to feed are more often abused by caregivers and may not grow as well as children who are perceived as easy to feed (Klein & Stern, 1971). Thus, maladaptive cycles can occur for a variety of reasons.

An understanding of the physical, social, and cultural mealtime environment is also important to develop a holistic perspective on the feeding process (Case-Smith & Humphry, 2000; Koontz-Lowman & Lane, 1999).

This involves an assessment of the physical environments in which children eat (e.g., home, school, day care, restaurants, and social gatherings). Preparation of meals and the feeding process are ways in which families communicate their values and priorities, in addition to being a method of meeting nutritional needs. Assessment should therefore include an understanding of the family's goals and priorities.

Knowledge of normal developmental patterns and the sequential advancement of oral sensorimotor skills is a prerequisite to understanding the assessment process (Chapter 2). Assessment of oral–motor and feeding activities follows directly from the knowledge of normal expectations and variations from those expectations.

This chapter presents issues related to the clinical examination of feeding and swallowing that is usually performed by a speech–language pathologist and/or an occupational therapist with specialized training in pediatric feeding and swallowing problems. Although the background of the oral–motor/feeding specialist may vary in different settings, the knowledge and skills employed must be extensive. The risks for serious physiologic consequences are great for children with feeding problems if accurate diagnoses are not made or if treatment is carried out in a fragmented or inappropriate fashion. This chapter is not intended as a procedural manual, but is designed to describe aspects of feeding and swallowing that need to be observed and evaluated. This should be conducted in conjunction with an interdisciplinary team of professionals who have the child's total well-being as the primary goal. The team approach is stressed throughout this chapter. Discussion will focus on criteria for referral; review of the medical, developmental, and feeding history; physical examination; and observation of a typical meal.

■ CRITERIA FOR REFERRAL

The most common criteria for referral of infants and children for an interdisciplinary team oral–motor and feeding evaluation are described in Table 7–1. In addition, problems such as emesis or vomiting, nasal regurgitation, and increased drooling may need investigation. Children delayed in certain developmental milestones may need evaluation. These include children who demonstrate an inability to take spoon feedings by 9 months of age, to chew table food and to self-feed with finger food or a spoon by 18 months, or to drink from a cup by 24 months.

Infants with cleft palate in isolation or with cleft lip or other craniofacial anomalies should be evaluated before the first oral feeding attempt so that appropriate adaptations can be made to facilitate efficient oral feeding (Chapter 12). Infants who demonstrate weak or incoordinated suck and swallow patterns in addition to a cleft are at risk for aspiration and poor

Table 7–1. Common Criteria for Referral of Infants and Children for Feeding and Swallowing Evaluation

- Sucking and swallowing incoordination
- Weak suck
- Breathing disruptions or apnea during feeding
- Excessive gagging or recurrent coughing during feeds
- New onset of feeding difficulty
- Diagnosis of disorders associated with dysphagia or undernutrition (Chapter 3)
- Weight loss or lack of weight gain for 2 to 3 months (undernutrition)
- Severe irritability or behavior problems during feeds
- History of recurrent pneumonia and feeding difficulty
- Concern for possible aspiration during feeds
- Lethargy or decreased arousal during feeds
- Feeding periods longer than 30 to 40 min
- Unexplained food refusal and undernutrition (failure to thrive) (Chapter 13)
- Drooling persisting beyond age 5 years (Chapter 11)
- Nasopharyngeal reflux with feeding
- Delay in feeding developmental milestones
- Children with craniofacial anomalies (Chapter 12)

weight gain. They may develop maladaptive compensatory strategies in a relatively short time period and need close follow-up. Infants should be followed with craniofacial teams for comprehensive care. Follow-up evaluations are helpful in preparation for feeding alterations that may be needed in relation to surgical procedures.

Children with a history of functional or borderline compensated feeding skills may be referred for clinic oral sensorimotor and feeding evaluation following changes in health status that have a negative impact on safety of oral feeding, nutrition, or feeding skills. For example, a typical child who has a severe head injury with respiratory complications requiring a tracheotomy is likely to have swallowing and feeding problems in the acute phase of recovery that will require thorough assessment and follow-up intervention. Another example is the child with cerebral palsy (CP) who seems to do well until an upper respiratory infection at age 9 years. This child may not return to the level of efficiency evidenced prior to the episode and will need a team approach to evaluate and make recommendations for means to maximize the safety of feeding. Regardless of the reason for the referral, the first step in the assessment is to review the family, medical, developmental, and feeding history.

■ REVIEW OF FAMILY, MEDICAL, DEVELOPMENTAL, AND FEEDING HISTORY

The assessment of oral sensorimotor and feeding problems begins with a thorough history. Information is obtained from the medical chart, medical and educational professionals, parents, and other caregivers. Family, prenatal, birth, and neonatal histories are all important. Formats may differ from one institution to another, but the history should encompass the range of information suggested in Appendix A. The oral sensorimotor/feeding specialist may not have to get all of the following information independently because much of it may be available in prior reports. Whenever possible, the clinician should try to get information directly from a primary source, rather than relying on other interpretations that may be subject to eror. When conflicting or incomplete information is present, it is best to take your own history from an appropriate source. Obviously, there are significant differences in both process and content in relation to the range of medical–surgical problems and the age at which a patient is seen initially.

Family and Social History

Primary caregivers and the composition of the immediate family unit are identified. The social history yields information that is critical to the overall management plan. Awareness of rapidly changing social situations is important because the recommendations will be affected for both short- and long-range planning. Cultural, educational, and socioeconomic differences also may impact on management decisions.

Family history may reveal similar problems in other family members, for example, neurologic problems, cleft palate or other craniofacial anomalies, or respiratory/breathing and feeding difficulties. Environmental factors likely to have an adverse effect on a child's respiratory status include smoking or the presence of pets in the home.

Medical and Developmental Prenatal, Birth, and Perinatal History

Prenatal History to Birth

Aspects of prenatal history relevant to feeding and swallowing problems include, but are not limited to, maternal infection, medications taken by mother during pregnancy, substance abuse by father or mother, radiation, toxemia, bleeding, thyroid disease, or polyhydramnios (excessive volume of amniotic fluid). Helpful information about the birth and perinatal period can include, but is not limited to, Apgar scores, cord pH, trauma during delivery, prolonged hypoxia or anoxia, intubation, other respiratory distress, surfactant therapy, and cardiac status.

The Apgar scale (Apgar, 1966) is used routinely as part of the immediate care of a newborn infant. This scale permits a quick and thorough examination of a neonate's response to the birth process and immediate adaptation to extra-uterine life. Assessment is done routinely at 1 min after birth and again at 5 min, with each assessment taking about 1 min to complete. Five characteristics are measured: heart rate, respiratory effort, muscle tone, reflex irritability, and color (Table 7–2). Each attribute is scored 0, 1, or 2, and those scores are summed for a maximum score of 10. Scores are usually interpreted as poor (0–3), fair (4–7), and good (7–10).

Apgar scores are frequently used as a control on the population of infants investigated in neonatal follow-up studies, although a direct association has not been established between any complication during the birth process and a bad neurologic outcome in term newborns (Nelson & Ellenberg, 1984). Most newborns with low 5-min Apgar scores will be neurologically abnormal.

Cord pH is obtained by fetal scalp blood sampling to determine the fetal acid–base status. This procedure is performed only after rupture of the membranes. A blood sample is obtained from the fetal presenting part (usually the scalp but sometimes the buttocks), and the fetal blood pH is determined. A pH of 7.25 or greater has been shown to correlate (with 92% accuracy) with a 2-min Apgar score of 7 or greater. A pH of less than 7.15 correlates with a

Table 7–2. Apgar Scoring at 1 and 5 Minutes Following Birth

Attribute	Score		
	0	**1**	**2**
Heart rate	Absent	Below 100	Above 100
Repiratory effort	Absent	Slow, irregular, hypoventilation	Steady, good cry
Muscle tone	Flaccid	Some flexion of arms and legs	Good flexion, active motion
Irritability	No response	Some motion; cry	Vigorous cry
Color	Blue or pale	Blue hands and feet; pink body	Pink overall

Note. Adapted from "The Newborn (APGAR) Scoring System: Reflections and Advice," by V. Apgar, 1966, *Pediatric Clinics of North America, 13,* p. 645.

2-min Apgar score of less than 7 (80% accuracy). Standard protocol uses the following results (Gomella, Cunningham, & Eyal, 1994, p.3):

- pH > 7.25: Normal result; fetus is probably normal.
- pH < 7.20: Abnormal result; fetus is acidotic. If this result occurs in absence of maternal acidosis, and a repeat test done 10 min after the first reveals the same or more acidotic pH, delivery is indicated.
- pH between 7.20 and 7.25: Test should be repeated. Decisions regarding delivery depend on the clinical situation.

One illustration is presented to show the usefulness of these measures as an aid in understanding conditions in the neonatal intensive care unit (NICU). Perinatal asphyxia exists when an antepartum event, labor, or a birth process diminishes the oxygen supply to the fetus. The diminished oxygen supply causes decreased fetal or newborn heart rate, resulting in impairment of exchange of respiratory gases, oxygen, and carbon dioxide and inadequate perfusion of the tissues and major organs. Incidence figures vary because of nonuniform clinical criteria on which definitions are based. Incidence of perinatal asphyxia is reported in most centers at about 1.0 to 1.5%. It occurs in about 9% of infants less than 36 weeks gestational age and in 0.5% of infants more than 36 weeks gestational age (Snyder & Cloherty, 1998). Interestingly, less than 10% of children with CP show evidence of perinatal asphyxia.

Perinatal asphyxia is diagnosed by four clinical criteria (American Academy of Pediatrics, American College of Obstetricians and Gynecologists, 1992): (a) profound metabolic or mixed acidemia (pH < 7.00) on umbilical cord arterial blood sample: (b) persistence of Apgar score of 0 to 3 for > 5 min; (c) clinical neurologic sequelae in the immediate neonatal period to include seizures, hypotonia, coma, or hypoxic-ischemic encephalopathy; and (d) evidence of multiorgan system dysfunction in the immediate neonatal period. No one factor is likely to correlate with a feeding and swallowing problem, but each one may aid in delineation of the problem.

Medical and Developmental History Specific to Neonates (First 28 Days)

Significant events pointing to neurologic dysfunction during the neonatal period include the need for prolonged resuscitation, altered states of consciousness, seizures, deficient movement, and disturbances of sucking and swallowing (Fenichel, 1990). Feeding deficits in these first few weeks of life may be markers for possible underlying neurologic problems. Because neurologic problems frequently manifest themselves in the neonatal period, information regarding arousal and alertness, respiratory status, rooting and other reflexes (see Chapter 3), medication, and nonnutritive sucking is sought. Prior medical tests and surgeries, if any, are noted.

Feeding History

Feeding history can differ among reporters because their perceptions about the child's skills and abilities vary (Reilly & Skuse, 1992). Children frequently demonstrate different behavior with different feeders in different environments. Variability is a real phenomenon and this will often complicate decision making for treatment plans. Caregivers' descriptions of feeding behaviors are usually accurate and reliable from each one's perspective. Nonetheless, denial of or lack of awareness of problems, especially with inconsistent reports from one observer to another, needs to be explored. For example, food refusal may be interpreted as a child being lazy or not hungry when, in fact, the child is saying "no" because of the discomfort related to silent aspiration, gastroesophageal reflux, or esophagitis.

When asked about concern for aspiration, caregivers of 16 of 48 children who demonstrated aspiration on fluoroscopy said they had no concern regarding possible aspiration because the child did not cough or gag when eating and drinking (Arvedson, Rogers, Buck, Smart, & Msall, 1994). Videofluoroscopic swallow study (VFSS) revealed silent aspiration for all but 2 (94%) of the children who aspirated. This finding emphasizes that with CNS damage, the probability of a cough response to aspiration is low. Caregivers cannot accept the lack of cough as a sign of safe feeding. Other signs and symptoms that may become evident by history include hoarseness or gurgly voice quality, respiratory stridor, recurrent pneumonias or upper respiratory tract infections, apnea, and cyanosis (Chapter 4) (Christie, 1984; Illingworth, 1969; Kramer, 1985).

Clinicians are wise to get information from more than one person and in multiple formats. Caregivers may complete a printed questionnaire before they come to the initial clinic evaluation. Clinicians can ask questions in an interview during the evaluation session. A combination of questionnaire and interview is likely to yield the most complete and comprehensive history. Insuring that the questions asked are clear and understandable requires knowledge of the caregivers' language, culture, and education.

Parents should be asked to describe feeding behaviors rather than answer simple questions that require "yes" or "no" responses. For example, "Describe what your baby does when the milk flow is too fast," gives more information than, "Does your baby choke when the milk flow is too fast?" The answer to "Tell me how your child chews" yields more useful information to the clinician than a simple question, such as, "Does she have trouble chewing?"

Table 7–3. Factors Included in a Feeding History for Oral and Nonoral Feeders

- Position(s) for feeding and seating arrangements
- Duration of feeding times (average and range)
- Intervals between feedings or meal times
- Tube feeding (type, partial or total nutrition, nighttime rate)
- Infants: Breast or bottle feeding (types of nipples, formula), burping ease
- Children who get food as well as liquid: Types of textures, use of utensils
- Child's participation in self-feeding process (total or assisted)
- Diet: At least a 3-day diet history is helpful including all food and liquid with amounts; permits dietitian to calculate nutritional value and calories
- Respiratory status: Aspiration pneumonia, bronchitis, asthma, etc. Noisy breathing, gurgly voice quality with feeding, coughing, choking
- Other signs of distress: Fussy during feeding, food refusal, falling asleep, arching, neck hyperextension
- Other factors: Tests (e.g., upper gastrointestinal study [UGI], scintiscan, pH probe, videofluoroscopic swallow study [VFSS]; surgical procedures, medical treatments, medications)
- Sleep patterns: Waking during the night, snoring, mouth breathing
- Cognitive and communication status: Verbal and nonverbal skill levels
- Behavior during meals: Stress at meal times, participation with family
- History of therapeutic intervention for developmental or feeding problems

Feeding history includes the questions relative to the factors shown in Table 7–3. These items are applicable even for infants and children who have never fed orally (Appendix A shows options). Duration of mealtimes should be explored thoroughly. Lengthy meal times can be a marker for feeding and swallowing problems. Longer feeding times do not compensate for the severity of feeding impairments in many multiply handicapped children (Gisel & Patrick, 1988). Meal times should take approximately 30 min in most cultures. If on a routine basis 45 to 50 min or more are required to complete a meal, changes need to be made to improve the efficiency. The risk for aspiration increases with the duration of meal times (Arvedson et al., 1994). Duration of meal times also must be considered in relationship to other activities that are important in each day. The child should not expend more energy eating than what is consumed. Some mothers have reported spending up to 7 hours a day feeding a handicapped child (Johnson & Deitz, 1985). Clinicians should question whether parental reports may be exaggerated in relation to the stress involved in meal times. Videotaped feeding sessions of 12 children with CP and oral sensorimotor dysfunction were compared with matched control subjects (age, gender, and race) (Reilly & Skuse, 1992). Duration of meals did not differ significantly, although parents of the children with CP had reported excessive time spent on meals.

The nutrition status (Chapter 6) and the interactive behaviors of the caregiver and child are also important factors (Chapter 13). The long-term prognosis for development of functional oral sensorimotor skills and safe oral feeding relates directly to the underlying health and neurologic status. The information gained through thorough history taking is invaluable in planning the rest of the evaluation. There is no single pediatric assessment scale that can be recommended to encompass all aspects of a clinic feeding and swallowing evaluation. Some published assessments are described in Appendix B. Clinicians frequently take portions of commercially available scales and modify them to meet the needs of their populations, institutions, or practice patterns.

■ PHYSICAL EXAMINATION

The clinical examination of feeding and swallowing in infants and children begins with overall observation of the individual that includes attention to posture and position, state of alertness, airway status, neurodevelopment, communication, oral sensorimotor status, whole body sensory awareness, and cognitive levels of functioning. The initial signs and symptoms of feeding difficulties may be markers for broader central or peripheral nervous system deficits and closely related to airway and gastrointestinal tract function. Clinicians must be able to interpret cues from the child indicating readiness to feed or not to feed as the case may be.

The overall goals of assessment are to determine the nature of the problem and the most effective methods of management. It must be realized, however, that assessment is an ongoing process. Furthermore, caregivers are an integral part of the assessment process as well as the treatment program.

Readiness for Feeding: Sensory and Posture Issues

Oral Sensory Assessment

Sensory factors are basic to motor function, and as a result of developmental processes, older infants and children acquire competence in the evaluation of the physical character of food and are able to ingest it voluntarily. Bosma (1986) stated that sensory information is generated primarily by voluntary motions of the tongue, lips, and mandible. A prefeeding examination includes observations of responses to visual and auditory stimuli, as well as to smell, touch, and taste. Stimuli can be varied on several parameters, for example, degree of brightness, loudness of sounds, and firm-to-light touch to the face and mouth.

A standardized oral sensory assessment presently is not available. Sensory histories include test items that assess oral sensory defensiveness (e.g.,

Blanche, Botticelli, & Hallway, 1995). Astute clinicians can obtain information through a feeding observation. Some examples of commercially available assessments are listed at the end of Appendix B. Children may demonstrate a hyporeactive, hyperreactive, or sensory-defensive response to sensory input (Table 7–4) (Blanche et al.; Morris & Klein, 1987, 2000; Palmer & Heyman, 1993). These disorders represent problems with sensory modulation, or the ability to receive and grade sensory input from the environment (Case-Smith & Humphry, 2000). These disorders interfere with a child's ability to discriminate oral sensory input accurately and may therefore impair oral–motor function. If sensory overload becomes too great,

Table 7–4. Characteristics to Aid in Differentiation of Children with Oral Sensory and Motor Disorders

Sensory Disorder	Motor Disorder
Demonstrates nipple confusion with breast-feeding and bottle-feeding	Inefficient suck with breast and bottle
Inability to differentiate different tastes in a bottle despite an intact suck	Differentiates tastes in a bottle
Manages liquids better than solid foods	Oral motor inefficiency or incoordination is noted with all textures
Able to sort food out in a mixed texture	Swallows food whole when offered mixed textures
Holds food under tongue or in cheek and avoids swallowing	Unable to hold and manipulate bolus on tongue; food falls out of mouth or into cheeks
Vomiting only certain textures	Vomiting is not texture specific
Gags when food approaches or touches lip	Gags after food is moved through oral cavity
Hypersensitive gag with solids; normal liquid swallow	Gags with liquids and solids after swallow is triggered
Tolerates own fingers in mouth, does not accept someone else's fingers	Tolerates others' fingers in mouth
Does not mouth toys	Accepts teething toys but is unable to bite them or maintain them in the mouth
Refuses toothbrushing	Accepts toothbrushing

Note. Adapted from "Assessment and Treatment of Sensory Moter-Based Feeding Problems in Very Young Children," by M. M. Palmer and M. B. Heyman, 1993, *Infants and Young Children, 6,* pp. 67–73.

coping strategies may include attempts to organize the environment by rhythmic behaviors, avoidance of eye contact, or inconsistent response to sensory input. Typical rhythmic behaviors, usually seen in older infants and children, are rocking, thumb or finger sucking, flapping hands or arms, and spinning objects (Morris & Klein, 1987). The interrelationships of sensory input and motor coordination of oral structures are complex.

Hyporeactive Responses

Children with hyporeactive responses to oral input may have diminished response to taste, temperature, or the proprioceptive input associated with chewing and sucking (Case-Smith & Humphry, 2000; Glass & Wolf, 1998). This may result in a craving for foods that provide increased oral input (e.g., strong flavors, crunchy textures, extreme temperatures), drooling, and an inclination to stuff too much food into the mouth. These children may also demonstrate poor sucking or chewing skills because they are not receiving appropriate sensory input to support refined skills.

Hyperreactive Responses

Children with hyperreactive responses to oral sensory input typically have a CNS disorder. They may have excessive response to taste, temperature, and touch in and around the oral region that manifests as an increase in hypertonicity or abnormal motor movements. For example, they may respond to sensory input, such as a strong taste, with a jaw thrust or a tongue thrust (Morris & Klein, 1987). Oral hypersensitivity may be a prominent symptom in children with respiratory difficulties, esophagitis, or gastroesophageal reflux disease/extra-esophageal reflux disease (GERD/EERD).[1] In some instances, the underlying physiologic disturbances may be marked by oral aversiveness. Thus, the importance of the interdisciplinary team is again emphasized, so that accurate diagnoses can be made as a basis for appropriate intervention.

Oral Sensory Defensiveness

Children with oral sensory defensiveness demonstrate an emotional response to sensory input in or around the oral region. Sensory defensiveness may be a part of a whole-body response to sensory input, or it may be

---

[1]Gastroesophageal reflux disease (GERD) refers to the abnormal regurgitation of acid into the esophagus causing symptoms. When the acid and other stomach contents emerge from the upper esophageal sphincter into the pharynx, larynx, mouth, and nasal cavities, the most commonly accepted term is extra-esophageal reflux disease or EERD (Sasaki & Toohill, 2000).

confined to the oral region. A whole-body response is often seen in children with developmental delay, learning disabilities, or autism (Wilbarger & Wilbarger, 1991). Children who have had aversive oral medical treatments or who have had a period of sensory deprivation due to gastrostomy tube feedings may have an emotional response that is confined to the mouth and oral region. Other children may have sensory defensiveness due to CNS impairment that influences the sensory innervation to the oral region (Case-Smith & Humphry, 2000). Children with sensory defensiveness may avoid many textures and tastes, demonstrate an aversion to tooth brushing, and never mouth toys. They may put their own fingers to their mouth but be defensive to oral input from another individual (Palmer & Heyman, 1993).

Sensory or Motor-Based Problems

It is often difficult to differentiate between a motor and a sensory-based feeding problem. Some children may demonstrate both sensory and motor problems in varying degrees. Some behaviors that can help to differentiate whether a child is demonstrating an abnormal oral–motor response, an abnormal swallow, or sensory based problems are listed in Table 7–4 (Palmer & Heyman, 1993).

Children with neuromuscular disorders may have sensorimotor dysfunction. Children who have a history of receiving invasive oral treatments related to conditions such as chronic lung disease, tracheoesophageal fistula, esophageal atresia, and cardiac defects also may demonstrate sensorimotor dysfunction (Palmer & Heyman, 1993). Some children with no documented neuromuscular or developmental disorder also may demonstrate problems in this area.

Some children with an abnormal response to sensory input during meal times have behavior problems related to eating and feeding. Children who have sensory issues (tactile defensiveness, hypersensitivity, or both) often produce avoidance responses to varied types of stimulation or exhibit a generalized irritability. The child's ability to self-calm and regulate is noted. Children who are irritable during mealtime or who frequently refuse various tastes and food textures may be responding to what they perceive as aversive sensory input. Adults may misinterpret these responses as negative or belligerent behaviors. Children with sensory problems also may learn to manipulate the mealtime environment to avoid unpleasant sensory experiences. Detailed discussion is found in Chapter 13.

Postural Control

A comprehensive assessment of feeding also should focus on a child's muscle tone, postural control, and overall fine and gross motor skill levels. The importance of good posture for safe and efficient feeding is well documented (e.g., Alexander, 1987; Glass & Wolf, 1998; Larnett & Ekberg, 1995; Macie & Arvedson, 1993; Morris & Klein, 1987, 2000; Morton, Bonas, Fourie, & Minford, 1993).

Abnormal Muscle Tone

Normal development of muscle tone has been described in Chapter 2. Clinicians need to understand abnormal muscle tone and postural control to make observations during the clinical assessment of feeding and swallowing. The emergence of abnormal motor skills in children with CNS dysfunction may result from poor internal control of proximal body parts due to abnormal muscle tone. Young infants with CNS dysfunction first develop hypotonia, which then results in an inadequate and unstable base for more refined extremity and oral sensorimotor movement. Children with abnormal muscle tone may develop abnormal sitting postures when they attempt to sit up. They may not have the internal control or the stable base necessary to adapt to a supporting surface. Therefore, they will demonstrate stereotypic, rather than normal, sitting postures. These abnormal stereotypic postures may include head–neck hyperextension, scapular adduction, and humeral adduction and internal rotation (Bly, 1994). Hypotonia of the trunk also may lead to a tendency to sit with an abnormal kyphotic posture, with the spine flexed forward. These abnormal postures provide a poor base of stability, thus interfering with the development of refined oral-motor function (Figure 7–2).

Older children with CNS disorders may demonstrate abnormal muscle tone including hypotonia, or low muscle tone (Capute & Accardo, 1991). This is characterized by decreased resistance to passive range of motion, increased joint range of motion, and poor ability to move up against gravity. Other children demonstrate hypertonic muscle tone, or spasticity (Figure 7–3). Increased resistance to passive joint movement and limitations in joint range of motion are identified. Children with spasticity also may demonstrate abnormal movement patterns and remnants of primitive postural reflexes. These children may develop joint deformities that include contractures. Children with athetosis demonstrate fluctuating muscle tone that manifests as random movement patterns. Based on the intricate relationship between overall body posture and oral sensorimotor function, children with CNS disorder and abnormal muscle tone are at risk for oral sensorimotor dysfunction.

Prefeeding Observations of Older Children

Problems with central alignment, tone, and positioning relate directly to the oral sensorimotor system. Observations are made about head and trunk control with the child in his or her usual sitting position in whatever seating system is used for feeding. Particular attention should be paid to the child's

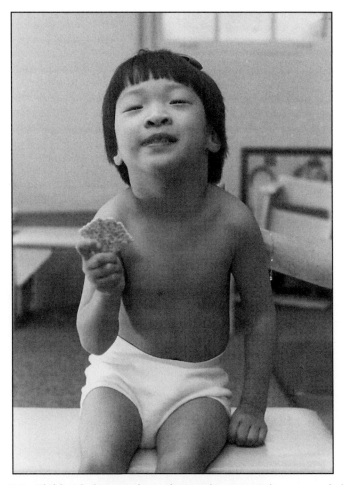

Figure 7–2. Child with decreased muscle tone (hypotonia), hyperextended neck, and trunk shifted to the left. She has difficulty in self-feeding.

posture and movement patterns. Presence of primitive reflexes, level of physical activity, and any type of independent oral stimulation (putting objects or fingers into the mouth) are noted. The clinician observes the child for overall affect, temperament, and responsiveness. Areas to evaluate include the level of alertness, head and mouth position, presence of drooling, and means of both verbal and nonverbal communication between parents and child. The clinician notes the child's use of eye contact, head turning, touch, and avoidance responses.

Posture influences the oral preparatory (or bolus formation), oral, pharyngeal, and esophageal phases of swallowing. Gross and fine motor skill

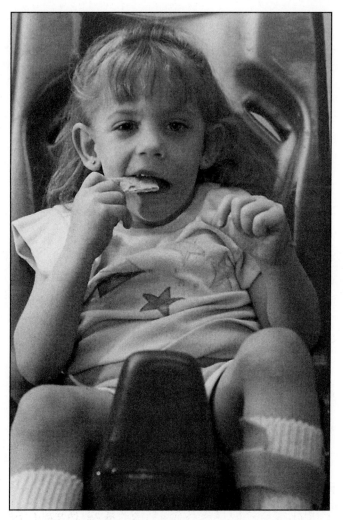

Figure 7–3. Child with cerebral palsy who has increased muscle tone (hypertonia) with increased flexion in upper extremities. She has difficulty in self-feeding and needs posterior support.

development, respiration and phonation, and oral sensorimotor/feeding skills are interrelated in intricate ways as discussed in Chapter 2.

Posture and the Oral Phase of the Swallow

Abnormal oral postures may be used to attempt to provide stability. The development of tongue retraction, an abnormal oral sensorimotor skill noted during feeding in a child with CP, may be directly related to abnormal posture and poor muscle tone (Alexander, 1987). The child may use an abnormal pattern of neck hyperextension and tongue retraction as an abnormal base of stability to lift and turn the head and open the mouth. A child with CP also may use humeral extension or scapular retraction as an abnormal base of stability. These maladaptive compensations promote poor tongue, jaw, cheek, and lip mobility.

Posture and the Pharyngeal Phase of the Swallow

Neck hyperextension influences the alignment of pharyngeal structures and places children at higher risk for aspiration during feeding. Postural control also is related to coordination between respiration and swallowing during feeding. A child must demonstrate stability through the spine and mobility in the rib cage for efficient respiration. This relationship of stability and mobility is crucial during the intricate coordination of breathing and swallowing that takes place during oral feeding (Oetter, Richter, & Frick, 1995).

Posture and the Esophageal Phase of the Swallow

GERD/EERD may be influenced by body posture. Orenstein and Whitington (1983) suggested that the supine position for infants may increase GERD/EERD. The American Academy of Pediatrics (2000) recommended that healthy infants be positioned in supine for sleep, including infants with GERD/EERD. There is no increase in deaths attributable to aspiration with change from prone to supine sleeping for infants in the United Kingdom (Fleming, 1994). Meyers and Herbst (1982) recommended placing the infant in a prone position with the head elevated 30° for 1 to 2 hours after feeding. Orenstein (1990) studied 100 infants under 6 months of age using esophageal pH probe studies in the flat prone position and in the prone position with 30° of head elevation. The flat prone position was as effective in preventing reflux as the prone position with head elevation for infants under 6 months of age. The head-elevated position may be beneficial for infants under 10 days of age, but not for older infants (Orenstein). Chapter 5 discusses management of GERD/EERD in greater detail.

Optimal Feeding Posture

The optimal sitting posture to support oral sensorimotor function includes the following (Alexander, 1987; Glass & Wolf, 1998) (Figure 7–4):

1. Neutral head position (symmetry, midline stability), with balance between flexion and extension
2. Neck elongation

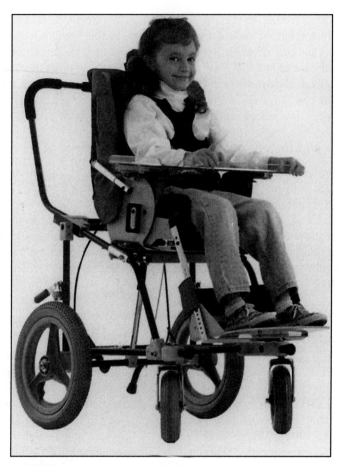

Figure 7–4. Child seated in a Kid-Kart system to demonstrate "optimal" positioning for feeding.

3. Symmetrical shoulder girdle stability and depression
4. Symmetrical trunk elongation
5. Pelvis stability, with the child's hips symmetrical in neutral position
6. Hips, knees, and ankles each at 90°, with neutral base of abduction and rotation
7. Symmetrical and stable positioning of the feet in neutral with slight dorsiflexion (never plantar flexed), supported by a firm surface

Suggestions that apply to many children include the use of minimal flexion of the cervical vertebrae that allows the shoulders to be slightly in front of the body. The thoracic portion of the spine can be extended to assist with thoracic cavity extension for maximizing respiratory function (Geyer & McGowan, 1995). Complications arise when children have significant scoliosis or kyphosis, making it more difficult to achieve an optimal position. Although this information is useful and makes intuitive and clinical sense, it is not based on empiric data. Further research is needed to provide more specific guidelines regarding the best posture for optimal oral sensorimotor function. It is likely that there is no single best posture and that variations are needed to meet the needs of individual infants and children.

■ EXAMINATION OF INFANTS

Premature Infants in the Neonatal Intensive Care Unit

Professionals who are called into the Neonatal Intensive Care Unit (NICU) to examine infants with sucking and swallowing problems must have extensive knowledge about the physiology of sucking and swallowing as well as etiologies and diagnoses of the infants. It is critical to understand the implications of various genetic, neurologic, pulmonary, cardiac, and gastrointestinal disorders that these often critically ill infants experience. Prognoses for short- and long-term oral feeding usually are directly related to the physical and physiologic status. It is as important for the feeding specialist to be able to state that an infant is not ready for oral feeding as it is to give guidance for ways to maximize oral feeding skills and safety in those infants who are stable and ready to feed orally.

The survival of very-low-birth-weight (VLBW) infants has increased from approximately 50% for infants weighing less than 800 g in the period 1986 to 1990 to 70% by 1994 for infants weighing less than 750 g. The survival rate up to 1980 was only 20%. Thus, only recently has the focus on evaluating infants in the NICU become widespread. In addition to knowledge about etiologies, clinicians need to have a reasonable fund of knowledge about embryology and genetics. Premature infants have immature postural tone, respiratory function, and structural alignment. Body position appears to affect blood gases and lung mechanics of VLBW infants during tube feedings. Prone position results in a significant increase in arterial oxygen saturation during nasogastric (NG) tube feeding (Mizuno & Aizawa, 1999). The prone position may allow for improvement in lung mechanics by decreasing energy expenditure for spontaneous breathing and may shorten the period of ventilator support for very-low-birth-weight infants with chronic lung disease. Infants usually need to be off ventilator support for the clinician to consider oral feeding. Basic guidelines related to respiratory rate are helpful to determine whether oral feeding should even be considered during an initial bedside examination:

- Postpone oral feeding if resting respiratory rate is > 70 breaths per minute (BPM) prior to feeding.
- Stop oral feeding if respiratory rate goes higher than 80–85 BPM during oral feeding.

Despite the presence of both swallowing (11 to 12 weeks) and sucking (18 to 24 weeks) behaviors in utero, suck–swallow and breathing are not expected to be well enough coordinated for successful oral feeding to meet nutritional needs until about 34 weeks gestational age in most premature infants. Some healthy preterm infants may demonstrate readiness for oral feeding by 32 weeks and, in some instances, even earlier. Once infants can tolerate enteral feedings, they usually get nutritional needs met via orogastric (OG) or NG tube feedings. Until premature infants demonstrate readiness for essentially all feedings orally, they continue with OG or NG tube feeds for assurance of meeting nutritional needs. "Normal" premature infants of 34 to 36 weeks gestation may demonstrate skills that show positive prognosis for becoming full oral feeders, but in fact they may not consistently take oral feedings efficiently until closer to 37 weeks gestation. Prior to that time, opportunities can be given for nonnutritive sucking on a pacifier or a caregiver's little finger, along with partial nipple feeds, as tolerated (Chapter 9).

Feeding specialists may be consulted for consideration of oral feeding for infants once they are medically and surgically stable. Specialists also may be consulted for infants who clearly are not ready to begin oral feeding but who should benefit from nonnutritive stimulation that can help to prepare them for oral feeding, to assist in normalizing all aspects of development, and, in some instances, help prepare families for the potential of long-term nonoral feeding needs. Early identification of neonates at risk for developing feeding problems in infancy is important for potential prevention of severe problems (Hawdon, Beauregard, Slattery, & Kennedy, 2000).

After a thorough reading of the medical chart, a clinician can begin the bedside assessment by making observations of the infant at rest to note the following:

- state, posture, and position;
- sensitivity to stimuli;
- respiratory status;
- heart rate; and
- oral-peripheral mechanism.

Any asymmetry of the extremities, trunk, and especially the face is noted. Infants with *increased* tone and hypersensitivity to stimuli tend to have uncoordinated sucking. In contrast, infants with *decreased* tone and lack of sensory arousal frequently have poor initiation of sucking with weakness. Open mouth posture that can indicate mouth breathing raises the possibility of low tone or upper airway obstruction, given that infants are described as primarily nasal breathers. Premature infants may be unable to integrate sensory input from the environment. The examiner must be alert to signals that indicate stress or lack of integration. These signals may include dusky skin color, irregular breathing patterns, overall agitated state, and reduced level of alertness.

Oral sensorimotor patterns of premature infants, as well as other physical and physiologic attributes, are different from term infants (Table 7–5; Figures 7–5 and 7–6). Infants with poor sucking abilities have been found to require significantly longer feeding times (Casaer, Daniels, Devlieger, DeCock, & Eggermont 1982). With gavage feeding or prolonged use of endotracheal tubes, oral function may not develop readily. In some infants, oral function can become disorganized with decreased sucking abilities. Coordinated nonnutritive sucking and swallowing are necessary but not sufficient for the development of an adequate suck/swallow/breathe pattern for nutritive purposes in infants.

Table 7–5. Physical and Physiologic Attributes of Premature and Term Infants for Feeding Readiness

Attribute	Premature Infants	Term Infants
Position/posture	Extensor	Flexor
Neck, trunk, & shoulder stability	Poor	Good
Set for sucking anatomically	Unfavorable	Favorable
Suck strength	Weak	Strong
Lip seal	Inadequate	Adequate
Cheek stability	Unstable	Good
Jaw stability for repetitive suck	Insufficient	Sufficient
Hunger and thirst signals	Inadequate	Adequate
Neurologic status	Disorganized, irritable	Organized
Suck/swallow/ breathe pattern	Dysrhythmic	Rhythmic
Oral–motor reflexes	Incomplete	Intact

Note. Adapted from *Pre-feeding Skills: A Comprehensive Resource for Feeding Development* (p.313), by S. E. Morris and M. D. Klein, 1987. Tucson, AZ: Therapy Skill Builders.

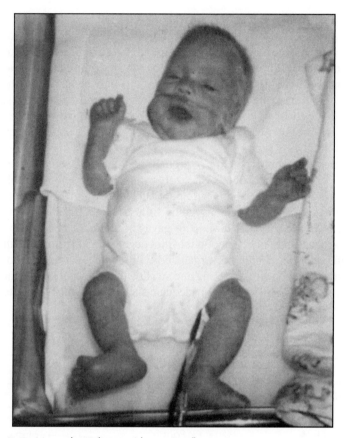

Figure 7–5. Normal newborn with passive flexor posture.

If the clinician does not find any contraindications to continuing the examination, the infant can be picked up and placed in an appropriate position for potential feeding. The infant may attain and maintain a calm, alert state if swaddled and held semiupright in a neutral posture that keeps the trunk, neck, and head in a straight line. Respiratory rate should stay in the range of 40 to 60 BPM, except possibly in infants with cardiac problems who are likely to have a more rapid respiratory rate. Check for rooting responses, which should be seen when infants are hungry as they search for the breast or other nipple. If rooting is not spontaneous, consider stroking rhythmically from ear to mouth in a firm but gentle way at a rate of 1 stroke per sec. This is the rate of nutritive sucking. The next step is evaluation of nonnutritive sucking.

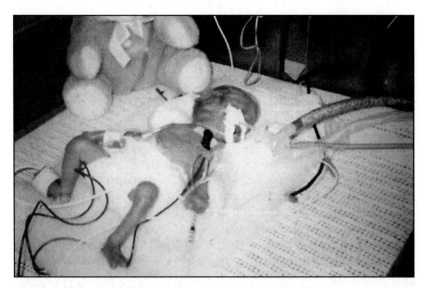

Figure 7–6. Premature infant with passive extensor posture.

Nonnutritive Sucking

Nonnutritive sucking is assessed as the examiner eases a gloved fifth finger slowly into the infant's mouth to the midtongue region. The finger should be placed no further posteriorly than the upper border of the soft palate so as not to elicit a gag reflex (McBride & Danner, 1987). This is accomplished with the infant held so that the head is in neutral position. Nonnutritive sucking or mouthing on the examiner's fifth finger for 1 min is measured in sucks per sec (Case-Smith, Cooper, & Scala, 1989). The rate should be 2 sucks per sec. If no sucking action is noted, try stroking the tongue or the hard palate from mid to front at 1 stroke per sec (nutritive sucking rate) 4 to 6 times, then stop and hold finger in the infant's mouth. Repeat after several seconds up to 10 to 12 times. Slow removal and replacement of the finger on the tongue at least twice allows for observation of initiation of movement, cupping of the tongue, and extension and retraction of the tongue.

The normal infant closes the mouth and will initiate a sucking action spontaneously and immediately. The tongue of an infant with hypotonia will feel soft and can be moved easily by the examiner, whereas the tongue of an infant with hypertonia may be firm and contracted. An excessive bite is present if the jaws clamp firmly against the finger and sucking does not begin. Nonnutritive sucking can be assessed immediately before an oral feeding or a nonoral tube feeding, as well as during a tube feeding. Breathing patterns are observed for any changes in rate and rhythm. The presence of any respiratory noises during nonnutritive suck and swallow are also noted. All signs of respiratory distress require in-depth evaluation before evaluation of nutritive sucking is undertaken (Chapter 4).

An adequate nonnutritive sucking pattern may not necessarily lead to adequate nutritive sucking for successful oral feeding. Nonetheless, some benefits of nonnutritive sucking have been demonstrated to facilitate a more rapid transition from gavage to oral feedings (Bernbaum, Pereira, Watkins, & Peckham, 1983), for increasing transcutaneous oxygen tension in infants between 32 and 35 weeks postconceptional age (Paludetto, Robertson, Hack, Shivpuri, & Martin, 1984), and for increasing weight gain with earlier discharge from hospital (Field et al., 1982).

Elicitation of the *Santmyer swallow* is another method for stimulating a swallow in infants (Orenstein, Giarrusso, Proujansky, & Kocoshis, 1988). This infant reflex is elicited by gently blowing a puff of air in the infant's face, which should then result in a swallow in infants ranging in age from 33 weeks gestation to 11 months. Children from 11 months to 2 years of age vary in their responses. Neurologically normal children older that 2 years of age should not show a *Santmyer swallow*. This stimulus may be useful in making initial observations about the timing of a swallow production because the response is an immediate primary peristaltic sequence with motility characteristics identical to spontaneous swallowing. The *Santmyer swallow* is useful during the placement of a nasogastric tube or a pH probe when a swallow is needed for tube placement (Orenstein et al.). It has also been used when evaluating swallowing function during esophageal manometry.

If the infant does not demonstrate a functional nonnutritive suck, the clinician should make recommendations for oral stimulation that may help prepare the infant for oral feeding. If the infant demonstrates a functional nonnutritive suck and has a stable airway, proceed with a feeding evaluation.

Nutritive Sucking and Swallowing

The feeding evaluation is most likely carried out with a nipple and bottle, unless the mother is in the NICU and prepared to breast-feed. If the infant has an OG or NG tube, it should be removed for the feeding evaluation when one anticipates that the infant may truly be ready for oral feeds. Infants with NG tubes are shown to have saturations significantly lower than those with OG tubes before, during, and after feedings (Daga, Lunkad, Daga, & Ahuja, 1999). If, however, history and physical findings suggest that the infant is not likely to take much liquid orally, it may be better for the infant to keep the tube in place. NG tubes do have deleterious effects in VLBW infants: e.g.

decreased nasal airflow, increased airway resistance, and abnormal airway distribution. An intermittent NG tube may create other problems: insertion stimulates the larynx and may cause a laryngospasm. Apnea and bradycardia are more likely, and pharyngeal and esophageal trauma are possible (Symington, Ballantyne, Pinelli, & Stevens, 1995). An NG tube that is in place before feeding can affect the start of the oral feeds with lower tidal volume and lower minute ventilation. An NG tube in place during feeding can affect the feeding by decreasing tidal volume, minute ventilation, pulse rate, oxygen saturation, force of sucking, and volume consumed (e.g., Daga et al.; Greenspan et al., 1990).

The evaluation of an oral feeding should be carried out with the infant feeding for at least 15 to 20 min, which is sufficient for a premature infant to take the full feeding if he or she is efficient. It is a time frame that allows a clinician to determine whether the infant becomes disorganized or fatigued as the feeding continues. These observations are important for potential recommendations about the oral feeding plan. The efficient feeder is likely to suck at a rate of 1 suck per sec, in bursts of anywhere from 10 to 30 suck/swallow sequences, then a pause of 1 to 2 seconds as the infant takes a breath and swallows an additional time or two. The pattern is repeated for the duration of the feeding. Sucking bursts are likely to get shorter near the end of the feeding. The infant may be tested with different nipples and containers when the initial nipple does not make the infant appear safe and efficient. Viscosity can be changed as one of the variables in flow rate. If the flow rate is too fast, the infant will have to work to slow it down. That may be more troublesome than if the infant has to work harder to suck and swallow the liquid. Most infant assessments consist of descriptive observations, which are compared with normal development. Deviations from normal are noted (see Appendix B).

Decisions about management recommendations (Chapter 9) have to take into account multiple factors related to underlying physical and physiologic status, as well as the performance during the feeding evaluation. Neonates, particularly VLBW infants, with disorganized or dysfunctional feeding are at high risk for longer term feeding problems that may include difficulties in making the transition to solid food at 6 months of age and for tolerating lumpy food by 12 months of age (Hawdon et al., 2000).

Infant Evaluation

Term and premature infants are different in a number of attributes that have an impact on oral feeding (Morris & Klein, 1987) (Table 7–5). By the time infants reach 39 to 40 weeks gestation or term, they demonstrate physiologic flexion of the limbs that contributes to successful oral feeding. Rhythmic suck/swallow/breathe coordination is another necessary characteristic.

Prefeeding Observation

The same principles used in the NICU hold for observation of infants before doing any feeding evaluation. It is always useful to approach infants with the intent of doing more watching than handling. The infant is first observed when awake and not being stimulated so that the level of spontaneous activity can be noted, as described above.

A complete assessment of oral structures and function is made before any introduction of liquid. Lip action is important for latching on to the breast and getting a seal for both breast and nipple feeding via bottle. Visual inspection of the structures in the mouth (tongue, palate, buccal musculature, and pharynx) permits identification of any structural abnormality that could interfere with sucking and swallowing.

A cleft of the palate, with or without cleft lip, may be observed (Chapter 12). A submucous cleft of the soft palate, characterized by notching at the junction of the hard and soft palate with a zona pellucida (indicating submucosal diastasis of palatal musculature) and a bifid uvula, may or may not be symptomatic in relation to feeding function (Figure 4–2). Shape and height of the hard palate are also noted. Children who were intubated orally for as few as 2 weeks during the newborn period may develop a persistent narrow groove in the midline of the hard palate. This complication is reported in up to 87.5% of orally intubated infants (Erenberg & Nowak, 1984) (Figures 7–7 and 7–8). Intraoral palatal prostheses can be fabricated to protect the palate during periods of prolonged endotracheal intubation (von Gunten, Meyer, & Kim, 1995). Palatal groove formation is also reported in infants who were fed for prolonged periods with OG tubes (Arens & Reichman, 1992). The palatal architecture is disrupted and these children exhibit a high incidence of enamel defects in primary dentition. Preventive measures include acrylic palatal appliances or preferential use of NG tubes. As children get older, food may get lodged in the groove. A high arched palate has no proven negative effects on oral–motor function. Tongue shape, placement "at rest," and movement patterns are observed before any food or liquid is presented.

The presence of rooting responses and the quality of tongue action can lead to inferences about the readiness to suck. The rooting response of a normal infant is a head turn toward the side being stroked, or the infant may make side-to-side head movements while turning toward the side where stroking occurred. The infant will search by moving the lips and head to try to take the stimulus into the mouth.

Laryngeal function for airway protection is inferred by perceptual observation of vocal quality. Voice quality may change when the child's position for feeding is changed. The clearest voice quality for a specific infant is usually noted when that infant is in the best position for feeding,

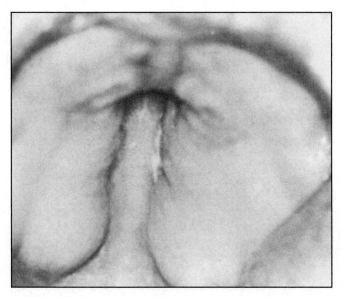

Figure 7–7. Groove formed in the midline of hard palate and alveolar ridge by orotracheal intubation in an infant born at 38 weeks gestation. Notching can be seen anterior to posterior in the alveolar ridge to the soft palate.

whether upright, side lying, or prone. A "gurgly" voice quality may indicate pooling or residue of material in the pharyngeal recesses; however, normal phonation is only an indirect indication of laryngeal function for airway protection during swallowing and not a guarantee that the pharyngeal recesses are free of residue or that aspiration is absent (Chapters 4 and 10).

Infant Nutritive Sucking Observation

The first oral feeding observation is performed after the infant's cardiac and respiratory status are stable, bowel sounds are adequate, and feedings can be done with minimal respiratory distress (Babson, Pernoll, & Benda, 1980). Three major concerns of the examiner are: (a) safe feeding with minimal risk for aspiration, (b) functional feeding with sufficient caloric intake to assure weight gain within a reasonable length of time at each feed, and (c) pleasurable feeding (Harris, 1986). Unless pleasurable feeding occurs regularly and efficiently, the infant is in danger of undernutrition or malnutrition. To reiterate, adequate weight gain is critical in the first months of life.

Observation of the infant feeding for at least 15 to 20 min is helpful because there are some infants who appear to have adequate coordination for

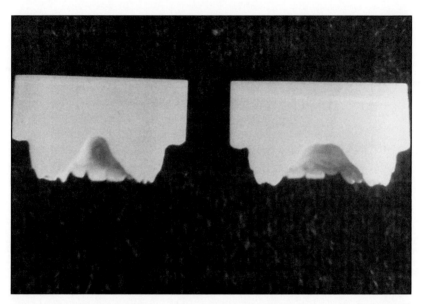

Figure 7–8. Plaster model of cross-section at the first permanent molar in a 7-year-old child. The left model shows the persistent V-shaped deformity in the hard palate associated with orotracheal intubation for a few weeks as an infant. The one on the right is normal.
Note: From "Pediatric Dentistry," by J. E. Bernat, 1992. In L. Brodsky, L. Holt, and D. H. Ritter–Schmidt (Eds.), *Craniofacial Anomalies: An Interdisciplinary Approach* (p. 157). St. Louis: Mosby Year Book. Copyright 1992 by the publisher. Reprinted by permission.

the first few minutes but then cannot sustain the necessary rhythmic suck/swallow/breathe patterns long enough to take sufficient quantity to meet nutritional needs. A rhythmic pattern of nutritive sucking is expected to occur at a rate of 1 suck per sec. The sucking sequence consists of "bursts" followed by a brief pause of 1 to 2 sec. The burst usually consists of 10 to 30 sucks in rapid succession. A typical healthy infant appears to be sucking nearly constantly, with frequent swallows and breaths allowing for a relatively large volume of food to be consumed in a short period of time without aspiration. The examiner watches for signs of increased cardiac or respiratory rate, dysrhythmia of cardiac and respiratory patterns, gagging, spitting, tongue thrusting, squirming and withdrawing, arching of the back or neck, and falling asleep. Lip closure, tongue action, cheek posture, and laryngeal movement are all observed. Because neurologically impaired infants with sucking difficulty are at increased risk for aspiration during feeds, suctioning capabilities should be readily available during the assessment.

The type of nipple and viscosity of the liquid have been shown to influence the sucking behavior of neonates. Nipple pliability and the size of the hole are both important (Adram, Kemp, & Lind, 1958; Dubignon & Campbell, 1968). Brown (1972) found that infants responded preferentially to a regular rounded nipple shape compared with a blunt Nuk-type nipple (Figure 7–9). On the other hand, clinical experience has shown that some infants do prefer Nuk-type nipples. Thus, the important thing to remember is that infants vary considerably in nipple preferences, so several types may need to be tried (Mathew, Belan, & Thoppil, 1992). It is also important that the underlying cause for the sucking difficulty be determined so the clinician knows it is safe to experiment with nipples and also containers (Figure 7–9). Case Study 1 in Chapter 8 is an example of an infant with focal spasm of the upper esophageal sphincter, for which a nipple change would be irrelevant to the basic problem. In fact, any attempt initially to feed this infant orally would be detrimental. Small amounts of liquid can be introduced gradually for practice, with close observation for nasopharyngeal reflux and possible aspiration. Thickened liquid may be preferable with greater potential for being propelled through the esophageal area of spasm. Nipple preference also may change over time, especially for those infants who start out with a small, soft preemie nipple and after a few weeks progress to a longer, firmer nipple.

Satiation also influences sucking. From the first day of life, the presence of milk in the stomach appears to be an inhibitor of nutritive sucking (Satinoff & Stanley, 1963). The sucking rate also varies with the concentration of sucrose. Burke (1977) found that swallowing activity increased relative to the number of sucks, and sucking rate slowed as amount and concentration of sucrose was increased. Infants have been found to suck at higher rates for formula with a higher relative viscosity (Kron, Stein, Goddard, & Phoenix, 1967). Thus, assessment at what would be the normal feeding time as well as the use of various nipples, containers, and even formulas may influence the outcome of the evaluation.

Examination of Infants on Nonoral Feeding

When an infant is getting nutritional needs met via OG or NG tube feedings, it is desirable to have the tube removed prior to assessment of oral nipple feeding. An OG tube can interfere with oral feeding because it prevents adequate lip closure and tongue movement, which in turn may interfere with effective buildup of intraoral pressure during sucking. It is not clear how any tube, whether OG or NG, may affect the pharyngeal area and in turn what effect that will have on the coordination of suck–swallow patterns, but assessment should be done in as normal conditions as possible. Some believe that the tube cannot be replaced immediately after the infant

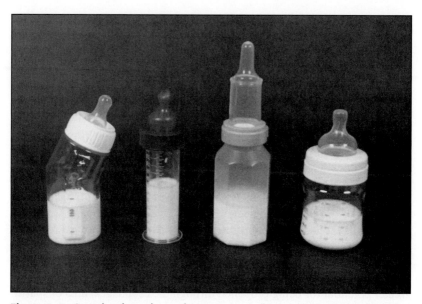

Figure 7–9. Sample of nipples and containers. Left to right: Angle bottle with a "standard" nipple, Volufeeder with a Nuk-type nipple, Haberman feeder, and Avent feeding system.

has taken some liquid because of increased risk for emesis. The feeding schedule may then be disrupted if the required amount cannot be given to the infant within approximately 30 min. Thus, there may be some patients for whom the initial assessment will be done with tube in place. Serial assessments may be needed over several feeding times, or even over several days, to monitor change in the infant, to establish an oral sensorimotor and feeding plan, and to assist in implementing recommendations.

One of the major considerations in determining when a tube-fed infant is ready for oral feedings is tolerance of bolus tube feedings in comparison with continuous tube feedings. Continuous feeds are delivered slowly over a period of hours when the infant's system cannot handle larger quantities in short time periods. In contrast, bolus feeds are usually given over a period of 15 to 20 min, with several hours between feedings so that normal hunger and wake cycles can be established. Advancing from one type of tube feeding to another and generally to oral feedings is addressed in Chapters 5 and 9.

Feeding Observation

Once the general physical examination with oral peripheral examination is completed, the clinician should observe a primary caregiver feeding the infant as typically as possible. Observations are made of child and of caregiver actions and interactions. A basic cranial nerve examination is carried out (Table 7–6). Therapeutic adjustments may be considered as the feeding session progresses, providing the infant appears to have a safe swallow (details in Chapter 9). The clinician may be able to suggest changes that could include position and posture, types of nipples, fluid viscosity, and ways to work through sensory issues. If there are concerns about risks for aspiration, safety of the airway, or possibilities of GERD/EERD, the clinician makes recommendations for additional consultations or testing. If there are concerns related to nutritional status, a dietitian should be consulted. The infant who is evaluated by an interdisciplinary team has the advantage of the dietitian being present for immediate consultation.

■ ASSESSMENT OF CHILDREN WHO ARE TRANSITIONAL FEEDERS OR OLDER

Assessment scales for children measure various aspects of feeding and swallowing at the impairment, activity, and participation levels. No one scale encompasses all aspects. Thus clinicians need to be selective for different

Table 7–6. Observations That Correlate to Cranial Nerve (CN) Function During Feeding Assessment

CN	Stimulus	Normal Response	Deficit Response
V	Food on tongue	Mastication initiated	Bolus not formed Mandible movements limited or incoordinated
VII	Sucking	Lips pursed to latch on to nipple	Lack of lip seal
	Food on lower lip	Lip closure	Lack of lip movement
	Smile	Retraction of lips	Asymmetry or lack of retraction
IX, X	Food posterior in mouth	Swallow < 2 sec	Delayed pharyngeal swallow
		Soft palate elevation and retraction	Nasopharyngeal reflux
XII	Food on tongue	Tongue shape, point and protrude	Lack of tongue movement or incoordination, excessive thrust, fasciculations

needs. Appendix B has brief descriptions of several assessment tools. This list is not inclusive, nor does it intend to be discriminatory, but rather to give the reader a sample of measures that incorporate the principles of WHO (1997).

Scales include, but are not limited to, the School Functional Assessment (Coster, Deeney, Haltiwanger, & Haley, 1998) and the Holistic Feeding Observation Form (Koontz-Lowman & Lane, 1999) at the participation level. Other measures include the WeeFIM-Functional Independence Measure for Children (Hamilton & Granger, 1991), the Pediatric Evaluation of Disability Inventory—PEDI (Haley, Coster, Ludlow, Haltiwanger, & Andrellos, 1992), SOMA: Schedule for Oral Motor Assessment (Reilly, Skuse, & Wolke, 2000), the Multidisciplinary Feeding Profile (MFP) (Kenny et al., 1989), and Oral-Motor/Feeding Rating Scale (Jelm, 1990).

A global approach is emphasized for problem solving and creativity to develop feeding strategies without a formal scale (Morris and Klein, 1987) and with The Developmental Pre-feeding Checklist (Morris and Klein, 2000). Both rational and intuitive approaches are used to obtain a global overview from which a sequential analysis is carried out to evaluate specific factors that may contribute to the feeding problem. The sequential analysis is essentially descriptive, comparing a child's strengths and deficits to normal development. These analyses stress the importance of considering a number of environments including learning, communication, physical, and sensory environments, along with normal oral-motor skills, limited oral-motor skills, and treatment possibilities.

Observations of the caregiver and the child form a basis for early identification of children in need of nonoral supplementary feeding of some type (Gisel and Patrick, 1988). In this assessment, specific negative actions by caregivers and the child are noted, and each one is given a score of 1. The lower the score, the more normal the feeding status. The early identification and rehabilitation of undernutrition may improve motor functioning for oral feeding and for other systems (Chapter 6).

Check-lists may be useful for systematizing observations (Herman, 1991; Warner, 1981). Published protocols include evaluation of many of the same variables, but, in general, interpretation guidelines are lacking. At present, no universally accepted standard exists for feeding assessment. Therefore, knowledge of normal development and experience with oral sensorimotor and feeding function provide reference points for clinicians to evaluate children with abnormal functioning.

Feeding Observation of Older Children

Although a feeding assessment in the child's home would be ideal, it is not always possible. In a clinic setting, the assessment begins with an observation of a primary caregiver carrying out the usual feeding procedures in as "normal" a routine as possible (Appendix A). The usual seating, positioning equipment, and feeding utensils should be at the assessment site whenever feasible. The peripheral oral sensorimotor examination is similar to that described for infants. Dentition and occlusion patterns are noted in children once they have teeth.

Open mouth posture is fairly common in multiply handicapped children. Drooling is a common occurrence with lack of consistent lip closure. Persistent drooling indicates a lack of or reduced frequency of swallowing of saliva. It is important to determine the underlying reasons for the open mouth posture, that is, whether it is related to respiratory or neuromuscular status. Intervention related to drooling will differ according to the underlying causes of specific problems (Chapter 11).

Cervical Auscultation

Cervical auscultation, using a stethoscope or microphone, may be useful as one part of the clinic evaluation to make inferences about the pharyngeal phase of the swallow. Infants and children with feeding problems may demonstrate voice or breathing patterns that reflect the presence of excessive secretions, liquid, or food in the larynx. A "gurgly" voice quality raises concern about risk for aspiration with indications that material has spilled into the upper airway. Awareness of the relationship of these vocal quality changes to impaired swallowing will alert the clinician to a need for additional diagnostic studies. Although these sounds are audible to a normal listener at times, a stethoscope may further aid in the assessment of less obvious difficulties.

Using a microphone attached to the neck, the clinician can use this noninvasive method to record sounds on a tape recorder, display them on an oscilloscope, and also record sounds on a digital signal processor. The optimal site for the microphone or the stethoscope is at the lateral aspect of the larynx. Vice and colleagues (Vice, Heinz, Giuriati, Hood, & Bosma, 1990) observed a single feed by six normal infants in the first 2 days of life. They found that swallow breath sounds were distinctively patterned, with discrete sounds preceding and following the bolus transit sounds.

A computer-facilitated evaluation of the pharyngeal phase of swallowing may be especially useful for evaluation of nipple-feeding competence in preterm infants and in infants with relatively subtle forms of CNS impairments. According to Vice et al. (1990), the acoustic observations reveal aspects of swallow and breathing not recognized previously. The swallow breaths form a consistent pattern with some variation in duration. The discrete sounds of successive swallows appear to be stable elements in the rhythmic sequences that are similar in pattern. Clinicians could learn to recognize abnormal bubbling sounds that are formed to clear the respiratory tract and are less extensive than a cough. These may be different from the sounds of laryngeal stridor and vocalization changes, but may be as important in identifying foreign substances in the upper airway. With experience, clinicians may be able to use the stethoscope alone to gain valuable information, even if the computerized analysis is not available. It is important to remember that, at best, auscultation is useful in screening and not appropriate for definitive diagnosis.

Feeding Evaluation of Older Children

Posture and positioning evaluation is the first step in assessing older children. Adjustments are made when necessary. For oral feeders, the clinician should observe a feeding with the child and a familiar feeder. Whenever possible, the child is seated in the chair that is typically used at mealtime. Differences in efficiency with varied textures and different amounts per bite or sip can be noted. Initial presentations of food and liquid should be of small amounts, usually about $\frac{1}{3}$ teaspoon or 2 cc's, on a spoon. Many children with disabilities who present for assessment are primarily on a pureed diet. The first food used in assessment is usually the texture reported to be the easiest for the child. Gradual changes can be made toward thinner liquids, which may be presented on a spoon at first, as the feeder can control the amount more precisely than with a cup. Thickened liquid may be used when the child shows slow initiation of tongue action and a delayed swallow. Swallowing of liquids should be observed with the familiar feeder presenting liquid in the typical routine, and also by the clinician who may want to have the child try to make some specific changes. This approach aids in prognosis.

Chewable food will be used if, by history and initial observations during the session, the child appears ready for it. There certainly may be times in which the child is assessed using chewable food even when it has never been given in the past. There is evidence that solid foods need to be introduced at appropriate times even with developmentally delayed children. The longer the delay, the more difficult it may become for these children to accept texture changes (Illingworth & Lister, 1964). The choice of food is guided by the need to minimize any risk for choking. Examples of chewable foods typically formed into a bolus with limited munching or chewing are graham crackers, plain sugar cookies, or cooked carrots. With these particular foods, the risk for choking or aspiration appears less than for foods that flake apart (potato chips, pretzels, saltine crackers) or those with skins or shells (hot dogs, corn, peas). It is also helpful to avoid small and hard textures that could be swallowed whole readily (peanuts, M & Ms, or solid hard candy).

Assessment of spoon-feeding helps delineate tongue, jaw, and lip movement problems. Familiar spoons or other utensils should be used first, then therapeutic spoons can be introduced to note differences in function. These oral sensorimotor motions may be exaggerated and thereby lead to disruption of rhythm and organization, both of which are critical to coordination of swallowing. Each task should yield information to assist in defining the structures involved most prominently in the incoordination and how that incoordination differs from the normal movement. Three examples illustrate these exaggerated movements: tonic bite, tongue thrust, and lip retraction. Although they are described as individual actions for a child, it is common for multiple exaggerated movements to be present within a single child.

A child with a tonic bite may clamp down on a spoon as it enters the mouth and not be able to release the bite. This disrupts the rhythm and leads to overall disorganization. Likewise, during play with the fingers in the mouth, the child with a tonic bite clamps down on the fingers resulting in an unpleasant experience. The likely result is less oral stimulation, thus beginning a cycle of avoidance. The combination of lack of pleasurable oral stimulation and reduced stimulation may increase the possibility of oral defensiveness. The spoon or fingers cannot be pulled out of the mouth easily, which may actually promote increased biting.

Tongue thrust and tongue retraction both interfere with efficient handling of food. Both tongue patterns indicate that the tongue cannot organize food into a bolus and propel it posteriorly for an efficient swallow. A tongue thrust interferes with placement of the food in the mouth, as well as the child's ability to suck, chew, and swallow. The forward propulsion of the tongue pushes food right back out of the mouth before any lip closure occurs. Tongue retraction is most noticeable "at rest" because the tongue is held posterior in the oral cavity. This retraction may be mistaken for tongue thrust because in both instances food gets pushed out of the oral cavity. The difference is that with tongue retraction, food can be placed into the front of the mouth easily, but once the mouth closes, the tongue, which has to move forward from its posterior position, pushes the food out.

Lip retraction is usually associated with sensory defensiveness or increased tone, resulting in excessive tension in the lips. This retraction makes it difficult to remove food from the spoon, to accomplish cup-drinking, and to suck through a nipple or a straw. Sensory defensiveness usually occurs in response to touch around or in the mouth. Light touch often results in a strong pulling away from the stimulus. Sensory defensiveness and increased tone may result in abnormal movements or posturing throughout the entire body.

One of the primary goals during the assessment is to determine whether the feeding difficulty is primarily a swallowing deficit, and if so, which phase(s) of swallowing appear impaired with an estimate of severity and specificity (Table 7–7). The clinical assessment yields more specific information about bolus formation (oral preparatory) and the oral phase of the swallow. At best, pharyngeal phase problems can only be inferred and

Table 7–7. Signs and Symptoms of Swallowing Problems in Bolus Formation, Oral, and Pharyngeal Phases With Possible Treatment Options

Phase of Swallow	Sign or Symptom	Treatment to Improve[a]
Oral preparatory or bolus formation	Food falls out of mouth	Posture and seating
	Pooling in anterior sulci	Sensory aspects of food
	Lack of tongue action to form bolus	Lip closure
		Rotary tongue & jaw action
	Lack of chewing	Sensory aspects of food
Oral	Pooling in lateral sulci	Lip closure and buccal tension
	Food pushed out of mouth	Tongue exercises to reduce thrusting
	Slow bolus formation	Tongue manipulation
	Piecemeal deglutition	Lateral tongue action and rotary jaw action
	Delayed swallow	Initiate tongue action quickly
Pharyngeal	Pooling in vallecula and pyriform sinuses	Posture and seating
		Improve timing of swallow production
	Residue in pharyngeal recesses after swallow	Multiple swallows per bite; alternate textures
	Gurgly voice quality	Improve vocal fold closure with voice therapy
	Aspiration on liquids, safe for thicker textures	Thicken liquids
	Aspiration on paste, safe with liquids	Make food thinner texture
	Choking on mixed textures in the same bite	Make each bite of a consistent texture; alternate per bite
	Swallow delayed a few seconds for best texture	Nonoral feedings
	Aspiration for all textures (frequent)	Nonoral feeding; oral stimulation without food except for tastes

[a]These treatment suggestions are explained in detail in Chapter 9.

frequently need instrumental assessment for delineation by objective measurement. For example, the clinician can look into the oral cavity and see material in the anterior or lateral sulci before, during, or after a swallow. Partial swallow of a bolus may result in residual that can be seen in the oral cavity. Tongue movements and jaw action can be viewed directly. Lip closure, or lack of closure, and liquid or food loss out of the mouth can be seen. Bolus formation time and oral skills, particularly for chewing, can be noted (Gisel, 1991). Children with CP are found to take significantly longer to chew hard solid food than typical children (Gisel, Alphonce, & Ramsay, 2000). Children with Down syndrome show patterns of chewing different from typical children (Gisel, Lange, & Niman, 1984). The number of swallows per bolus can be estimated when the clinician can see, feel, or hear that there is hyoid and laryngeal elevation. The time before seeing laryngeal elevation can be measured to provide estimate of delay in pharyngeal swallow onset. Head and neck position changes and facial grimacing are visible.

Pharyngeal phase problems can be inferred by noting a significant delay in production of a swallow, gurgly voice quality, cough, and increased respiratory effort or respiratory distress. The longer the delay in production of a swallow, the more consistent a gurgly voice quality, and the more swallows needed per bolus with any respiratory distress, the greater the probability of a significant pharyngeal phase problem. Such a problem should be delineated objectively with an instrumental assessment, for example, flexible endoscopic examination of swallowing (FEES) (Leder & Karas, 2000; Willging, 1995; Willging, Miller, Hosan, & Rudolph, 1996) or VFSS to make the most effective and coordinated recommendations for management (Arvedson & Lefton-Greif, 1998; Arvedson et al., 1994; Fox, 1990; Griggs, Jones, & Lee, 1989; Logemann, 1983, 1998) (Chapter 8).

Clinicians need to differentiate immature but essentially normal patterns, from abnormal patterns because the prognosis for improvement and the recommendations for treatment strategies differ for these two situations. Children with immature oral skills are easier to manage than those who have abnormal patterns. It is common that an individual child may show both immature and abnormal patterns, however, which complicates the decision-making process. Once observations are completed, clinicians must make decisions whether the child's patterns would be appropriate if the child were younger or if the actions are deviant regardless of age. These patterns are likely to be distinguishable in suck–swallow sequencing, jaw control or stability, tongue mobility, lip closure, dissociation of tongue and jaw and cheek movements during drinking and chewing (Lane & Cloud, 1988; Morris & Klein, 1987, 2000; Ottenbacher et al., 1983; Stratton, 1981).

Children may signal aversive responses by food refusal in a variety of ways. Some children hyperextend the head and neck, turn the head, spit food out of the mouth, or close the mouth tightly so food cannot be placed into it. Some children are observed to take their hands and push at the sides of their neck during and after feeding. VFSS frequently reveals residue in the pharyngeal recesses in these children. It appears that the child may be trying to eliminate that material. Unfortunately, caregivers and professionals commonly see this activity as a behavioral habit. The child is not likely to be effective in moving the material because of the location. The residue places the person at considerable risk for aspiration after swallowing. The child may use food refusal as a behavior. The history and physical findings frequently determine an underlying physiologic basis that is prominent, or at least was prominent in the past. Because of the complex factors involved with food refusal in most children, interdisciplinary team evaluations are particularly valuable.

Completion of the Clinical Assessment and Follow-Up

Once the clinical assessment has been completed, additional information may be sought through radiologic, metabolic, respiratory, and other diagnostic studies. The interdisciplinary team should compile findings from all assessments for appropriate coordinated recommendations to be made. Physician input is of utmost importance in developing the management plan for children with defined medical and health risks.

Treatment options are discussed in detail in Chapter 9. The options vary according to the etiologies and observations made during assessment. Seating and positioning changes may be made under the direction of seating specialists. Texture variations may be made. Amount per bolus and timing of bolus presentations can be altered. Utensils may be changed. Oral sensorimotor practice may be carried out with or without food. Children may receive full oral feedings, a combination of tube and oral feedings, or nutritional needs may be met entirely by tube feeding. When a child is fed nonorally, an oral stimulation program may be done with no food or with very small amounts for practice and pleasure, but not with a focus on feeding. Case studies exemplifying the integration of assessment and management concerns are found in Chapter 9.

Assessment With Tracheotomy

The degree and type of difficulty with sucking and swallowing relates most closely to the underlying reasons for a tracheotomy. Nonetheless, the tracheotomy tube itself will result in some restriction of laryngeal elevation and may thus interfere with swallowing. Long-term tracheotomy may affect swallowing in young children (Abraham & Wolf, 2000). The placement of the infant's larynx high in the neck makes tracheotomy less likely to be a major factor in swallowing problems for infants compared with older children or adults. In addition, airway protection capabilities should be verified before giving any liquid. The methylene blue dye test is not considered sufficiently sensitive to screen for aspiration. Glucose strips may be a better screening alternative, particularly when looking for refluxate in the trachea in children on OG or NG enteral feeds. Accurate diagnosis requires instrumental testing via endoscopy or fluoroscopy. Endoscopy is the procedure of choice when concerns are raised for the safety of swallowing oral secretions and mucous. When oral secretions are suctioned out the tracheotomy tube, aspiration is diagnosed. The presence of any liquid or food taken in orally that appears in the tracheotomy tube should prompt feeders to discontinue oral feeds until the problem is thoroughly investigated (Chapter 4). Findings on instrumental examinations are usually helpful to clinicians and parents as they formulate a treatment plan.

Assessment with Children Exhibiting Primarily Behavior or Sensory Related Problems

See Chapter 13 for assessment and management. Readers are reminded that the physical and physiologic underpinnings to food refusal are real and need to be delineated.

■ CONCLUSION

The clinical evaluation of feeding and swallowing problems in infants and children is an ongoing process. The initial evaluation is critical in establishing baselines of function in all aspects so decisions can be appropriate and timely when there is need for additional information or when management plans can be formulated. The management issues will be discussed in Chapter 9. Once management decisions are made and intervention processes are put in place, evaluation continues to be an integral part for clinicians and caregivers. They monitor health status and progress toward achieving desirable outcomes that include stable health, adequate nutrition, optimal oral sensorimotor skills, and highest level functioning for all children within their environments.

■ APPENDIX A

Oral–Motor and Feeding Evaluation

Name _____ Chart Number _____

Date of evaluation _____ Referral _____

Date of birth _____ Diagnosis _____

C.A. _____ Adjusted age _____ Clinician _____

Summary_____

_____

Put a (✔) to indicate presence of any factor; describe briefly.

NA = not applicable

HISTORY

    I. Family and Social History

        _____ Primary caregivers: _____ Parent _____ Babysitter _____ Foster parent

        other_____

        _____ Other persons in the home_____

        _____ Neurologic problems_____

        _____ Cleft palate or other craniofacial anomalies _____

        _____ Feeding problems in family _____

        _____ Respiratory/breathing problems (asthma, allergies) _____

        _____ Environmental factors (smoking, pets) _____

    II. Prenatal history

        _____ Medications_____

        _____ Substance abuse (smoking, alcohol, other drugs)

            Mother_____

            Father_____

        _____ Maternal infection_____

        _____ Radiation _____

        _____ Toxemia_____

        _____ Bleeding _____

        _____ Thyroid disease _____

        _____ Polyhydramnios_____

        _____ Other factors _____

III. Birth history
_____ Birth weight _____ Gestational age
_____ Trauma _____
_____ Apgar scores _____
_____ Intubation _____
_____ Prolonged hypoxia or anoxia/respiratory distress _____
_____ Surfactant therapy _____
_____ Cardiac problems _____
_____ Other complications _____

IV. Neonatal period (first 28 days)
_____ Alert _____ Lethargic, difficult to rouse_____
_____ Respiratory problems
_____ Supplemental ventilation _____
_____ Respiratory distress syndrome _____
_____ Apnea and bradycardia_____
_____ Breathing rate and effort
_____ Stridor_____
_____ Stertor_____
_____ Rooting reflex intact _____ Absent _____ Inconsistent
_____ Bubbling secretions ___ Intermittent ___ Frequent ___ Excessive
_____ Medication_____
_____ Weak or dysrhythmic nonnutritive suck (pacifier or finger)_____

V. Feeding history—describe each factor
Position: _____ Cradle held _____ Upright held _____ Upright in chair
Duration: _____ 20 minutes _____ 30–40 minutes _____ More than 45 minutes
Intervals: _____ 2 hours _____ 3 hours _____ 4 hours _____ Other
Tube feedings: _____ If yes, type _____
        How long? _____ weeks _____ months
Sucking
        _____ Breast _____ Bottle (_____ nipple type _____ formula)
        Lip seal: ____No liquid loss _____Liquid loss at corners of mouth
        _____ Excessive vertical jaw action _____ Hard to burp
Textures in diet
_____ Liquid
_____ Puree
_____ Lumpy puree or ground textures
_____ Solid
Diet (per 24 hour day)
Quantity of food _____
Quantity of liquid (oz/cc) _____
Vitamin/mineral supplement _____

Appetite: _____ Good _____ Inconsistent _____ Poor
Food allergies or intolerance _____
Gagging or emesis: ___ During feed ___ After feed (at least 30 minutes)
Preferred food temperature: _____ Warm _____ Cold
Preferred liquid temperature: _____ Warm _____ Cold
Location for feeding: ____One place _____ Several places
Utensils
_____ Bottle and nipple _____ Cup _____ Straw
_____ Spoon _____ Fingers
Respiratory status
_____ Supplemental ventilation
_____ Aspiration or pneumonia
_____ Bronchitis or chronic upper respiratory infection
_____ Allergies or asthma
_____ Noisy breathing: _____ With feeds _____ Apart from feeds
_____ Gurgly voice quality: _____ During feeds _____ After feeds
_____ Coughing or choking: _____ During feeds _____ After feeds
_____ Trouble breathing during feeds
Other signs of distress
_____ Fussing during feeding
_____ Head turning to avoid feeding
_____ Falling asleep during feeding
_____ Postural changes: _____ Stiffening _____ Hyperextending

VI. Other factors
Past medical/surgical history
_____ Upper GI or scintiscan: _____
_____ Videofluoroscopic swallow study: _____
_____ Surgical procedures—describe _____
Sleep
_____ Waking in night
_____ Snoring
_____ Mouth breathing
Communication—primary mode
_____ Nonverbal
_____ Verbal: ____ Intelligible (more than 50%) ___ Unintelligible
Therapeutic Intervention
_____ Occupational Therapist
_____ Speech–Language Pathologist
_____ Physical Therapist
_____ Special Education
_____ Other _____
Miscellaneous comments: _____
_____

PHYSICAL EXAMINATION

I. Prefeeding observations

  A. Position at rest

    _____ Prone _____ Supine _____ Side lying

    _____ Independent sitting _____ Supported sitting

    _____ Flexion _____ Hyperextension

    _____ Trunk asymmetry _____ Limb asymmetry

    _____ Variable: _____

  B. Level of arousal and alertness

    _____ Sustained for at least 10 minutes

    _____ Intermittent and fluctuating

    _____ Falls asleep within 4–5 minutes

  C. Muscle tone and movement patterns

    _____ Tone normal ____ Hypertonicity ____ Hypotonicity

    ____ Variable

    _____ Proximal stability: _____ Adequate _____ Deficient

    If deficient, _____ Location (trunk, waist, shoulder)

    _____ Distal mobility: _____ Adequate _____ Deficient

    If deficient, _____ Location (arms, legs)

  D. Irritability (state)

    _____ Usually quiet

    _____ Infrequent and calms easily

    _____ Frequent, but calms with holding

    _____ Frequent, difficult to quiet

  E. Airway status

    _____ No problem

    _____ Stridor _____ Stertor

    _____ Dusky spells ____with feeding _____ apart from feeding

    _____ Oxygen dependent

    _____ Tracheotomy: _____ Size _____ Type _____ Speaking valve

    _____ Ventilator dependent

  F. Communication

    _____ Nonverbal _____ Verbal: _____ Intelligible _____ Babbles

    _____ Vowel vocalizations only

    _____ Voice quality normal _____ Abnormal

    _____ Breathy _____ Shrill _____ Hypernasal

    _____ Gurgly _____ Weak _____ Hyponasal

    _____ Pitch normal _____ High ____Low

    _____ Volume normal _____Weak _____Overloud

  G. Face and mouth—structure and function

    _____ Facial symmetry _____ Facial asymmetry

    _____ Mandible normal _____ Small

_____ Cheek tone normal _____ Reduced
_____ Lips closed _____ Lips open
_____ Tongue symmetrical _____ Tongue asymmetrical
_____ Tongue protrusion midline _____ Tongue protrudes to one side
_____ Tongue soft (hypotonic) ____ Tongue contracted (hypertonic)
_____ Hard palate symmetrical ____ High arch
_____ Narrow _____ Cleft
_____ Soft palate normal _____ Cleft
_____ Jaw stability normal _____ Jaw instability
_____ Gag reflex
_____ Rooting reflex
_____ Bite reflex
_____ Nonnutritive suck/swallow coordinated _____ Incoordinated

H. Drooling
_____ Seldom _____ Variable _____ Frequent _____ Constant
_____ Minimal _____ Moderate _____ Severe _____ Profuse
_____ To lip _____ To chin _____ To clothes _____ To table
_____ Bib or clothing changes each day: _____ How many
_____ Awareness: _____ High _____ Occasional _____ Never

II. Nonnutritive sucking
_____ Responsive to stroking around mouth: ____ Eager
_____ Inconsistent
_____ Rooting when stroked near corners of mouth
_____ Always _____ Inconsistent _____ Never
_____ Sucking on little finger: _____ Rhythmic _____ Dysrhythmic

III. Oral–motor function and feeding assessment
A. Movement of oral structures (check if present)
_____ Lips: _____ Retraction _____ Pursing
_____ Tongue:_____ Elevation _____ Protrusion _____ Lateralization
_____ Rapid movement
_____ Soft palate: _____ Elevation/retraction during phonation
_____ Mandible: _____ Vertical movement _____ Rotary movement
B. Protective mechanisms—upon command, no food
_____ Swallow _____ Cough _____ Gag
C. Primary feeder with infant—describe:
Communication/interaction _____
Positioning _____
Utensils _____
Amount per meal _____
Length of meal (minutes)_____
Avoidance/refusal _____

D. Feeding assessment: Check (✔) all that apply

_____ Breast-feeding: _____ Latch readily _____ Poor latch

_____ Suck/swallow/respiratory sequence: _____ Normal
_____ Incoordinated

_____ Suckling bursts: _____ Appropriate pauses _____ No pause

_____ Flow rate: _____ Normal (bubbles with each suck–bottle)
_____ Poor

_____ Lip closure: _____ Normal _____ Open mouth

_____ Loss of liquid: _____ Minimal _____ Moderate

_____ Tongue movement: _____ Normal _____ Lateral _____ Thrusting

_____ Laryngeal elevation: _____ During swallow _____ Absent

_____ Pocketing of food/liquid: _____ Cheeks _____ Front of mouth

_____ Nasopharyngeal reflux: _____ Liquid only _____ Food

_____ Changes in respiratory function
     _____ Noisy breathing
     _____ Chest retractions
     _____ Inconsistent rate of breathing or dysrhythmia
     _____ Nasal obstruction
     _____ Bradycardia _____ Apnea _____ Cyanosis
     _____ Desaturation (usually measured by pulse oximetry)
_____ Alert for entire feed _____ Lethargy noted
_____ Coughing _____ Choking _____ Gagging _____ Spitting
_____ Emesis (vomiting): _____During feeding
     _____ Apart from feeding
_____ Spoon feeding: _____ Sucks food off spoon _____ Closes lips
     _____ Upper lip active _____ Upper lip no movement
_____ Chewing: _____ Suck–swallow _____ Munching
     _____ Rotary jaw _____ Lateral tongue _____ Abnormal
_____ Straw drinking: _____ Anticipates _____ Lip seal
     _____ Successful _____ Unsuccessful
_____ Associated movements
     _____ Arching back, neck or head
     _____ Squirming or withdrawing
     _____ Falling asleep
     _____ Other _____
_____ Feeding time less than 30 minutes _____ More than 30 minutes

E. Changes made during assessment with positive outcome _____
_____

F. Changes made during assessment with negative outcome_____
_____

■ APPENDIX B. ASSESSMENT SCALES AND MEASURES OF VARIOUS ASPECTS OF FEEDING AND SWALLOWING IN CHILDREN: IMPAIRMENT, ACTIVITY, AND PARTICIPATION LEVELS

Assessment Scales for Infants

The Neonatal Oral–Motor Assessment Scale (NOMAS) (Braun & Palmer, 1986)

This scale is an attempt to identify and quantify normal and deviant oral sensorimotor patterns in neonates. It was revised to improve clarity and sensitivity of responses (Case-Smith, 1988) and yields semiquantitative information in the identification of oral–motor dysfunction by 40 weeks gestational age. It rates individual tongue and jaw responses during nonnutritive and nutritive sucking and is found to differentiate tongue from jaw movements and oral–motor disorganization from dysfunction. It assesses both abnormal and normal oral sensorimotor function that can be accompanied by hypotonia. Oral sensorimotor dysfunction associated with generalized hypotonia suggests to Braun & Palmer that these infants have a significant "cerebral" involvement.

Revised Version of the NOMAS (Case-Smith, Cooper & Scala, 1989)

This version identifies different oral–motor behaviors in efficient and inefficient feeders based on a sample of high-risk premature neonates. Inefficient feeders showed lack of rhythm, disorganization in jaw and tongue movements, and pauses of more than 6 sec between sucking bursts. These responses in the inefficient feeders appear closely related to abnormal respiratory patterns, and emphasize the necessity of a stable airway for efficient oral feeding. Poor feeders showed no difficulty in initiating movement or in swallowing liquid, but they had difficulty maintaining a rhythmic pattern with a consistent rate of sucking.

Assessments for Children

School Functional Assessment (Coster, Deeney, Haltiwanger, & Haley, 1998)

This standardized evaluation includes test items on a child's participation and functional skills in the school environment. This tool has established levels of reliability and validity and can be used with children in elementary school (grades K–6). It measures the child's participation in many school environments and includes test items related to mealtime and snack time. It considers the level of physical assistance the child needs, as well as the adaptive equipment he or she may use during the meal.

The Holistic Feeding Observation Form (Koontz-Lowman & Lane, 1999)

This interview and observation guide is designed to evaluate all aspects of the eating and feeding process, including the social and physical environment, as well as specific sensory, communication, and motor skills. This tool can guide the clinician in developing a collaborative treatment plan with families and Early Intervention or school-based personnel. Specific questions regarding posture and seating, respiratory issues, communication and behavior, sensory development, and oral–motor development are designed to guide the clinician during a feeding observation and during the treatment planning process.

WeeFIM—Functional Independence Measure for Children (Hamilton & Granger, 1991)

WeeFim is a functional assessment for children with physical disabilities with developmental ages of 6 months to 6 years. It measures a wide range of functional skills including feeding skills.

The Pediatric Evaluation of Disability Inventory—PEDI (Haley, Coster, Ludlow, Haltiwanger, & Andrellos, 1992)

The PEDI is a norm-referenced and criterion-referenced scale based on a parent interview that measures functional skills and caregiver assistance for children ages 6 months to 7 years. It also includes many test items that measure feeding skills.

SOMA: Schedule for Oral Motor Assessment (Reilly, Skuse, & Wolke, 2000)

This assessment addresses functional oral–motor skills at the impairment, activities, and limitation levels. It is a standardized oral–motor scale with established levels of reliability and validity, designed to screen for subtle degrees of oral–motor dysfunction. It can be used as a screening tool for children with developmental abilities from 6 months to 2 years of age. The standardized presentation of textures includes puree, semisolids (lumpy spoon food), solids (dried fruit), biscuits, and liquids in a bottle, trainer cup, and open cup. The clinician scores from videotape. It includes score sheets and administration and scoring manual with specific instructions to measure jaw function, tongue function, lip function, and swallowing function that are overtly visible during a clinical examination.

The Multidisciplinary Feeding Profile (MFP) (Kenny et al., 1989)

This is the first statistically developed protocol for patients who are dependent feeders and is shown to be reliable for children with neurologic deficits who cannot feed themselves. The range of clinical data makes it a comprehensive feeding-disorder assessment package with a multidisciplinary base. It can be completed in 30 to 45 minutes and provides scaled numerical ratings for a variety of components including physical/neurologic factors (posture, tone, reflexes, and motor control), oral–facial structure, oral–facial sensory inputs, oral–facial motor function, ventilation/phonation, and a functional feeding assessment. The scaled numerical ratings do *not* lead to a definition of the level of severity of feeding problems. Although content validity was not assessed objectively, the investigators consider the MFP scale to be content-valid, based on their experience, and reliable, based on consistency of results with repeated measurements.

Oral–Motor/Feeding Rating Scale (Jelm, 1990)

This scale measures oral–motor skills at the impairment level and at the activities level. It is useful for children as young as 12 months, with some portions useful for older children or adults. This scale examines specific movements and uses a 6-point (0–5) scale in eight function areas and three specific oral–motor movements. The eight function areas include breast-feeding, bottle-feeding, spoon-feeding, cup-drinking, biting a soft cookie, biting a hard cookie, chewing, and straw drinking (not evaluated until children are 3 years of age because of wide variation in movements in younger children). The three specific oral–motor movements are lip/cheek, tongue, and jaw movement. It provides an overview of abilities in related areas of feeding function to include self-feeding, adaptive feeding equipment, diet adaptations, position, sensitivity, food retention, swallowing, and orofacial structures.

■ REFERENCES

Abraham, S. S., & Wolf, E. L. (2000). Swallowing physiology of toddlers with long-term tracheostomies: A preliminary study. *Dysphagia, 15,* 206–212.

Adram, G. M., Kemp, F. H., & Lind, J. (1958). A cineradiographic study of infant bottle feeding. *British Journal of Radiology, 31,* 11–22.

Alexander, R. (1987). Oral-motor treatment for infants and young children with cerebral palsy. *Seminars in Speech and Language, 8,* 87–100.

Altman, P. L., & Dittmer, D. S. (Eds.). (1968). *Metabolism.* Bethesda, MD: Federation of Societies for Experimental Biology.

American Academy of Pediatrics, Task Force on Infant Positioning and SIDS. (2000). Changing concepts of sudden infant death syndrome: Implications for infant sleeping environment and sleep position. *Pediatrics, 105,* 650–656.

American Academy of Pediatrics, American College of Obstetricians and Gynecologists. (1992). Relationship between perinatal factors and neurologic outcome. In R. L. Poland & R. K. Freeman (Eds.), *Guidelines for perinatal care* (3rd ed.; 221). American Academy of Pediatrics.

Apgar, V. (1966). The newborn (APGAR) scoring system: Reflections and advice. *Pediatric Clinics of North America, 13,* 645.

Arens, R., & Reichman, B. (1992). Grooved palate associated with prolonged use of orogastric feeding tubes in premature infants. *Journal of Oral Maxillofacial Surgery, 50,* 64–65.

Arvedson, J. C., & Lefton-Greif, M. A. (1998). *Pediatric videofluroscopic swallow studies: A professional manual with caregiver guidelines.* San Antonio, TX: Communication Skill Builders.

Arvedson, J., Rogers, B., Buck, G., Smart, P., & Msall, M. (1994). Silent aspiration prominent in children with dysphagia. *International Journal of Pediatric Otorhinolaryngology, 28,* 173–181.

Babson S. G., Pernoll, M. L., & Benda, G. I. (1980). Nutritional requirements and oral feeding of the low birth weight infant. In S. G. Babson, M. L. Pernoll, & G. I. Benda (Eds.), *Diagnosis and management of the fetus and neonate at risk.* St. Louis: C.V. Mosby.

Bernbaum, J. C., Pereira, G. R., Watkins, J. B., & Peckham, G. J. (1983). Nonnutritive sucking during gavage feeding enhances growth and maturation in premature infants. *Pediatrics, 71,* 41–45.

Blanche, M. A., Botticelli, T. M. & Hallway, M. (1995). *Combining neurodevelopmental treatment and sensory integration principles: An approach to pediatric therapy.* San Antonio, TX: Therapy Skills Builders.

Bly, L. (1994). *Motor skills acquisition in the first year.* Tucson, AZ: Therapy Skills Builders.

Bosma, J. F. (1986). Development of feeding. *Clinical Nutrition, 5,* 210–218.

Braun , M. A. & Palmer, M. M. (1986). A pilot study of oral sensorimotor dysfunction in "at-risk" infants. *Physical & Occupational Therapy in Pediatrics, 5,* 13–25.

Brown, J. (1972). Instrumental control of sucking response in human newborns. *Journal of Experimental Child Psychology, 14,* 66–80.

Burke, P. M. (1977). Swallowing and the organization of sucking in the human newborn. *Child Development, 48,* 523–531.

Capute, A. J., & Accardo, P. G. (1991). Cerebral palsy: The spectrum of motor dysfunction. In A. J. Capute & P. G. Accardo (Eds.), *Developmental disabilities in infancy and childhood* (335–348). Baltimore: Paul H. Brooks.

Casaer, P., Daniels, H., Devlieger, H., DeCock, P., & Eggermont, E. (1982). Feeding behavior in preterm neonates. *Early Human Development, 7,* 331–346.

Case-Smith, J. (1988). An efficacy study of occupational therapy with high-risk neonates. *American Journal of Occupational Therapy, 42,* 499–506.

Case-Smith, J., Cooper, P., & Scala, V. (1989). Feeding efficiency of premature neonates. *American Jouranl of Occupational Therapy, 43,* 245–250.

Case-Smith J., & Humphry, R. (2000). Feeding intervention. In J. Case-Smith (Ed.), *Occupational therapy for children* (4th ed.; 453–488). St. Louis: Mosby.

Christie, D. L. (1984). Pulmonary complications of esophageal disease. *Pediatric Clinics of North America, 31,* 835–849.

Coster, W., Deeney, T., Haltiwanger, J., & Haley, S., (1998). *School Function Assessment (SFA).* San Antonio, TX: Therapy Skill Builders.

Daga, S. R., Lunkad, N. G., Daga, A. S., & Ahuja, V. K. (1999). Orogastric versus nasogastric feeding of newborn babies. *Tropical Doctor, 29,* 242–243.

Dubignon, J., & Campbell, D. (1968). Intra-oral stimulation and sucking in the newborn. *Journal of Experimental Child Psychology, 6,* 154–166.

Erenberg, A., & Nowak, A. J. (1984). Palatal groove formation in neonates and infants with orotracheal tubes. *American Journal of the Disabled Child, 138,* 974–975.

Fenichel, G. M. (1990). *Neonatal neurology* (3rd ed.; 4). New York: Churchill Livingstone.

Field, T., Ignatoff, E., Stringer, S., Brennan, J., Greenberg, R., Widmayer, S., & Anderson, G. C. (1982). Nonnutritive sucking during tube feedings: Effects on preterm neonates in an intensive care unit. *Pediatrics, 70,* 381–384.

Fleming, P. J. (1994). Understanding and preventing sudden death syndrome. *Current Opinions in Pediatrics, 6,* 158–162.

Fox, C. A. (1990). Implementing the modified barium swallow evaluation in children who have multiple disabilities. *Infants and Young Children, 3,* 67–77.

Geyer, L. A., & McGowan, J. S. (1995) Positioning infants and children for videofluoroscopic swallowing function studies. *Infants and Young Children 8(2):*58–64.

Gisel, E. G. (1991). Effect of food texture on the development of chewing of children between six months and two years of age. *Developmental Medicine and Child Neurology, 33,* 69–79.

Gisel, E. G., Alphonce, E., & Ramsay, M. (2000). Assessment of ingestive and oral praxis skills: Children with cerebral palsy vs. controls. *Dysphagia, 15,* 236–244.

Gisel, E. G., Lange, L. J., & Niman, C. W. (1984). Chewing cycles in 4- and 5-year old Down's syndrome children: A comparison of eating efficacy with normals. *American Journal of Occupational Therapy, 38,* 666–670.

Gisel, E. G., & Patrick, J. (1998). Feeding and oral-motor skills. In Case-Smith, J. (Ed.). *Pediatric occupational therapy and early intervention* (2nd ed.; 127–163). Woburn, MA: Butterworth-Heinemann.

Glass, R. P., & Wolf, L. S. (1998). Feeding and oral-motor skills. In Case-Smith, J. (Ed.). *Pediatric occupational therapy and early intervention* (2nd ed.; 127–163). Woburn, MA: Butterworth-Heinemann.

Gomella, T. L., Cunningham, M. D., & Eyal, F. G. (Eds.). (1994). *Neonatology: Management, procedure, on-call problems, diseases and drugs* (3rd ed.). Stamford, CT: Appleton & Lange.

Greenspan, J. S., Wolfson, M. R., Holt, W. J., et al. (1990). Neonatal gastric intubation: Differential respiratory efforts between nasogastric and orogastric tubes. *Pediatric Pulmonology, 8,* 254–258.

Griggs, C. A., Jones, P. M., & Lee, R. E. (1989). Videofluoroscopic investigation of feeding disorders in children with multiple handicap. *Developmental Medicine and Child Neurology, 31,* 303–308.

Groher, M. E. (Ed.). (1997). *Dysphagia: Diagnosis and management* (3rd ed.). Stoneham, MA: Butterworth-Heinemann.

Haley, S. M., Coster, N. J., Ludlow, L. H., Haltiwanger, J., & Andrellos, P. (1992). *Pediatric Evaluation of Disability Inventory (PEDI).* San Antonio, TX: Therapy Skill Builders.

Hamilton, B. B. & Granger, C. V. (1991). Wee-FIM—Functional Independence Measure for children.

Harris, M. (1986). Oral sensori-motor management of the high-risk neonate. *Occupational Therapy in Pediatrics, 6,* 231–253.

Hawdon, J. M., Beauregard, N., Slattery, J., & Kennedy, G. (2000). Identification of neonates at risk for developing feeding problems in infancy. *Developmental Medicine and Child Neurology, 42,* 235–239.

Herman, M. J. (1991). Comprehensive assessment of oral sensori-motor dysfunction in failure-to-thrive-infants. *Infant-Toddler Intervention, 1,* 109–123.

Illingworth, R. S. (1969). Sucking and swallowing difficulties in infancy: Diagnostic problems of dysphagia. *Archives of Diseases in Children, 44,* 238.

Illingworth, R. S., & Lister, J. (1964). The critical or sensitive period, with special reference to certain feeding problems in infants and children. *The Journal of Pediatrics, 65,* 840–848.

Jelm, J. M. (1990). *Oral sensori-motor/feeding rating scale.* Tucson, AZ: Therapy Skill Builders.

Johnson, C. B., & Deitz, J. C. (1985). Time and use of mothers with preschool children: A pilot study. *American Journal of Occupational Therapy, 39,* 578–583.

Kenny, D., Koheil, R., Greenberg, J., Reid, D., Milner, M., Roman, R., & Judd, P. (1989). Development of a multidisciplinary feeding profile for children who are dependent feeders. *Dysphagia, 4,* 16–28.

Klein, M., & Stern, L. (1971). Low birth weight and the battered child syndrome. *American Journal of Disabled Child, 122,* 15–18.

Koontz-Lowman, D., & Lane, S. J. (1999). Children with feeding and nutritional problems. In S. M. Porr & E. B. Rainville (Eds.), *Pediatric therapy: A systems approach* (379–423). Philadelphia: F. A. Davis.

Kramer, S. S. (1985). Special swallowing problems in children. *Gastrointestinal Radiology, 10,* 241–250.

Krick, J., & Van Duyn, M. S. (1984). The relationship between oral sensorimotor involvement and growth: A pilot study in a pediatric population with cerebral palsy. *Journal of the American Dietetic Association, 84,* 555–569.

Kron, R. E., Stein, M., Goddard, K. E., & Phoenix, M. (1967). Effect of nutrient upon the sucking behavior of newborn infants. *Psychosomatic Medicine, 29,* 24–32.

Lane, S. J. & Cloud, H. H. (1988). Feeding problems and intervention: An approach. *Topics in Clinical Nutrition, 3,* 23–32.

Langmore, S. E., & Logemann, J. A. (1991). After the clinical bedside swallowing examination: What next? *American Journal of Speech-Language Pathology, Sept.,* 13–19.

Larnett, G., & Ekberg, O. (1995). Positioning improves the oral and pharyngeal swallowing function in children with cerebral palsy. *Acta Pediatrics, 84,* 689–692.

Leder, S. B., & Karas, D. E. (2000). Fiberoptic endoscopic evaluation of swallowing in the pediatric population. *The Laryngoscope, 110,* 1132–1136.

Logemann, J. A. (1983). *Evaluation and treatment of swallowing disorders.* Austin, TX: PRO-ED.

Logemann, J. A. (1993) *Manual for the videofluorographic study of swallowing* (2nd ed.). Austin, TX: PRO-ED.

Logemann, J. A. (1998). *Evaluation and treatment of swallowing disorders* (2nd ed.). Austin, TX: PRO-ED.

Macie, D., & Arvedson, J. (1993). Tone and positioning. In J. Arvedson & L. Brodsky (Eds.), *Pediatric swallowing and feeding: Assessment and management* (209–247). San Diego, CA: Singular Publishing Group.

Mathew, O. P., Belan, M., & Thoppil, C. K. (1992). Sucking patterns of neonates during bottle feeding: Comparison of different nipple units. *American Journal of Perinatology, 9,* 265–269.

McBride, M. E., & Danner, S. C. (1987). Sucking disorders in neurologically impaired infants: Assessment and facilitation of breastfeeding. *Clinics in Perinatalogy, 14,* 109–130.

Meyers, W. F. & Herbst, J. T. (1982). Effectiveness of positioning therapy for gastroesophageal reflux. *Pediatrics, 69,* 768–772.

Mizuno, K. & Aizawa, M. (1999). Effects of body position on blood gases and lung mechanics of infants with chronic lung disease during tube feeding. *Pediatrics International, 41,* 609–614.

Morris, S. E., & Klein, M. D. (1987). *Pre-feeding skills: A comprehensive resource for feeding development.* San Antonio, TX: Therapy Skill Builders.

Morris, S. E., & Klein, M. D. (2000). *Pre-feeding skills: A comprehensive resource for mealtime development.* (2nd ed.). San Antonio, TX: Therapy Skill Builders.

Morton, R., Bonas, R., Fourie, B., & Minford, J. (1993). Videofluoroscopy in the assessment of feeding disorders or children with neurological problems. *Developmental Medicine and Child Neurology, 35,* 388–395.

Nelson, K. B., & Ellenberg, J. H. (1984). Obstetrical complications as risk factors for cerebral palsy or seizure disorders. *Journal of American Medical Association, 251,* 1843–1848.

Oetter, P., Richter, E., & Frick, S. (1995). *M.O.R.E.: Integrating the mouth with sensory and postural functions* (2nd ed.). Hugo, MN: PDP Press.

Orenstein, S. R. (1990). Prone positioning in infant gastroesophageal reflux: Is elevation of the head worth the trouble? *The Journal of Pediatrics, 117,* 184–187.

Orenstein, S. R., Giarrusso, V. A., Proujansky, R., & Kocoshis, S. A. (1988). The Santmyer swallow: A new and useful infant reflex. *Lancet, 1,* 345–346.

Orenstein, S. R., & Whitington, P. F. (1983). Positioning for prevention of infant gastroesophageal reflux. *Jouranl of Pediatrics, 103,* 534–537.

Ottenbacher, K., Bundy, A., & Short, M. A. (1983). The development and treatment of oral sensori-motor dysfunction: A review of clinical research. *Physical and Occupational Therapy in Pediatrics, 3,* 1–13.

Palmer, M. M., & Heyman, M. B. (1993). Assessment and treatment of sensory motor-based feeding problems in very young children. *Infants and Young Children, 6,* 67–73.

Paludetto, R., Robertson, S. S., Hack, M., Shivpuri, C. R., & Martin, R. J. (1984). Transcutaneous oxygen tension during nonnutritive sucking in preterm infants. *Pediatrics, 74,* 539–542.

Reilly, S., & Skuse, D. (1992). Characteristics and management of feeding problems of young children with cerebral palsy. *Developmental Medicine and Child Neurology, 34,* 379–388.

Reilly, S., Skuse, D., & Wolke, D. (2000). *SOMA: Schedule for Oral Motor Assessment.* Eastgardens, New South Wales: Whurr.

Sasaki, C. T., & Toohill, R. J. (2000). Ambulatory pH monitoring for extraesophageal reflux—Introduction. *Annals of Otology, Rhinology, & Laryngology, 109*(Suppl.10), 2–3.

Satinoff, E., & Stanley, W. C. (1963). Effect of stomach loading on sucking behavior in neonatal puppies. *Journal of Comparative Physiological Psychology, 56,* 66–68.

Snyder, E. Y. & Cloherty, J. P. (1998). Perinatal asphyxia. In Cloherty, J. P., & Stark, A.R., *Manual of neonatal care* (4th ed.; 515). Philadelphia: Lippincott-Raven Publishers.

Stratton, M. (1981). Behavioral assessment scale of oral functions in feeding. *The American Journal of Occupational Therapy, 35,* 719–721.

Symington, A., Ballantyne, M., Pinelli, J., & Stevens, B. (1995). Indwelling versus intermittent feeding tubes in premature neonates. *Journal of Obstetric and Gynecologic Neonatal Nursing, 24,* 321–326.

Vice, F. L., Heinz, J. M., Giuriati, G., Hood, M., & Bosma, J. F. (1990). Cervical auscultation of suckle feeding in newborn infants. *Developmental Medicine and Child Neurology, 32,* 760–768.

von Gunten, A. S., Meyer, J. B., & Kim, A. K. (1995). Dental management of neonates requiring prolonged oral intubation. *Journal of Prosthodontics, 4,* 221–225.

Warner, J. (1981). *Helping the handicapped child with early feeding.* Winslow, Buckingham, England: Winslow Press.

Wilbarger, P. & Wilbarger, J. L. (1991). *Sensory defensiveness in children ages 2–12.* Santa Barbara, CA: Avanti Educational Programs.

Willging, J. P. (1995). Endoscopic evaluation of swallowing in children. *International Journal of Pediatric Otorhinolaryngology, 32* (Suppl.), S 107–S108.

Willging, J. P., Miller, C. K., Hogan, M. J., & Rudolph, C. D. (1996). Fiberoptic endoscopic evaluation of swallowing in children: A preliminary report of 100 procedures *Dysphagia, 11,* 162.

World Health Organization. (1997). *International Classification of Imapairment, Disability, and Handicap* (ICIDH2). Geneva, Switzerland.

■ CHAPTER 8

Instrumental Evaluation of Swallowing

Joan Arvedson, Linda Brodsky, and Steven Christensen

■ SUMMARY

Evaluation of feeding and swallowing often requires the use of additional studies that focus on various functional and structural aspects of swallowing. Three imaging studies have been developed to help visualize, both directly and indirectly, the swallowing mechanism in all four phases. These are videofluoroscopic swallow study (VFSS), flexible endoscopic evaluation of swallowing (with sensory testing) (FEES[ST]), and ultrasonography (US) of the oral and pharyngeal cavities.

Although clinical evaluation is of paramount importance, additional studies are invaluable in answering specific questions as to the safety for feeding and to the relative contribution of various structures or physiologic processes to feeding and swallowing difficulties, particularly risks for aspiration. Furthermore, effectiveness of therapy over time can be measured objectively and often quantitatively. This approach is requisite for increasing our understanding of disease processes and their clinical manifestations that are still poorly understood.

A description of each procedure is followed by a discussion of its technical performance. Special considerations in the preparation for, or the interpretation of, each study are described. The relative advantages and disadvantages of each are detailed. Finally, the pearls and pitfalls of interpretation and clinical correlation are discussed. Case studies highlight some of these issues.

■ INTRODUCTION

Comprehensive evaluation to recommend individualized management for infants and children with swallowing problems frequently requires the use of specialized imaging studies. VFSS, FEES, and US are the studies most often used. Each one has its proponents, but all provide useful information for the various clinical situations encountered when infants and children have abnormal feeding and swallowing. Other instrumental procedures routinely used in the evaluation of pediatric patients with dysphagia include upper gastrointestinal (UGI) study, scintiscan, 24-hour dual-channel pH monitoring, flexible fiberoptic nasopharyngolaryngoscopy[1] (FFNL), direct rigid laryngoscopy, bronchoscopy, and esophagoscopy (Chapters 4 and 5). In addition, manometry and electromyography (EMG) are useful in some instances.

Clinical assessment of oral sensorimotor function and swallowing is aided immeasurably by the additional *objective* information provided in specific situations (ASHA, 2000a; Benson & Lefton-Greif, 1994; Langmore & Logemann, 1991). These objective measures are particularly important in evaluating the pharyngeal and esophageal phases of swallowing in terms of both structure and function, not usually attainable by clinical examination alone. An example is the well-known fact that the risk for aspiration is greatly increased in most multiply involved children, although many have no observable clinical indications (coughing or choking), especially in children with neurologic impairment. Thus, the clinical assessment is inadequate in a high proportion of patients. Inaccurate or incomplete information will render recommended treatment strategies to be ineffective at best and potentially harmful at worst.

The instruments chosen to conduct an evaluation will depend on the anatomic areas and functional processes that need to be assessed. Instrumental measurement and scanning techniques are not used in isolation, but as part of a comprehensive evaluation with a thorough clinical examination of oral and pharyngeal functioning. Several different studies may be performed, each of which may be useful for the evaluation of oral, pharyngeal, laryngeal, upper esophageal, and respiratory function related to normal and abnormal swallowing. Most of these procedures have been developed for use with adults; however, more data are becoming available for their use with children (Arvedson, Rogers, Buck, Smart, & Msall, 1994; Bosma, Hepburn, Josell, & Baker, 1990; Hartnick, Miller, Hartley, & Willging, 2000; Kramer & Eicher, 1993; Langmore, Schatz, & Olson, 1991; Link, Willging, Miller, Cotton, & Rudolph, 2000; Liu, Kaplan, Parides, & Close, 2000; McConnell, Hester, Mendelsohn, & Logemann, 1988; McConnell, Mendelsohn, & Logemann, 1986; Palmer, 1989; Perlman, Luschei, & DuMond, 1989; Vice, Heinz, Giuriati, Hood, & Bosma, 1990; Willging,

---

[1]The terms flexible fiberoptic nasopharyngoscopy, flexible fiberoptic nasopharyngolaryngoscopy, and flexible fiberoptic laryngoscopy are used interchangeably.

2000). This chapter will present information related to US, FEES(ST), and VFSS. Each procedure's usefulness, indications, procedural considerations, and, perhaps most importantly, interpretation are discussed. It must be stressed that each study provides supplemental information, and the findings must be considered as only one part of the evaluation, for each study is only a glimpse of the swallowing mechanism at one point in time.

■ ULTRASONOGRAPHY (US)

US uses reflected sound as an imaging tool. This tool has been applied to visualize temporal relationships between movement patterns of oral and pharyngeal structures in infants (Bosma et al., 1990; Smith, Erenberg, Nowak, & Franken, 1985; Weber, Woolridge, & Baum, 1986) as well as in older children and adults (Fanucci, Cerro, Ietto, Brancaleone, & Berardi, 1994; Shawker, Sonies, Hall, & Baum, 1984; Shawker, Sonies, Stone, & Baum, 1983; Stone & Shawker, 1986; Sonies, 1990; Yang, Loveday, Metreweli, & Sullivan, 1997). US is most helpful in describing the oral preparatory and oral phases of swallowing, particularly in young infants (Bosma et al.).

US technicians and speech–language pathologists (SLPs) frequently carry out the study jointly. SLPs working in this area must be proficient in diagnosing oral and pharyngeal dysfunction and its relationship to swallowing to select appropriate patients for US study (ASHA, 1992). Clinicians involved in real-time US need to obtain appropriate training and knowledge in operating US systems, positioning patients, choosing bolus materials, and interpreting the results. Extensive knowledge of ultrasound imaging physics is not required.

Ultrasound is defined as sound propagated at frequencies above those audible to the human ear, that is, over 20 kHz. The frequencies used for diagnostic imaging range between 2 and 10 MHz, a 1,000-fold increase above the audible range (Sonies, 1987). During US imaging, a transducer is used both to generate sound waves and to receive ultrasound echoes. These echoes are then electronically converted into a computer generated image. An ultrasound beam, directed into a soft tissue medium, vibrates tissue particles in that medium. Body tissues (such as fat, muscle, fascia) and fluids (blood, cerebral spinal fluid, and water) have different densities and reflect echoes back to the transducer at different intensities, making different tissues or other substances distinguishable from each other at their interface. US is limited in that the sound echoes will not pass through bone.

Real-time US imaging displays the movement of anatomic structures. The image shows up in a variety of shades of gray, ranging from black to white. The shades of a gray scale correspond to predetermined values of the sound wave's intensity. The area beyond any bone is projected as black because the sound wave is reflected completely, leaving the area beyond the bone echo-free. Air, water, and the front surface of a bone project as white because they are highly reflective mediums. Muscles, glands, and other soft tissues project as shades of gray.

Auscultation of the larynx, using a stethoscope or microphone, is very different from US. The patterns of sound emissions auscultated during respiration, swallowing, and feeding may, however, have predictive value of aspiration and other coordination patterns of breathing and swallowing. As a noninvasive method, it has some use for screening and in monitoring treatment. The use of computer capture and electronic storage and display of data may prove to have some future clinical potential (Vice et al., 1990). (Further discussion of the use of auscultation can be found in Chapter 10.)

US Imaging Procedure

The oral cavity is well suited to ultrasound imaging because it is filled with air, soft tissue, and lubricated mucosal surfaces. The tongue in particular is surrounded by air, and its movements are defined during speech and by a liquid bolus during swallowing. Submental transducer placement creates scans in either the sagittal or the coronal planes (Fuhrmann & Diedrich, 1994; Yang, Loveday, Metreweli, & Sullivan, 1997). Submental views are best for imaging the tissue to air interface at the dorsum of the tongue. The sagittal view is best to show the genioglossus muscles; their midline septum is best seen in the coronal view (Bosma et al., 1990). Using a buccal window, a transverse plane may also be imaged. This view is particularly useful in infants who do not yet have teeth (Bosma et al.; Smith et al., 1985).

Tongue action can be observed during the oral preparatory and oral phases of swallowing. Nipple placement (breast and bottle) can be readily assessed with the mother and infant in natural feeding positions (Nowak, Smith, & Erenberg, 1994). For bottle- or breast-feeding infants, the transverse submental plane reveals the tongue grooving around the nipple. In infants and older children, the sagittal plane (viewed through the submentally placed probe) is useful to view the oral phase of the swallow as tongue action moves the bolus posteriorly toward the oropharynx (Figure 8–1A–C). The area just beyond the nipple edge corresponds to a portion of the tongue. Milk appears white in the image. Because the acoustic properties of water and other food differ, a bolus can be seen during preparation and transport toward the pharynx. The horizontal transbuccal plane cannot be used once teeth are present because teeth prevent passage of sound and obscure the view.

Suckle feeding is uniquely characteristic of mammals. It is biphasic, rhythmic, and coordinated, centered on the medial portion of the tongue (Bosma et al., 1990). The peristaltic wave begins with an initial discrete indentation in the superior margin in the medial portion of the tongue. The

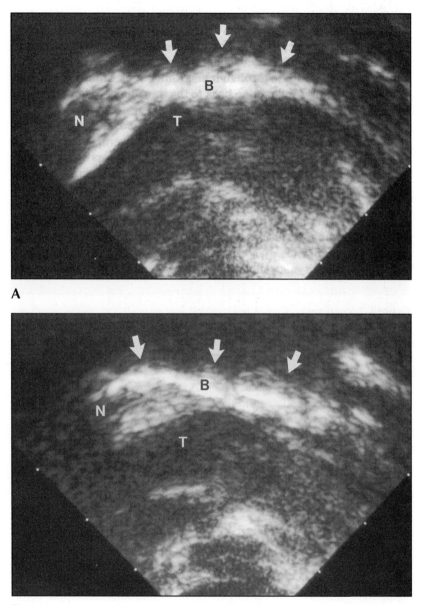

A

B

Figure 8–1. Ultrasound image in longitudinal submental plane of normal infant breast-feeding, showing progression of milk bolus posteriorly toward the orophayrnx. **A.** Tongue (T), palate (arrows) and mother's nipple (N) can be seen with milk bolus (B) anteriorly in the infant's mouth. **B.** Active sucking with milk bolus (B) moving posteriorly; N = nipple, T = tongue.

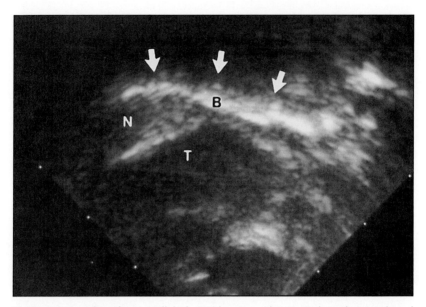

Figure 8–1 (continued). C. Milk bolus (B) has moved posteriorly in the mouth and is about to be swallowed; N = nipple, T = tongue.

tongue tip moves up toward the palate and compresses the nipple. The expressed milk is propelled into the pharynx. Lateral tongue position is stable and elevated, with the midtongue approximating the level of the lateral tongue posterior to the nipple (Bosma et al.). Simultaneous imaging of not only the tongue, but also the hyoid, mandible, and lower lip during US can provide valuable information for dysfunctional feeding in infants.

US imaging is particularly useful when there is concern for an oral phase problem during breast-feeding. Both mother and infant can be observed for extended time periods to define the oral phase without concern for radiation exposure, in contrast to VFSS (see below). For example, when a breast-feeding infant fails to initiate sucking readily or shows incoordinated sucking, it is possible to observe whether the difficulty is with the infant's suck–swallow patterns or the maternal milk supply (Smith et al., 1985). With premature infants, US may provide information to assess the infant's readiness for oral feedings. Muscle interactions and nipple deformation must be functional for successful oral feeding; these are both clearly seen with US.

Older infants and children can be assessed with transverse and longitudinal submental planes. In studying dysgnathia, Fuhrmann and Diedrich (1994) described five distinct steps or "stages" in the oral phase of a normal swallow induced with 2 ml of saline (approximating the volume of saliva in a single swallow) in normal children and children with various malocclusions. The normal swallow, stage 1, termed the *water collection stage,* showed water flowing into the anterior part of the floor of the mouth while the tip of the tongue is retracted slightly. In the *water elevation stage* (stage 2), the tongue tip moves upward to contact the palate at the level of the incisive papillae and assumes a "scoop shape." The dorsum of the mid-tongue is lowered. Stage 3 is termed the *transport stage* during which complete apposition of the tongue surface to the palate occurs and peristaltic motion of the soft palate and tongue propel the bolus posteriorly. The *late transport stage* (stage 4) sees the tongue dorsum lowered, tongue muscle contraction, and any remaining water flowing into the pharynx. In stage 5, the tongue goes back to resting position.

Whereas the oral phase of swallowing is visualized well using US, disordered oropharyngeal swallows are less well imaged. It is the oral preparatory and oral phases of swallowing, however, that are under voluntary control and therefore have the greatest potential to be altered with oral sensorimotor or other behavior based therapies.

Advantages and Disadvantages of US

The advantages and disadvantages of US are found in Table 8–1. US is most useful for the oral preparatory phase, also known as the bolus formation phase. In young infants, oral transit begins with expression of liquid from a nipple. The ability to capture tongue–palate–hyoid bone coordination during bolus transport is particularly important in assessing the role of laryngeal elevation in aspiration.

Interpretation—Pearls and Pitfalls

To give sound nutritional advice, the feeding potential of the infant must be established. Failure to have an effective and efficient suck/swallow/breathe pattern is usually due to multiple causes, at least a few of which are due to oral preparatory and oral phase dysfunction during swallowing. When an infant or child handles the bolus normally, the tongue is symmetrical, and a V-shaped groove is seen in the center of the tongue (coronal plane). A lateral seal is seen where the lateral tongue borders contact the hard palate. Effective bolus transport is accompanied by a "stripping wave" seen in the midline sagittal plane. Simultaneously, the lateral seal is preserved (coronal plane). Dysfunctional oral preparatory and oral phases of swallow image as asynchronous or asymmetric activity (Yang et al., 1997).

Unique to US is an excellent view of the elevation of the hyoid bone as a marker of laryngeal elevation, an important activity for airway protection from aspiration. Well seen in the sagittal plane, the hyoid bone is monitored

Table 8–1. Advantages and Disadvantages of Ultrasound (US)

Advantages
- Excellent soft tissue delineation in oral cavity
- Provides dynamic views of oral preparatory phase and oral phase of swallowing
- Multiplanar—sagittal, coronal, and, in infants, transverse
- Can evaluate structures at rest, bolus control, and swallow
- Captures tongue, palate, and hyoid activity for assessment of laryngeal elevation with initiation of pharyngeal swallow
- No radiation exposure
- Swallows can be sampled repeatedly and for prolonged periods of time
- Requires no contrast, uses "real" food or liquid
- Equipment is available at major medical centers
- Body positioning for patient and mother is not problematic

Disadvantages
- Limited to oral preparatory phase and oral phase swallowing
- Cannot detect laryngeal penetration or aspiration directly
- Structural landmarks are difficult to identify and may need to be created
- Availability of trained personnel may be limited
- Laryngeal structures cast shadow that obscures view of the airway
- Has not yet gained widespread clinical use because of limited data and trained personnel

during bolus propulsion and should be elevated at the end of stage 4 of the oral phase when the pharyngeal swallow is triggered or "at the onset" of the pharyngeal swallow. Absence of hyoid elevation may indicate a sensory deficit or fixation from tracheotomy. Young infants display only limited elevation of the hyoid bone. Some show anterior displacement. Uncoordinated hyoid bone movement may indicate abnormal motor or reflex activity (Yang et al., 1997).

As sophistication in the diagnosis and treatment of feeding and swallowing disorders continues to evolve, US is likely to emerge as a more widely used imaging tool for clinic purposes. Coordination and comparison with other imaging procedures, such as VFSS and FEES(ST), will be necessary to gain maximal information from this imaging modality.

■ FLEXIBLE ENDOSCOPIC EVALUATION OF SWALLOWING (FEES) WITH SENSORY TESTING (FEES(ST))

Flexible nasopharyngoscopy uses FFNL to view the upper aerodigestive tract directly in infants and children. The anatomic and physiologic information gained for assessment of the hypopharynx and larynx is critical to accurate diagnosis in almost all presentations of pediatric dysphagia. Use of FFNL to evaluate swallowing in adults—FEES (the early studies did not include sensory testing)—was described more than a decade ago (Bastian, 1991; Langmore et al., 1991; Langmore, Schatz, & Olsen, 1988; Liu et al., 2000). Its use in the evaluation of laryngeal sensation (Aviv, 2000a; Aviv et al., 2000) and swallowing dysfunction in infants and children in a variety of clinical settings followed shortly (Aviv, 2000a; Aviv et al.; Aviv et al., 1998; Hartnick et al., 2000; Leder & Karas, 2000; Link et al., 2000; Migliore, Scoopo, & Robey, 1999; Willging, 1995; Willging, 2000; Willging, Miller, Hogan, & Rudolph, 1996).

The endoscopic method for evaluation of swallowing provides information about the events occurring immediately before and immediately after the pharyngeal swallow. Advances in digital photography and digital video imaging have revolutionized the use of this tool as safe, highly informative, and useful in both the diagnosis and treatment of swallowing dysfunction in patients of all ages, beginning with premature infants. In some instances, FEES may be an adjunct to VFSS (Bastian, 1991). Integration of FEES with a VFSS from the same patient has been facilitated by technology advances (e.g., Swallowing Work Station, Kay Elemetrics, Lincoln Park, NJ and Clark® TUT® Image Capture and Processing System, Clark Research and Development, Inc., Folsom, LA).

FEES(ST) Procedure

Optimally, FEES(ST) is best performed by a team consisting of a pediatric otolaryngologist and an SLP. The physician is skilled at passing the FFNL and has the comprehensive knowledge base to assess the anatomic, physiologic, and functional abnormalities found in the nasal, pharyngeal, and laryngeal regions. The SLP has specialized knowledge and experience in swallowing and communication and is able to focus on the oral sensorimotor status of the child and functional aspects of swallowing. This interdisciplinary team approach capitalizes on the expertise of professionals in these two allied fields, thereby providing a more comprehensive evaluation of the child's swallowing ability (ASHA, 2000b).

The child is in his or her normal posture for feeding. The FFNL is passed transnasally to view the pharynx and larynx. In general a 2.7 mm nasopharyngoscope will pass readily in almost all infants; a 3.0 or 4.0 mm nasopharyngoscope is attempted in older children.[2] Topical anesthesia is

---

[2] A 1.0 mm nasopharyngoscope is available but very fragile, gives limited visualization, and is very expensive. Thus, not many centers have invested in this scope.

used by some, taking great care to limit the area anesthetized to the nasal cavity so as not to interfere with the study. In some instances, the FFNL is used without administration of topical anesthesia to the nasal mucosa (Leder & Karas, 2000). When anesthesia is used, it is given as a spray from an atomizer or on a cotton pledgette. A mixture of 2% tetracaine and $\frac{1}{2}$% neosynephrine or oxymetazoline (1:1 mixture) is delivered to the nose. Tetracaine doses of 0.3 mg/kg are used for children under the age of 4 years (Willging, 2000). After about 5 minutes, the FFNL can be passed transnasally into the hypopharynx while the child is held in the caregiver's lap or is sitting on a regular chair or in a wheelchair (Figure 8–2). A Pedi-Endo Pacifier™ (Hood Laboratories, Pembroke, MA) is available and useful for some infants and toddlers who can be calmed before and during endoscopy (Figure 8–3). This pacifier allows feeding through or sucking while the physician passes an endoscope orally through the silicone pacifier with minimal disruption to the infant. Formula or other colored liquid can be introduced via a separate channel with a luer-lock syringe adapter for swallowing evaluations. The nasopharynx is not available for visualization with this procedure. Evaluation of structure and function is completed as described in Chapter 4.

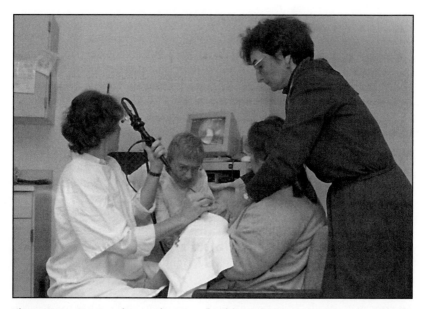

Figure 8–2. Young infant undergoing flexible endoscopic examination of swallowing, held in mother's lap.

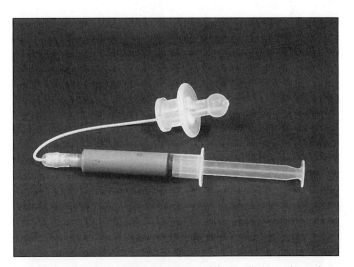

Figure 8–3. Pedi-Endo Pacifier™ with syringe filled with formula and green food coloring.

Swallowing is evaluated first for handling of secretions by placing a small amount of food coloring on the tongue. This technique also is used for children who are unable to initiate a swallow. If aspiration of oral secretions is witnessed, the test may be terminated. If the child can take food or liquid, the SLP gives various food textures to the patient to swallow. The entire examination is recorded on videotape or CD-ROM for documentation and review (Figure 8–4).

FEES/ST combines the standard endoscopic evaluation of swallowing with a technique that determines laryngopharyngeal sensory discrimination thresholds. The FFNL is placed 2 to 4 mm above the area to be tested. A 50-msec air pulse, 3 to 10 mm Hg pressure, is delivered to the arytenoid mucosa via a side port built into the nasopharyngoscope (FNL 10 AP Laryngoscope, Pentax Precision Instrument Corp, Orangeburg, NY) (Liu et al., 2000). Innervation of the laryngeal adductor reflex (LAR) by the superior laryngeal nerve is tested (Link et al., 2000; Liu et al.). Link and associates demonstrated feasibility in 92% of the 100 pediatric patients they attempted. A threshold of < 4 mm Hg was found only in patients who exhibited no aspiration. A threshold above 10 mm Hg was seen only in severe laryngeal penetration or aspiration. Elevated levels (between 4 and 10 mm Hg) were seen in a wide variety of clinical situations and correlated well to hypopharyngeal pooling of secretions, laryngeal penetration, and aspiration. Thus, FEES/ST appears safe and provides useful information

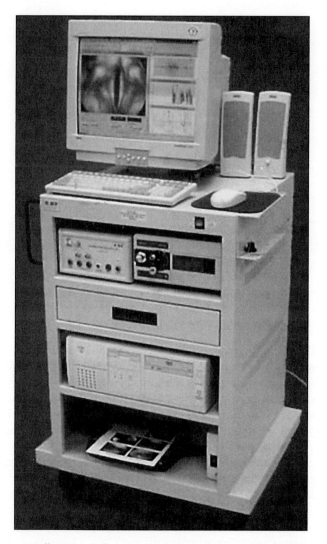

Figure 8–4. Swallowing work station, Key Elemetrics, used for FEESST and VFSS.

regarding sensory function. Findings should help to clarify safety of oral feeding, particularly in children with neurologic impairments and developmental disabilities. Understanding the sensory contribution will help supplement the extensive imaging information already available for the motor contribution in dysphagia.

Advantages and Disadvantages of FEES(ST)

The advantages and disadvantages of FEES(ST) are found in Table 8–2. The best results are gained when a reasonable amount of cooperation can be elicited from the patient. Examiner experience and patient preparation are important in gaining cooperation in children (3 years and older) (Link et al., 2000; Willging, 2000). Computer capture of both FEES and VFSS is facilitated by use of the Swallow Station. Bedside endoscopic swallow evaluations are performed easily and the system is used in the radiology suite (Figure 8–5).

Interpretation—Pearls and Pitfalls

Swallowing function parameters evaluated include pharyngeal pooling of secretions, premature spillage, laryngeal penetration, aspiration, residue, vocal fold mobility, gag reflex, and LAR (Gisel, Birnbaum, & Schwartz, 1998; Willging, 2000). FEES is more sensitive in establishing persistent residue and abnormal pooling than are other tests. Particularly when airway concerns are an issue, FEES is preferable to VFSS to assess airway safety even before oral intake during a VFSS (see Case Study in Chapter 10).

Table 8–2. Advantages and Disadvantages of Flexible Endoscopic Evaluation of Swallowing With Sensory Testing (FEES(ST))

Advantages
- Can be taken to the patient in any location
- Readily available
- Immediate examination can be performed (no scheduling needed)
- No radiation exposure
- Position of patient is flexible and not critical to results
- Observation of structure and function of hypopharynx and larynx possible
- May be repeated frequently
- Study may take as long as needed
- Tests sensory component

Disadvantages
- Incomplete examination of pharyngeal phase of swallow
- Only visualize immediately before or after a swallow
- Cannot assess oral or esophageal phases of swallow
- Unable to evaluate coordination of pharyngeal motility with tongue action, laryngeal elevation, and upper esophageal relaxation
- Minimally invasive
- Literature comparing it to videofluoroscopic swallow study is limited

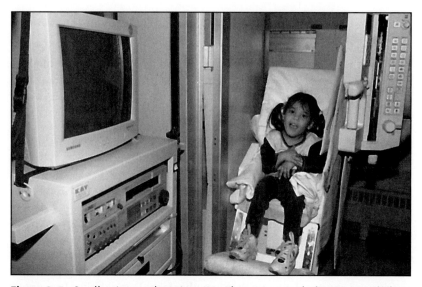

Figure 8–5. Swallowing work station, Key Elemetrics, ready for use in radiology suite with child in position for lateral view.

As stated above, examiner experience in a nonthreatening atmosphere is important to achieve successful results. In addition, patient and parental preparation are usually time-consuming but well worth the effort. This includes approximately 30 to 40 min to discuss the procedure with child and family and for follow-up play therapy with some children to minimize the anxiety level in preparation for the study.

Adequate anesthesia appears to be helpful to enable most children to complete the study. Lack of pain or discomfort enhances the child's trust in the physician and improves the quality of the study. If the anesthesia is given carefully, it should not compromise either the airway or the study results. Just as with VFSS, studies with uncooperative patients are subject to the same cautions and difficulties. The most informative studies mimic the usual swallowing pattern for the patient. Nonetheless, non-cooperative children and of course infants can be studied, and a modicum of information will be gained.

When an infant or child cannot be taken to a radiology fluoroscopy suite, FEES is performed at the bedside with video recording (see Figure 8–4). Children with difficulties in transferring to alternate seating systems, such as those with severe scoliosis or kyphosis who cannot be examined in the radiology suite, are excellent subjects. Children with muscular dystrophy or other neuromuscular conditions can be examined as they maintain their typical posture for feeding in whatever seating systems are useful in the home and school environments.

■ VIDEOFLUOROSCOPIC SWALLOW STUDY (VFSS)

Videofluoroscopy is the primary imaging technique for detailed dynamic assessment of oral, pharyngeal, and upper esophageal phases of a swallow. Other names for VFSS are found in Table 8–3. A comprehensive look at the esophageal phase (i.e., an esophagram) requires additional study conducted by the radiologist. The esophagus is only scanned with VFSS, which uses barium contrast and dynamic video recording of the swallow process.[3] VFSS is useful for both diagnostic purposes and to assist in management decisions. Differences in handling a variety of textures, assessment of compensatory techniques, and re-education procedures are demonstrated (Logemann, 1993; Siebens & Linden, 1985).

VFSS is used as part of a comprehensive diagnostic evaluation of infants, including premature infants, and children with swallowing difficulties. Although somewhat of a misnomer, the VFSS is often referred to as the "gold standard." This is an exaggeration because the findings reveal only a brief window in time in a somewhat artificial setting. Nonetheless, the information obtained when the study is carried out effectively with a cooperative patient is valuable as an important "piece of the puzzle."

VFSS has enjoyed widespread utilization since the early 1980s (Logemann, 1983). The multiple names for this procedure underscore the variations

Table 8–3. Alternate Terms for the Videofluoroscopic Swallow Study

- Modified barium swallow (MBS)
- Oral–pharyngeal motility study
- Videofluoroscopic swallowing function study/examination
- Videoradiographic swallow study
- Videofluorographic swallow study
- Three-phase swallow study
- Rehabilitation swallow study

---

[3]It is of historic interest that cineradiography, the procedure that preceded videofluoroscopy, was recorded on motion-picture film, resulting in a sharp image that could be analyzed frame-by-frame at 60 frames per second. Disadvantages of cineradiography include radiation exposure greater than with VFSS, lack of voice recordings, significant time for the study, and high cost of film development. Thus, cineradiography is no longer used routinely.

that exist in its performance. Lack of standardization of positioning, amount and order of bolus presentation (food and liquid), utilization of information needed for management decisions, and approach to special clinical situations are a few of the areas requiring greater attention to standardization.

Despite these variations, a number of characteristics identified during VFSS have impact on the oral, pharyngeal, and esophageal phases of the swallow, but VFSS is best for evaluation of the pharyngeal phase of the swallow. Other information gained is listed in Table 8–4 (Arvedson et al., 1994; Sorin, Somers, Austin, & Bester, 1988). A bolus can be followed through the upper esophageal sphincter (UES) and the esophagus. Cricopharyngeal opening, esophageal motility, and transit time are screened.

During a clinical bedside feeding observation, clinicians can only make inferences about potential for aspiration, especially in persons with neurologic deficits. Approximately 40 to 42% of aspiration is not detected in adults or children at the bedside clinical assessment (Logemann, 1983; Splaingard, Hutchins, Sulton, & Chaudhuri, 1988). A high incidence of silent aspiration has been found during radiographic studies involving children with multiple disabilities (Arvedson et al., 1994; Griggs, Jones, & Lee, 1989; Helfrich-Miller, Rector, & Strakes, 1986; Mirrett, Riski, Glascott, & Johnson, 1994). Of 186 children with swallowing dysfunction who underwent initial videofluoroscopic swallow studies at the Children's Hospital of Buffalo from 1989 through 1991, 48 children (26%) aspirated on at least one texture, most commonly liquid. Of those who aspirated, almost all (94%) had silent aspiration (Arvedson et al.).

Table 8–4. Structural and Functional Information Gained from Videofluoroscopic Swallow Studies

- Oral-phase bolus handling
- Velopharyngeal function, nasopharyngeal reflux
- Laryngeal elevation and hyoid bone movement
- Vocal fold function for airway protection
- Pharyngeal motility
- Pharyngeal transit time
- Pooling of secretions and contrast material in the valleculae and pyriform sinuses before swallows
- Number of swallows necessary to clear material per bolus
- Residue of secretions and contrast material in valleculae and pyriform sinuses after swallows
- Presence and timing of aspiration in relation to the swallow of varied textures
- Coordination of laryngeal elevation with onset of pharyngeal phase

Most children are referred for VFSS because they demonstrate clinical presentations that suggest dysphagia or they have diagnostic conditions that are associated with increased risk for dysphagia (ASHA, 2000a; Table 1–1). Some children present with signs that raise concerns about the presence of dysphagia, although no identifiable etiology is yet available to explain the presence of the signs or symptoms. Other children may present with limited or no clinical evidence of dysphagia but have risks based on previously established diagnoses or past medical history. Findings in the clinical assessment could lead to a physician's order for a swallow study, but one must not conclude that the mere presence of one or more of these signs and symptoms necessarily means that a swallow study should be done. The information obtained from the study must result in diagnostic clarity or impact current management recommendations.

VFSS Imaging Procedure

Findings from the clinical examination, as discussed in the previous chapter, are helpful in planning for VFSS. The goal is to obtain maximal pertinent information in minimal time. Attention needs to be paid to the child's posture, positioning, and sensitivity to oral stimulation (Zerilli, Stefans, & DiPietro, 1990). Other considerations include the array of food textures in the child's diet, method of presentation of liquids and solids, and presentation order of textures. Steps to insure an optimal examination include:

1. preparation of patients and caregivers for VFSS,
2. attention to physical setup for VFSS in pediatrics, including seating and postural considerations, and
3. performance of the VFSS, particularly coordination with the radiologist.

This chapter is not intended to be a procedural manual. Readers desiring detailed information can refer to Arvedson and Lefton-Greif (1998).

Preparation of Patients and Caregivers for VFSS

Caregivers should receive sufficient verbal and written information prior to the VFSS so they understand the reasons for the study, the way in which it will be done, and what information will be gained. Caregivers can then help to prepare the child for optimal cooperation. Parents may be helpful in the radiology suite with the child; in some instances, presence of a familiar feeder can be critical for success of the study. Clinicians need to work closely with the radiology department in their facility to achieve a well-functioning radiology–SLP team for VFSS.

The child should be awake, alert, and hungry. Parents are encouraged to withhold food and liquid for several hours before the examination. A hungry child is more likely to accept the barium-impregnated food and liquid. On the other hand, the child should not be so hungry that fussiness results; thus, scheduling the VFSS as close as possible to a regular feeding time is advisable. Timely appointments and a nonthreatening, playful atmosphere also help. Pacifiers, swaddling, or partial undressing may soothe infants. Caregivers can bring familiar foods, containers, and utensils. They also may bring favorite toys, audio-taped music, blankets, and other "comfort items." A cooperative child is necessary for an interpretable study. Fussy, crying children are at increased risk for aspiration because of incoordination of swallowing if they take food or liquid while they are crying. Findings cannot be interpreted reliably if the child's responses are not typical of behavior during routine mealtimes. Children who are lethargic are also at high risk for aspiration; however, children who are typically in a somewhat lethargic state while eating orally may undergo VFSS so clinicians can assist with management decisions.

Additional considerations are needed when a child has a feeding tube. Regardless of the type of feeding tube, VFSS should be done only after the child demonstrates experience with some food or liquid orally, at the very least in the context of oral sensorimotor/swallow practice. For children who are total nonoral feeders, the medical and clinical assessment will determine if oral–motor practice can include tastes of food or liquid that will help to prepare the child for a study. These children are usually referred for testing because questions are raised as to the possibility of management changes, such as increased or decreased amounts of oral feeding or texture changes.

Parents are reminded that this sample of swallows is strictly oral. A bolus of at least 2 to 3 cc, reflecting the amount of saliva in a typical swallow, is usually adequate to observe swallow function; an ability to consume 15 to 30 cc, more closely approximating an actual feed, is preferred. Children who do not have even oral tastes in their repertoire are not likely to complete a safe, valid, or reliable study.

A nasogastric (NG) tube should be removed whenever possible. The effects of NG tubes on swallowing function are not clearly understood. A child with an NG tube may experience changes in respiratory effort and oxygen saturation levels or in the timing and adequacy of velopharyngeal closure. The presence of NG tubes may increase the probability of gastroesophageal reflux (GER). A nasoduodenal (ND) tube is left in place for a child who is clearly not ready to do major oral feeding because an ND tube has to be reinserted under fluoroscopy.

Schedules may need to be adjusted for medications that are given in relation to mealtimes so they fit in to the timing of the VFSS (e.g., medications for seizure control and for gastroesophageal reflux). If medications make a child lethargic, scheduling times may need to be adjusted. Overall, caregivers should keep their children as close as possible to regular routines.

Physical Setup for VFSS

Fluoroscopy is a radiographic technique that permits dynamic imaging as movement is observed in real time via images that are transmitted directly to a videotape (or CD-ROM with new technology), which then becomes the permanent record. Basic equipment does not differ in relation to the age of the patient. The equipment consists of (a) a standard, tiltable fluoroscopic table, (b) an image intensifier tube that picks up the X-ray beam, (c) a video monitor, and (d) a videotape recorder (VCR) wired into the monitor for viewing the fluoroscopic image and tape recording simultaneously (Figure 8–6).

The VCR is typically wired into the controls of the fluoroscopy unit so the radiologist can activate the VCR and the fluoroscopy unit simultaneously. The simultaneous activation of videotape and fluoroscopy unit allows for accurate viewing with no gaps. Most VCR setups use $\frac{1}{2}$-inch videotapes, some super VH and some regular VH tapes, although $\frac{3}{4}$ inch tapes may still be used in some places. The high-quality taping with portable systems (e.g., Swallowing Work Station and Clark® TUT® Image Capture and Processing

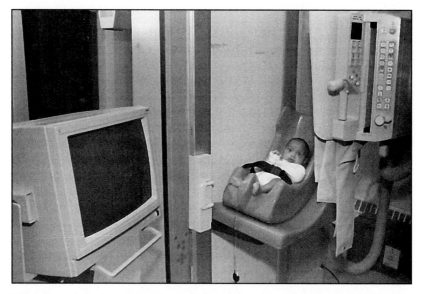

Figure 8–6. Infant positioned in small Tumbleform seat between the upright table and the image intensifier tube prior to videofluoroscopic swallow study.

System) allows for analysis with greater precision than possible a number of years ago. Almost any recorder can be used to record the image from fluoroscopy. Every study should have videotape recording with audio. (If a microphone is not built into the tape-recording system, it should be readily available and accessible for every study. If a headset is needed for audio replay, it should be stored with the microphone.) Digital systems are available and likely to become more commonly used in the near future. The simultaneous audio recording is essential to record instructions, describe events by the clinician, hear the patient's responses (particularly useful in relation to aspiration timing and presence or absence of a cough), and assessment of vocal quality (e.g., breathy, gurgly, dysphonic).

In clinical research facilities, the basic set up includes VCR equipment with a high-resolution frame-pause, slow-motion forward and reverse, and single-frame advance capability (Arvedson & Lefton-Greif, 1998; Logemann, 1993). Accessory equipment includes video counter timer to number each frame or field of the videotape, video character generator to print patient identifying information on the video image, and a video printer to produce a hard copy of a select video frame. The increased emphasis on efficacy of treatment and outcomes behooves all clinicians to use research thinking processes and problem-solving skills for data collection.

Radiation Safety

Radiation safety must be a high priority (Jones, Kramer, & Donner, 1985). Two rules of reason can be applied to patients undergoing radiation exposure for medical purposes (Tolbert, 1996). The first rule relates to medical necessity, which considers the importance of specific information required from an imaging procedure. This supports the earlier discussion about the importance of defining the questions to be answered before considering referral for VFSS. The second rule relates to the principle of keeping exposure levels "as low as reasonably achievable (ALARA)" (Tolbert, p. 4). In all instances ALARA means limiting exposures to that amount needed to achieve the purpose of the procedure (Tolbert).

All procedures are carried out in ways that minimize dose risks to the patient and others in the radiology suite. Dose is the amount of radiant energy that gets into the tissues of the body. The risk of harm at doses typically used during diagnostic X-ray procedures is not known precisely and probably cannot be determined with certainty. All persons are exposed to variable amounts of natural environmental radiation. Dose can be minimized by keeping the exposure time as short as possible ("fluoro-on" time). The use of shorter screening times, careful collimation of the beam to the area of interest, and reduction in the number of radiographs taken, if any, are all useful in reducing radiation dose (Beck & Gayler, 1990). In most instances, the videotape is the record, and no radiographs are needed. The method used for recording images is the major influence on radiographic doses (Martin & Hunter, 1994; Nicholson, Thornton, & Akpan, 1995).

The fluoroscopic tube needs to encompass the lips anteriorly, the palate superiorly, the posterior pharyngeal wall posteriorly, and the bifurcation of the airway and the esophagus inferiorly. The field should be coned to keep the ocular lens out of the field and to minimize radiation exposure to the difficult to shield thyroid gland. Radiologists are constantly challenged by active, moving children and frequently must follow that moving target with the imaging field. Magnification at the level of the larynx and at the entrance to the esophagus may be important when aspiration is suspected. The only practical way to minimize the dose to this area is to limit the fluoroscopy time.

Every swallow study should be monitored to conform to radiation safety standards and to minimize the duration of the study, as well as the amount of surface area exposed. *Guidelines of Radiation Safety* issued by the National Institutes of Health (NIH) recommend 5 rem/year for all diagnostic procedures after age 18 years and 3 rem to any tissue in a 13-week time period. Swallow studies are limited to a dosage of between 270 to 660 mrad/study, with a 10% reduction in that level recommended for children less than 18 years of age (Sonies, 1991). Careful planning will assure that no unnecessary time is spent with the child under fluoroscopy. Most studies with infants can be completed in 60 to 90 sec, and in some cases the examination can be performed in less time. Limiting exposure time and shielding of the reproductive organs should be used at all times (Sivit, 1990). Beck and Gayler (1990) also stated that initial diagnostic studies should rarely exceed 2 min of "fluoro-on" time. Even with the most difficult older patient, clinicians are urged to keep total fluoroscopy time to no more than 2 to 3 min with rare exceptions. Therapeutic maneuvers that include change in head position or evaluation of different bolus consistencies and volumes take longer. Thus, therapeutic maneuvers should be used sparingly and only when there is anticipation that such maneuvers can be incorporated into recommendations.

Seating and Positioning

Primary caregivers work with clinicians to get the child into the *typical* feeding position. If the position is different from an *optimal* position, the child can be observed in both positions. In general, the child's posture should be one that attains central alignment (Chapter 7). No single definition of optimal position can be stated because individual exceptions may be needed. Commercial seating and multiple positioning options are available for infants and children (Table 8–5). Seating possibilities for infants and children necessarily are varied to meet the specific needs of that child (Figures 8–6 and 8–7).

Table 8–5. Positioning and Equipment Options for Videofluoroscopic Swallow Study in Pediatrics

Patient Ages/Sizes	Equipment	Advantages	Disadvantages
Infants, no motor deficits or hypotonia	Infant seat	Easy to put in place Lightweight to store Support with towels	PA view difficult Potential metal parts Must be secured to table or foot plate
	Tumbleform (small size)	Base to adjust angle for feeding Attaches to footplate Inserts into other systems	Limited support of head and neck PA view difficult
	Infantascope or cradle	Rotating base	Limited support of head and neck
Infants + children (newborn to 60 in. and to 75 lbs)	MAMA system	Wide age group Cushion insert Single unit system on wheels	Lacks head support Seat too low to image down to lower esophageal sphincter and may need platform to raise seat
Infants + children with scoliosis	Side-lying on table	Custom made devices only	Not typical feeding position For selected patients
Toddlers	Tumbleform (medium size)	See above	See above
	MAMA system	See above	See above
	McMullen Dysphagia chair	Pediatric insert Has head support Straps to secure upper body Swivel base for PA view	Lacks trunk support

PA = Posterior-anterior, MAMA = Multiple Application Multiple Articulation (MAMA Systems, Inc., Oconomowoc, WI)

(continues)

Table 8–5. *(continued)* Positioning and Equipment Options for Videofluoroscopic Swallow Study in Pediatrics

Patient Ages/Sizes	Equipment	Advantages	Disadvantages
Older children	Footplate, stand or sit	No equipment needed	Requires independent standing or sitting
			Few qualify
	Tumbleform (large size)	See above	Limited body support
	MAMA system	See above	Bigger children may not fit
			See above
	Wheelchair	Allows child to stay in typical position for feeding	Usually too wide and low for adequate imaging in pediatric settings
			Metal parts
	Hausted chair	Hydraulic base to modify height	No head and trunk support
		Infant seat/wheelchair insert possible	
	McMullen Dysphagia chair	See above	See above
	Amigo Escort	Electric base to modify height	Lacks trunk support
All ages	Custom-built chairs	Designed to meet specific needs	

Note. From *Pediatric Videofluoroscopic Swallow Studies: A Professional Manual With Caregiver Guidelines,* p. 83, by Arvedson, J. C., & Lefton-Greif, M. A., 1998. San Antonio, TX: Communication Skill Builders. Copyright 1998 by The Psychological Corporation. Reprinted with permission.

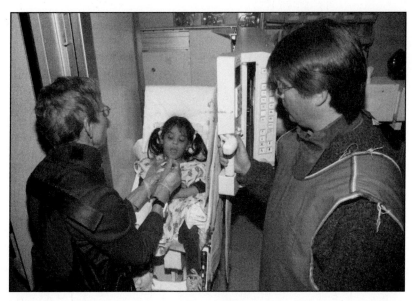

Figure 8–7. Videofluoroscopic swallow study in progress for a 3-year-old with cerebral palsy seated in the MAMA chair. Note thyroid collars on radiologist and SLP, also surgical leaded gloves and badges. Badges are at level of throat, under the lead apron, and on the feeder's wrist.

Seating systems can be adapted in a variety of ways to meet the needs of most children. Creativity by clinicians is encouraged. Basic stability and central alignment of the infant or child must be maintained with whatever modifications are made. A child with poor head or trunk control may need additional stabilization of the head to attain neutral midline position (e.g., Hensinger collar, a sponge, or head master collar [see Figure 9–9] can support the neck and head). Rolled towels or cushions can be placed alongside the head or trunk. One has to make sure that the child can tolerate restrictions of movement.

The position may need to be changed during an examination when difficulties become apparent or when the child is moved from the typical to the optimal position. An infant may take nipple feeds in a semireclined position and then be moved into upright position for spoon-feeding.

Children may vary considerably in what is perceived by caregivers and clinicians to be an optimal position for eating. Some children may be supported more effectively to maintain central alignment in a seat at a semireclining angle of approximately 35 to 45° than in upright posture. Infants have been studied via videofluorosopy in a reclining position resembling that of nursing infants on the side or bottle-fed infants in reclining position (Newman, Cleveland, Blickman, Hillman, & Jaramillo, 1991). A side-lying position may be necessary for a premature or very young infant (Fox, 1990), for a child who has a unilateral vocal fold paralysis with the non-paralyzed side down, or for a child with severe muscle tone imbalance (Geyer & McGowan, 1995; Ward, 1984). Bottle-fed infants are not usually fed in side-lying position, so this may not be helpful for those infants. An infant with Pierre Robin sequence may be able to bring the tongue forward in the oral cavity for more efficient sucking action and to aid in maintaining airway patency while in a modified prone position. It is best to simulate the normal or desired feeding position as closely as possible.

Given the space limitations between the upright table and the fluoroscopy unit in most pediatric radiology suites (typically 15 to 18 inches), the child is transferred into a special seating arrangement. The seating system needs to be as close as possible to the imaging equipment to maximize the quality of the image and reduce the amount of image magnification. Wheelchairs, even those for small children, are usually too wide to fit between the table and the fluoroscopic tube, and they are too low to allow for viewing the oral cavity, pharynx, and especially the esophagus. Portable fluoroscopy units are used in some adult facilities (e.g., long-term care facilities), but they may or may not be appropriate for infants and young children. C-arm units may be adaptable for older children who need to remain in their own wheelchairs. Other adaptations may be possible, depending on specification of equipment in radiology suites.

The caregiver may need to participate in the feeding. In *rare* instances, children resist separation to such a degree that it may be necessary to have the child seated on a caregiver's lap. The caregiver is shielded and seated for a lateral view with the child's back to the caregiver. In this way, the caregiver is not in the view, but the child is well positioned for a lateral view. It is not possible to cradle an infant in the caregiver's arms because the caregiver would block the pharyngeal view of the infant. Creativity may be needed to make the study successful with fearful children, or those who have severe motor deficits. It is also true that some children respond in more cooperative ways when parents are waiting outside the door of the radiology suite.

Individual variability requires the availability of different types and sizes of seating systems. Positioning options are discussed with advantages and disadvantages in Table 8–5. For example, the hypotonic child may need inhibition of abnormal patterns of fixation, promotion of alignment and stability, maintenance of upright posture for feeding, and promotion of symmetry and midrange control. The hypertonic child may need inhibition of excessively increased tone, inhibition of proximal fixation, and facilitation of movement. The success of the procedure depends greatly on having the patient in the most stable seating or positioning system possible (Arvedson & Lefton-Greif, 1998). Interpretation of the study will need qualification if the examiner questions the adequacy of the positioning. The child who walks into the radiology suite, stands in place or sits on the foot-plate, and eagerly takes the food and liquid presented is relatively rare.

Once the child is positioned appropriately and appears ready to take food and liquid, the study begins. Children with tracheotomy may need suctioning before taking food and liquid. Suctioning capabilities should be available throughout the study. If the child uses a speaking valve, testing should be done with and without the valve. A brief practice period of oral stimulation by a caregiver or a clinician familiar to a child may be helpful when a child shows oral defensiveness or tactile hypersensitivity. In sum-mary, adequate positioning is critical to the success of the VFSS.

Carrying Out VFSS

Typically, the VFSS is conducted by a team: a radiologist or another physi-cian who is knowledgeable regarding radiation safety and techniques, an X-ray technologist, and a speech–language pathologist (ASHA, 1992). The speech–language pathologist must demonstrate appropriate knowledge and skills to ensure that every decision made will benefit every patient who undergoes a VFSS (ASHA, 1990). In some institutions, a qualified speech–language pathologist and a radiology technician conduct the study as a team with consultation as needed from the physician. With high-risk infants and children, however, a physician should be directly involved in conducting this diagnostic study. The radiologist operates the fluoroscopic unit, identifies structural abnormalities, and when necessary, terminates a procedure that has unacceptable risks to the patient's health and safety.

The basic technique for videofluoroscopic swallow studies has been described previously in detail (Arvedson & Lefton-Greif, 1998; Logemann, 1983, 1993, 1998). The use of swallows of small amounts of barium--impregnated food and liquid differs from the standard barium swallow (or esophagram), in which only liquid barium is used to document the anatomy and physiology of the gastrointestinal system, usually with the patient in supine position. Compensatory techniques are not attempted. In contrast, the VFSS is usually conducted with the patient in upright (or at least semi-upright) position with compensatory techniques attempted in many instances to obtain structural and functional information (Table 8–4).

Caregivers are asked to bring samples of food that are in the child's usual diet, and especially those food textures for which they have the great-est concern related to coughing and gagging, food refusal, increased time for feeding, or increased need for suctioning. This process allows for iden-tification of foods that can be ingested safely. Barium impregnated food and liquid become the test material, with as close approximation as possible to foods that normally appear in the diet. Although every effort is made to assess the child in the most normal oral feeding situation, there may be times when other approaches are necessary, especially in the presence of severe oral sensorimotor dysfunction.

Barium sulfate products are used because of their high molecular density that acts as a positive contrast agent for radiographic studies. Barium sulfate is effectively inert and therefore not absorbed or metabolized by the body. It is eliminated unchanged from the body. Barium sulfate products should not be used in patients with known or suspected gastrointestinal tract perforation, known or suspected colonic obstruction, or hypersensitivity to barium sulfate formulations. Caregivers should inform their physician if the child is allergic to any drugs, food, or if there has been any prior reaction to barium sulfate products or dyes used for radiology procedures. Commercial barium sulfate materials should be latex-free (e.g., E-Z-EM products, E-Z-EM, Inc, Westbury, NY).

Children who eat and drink varieties of food and liquid usually get samples of liquid, smooth and lumpy puree, and chewable food impregnated with barium sulfate (Figure 8–8). Objectivity and standardization of

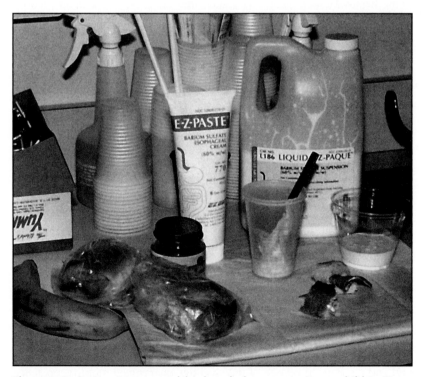

Figure 8–8. Barium impregnated food ready for presentation to child in Figure 8–7. Food was brought from home. Liquid will be given via cup.

rheologic properties and viscosity are needed (Cichero, Jackson, Halley, & Murdoch, 2000; Mann & Wong, 1996). The usual procedure is to start with the texture perceived by the caregiver to be the least problematic and progress to the texture of greatest concern. The order may be reversed in some instances, particularly with children who are tactilely defensive, because they may allow only a minimum number of bolus presentations. Procedural adjustments are made to meet the primary goal of obtaining maximal information in minimal time.

The order of presentation of liquid and food may change on the basis of history and prior observations about how the child handles various textures. Detailed information and tables regarding feeding supplies, contrast materials, textures and barium recipes for infants, procedural considerations for infants (assessed with liquid only) and children in transition feeding stages (6- to 36-month developmental ages) are available (Arvedson & Lefton-Greif, 1998).

Bolus size and timing of presentations can be varied because children's abilities may differ. Some children show improved timing and coordination of the swallow with larger boluses when they are presented with only a brief pause between presentations. Infants are usually given liquid barium of different viscosities through a nipple. When infants cannot produce rhythmic suck–swallow patterns sufficient to take enough liquid for swallowing, approximately 2 ml of liquid may be presented via syringe or spoon. The infant can be given the barium with a nipple alternating with a pacifier so documentation can be made of both nonnutritive sucking and swallowing of liquids with subsequent clearing of the oral and pharyngeal cavities (Fox, 1990). Breast-feeding infants present particular challenges because it is not possible to make the liquid barium as thin as breast milk and still have sufficient contrast to meet the purposes of the study. The nipple is another consideration that complicates interpretation because no commercially available nipple truly duplicates a breast for infant sucking.

In older children, liquid barium is usually presented first via spoon, and then larger quantities are given using a cup or a straw. Clinicians must remember that if residue is seen with the thicker material, the child's handling of subsequent boluses of thin or very thin liquid may be more difficult. Changing the order of consistencies may make it difficult for observers to determine the basis for any aspiration events. It is emphasized that clinicians must be astute observers, "on-line" decision makers, and have pertinent data regarding history and current status.

Both the speech–language pathologist and radiologist make observations relating to the evaluation. Timing of the swallow, coordination in oral and pharyngeal phases of the swallow, pharyngeal motility, presence or absence of material pooled in the pharyngeal recesses before a swallow or residue in the pharyngeal recesses after the swallow, and esophageal transit time are all studied. Occurrence of aspiration before, during, or after swallows of varied textures is documented.

In some children, it is not uncommon that aspiration may occur on the first one or two swallows. With additional swallows or different textures, improved timing and coordination with less or no aspiration is seen. Other children may show increased aspiration as the study progresses. Given that the study samples only a few swallows when a child has not eaten for at least a few hours, it is not possible to evaluate the changes that may occur when a child becomes fatigued near the end of a regular meal time. Another sample of swallows at that time would be useful for some children with multiple handicaps.

The lateral view gives the most useful information for pediatric patients, where asymmetry of head and neck structures is not a factor. Structural and functional information is obtained for multiple dimensions (Table 8–4). This view permits observations of lips, tongue, palate, epiglottis, laryngeal structures, and upper esophagus (Figures 8–9, A–C). Pharyngeal motility can be observed along with the opening of the UES. Table 8–6 summarizes radiographic findings and their associated swallow abnormalities. Pooling of barium in the valleculae or pyriform sinuses often results from delayed onset of the pharyngeal swallow and, in some instances, reduced pharyngeal motility. The pooling may be texture-related in some children. Oral and pharyngeal transit time can be measured. Nasopharyngeal reflux can be observed (Figure 8–10). Texture dependent aspiration can be seen (Figure 8–9C). Residue in pharyngeal recesses after swallows is likely to result from reduced tongue base and pharyngeal strength and pharyngeal motility (Figure 8–9B). Upper esophageal function and dysfunction can be observed (Case Study 1). Although esophageal transit time can be estimated or measured and immediate gastroesophageal reflux can be observed, VFSS is not the study of choice to specifically evaluate these problems (esophogram or UGI would be likely).

Clinicians must make decisions about the number of swallows needed for any specific texture, remembering that a major purpose is to examine the pharyngeal phase and not what happens with every texture or consistency that a child takes. *Every additional swallow observed creates an increase in radiation exposure.* In most infants and young children, the entire oral and pharyngeal regions of interest can be observed in one view. Esophageal transit is observed as one pass is made to the lower esophageal sphincter. Treatment recommendations differ depending on number and type of findings, including whether aspiration occurs before, during, or after swallows, and also on which textures. Recommendations also differ according to the status of pharyngeal motility.

The posterior-anterior (PA) view is helpful in documenting asymmetry in the passage of the bolus through the pharynx, especially by observation

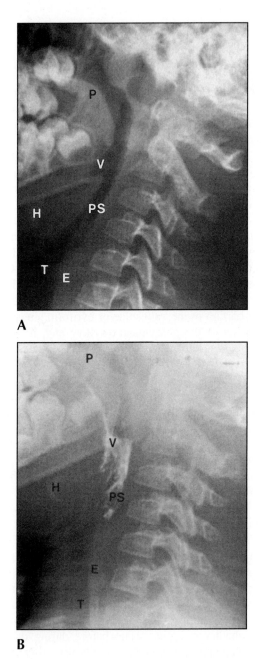

A

B

Figure 8–9. **A.** Lateral view of oral and pharyngeal structures on presentation of bolus: soft palate (P), vallecula (V), hyoid bone (H), pyriform sinus (PS), esophagus (E), and trachea (T). **B.** Lateral view of pharyngeal phase of swallow showing pooling of barium in vallecula (V) and pyriform sinus (PS) before swallow.

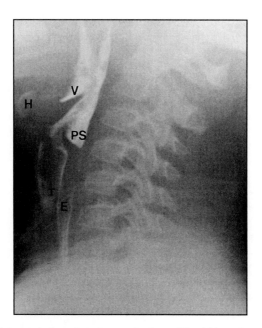

Figure 8–9. C. Lateral view showing aspiration of liquid into the trachea (T) that occurred after the swallow from of residue in the pyriform sinuses (PS) due to reduced pharyngeal motility.

of material moving through the valleculae and pyriform sinuses. The A-P view is more difficult to obtain in children with poor head control, but it may be important to visualize swallows when children assume different head positions to determine if certain changes can enhance effectiveness and safety (e.g., flexed or extended and in varied body positions). Further assessment of the upper esophageal sphincter can also be made with the A-P view (Figure 8–11A).

Aspiration is one of the major clinical problems evaluated with VFSS. Modifications of bolus size, texture, and temperature of food and liquid used during the videofluoroscopic procedure help clinicians make recommendations for avoiding or compensating for aspiration. These differences may become evident only with dynamic imaging. In children with neurologic impairment, texture may make a significant difference. Persons with neurologic impairments are usually most efficient at handling food that maintains a homogeneous consistency, resists separation into particles, remains discrete despite changing shape as it is propelled through the pharynx, and does not adhere to the mucosa, such as pudding. Liquids frequently are handled less safely than other boluses (Arvedson et al., 1994; Siebens & Linden, 1985). Some children may have greater success with food of different temperatures, for example cold versus warm food; however, data are lacking.

Table 8–6. Radiographic Findings Related to Phase of Swallowing

Phase	Observed Action	Radiographic Finding
Bolus formation	• Lack of lip closure • Tongue incoordination or weakness; reduced oral sensitivity • Limited mandibular movement	• Food falls out of mouth • Food stays on tongue or goes into sulci • Lack of bolus formation • Adherence to hard palate • Piecemeal deglutition • Aspiration before swallow, especially liquids and thin texture
Oral	• Limited tongue action • Tongue thrust • Reduced tongue elevation • Tongue incoordination	• Delayed oral transit time • Food pushed out of mouth • Piecemeal deglutition • Aspiration before swallow, especially thick textures • Aspiration before swallow, thin textures
Onset or trigger of pharyngeal swallow	• Delayed onset • Failure to initiate swallow	• Pooling in valleculae and pyriform sinuses • Pooling & residue in pharyngeal recesses • Aspiration is a high probability
Pharyngeal	• Nasopharyngeal reflux • Slow swallowing • Gurgly voice quality • Coughing or gagging (silent aspiration common) • Apnea • Breathy, hoarse voice, reduced laryngeal closure, reduced laryngeal elevation	• Velopharyngeal incoordination • Insufficient or delayed velar retraction and/or velar elevation • Delayed pharyngeal transit time • Reduced pharyngeal motility, laryngeal penetration • Pooling in pharyngeal recesses, aspiration before swallow • Residue in pharyngeal recesses, aspiration after swallow • Aspiration during swallow
Esophageal	• Delayed swallow, cough, gurgly • Emesis, pain, cough, apnea, or no observable symptom • Globus sensation (often reported in pharynx)	• Cricopharyngeal dysfunction • Reduced esophageal motility • Gastroesophageal reflux • Obstruction, stricture • Tracheoesophageal fistula • Esophagitis

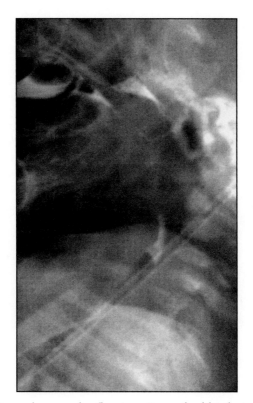

Figure 8–10. Nasopharyngeal reflux in a 2-month-old infant with DiGeorge syndrome.

Differences in efficiency of swallowing liquids can be noted whether liquid is presented via nipple, spoon, cup, or syringe. Changes in head and neck position can be observed as the child takes liquid in a variety of ways. Hyperextension of the neck may be an interfering factor because swallowing is normally done with the neck in midline or slight flexion. Neck flexion may facilitate laryngeal elevation by decreasing the tension and increasing the length of the inferior group of muscles from the sternum and clavicles. Nonetheless, the possibility that a child uses neck hyperextension as a compensatory action for a swallowing difficulty, particularly aspiration, must be considered. Recommendations for changing head and neck position are made on the basis of videofluoroscopic findings (Morton, Bonas, Fourie, & Minford, 1993), along with the clinical observations and reports from caregivers. There is no one right position for all children.

Swallowing and respiratory coordination are examined closely. Attempts have been made to correlate respiratory sounds with swallow

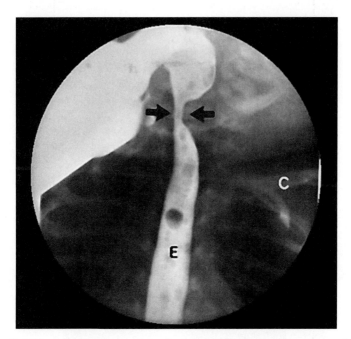

Figure 8–11A. Anteroposterior view of a 4-day-old infant with upper esophageal spasm or narrowing (arrows) of upper esophageal sphincter; esophagus (E) and clavicles (C) are labeled for orientation.

activity (Selley, Ellis, Flack, Bayliss, & Pearce, 1994) and to relate VFSS findings to pulse oximetry (Sellars, Dunnet, & Carter, 1998). No clear-cut relationship is reported for adults, nor has clinical experience found a direct relationship with infants and children. Infants and children without sufficient cognitive levels to comprehend and follow verbal directions to cough, clear their throat, or hold their breath and then swallow may not be able to benefit directly from intervention involving therapeutic maneuvers. Vocal quality is noted. Gurgly phonation during and immediately after swallows is an indication of residue spilling into the laryngeal vestibule, which relates to heightened risk for aspiration. Breathy voice quality raises suspicions for incomplete vocal fold closure and a heightened risk for aspiration. Thus, videofluoroscopic findings may assist clinicians to determine beneficial management strategies.

Advantages and Disadvantages of VFSS

The advantages and disadvantages of VFSS are listed in Table 8–7. As discussed, the best results are gained when patient cooperation is maximized,

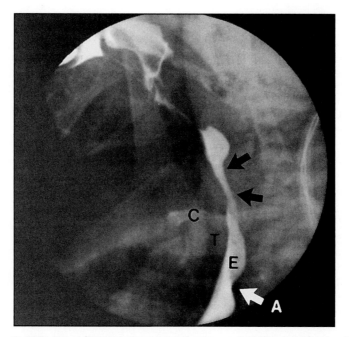

Figure 8–11B. Lateral view of narrowed upper esophageal sphincter (black arrows), trachea (T), barium-filled esophagus (E), clavicles (C), and posterior impression of an incidental right subclavian artery (A + white arrow).

the study is carefully planned based on clinical examination, and equipment and personnel are appropriate for performance of the study.

Interpretation—Pearls and Pitfalls

Accuracy of interpretation is critical. However, inter- and intrarater reliability are reported to be variable (Kuhlemeier, Yates, & Palmer, 1998; Wilcox, Liss, & Siegel, 1996). Training is shown to improve accuracy of findings (Logemann, 1993; Logemann, Lazarus, Keely, Sanchez, & Rademaker, 2000). Although the interpretation of findings should be carried out jointly by the SLP and radiologist, review by other specialists, such as the otolaryngologist or gastroenterologist, is not uncommon. The detailed report of findings is usually prepared by the SLP. Findings from VFSS can be discussed from a variety of viewpoints. This section summarizes findings in relation to phases of swallowing—oral, pharyngeal, and esophageal (Table 8–6). Bolus formation, or oral preparation, is discussed briefly for completeness, but the VFSS is not carried out to define the oral preparatory

Table 8–7. Advantages and Disadvantages of Videofluoroscopic Swallow Study

Advantages
- Tests overall swallowing ability including oral, pharyngeal, and upper esophageal phases
- Pharyngeal phase, especially motility and coordination, readily seen
- Coordination of pharyngeal motility with tongue action and with upper esophageal sphincter action can be evaluated
- Residue in the pharyngeal recesses and pyriform sinuses is seen
- Function deficits can be correlated with degree of aspiration
- Oral and pharyngeal transit times can be calculated
- Extensive literature correlates VFSS findings to clinical information
- Available in most institutions

Disadvantages
- Uses ionizing radiation, therefore studies must be short
- Equipment for positioning can be cumbersome
- Patient must be taken to radiology suite (portable units in some places)
- Requires trained personnel
- Requires the use of barium contrast material which alters the taste and texture of liquids and solid foods
- Aspiration risk may be unrecognized and result in airway problems at the time of the study

phase, which can be better imaged with US and described well in the clinical examination of swallowing and feeding.

Food intake requires effective lip closure and bolus formation—if these are lacking, food falls out of the mouth. Tongue hypotonia, uncoordinated tongue movement, reduced oral sensation, and buccal hypotonia all may interfere with the ability to form a bolus. Limited mandibular movement results in piecemeal deglutition. The ability to hold material and form a bolus of any texture in preparation for the posterior propulsion is affected. As food or liquid spreads throughout the oral cavity, VFSS images show pooling in the frontal and lateral sulci, adherence to the hard palate, piecemeal posterior movement to the back of the tongue, and food or liquid falling into the pharyngeal recesses before production of a swallow. Thus, a child may aspirate as material gets into the open airway before a swallow is produced; thin liquids pose the greatest risk.

In infants and young children, abnormal delay in onset of pharyngeal phase increases the risk for aspiration consequences. Unlike adults and older children, infants and young children usually collect the bolus in the valleculae before onset of the pharyngeal swallow. If the bolus is held in the pharynx before the initiation of a swallow, aspiration risk increases. Infants in whom the cough reflex is less developed have a high probability for silent aspiration. Aspiration may occur before the swallow, with the airway open until a swallow is produced.

Delay in onset of pharyngeal phase needs to be differentiated from a cricopharyngeal disorder or delayed opening of the cricopharyngeus, also known as the upper esophageal sphincter (UES) or pharyngoesophageal sphincter (PES). The lack of opening in the UES is more likely to relate to neurologic control of brain-stem function than to a true structural disorder. Exceptions do occur, and clinicians must be able to differentiate the types.

Slow pharyngeal transit time and reduced pharyngeal motility, in particular, place a child at high risk for aspiration, even if tongue action is adequate in the oral phase. Nonetheless, the vast majority of children with neurologic impairments show at least some oral preparatory phase and oral phase problems along with significant pharyngeal phase deficits. Nasopharyngeal reflux may indicate dysfunctional velopharyngeal closure or timing problems. Incoordination of pharyngeal phase and reduced pharyngeal motility often result in material remaining in the valleculae and pyriform sinuses after the swallow (residue), more commonly seen with thicker boluses. Aspiration of the residue occurs when material spills into the airway after the swallow. Reduced pharyngeal motility is seen often in children with multiple handicaps who aspirate on paste in more cases than on liquid (Griggs et al., 1989).

Unilateral signs and symptoms are less common in children than in adults. Children who have had strokes or who have brain-stem tumors may show unilateral signs. In those circumstances, an A-P view is important. Although reduced laryngeal elevation is relatively uncommon in young infants as the larynx is positioned high in the neck, vocal fold closure may be incomplete or incoordinated and thus would result in aspiration most commonly seen during a swallow. The aspiration events are typically silent, but in some instances observable actions could include coughing, gagging, or breathy and hoarse voice quality. Clinicians heighten their index of suspicion as the number of health-related variables and observable signs increase.

Cricopharyngeal dysfunction is relatively rare in infants and children, but cricopharyngeal spasm, pharyngoesophageal spasm, or cricopharyngeal achalasia may occur. These relatively isolated findings are likely to be a marker for broader disabilities that may emerge as the child grows. Figure 8–11 A&B shows a 4-day-old infant with fluoroscopic findings consistent with an upper esophageal swallow deficit. Children with Arnold Chiari malformations are reported to have neurogenic dysphagia with a combination of diffuse pharyngoesophageal dysmotility, cricopharyngeal achalasia, nasal regurgitation, tracheal aspiration, and gastroesophageal reflux. (Pollack, Pang, Kocoshis, & Putnam, 1992; Putnam et al., 1992).

The esophageal phase of the swallow can be impaired because of a number of neurologic conditions or structural anomalies. Some of the more common possibilities in infants and children include reduced esophageal motility or dysmotility, obstruction or stricture, tracheoesophageal fistula, or esophagitis. Gastroesophageal reflux frequently contributes to esophagitis and worsens swallowing function (discussed in detail in Chapter 5).

When aspiration occurs during VFSS, a chest film is taken immediately following the study to document areas with contrast present, as well as any other lung findings. Postural drainage and chest percussion may be used for some children if significant aspiration has occurred. Suctioning capabilities and appropriate personnel should be available for infants and children with tracheostomies and those with other major respiratory concerns.

Review of Findings

The videotape is reviewed by the SLP with caregivers following the study. The SLP makes recommendations and writes the report reflecting the team analysis (radiologist and SLP; at times other physicians including a developmental pediatrician or neurologist, pulmonologist, gastroenterologist, or otolaryngologist). Caregivers find the video image particularly helpful when a child aspirates silently. The video lets them see material in the airway, and the audio lets them hear that the child did not cough.

Caregivers are alerted that constipation is a possible side effect of the barium sulfate ingestion. Thus, recommendations are made for additional fluid intake and, in some instances, a laxative or suppository. Because the amount of barium contrast material is relatively small, constipation problems are not common. Allergic reactions are rare but should be mentioned.

Children with complex problems may undergo team consultation and interdisciplinary recommendations. The videotape is available for review during follow-up clinic visits or other conferences. With caregivers' permission, the taped study can be made available to a professional staff in an intervention program or school so that the team can carry out the management decisions more effectively. Findings from any particular diagnostic test are useful only when considered within the total context of the child. When caregivers fully understand and appreciate the results, they can incorporate recommendations into the child's daily activities.

Patients who are older, particularly with higher cognitive function, find the feedback helpful when the videotape is used in the treatment process. That feedback is not likely to be helpful with a young child or one with significant cognitive deficits and severe neurogenic dysphagia. Additionally, videotaped examples of findings that demonstrate normal swallows and abnormal swallows from various etiologies can be helpful in training. This training should be useful for graduate students as they prepare to become professionals in this high-risk area of patient care and for professionals already involved with pediatric feeding and swallowing.

Severity Classification

Classification of severity of swallowing and feeding problems in children would be helpful to compare findings among evaluators in multiple institutions, to monitor changes over time through various intervention and management strategies, and to measure outcomes. The most basic question is whether a person is safe for oral feeding of any texture. Based on studies with adults, Logemann (1983) first stated that if a radiographic study indicates that a person takes more than 10 sec to swallow every consistency of food tried, tube feedings will be needed to supplement oral feedings to provide adequate nutrition. Furthermore, patients who aspirate more than 10% of each bolus, regardless of texture, should not be feeding orally. Measurement is more difficult for children with neurologic deficits, especially for those who lose part of each bolus out of the mouth or produce multiple swallows for each bolus.

Classification systems have been developed primarily for use with adults. Splaingard and colleagues (1988) proposed a classification system using descriptive terms for a 5-point severity scale (Table 8–8). The Penetration-Aspiration Scale, an 8-point scale, was developed to quantify selected penetration and aspiration events observed during videofluoroscopic swallowing evaluations (Rosenbek, Robbins, Roecker, Coyle, & Wood, 1996). Thus far, data are available only for adults. This type of scale has potential for improved precision in describing the accidental loss of food or liquid into the airway while eating or drinking, which is perhaps the most clinically significant consequence of dysphagia as suggested by Rosenbek and colleagues. A radiologic rating of swallowing abnormalities developed at Duke University Medical Center for adults has a 5-point

Table 8–8. Severity Scale for Swallowing Problems

Severity Classification	Swallow Delay	Oral/ Pharyngeal Motility Reduced	Pharyngeal Pooling	Residue Postswallow	Aspiration
Normal	No	No	No	No	No
Mild	Slight	No	No	No	No
Moderate	Yes	Yes	Suspected	Yes	No
Severe	Yes	Yes	Yes	Yes	Trace
Profound	Severe, or absent swallow	Yes	Yes	Yes	>10%

Note. Adapted from "Aspiration in Rehabilitation Patients: Videofluoroscopy vs. Bedside Clinical Assessment" by M. L. Splaingard, B. Hutchins, L. D. Sulton, and G. Chaudhuri, 1988, *Archives of Physical Medicine and Rehabilitation, 69,* pp. 637–640.

severity scale for rating each of 6 aspects: oral-preparatory phase, reflex initiation phase, pharyngeal phase, pharyngeal appearance observed in anterior–posterior projection, aspiration, and pharyngeal–esophageal phase screening (Horner, Riski, Ovelmen-Levitt, & Nashold, 1992). The latter two scales have not been validated for the pediatric population.

There is limited research on application of videofluoroscopic findings to management decisions for the pediatric population. Findings that represent a limited sample in a brief period of time on one occasion must be placed into context with history and clinical findings. VFSS is found to be important in assessment of the risk for pneumonia in children with suspected dysphagia (Taniguchi & Moyer, 1994). These authors found that at age 1 year or less, the presence of gastroesophageal reflux, and an underlying diagnosis (e.g., cerebral palsy, traumatic brain injury, other central nervous system disorders, and failure to thrive) were also significant factors in predicting the risk of pneumonia.

Studies in adults have found that combined clinical and radiographic examination correlate well in relationship to feeding recommendations (Ott, Hodge, Pikna, Chen, & Gelfand, 1996). Mirrett and colleagues (1994) presented data to suggest that early diagnostic evaluation, including baseline and comparative VFSS, could be helpful in managing feeding difficulties in children with severe spastic cerebral palsy. Prevention of chronic aspiration, malnutrition, and unpleasant feeding experiences may thus be avoided. Griggs and colleagues (1989) spent 6 months studying 10 multiply handicapped individuals with feeding disorders, aged 9 months to 24 years. They found that severity qualitatively described on fluoroscopy related directly to "nourishment" status as measured by weight in relation to the expected mean for chronologic age. The researchers concluded that feeding techniques, textures, and position changes could be altered to meet each individual's needs more accurately than was possible with clinical bedside assessment alone.

Helfrich-Miller and colleagues (1986) reported on six profoundly retarded children with cerebral palsy who had videofluoroscopic findings of delayed swallowing and lingual dysfunction. Treatment programs developed on the basis of the videofluoroscopic findings included dietary modifications, oral–motor treatment, and thermal stimulation. VFSS was found to be more consistent than bedside assessments and allowed for the development of more systematic and safer treatment plans.

Repeat Studies

A frequently asked question is, "When do you repeat a VFSS?" The simple answer is "as seldom as possible." The same criteria that were used in decisions for an initial study are used for any follow-up study. A significant change in health status, recurrence of previous signs and symptoms, prior history of silent aspiration, or failure to grow may indicate possible need to change diet textures or some other aspect of intervention. Swallow status is one of the variables which then must be reevaluated. Improved oral sensorimotor functioning in children with profound mental retardation and neurologic impairments has not proven to correlate with improved pharyngeal functioning. Nonetheless, fluoroscopic findings have revealed improved pharyngeal transit time for paste consistencies and reduced aspiration following treatment with thermal stimulation (Helfrich-Miller et al., 1986). VFSS findings are useful when concerns relate to pharyngeal phase function and the need to define status for possible changes in management.

Management options may include changes in diet textures, positioning and seating, specialized feeding tools and techniques, behavioral modification, direct oral sensorimotor practice, sensory based approaches, or specific instructions related to coughing, breathing, or timing of the swallow. Alternate methods of nonoral feeding may need to be considered, with plans for oral sensorimotor stimulation with or without food to be included in the practice. These management options are discussed in detail in the next chapter.

■ CASE STUDIES

Case Study 1

"John" was born at term following an uncomplicated pregnancy. He was suctioned vigorously because of meconium aspirates but did not require intubation. He was transferred to the regional neonatal intensive care unit on day 2 of life because of cyanosis during oral feeding attempts. He coughed and gagged with feeds. He also had a weak, breathy, and hoarse cry. He had normal vocal fold function with FFNL; with direct rigid laryngoscopy, the arytenoids were characterized by mild edema. A VFSS revealed insufficient opening of the upper esophageal sphincter and what appeared to be a focal spasm high in the esophagus, but just below the cricopharyngeal sphincter, with nasopharygneal reflux (Figure 8–11A, B). No tracheal aspiration was evident on the initial study. Physicians recommended no direct medical or surgical intervention for at least several weeks but close monitoring because time and growth may allow for spontaneous resolution.

Feedings were given via NG tube. Oral sensorimotor assessment revealed normal nonnutritive sucking and oral sensation. This infant did not tolerate more than a drop of 5% glucose solution on the end of his mother's finger or on the pacifier without coughing, gagging, and becoming cyanotic. Additional diagnostic work-up included computerized tomographic scan of the head, which was normal. No liquid feedings could be attempted in the neonatal period. He was discharged to home on NG feedings to be reevaluated several weeks later. Parents continued to provide oral–motor stimulation for nonnutritive sucking, and very small amounts of liquid for test and practice purposes. After a few weeks, thickened liquid was presented in small amounts via syringe for practice with close monitoring to minimize stress. Esophageal dilation occurred at about 4 months of age. He gradually increased volumes with oral feeding and was a total oral feeder by 6 months.

Continued developmental examinations revealed hypotonia, which became more evident as he got older. Speech was characterized by hypernasality due to velopharyngeal insufficiency and also a flaccid dysarthria. He continued to have difficulty swallowing, noted with gulping and multiple swallows needed for thin liquids. Follow up VFSS at age 3 years revealed similar upper esophageal deficits and nasopharyngeal reflux, although he was a functional oral feeder with no aspiration. Multiview videofluoroscopic speech study also revealed velopharyngeal insufficiency. John needed coaxing and preparation for FFNL in voice clinic with otolaryngologists and SLPs. Findings were consistent with perceptual speech motor findings and the fluoroscopy. In addition on endoscopy, a prominent pulsating carotid artery was evident. A diagnosis of velocardiofacial syndrome was confirmed by genetics work-up.

Comment

This child is a good example of the importance of delineating pharyngeal and esophageal phases of swallowing to make appropriate oral–motor and swallowing recommendations. There is no direct oral sensorimotor treatment that can alter esophageal functioning. Nonnutritive sucking experience can be provided, with continued assessment to monitor change and potential for oral feeding. The importance of a thorough diagnostic work-up with feeding problems in the neonatal period cannot be overemphasized. Parents need as much objective information as possible when they cannot feed their newborn in the expected ways. Follow-up over time is also vital. Significant feeding and swallowing problems in the neonatal period are often markers for more global developmental problems. Although the genetics diagnosis should have been made earlier, in this instance, the parents stated that the diagnosis would have been even harder to accept had it been made earlier. Sensitivity and communication with parents are sometimes as important as actual findings.

Case Study 2

"Sonia" is a 29 weeks gestation, premature quintuplet, born by Caesarian section. Her mother had a history that included cocaine addiction. This infant showed signs of respiratory distress with nipple feeds at the time of bedside evaluation when she was 35 weeks gestational age. She had been bottle feeding for nearly 2 weeks; however, intermittent symptoms of respiratory distress continued to occur. NG tube feedings supplemented her oral feedings.

Additional medical problems included respiratory distress syndrome and a Grade II intraventricular hemorrhage (IVH). The bedside evaluation revealed variable functional sucking and swallowing with incoordination of suck/swallow/breathe sequencing resulting in long, stressful feeding times. VFSS was performed to evaluate for aspiration risks. The VFSS demonstrated no aspiration and no pharyngeal phase deficits, except for trace and intermittent nasopharyngeal reflux, which is considered within normal limits for young infants. Thus, she appeared safe to proceed with oral feeding. She became a full oral feeder within 10 days and was discharged to a foster family.

Comment

This infant demonstrates the importance of defining the pharyngeal physiology when there are clinical signs of respiratory concerns that may interfere with safe oral feeding. Nurses were able to implement guidelines for maximizing efficiency of nipple-feeding with greater confidence once they had the VFSS findings. The foster parents were trained to carry out feedings with the best techniques for posture, position, monitoring of flow rate, and pacing as needed. This infant grew well over the next several months of life and made good developmental progress as anticipated for infants with Grade II IVH.

■ REFERENCES

Arvedson, J., & Lefton-Greif, M. A. (1998). *Pediatric videofluoroscopic swallow studies: A professional manual with caregiver guidelines.* San Antonio, TX: Communication Skill Builders.

Arvedson, J., Rogers, B., Buck, G., Smart, P., & Msall, M. (1994). Silent aspiration prominent in children with dysphagia. *International Journal of Pediatric Otorhinolaryngology, 28,* 173–181.

American Speech–Language–Hearing Association (1990). Knowledge and skills needed by speech-language pathologists providing services to dysphagic patients. *ASHA, 32*(Suppl. 2), 7–12.

American Speech–Language–Hearing Association (1992). Instrumental diagnostic procedures for swallowing. *ASHA, 34*(Suppl. 7), 25–33.

American Speech–Language–Hearing Association (2000a). Clinical indicators for instrumental assessment of dysphagia (guidelines). *ASHA,* (Suppl. 20), 18–19.

American Speech–Language–Hearing Association (2000b). Roles of the speech–language pathologist and otolaryngologist in the performance and interpretation of endoscopic examinations of swallowing (position statement). *ASHA*, (Suppl. 20), 17.

Aviv, J. E. (2000a). Clinical assessment of pharyngolaryngeal sensitivity. *American Journal of Medicine, 108(4a),* 68s–72s.

Aviv, J. E. (2000b). Prospective, randomized outcome study of endoscopy versus modified barium swallow in patients with dysphagia. *The Laryngoscope, 110,* 563–574.

Aviv, J. E., Kaplan, S., Thomson, J. E., Spitzer, J., Diamond, B., & Close L. G. (2000). The safety of flexible endoscopic evaluation of swallowing with sensory testing (FEESST): An analysis of 500 consecutive evaluations. *Dysphagia, 15,* 39–44.

Aviv, J. E., Kim, T., Thomson, J. E., Sunshine, S., Kaplan, S., & Close L. G. (1998). Fiberoptic endoscopic evaluation of swallowing with sensory testing (FEESST) in healthy controls. *Dysphagia, 13,* 87–92.

Bastian, R. W. (1991). Videoendoscopic evaluation of patients with dysphagia: An adjunct to the modified barium swallow. *Otolaryngology Head Neck Surgery, 104,* 339–350.

Beck, T. J., & Gayler, B. W. (1990). Image quality and radiation levels in videofluoroscopy for swallowing studies: A review. *Dysphagia, 5,* 119–128.

Benson, J. E., & Lefton-Greif, M. A. (1994). Videofluoroscopy of swallowing in pediatric patients: A component of the total feeding evaluation. In D. N. Tuchman & R. S. Walter, (Eds.), *Disorders of feeding and swallowing in infants and children: Pathophysiology, diagnosis, and treatment* (187–200). San Diego, CA: Singular Publishing Group.

Bosma, J. F., Hepburn, L. G., Josell, S. D., & Baker, K. (1990). Ultrasound demonstration of tongue motions during suckle feeding. *Developmental Medicine and Child Neurology, 32,* 223–229.

Cichero, J. A. Y., Jackson, O., Halley, P. J., & Murdoch, E. B. (2000). How thick is thick? Multicenter study of the theological and material property characteristics of mealtime fluids and videofluoroscopy fluids. *Dysphagia, 15,* 188–200.

Fanucci, A., Cerro, P., Ietto, F., Brancaleone, C., & Berardi, F. (1994). Physiology of oral swallowing studied by ultrasonography. *Dentomaxillofacial Radiology, 23,* 221–225.

Fox, C. A. (1990). Implementing the modified barium swallow evaluation in children who have multiple disabilities. *Infants and Young Children, 3,* 67–77.

Fuhrmann, R. A. W., & Diedrich, P. R. (1994). B-mode ultrasound scanning of the tongue during swallowing. *Dentomaxillofacial Radiology, 23,* 211–215.

Geyer, L. A., & McGowan, J. S. (1995). Positioning infants and children for videofluoroscopic swallowing function studies. *Infants and Young Children, 8,* 58–64.

Gisel, E. G., Birnbaum, R., & Schwartz, S. (1998). Feeding impairments in children: Diagnosis and effective intervention. *International Journal of Orofacial Myology, 24,* 27–33.

Griggs, C. A., Jones, P. M., & Lee, R. E. (1989). Videofluoroscopic investigation of feeding disorders in children with multiple handicap. *Developmental Medicine and Child Neurology, 31,* 303–308.

Hartnick, C., Miller, C., Hartley, B., & Willging, J. (2000). Pediatric fiberoptic endoscopic evaluation of swallowing. *Annals of Otorhinology and Laryngology, 109,* 996–999.

Helfrich-Miller, K. R., Rector, K. L., & Strakes, J. A. (1986). Dysphagia. Its treatment in the profoundly retarded patient with cerebral palsy. *Archives of Physical Medical Rehabilitation, 67,* 520–525.

Horner, J., Riski, J.E., Ovelmen-Levitt, J., & Nashold, B. S. (1992). Swallowing in torticollis before and after rhizotomy. *Dysphagia, 7,* 117–125.

Jones, B., Kramer, S. S., & Donner, M. (1985). Dynamic imaging of the pharynx. *Gastrointestinal Radiology, 10,* 213–224.

Kramer, S. S., & Eicher, P. M. (1993). The evaluation of pediatric feeding abnormalities. *Dysphagia, 8,* 215–224.

Kuhlemeier, K. V., Yates, P., & Palmer, J. B. (1998). Intra- and inter-rater variation in the evaluation of videofluorographic swallowing studies. *Dysphagia, 13,* 142–147.

Langmore, S. E., & Logemann, J. A. (1991). After the clinical bedside swallowing examination: What next? *American Journal of Speech-Language Pathology, Sept. 1991,* 13–19.

Langmore, S. E., Schatz, K., & Olsen, N. (1988). Fiberoptic endoscopic examination of swallowing saftey: A new procedure. *Dysphagia, 2,* 216–219.

Langmore, S. E., Schatz, K., & Olsen, N. (1991). Endoscopic and videofluoroscopic evaluations of swallowing and aspiration. *Annals of Otolaryngology, Rhinology, and Laryngology, 100,* 678–681.

Leder, S. B., & Karas, D. E. (2000). Fiberoptic endoscopic evaluation of swallowing in the pediatric population. *The Laryngoscope, 110,* 1132–1136.

Link, D. T., Willging, J., Miller, C. K., Cotton, R., & Rudolph, C. D. (2000). Pediatric laryngopharyngeal sensory testing during flexible endoscopic evaluation of swallowing: Feasible and correlative. *Annals of Otology Rhinology and Laryngology, 109,* 899–905.

Liu, H., Kaplan, S., Parides, M., & Close, L. (2000). Laryngopharyngeal sensory deficits in patients with laryngopharyngeal reflux and dysphagia. *Annals of Otorhinology and Laryngology, 109,* 1000–1006.

Logemann, J. (1983). *Evaluation and treatment of swallowing disorders.* Austin TX: PRO-ED.

Logemann, J. A. (1993). *Manual for the videofluorographic study of swallowing* (2nd ed.). Austin, TX: PRO-ED.

Logemann, J. A. (1998). *Evaluation and treatment of swallowing disorders* (2nd ed.). Austin, TX: PRO-ED.

Logemann, J. A., Lazarus, C. L., Keely, S. P., Sanchez, A., & Rademaker, A. W. (2000). Effectiveness of four hours of education in interpretation of radiographic studies. *Dysphagia, 15,* 180–183.

Mann, L. L., & Wong, K. (1996). Development of an objective method for assessing viscosity of formulated foods and beverages for the dysphagic diet. *Journal of the American Dietetic Association, 96,* 585–588.

Martin, C. J., & Hunter, S. (1994). Reduction of patient doses from barium meal and barium enema examinations through changes in equipment factors. *British Journal of Radiology, 67,* 1196–1205.

McConnell, F. M. S., Hester, T. R., Mendelsohn, M. S., & Logemann, J. A. (1988). Manufluorography of deglutition after total laryngopharyngectomy. *Plastic and Reconst Surg, 81,* 946–351.

McConnell, F. M. S., Mendelsohn, M. S., & Logemann, J. A. (1986). Examination of swallowing after total laryngectomy using manofluorography. *Head & Neck Surgery, 9,* 3–12.

Migliore, L. E., Scoopo, F. J., & Robey, K. L. (1999). Fiberoptic examination of swallowing in children and young adults with severe developmental disability. *American Journal of Speech-Language Pathology, 8,* 303–308.

Mirrett, P. L., Riski, J. E., Glascott, J., & Johnson, V. (1994). Videofluoroscopic assessment of dysphagia in children with severe spastic cerebral palsy. *Dysphagia, 9,* 174–179.

Morton, R. E., Bonas, R., Fourie, B., & Minford, J. (1993). Videofluoroscopy in the assessment of feeding disorders of children with neurological problems. *Developmental Medicine and Child Neurology, 35,* 388–395.

Newman, L. A., Cleveland, R. H., Blickman, J. G., Hillman, R. E., & Jaramillo, D. (1991). Videofluoroscopic analysis of the infant swallow. *Investigative Radiology, 26,* 870–873.

Nicholson, R. A., Thornton, A., & Akpan, M. (1995). Radiation dose reduction in paediatric fluoroscopy using added filtration. *British Journal of Radiology, 68,* 296–300.

Nowak, A. J., Smith, W. L., & Erenberg, A. (1994). Imaging evaluation of artifical nipples during bottle feeding. *Archives of Pediatrics and Adolescent Medicine, 148,* 40–42.

Ott, D. J., Hodge, R. G., Pikna, L. A., Chen, M. Y. M., & Gelfand, D. W. (1996). Modified barium swallow: Clinical and radiographic correlation and relation to feeding recommendations. *Dysphagia, 11,* 187–190.

Palmer, J. B. (1989). Electromyography of the muscles of oropharyngeal swallowing: Basic concepts. *Dysphagia, 4,* 192–198.

Perlman, A. L., Luschei, E. S., & DuMond, C. E. (1989). Electrical activity from the superior pharyngeal constrictor during reflexive and non-reflexive tasks. *Journal of Speech and Hearing Research, 32,* 749–754.

Pollack, I. F., Pang, D., Kocoshis, S., & Putnam, P. (1992). Neurogenic dysphagia resulting from Chiari malformations. *Neurosurgery, 30,* 709–719.

Putnam, P. E., Orenstein, S. R., Pang, D., Pollack, I. F., Proujansky, R., & Kocoshis, S. A. (1992). Cricopharyngeal dysfunction associated with Chiari malformations. *Pediatrics, 89,* 871–876.

Rosenbek, J. C., Robbins, J., Roecker, E. B., Coyle, J. L., & Wood, J. L. (1996). A penetration-aspiration scale. *Dysphagia, 11,* 93–98.

Sellars, C., Dunnet, C., & Carter, R. (1998). A preliminary comparison of videofluoroscopy of swallow and pulse oximetry in the identification of aspiration in dysphagia patients. *Dysphagia, 13,* 82–86.

Selley, W. G., Ellis, R. E., Flack, F. C., Bayliss, C. R., & Pearce, V. R. (1994). The synchronization of respiration and swallow sounds with videofluoroscopy during swallowing. *Dysphagia, 9,* 162–167.

Shawker, T. H., Sonies, B. C., Hall, T. E., & Baum, B. J. (1984). Ultrasound analysis of tongue, hyoid, and larynx activity during swallowing. *Investigative Radiology, 19,* 82–86.

Shawker, T. H., Sonies, B. C., Stone, M., & Baum, B. J. (1983). Real-time ultrasound visualization of tongue movement during swallowing. *Journal of Clinical Ultrasound, 11,* 485–490.

Siebens, A., & Linden, P. (1985). Dynamic imaging for swallowing re-education. *Gastrointestinal Radiology, 10,* 251–253.

Sivit, C. J. (1990). Role of the pediatric radiologist in the evaluation of oral and pharyngeal dysphagia. *Journal of Neurologic Rehabilitation, 4,* 103–110.

Smith, W. L., Erenberg, A., Nowak, A., & Franken, E. A. (1985). Physiology of sucking in the normal term infant using real-time US. *Radiology, 156,* 379–381.

Sonies, B. (1987). Ultrsound imaging of the oral area: Clinical application and implications for rehabilitation. *Rehabilitation Report, 3,* 1–3.

Sonies, B. (1990). Ultrasound imaging and swallowing. In M. Donner & B. Jones (Eds.), *Normal and abnormal swallowing: Imaging in diagnosis and therapy* (109–119).

Sonies, B. (1991). Instrumental procedures of dysphagia diagnosis. *Seminars in Speech and Language, 12,* 185–197.

Sorin, R., Somers, S., Austin, W., & Bester, S. (1988). The influence of videofluoroscopy on the management of the dysphagic patient. *Dysphagia, 2,* 127–135.

Splaingard, M. L., Hutchins, B., Sulton, L. D., & Chaudhuri, G. (1988). Aspiration in rehabilitation patients: Videofluoroscopy vs bedside clinical assessment. *Archives of Physical Medicine and Rehabilitation, 69,* 637–640.

Stone, M., & Shawker, T. H. (1986). An ultrasound examination of tongue movement during swallowing. *Dysphagia, 1,* 78–83.

Taniguchi, M. H., & Moyer, R. S. (1994). Assessment of risk factors for pneumonia in dysphagic children: Significance of videofluoroscopic swallowing evaluation. *Developmental Medicine and Child Neurology, 36,* 495–502.

Tolbert, D. (1996). Sources of radiation exposure. In M. L. Janower and O. W. Linton, (Eds.), *Radiation risk: A primer* (3–4). Reston, VA: American College of Radiology.

Vice, F., Heinz, J., Giuriati, G., Hood, M., & Bosma, J. (1990). Cervical auscultation of suckle feeding in newborn infants. *Developmental Medicine and Child Neurology, 32,* 760–768.

Ward, D. E. (1984). *Positioning the handicapped child for function.* Chicago: Phoenix Press.

Weber, F., Woolridge, M. W., & Baum, J. D. (1986). An ultrasound study of the organization of sucking and swallowing by newborn infants. *Developmental Medicine and Child Neurology, 28,* 19–24.

Wilcox, F., Liss, J. M., & Siegel, G. M. (1996). Interjudge agreement in videofluoroscpoic studies of swallowing. *Journal of Speech and Hearing Research, 39,* 144–152.

Willging, J. P. (1995). Endoscopic evaluation of swallowing in children. *International Journal of Pediatric Otorhinolaryngology, 32,* s107–s108

Willging, J. P. (2000). Benefit of feeding assessment before pediatric airway reconstruction. *The Laryngoscope, 110,* 825–834.

Willging, J. P., Miller, C. K., Hogan, M. J., & Rudolph, C. D. (1996). Fiberoptic endoscopic evaluation of swallowing in children: A preliminary report of 100 procedures. *Dysphagia, 11,* 162.

Yang, W. T., Loveday, E. J., Metreweli, C., & Sullivan, P. B. (1997). Ultrasound assessment of swallowing in malnourished disabled children. *British Journal of Radiology, 709,* 992–994.

Zerilli, K. S., Stefans, V. A., & DiPietro, M. A. (1990). Protocol for the use of videofluoroscopy in pediatric swallowing dysfunction. *American Journal of Occupational Therapy, 44,* 441–446.

CHAPTER 9

Management of Feeding and Swallowing Problems

Joan Arvedson, Linda Brodsky, and Donna Reigstad

■ SUMMARY

Management of feeding and swallowing problems for infants and children is based on adequate nutrition and gastrointestinal function, stable pulmonary function, and developmentally appropriate oral sensorimotor and feeding skills. Optimally, this occurs within the context of maximal participation in the social and communication activities associated with mealtimes for child and parent. When children cannot safely meet their nutritional needs by oral feeding, supplemental nutrition routes are needed. Nonoral feeding should not be seen as a failure or last resort, but should be approached as a means for maximizing safety, growth, and development.

Primary to a successful oral sensorimotor and swallowing program is as healthy a child as possible. Medical, surgical, and nutritional considerations are all important and are detailed in other chapters. Positioning, seating, muscle tone, and sensory issues all need to be addressed during therapy. Underlying disease state(s), chronologic and developmental age of the child, social and environmental arena, and psychologic and behavioral factors all impact on treatment recommendations.

■ INTRODUCTION

Although the field of swallowing and feeding problems in children is still in its infancy, evidence-based practice is encouraged for all clinicians involved in the assessment and management of these high-risk infants and children. Limited studies are available that focus on the many situations encountered in this varied and challenging population. The best professionals use their individual expertise along with the best available external evidence for care of all persons (Letts & Bosch, 2001).

Professionals practicing evidence-based medicine will identify and apply the most efficacious interventions to maximize the quality and quantity of life for individuals. In relation to the discussion of management for these high-risk children, the best evidence for any and all therapies will be presented. Systematic reviews of therapy have become the focus of an international group of clinicians, methodologists, and consumers who have formed the Cochrane Collaboration.[1] Clinicians are urged to collect data in their own settings and to participate in multicenter clinical trials whenever possible. It is through careful observation, reporting, and collaboration that advances in both diagnosis and treatment can be made.

This chapter addresses management related to oral sensorimotor treatment and to other approaches that may have a positive effect on oral sensorimotor function in infants and children who have feeding and swallowing problems. The majority of affected children have multiple diagnoses that include at least some degree of neurologic incoordination or weakness. The importance of interdisciplinary communication and team decision making is emphasized repeatedly throughout this book, and its application is further elaborated in this chapter. Discussion will cover principles of an oral sensorimotor program, postural and positioning intervention, oral feeding with infants, transition feeding, oral sensory approach to feeding, treatment related to specific anatomic structures, regression in oral feeding, treatment with tube-fed infants and children, and treatment of children with specific diagnoses. Case reports demonstrate the complexities of feeding in individual children who are best served by an interdisciplinary team.

■ GENERAL PRINCIPLES OF AN ORAL SENSORIMOTOR PROGRAM

General Principles

Oral sensorimotor function refers to all aspects of movement of the structures in the oral cavity and pharynx, down to the level of the upper esophageal sphincter (UES) through which food enters the esophagus. The

---

[1]Cochrane Database of Systematic Reviews. Available from BMJ Publishing Group, P.O. Box 295, London WC1H 9TE, UK. Tel: +44 (0)20 7383 6185/6245; Fax +44 (0)20 7383 6662. Reviews are published on computer disk and CD, on the Internet, and in a variety of other forms.

primary functions of the oral sensorimotor system relate to swallowing and to communication.

Different oral sensorimotor programs have different goals that include the following:

1. to develop coordinated movements of the mouth, respiratory, and phonatory systems for communication (Morris & Klein, 1987, 2000);
2. to improve coordination of oral–motor movements to enhance feeding skills (Arvedson, 1993; Case-Smith & Humphry, 2000; Glass & Wolf, 1998; Wolf & Glass, 1992);
3. to have more normal sensory oral experiences during mealtime (Klein & Morris, 1999; Morris and Klein, 1987, 2000; Palmer & Heyman, 1993); and
4. to improve whole body sensory processing (Oetter, Richter, & Frick, 1995; Wilbarger & Wilbarger, 1991).

Oral sensorimotor stimulation and treatment programs have oral feeding as one of the major goals. This approach is multimodal to encourage coordinated timing and sufficient muscle strength for food and liquid to be swallowed safely without aspiration. Oral sensorimotor treatment can include direct "exercises" of the oral mechanism, as well as indirect approaches that may lead to improvement in oral sensorimotor coordination and safety of swallowing (Table 9–1).

Table 9–1. Direct and Indirect Approaches to Improve Oral Sensorimotor Function in Infants and Young Children With Feeding and Swallowing Problems

Type of Approach	Purpose
Direct	
Oral "exercises"	Stimulate structures for function
	Encourage mouth exploration
	Caution: Invasive and may be aversive; may increase secretions
Indirect	
Alterations in environment	Reduce distractions
	Improve ability to focus
	Caution: Limited social interactions
Position and seating	Better support for feeding
	Improve trunk and head control
Communication signals	Touch and verbal cueing for visually impaired
	Touch and visual cueing for hearing impaired
Food changes	Alter texture, taste, and temperature of food
	Change timing intervals for food presentation
	Vary size of bolus

A total oral sensorimotor and behavioral management program as advocated in this interdisciplinary-team-focused approach transcends the limitation of and is very different from a feeding therapy program. Although a feeding therapy program may include certain aspects of a total oral sensorimotor and behavioral management programs in some instances, the differences are substantial (Morris, 1989).

Feeding therapy is not advocated as an isolated approach because the primary goal of feeding therapy is oral feeding. That focus may not only be inappropriate for some children, it may actually be detrimental. When the focus is on feeding alone, important steps in achieving fundamental skills required for normal oral feeding will be bypassed. A "feeding therapy" approach results in a sense of failure when successful oral feeding is not accomplished within a short time. Food and liquid may be introduced before the necessary respiratory, oral, and pharyngeal skills are achieved. When the mechanics of sucking, chewing, and swallowing are emphasized, clinicians and family may overlook associated activities important in the development of communication and positive psychosocial interaction so basic in the development of feeding (Koontz-Lowman & Lane, 1999; Morris & Klein, 1987, 2000).

In contrast, oral sensorimotor treatment has primary goals that include the development of coordinated movements of the mouth, respiratory, and phonatory systems for both communication and oral feeding (Morris & Klein, 1987, 2000). Oral sensorimotor programs that address several concerns are well documented (e.g. Alexander, 1987; Arvedson, 1993; Morris & Klein, 1987, 2000; Ottenbacher, Scoggins, & Wayland, 1981; Riordan, Iwata, Wohl, & Finney, 1980; Sobsey & Orelove, 1984).

Some evidence-based reports are available, even though most program treatment guidelines are not empirically based. Children with cerebral palsy (CP) and moderate eating impairment appear to maintain weight for age at the lower end of expected norms with oral sensorimotor treatment (OST) but have prolonged mealtimes (Gisel, 1996). Oral caloric supplementation is suggested to provide energy for growth. A different group of children with CP and moderate eating impairment showed no change in eating efficiency with OST. Although they had less spillage, weight remained at the lowest level of age norms (Gisel, Applegate-Ferrante, Benson, & Bosma, 1995). Efficacy of treatment data are needed to answer many questions for different ages, populations, and problems.

Focusing on the total child places oral feeding as a by-product and not a direct major goal of the program. Communication is enhanced in the oral sensorimotor approach. A systematic developmental approach that heightens sensory awareness, perception, and discrimination within the mouth reinforces other developmental achievements. Oral movement is used to explore and understand the world through body parts, toys, clothing, sounds, food, and liquids. The interactive use of touch and movement is emphasized, along with developing maximal total communication skills. Food and liquid are not essential for practice because the goals of oral sensorimotor development can be met in many ways, although food may be introduced for experiences of smell, taste, texture, and temperature variations. The entire experience must be noninvasive and nonstressful to the child. When the child signals discomfort or stress, caregivers must take that information and translate it into "stop." It is critical that caregivers and professionals keep in mind the communication aspects of any therapeutic activity.

The relationships of oral–motor development to feeding and to speech seem logical and appear to be supported on the basis of clinical experience, but data-based research is lacking either to support or refute a causal relationship between the development of the sensorimotor control of feeding and early speech patterns. As speech and feeding skills emerge, three parallel tracks are seen with: (a) increased number and variety of oral movements and positions, (b) expansion of simple movements with smooth integration of earlier movement patterns, and (c) separation or differentiation of movement of two or more components of the system (Morris, 1985). The acquisition and maturation of movement skills appear to underlie both early sound production and feeding abilities.

Principles Directly Relevant to Management Plans

The discussion regarding specific feeding and swallowing interventions highlights some areas of current management. It is not meant to be a "cookbook" for oral sensorimotor treatment because this would be impossible, given the multitude of factors that impact on treatment decisions in infants and children who are constantly growing and changing. The most important skill that the clinician can bring to intervention with infants and young children is the ability to analyze and synthesize all relevant information related to underlying medical and health status, family dynamics, social and cultural aspects, and skill levels of the child. This ability allows clinicians to put together a plan that truly takes into account the total child. (Characteristics that aid in differentiation of children with oral sensory deficits from those with primary oral motor deficits are described in Chapter 7, Table 7–4.)

Oral sensorimotor treatment may be particularly important for children who are fed nonorally. Purposeful swallowing when a stimulus is presented (e.g., drop of juice clinging to a pacifier, a spoon dipped into puree) may help a child to handle her own secretions more effectively and safely. The risk for aspiration of one's own secretions is frequently relatively high when stimulation is lacking for swallowing boluses of food. It is important to try to determine the optimal amount and frequency of oral sensorimotor stimulation for each child. In general, a belief that any stimulation is positive, or that more is better, may actually be erroneous (Korner, 1990). Excessive stimulation may lead to harm in some instances.

Intervention for children with feeding and swallowing deficits must be based on accurate diagnosis and not just a series of oral sensorimotor techniques for specific signs that a child exhibits. For example, a child who demonstrates open mouth posture may be harmed by exercises aimed at getting the lips together when the underlying reason he or she has the mouth open is to assist breathing. A subtle upper airway obstruction may be manifested only by the open mouth posture. In this instance, the medical examination and follow-up management must be undertaken before one could expect results with an oral sensorimotor program. On the other hand, if the underlying condition is hypotonia without airway obstruction, oral sensorimotor exercises may assist the child to develop a more effective tongue-base propulsion to produce a swallow with the lips closed.

The basic principles recognized by many pediatric feeding and swallowing specialists include the following:

1. the relationship between child and caregiver is an important part of a feeding evaluation and subsequent follow-up management plans;
2. the child and family should be included in treatment planning and implementation;
3. oral, respiratory, and neurologic systems within a child should be examined carefully;
4. tone and movement patterns throughout the entire body must be changed before making specific changes to the oral sensorimotor system (Morris & Klein, 1987, 2000);
5. tone and movement patterns in the jaw, tongue, lips, and palate must be altered when necessary to reduce the impact of oral reflexes that may interfere with feeding;
6. normal patterns of movement must be facilitated to replace abnormal movement patterns that interfere with function;
7. normalizing the ability to accept and to integrate visual, auditory, tactile, balance, taste, and temperature information is necessary before direct facilitation of new oral feeding pattern attempts can be made; and
8. oral sensorimotor treatment may be included during a child's typical daily activities to include play, mealtime, and toothbrushing.

The acquisition of functional motor skills is achieved primarily through appropriate sensory input. When children have reduced sensory input or disordered response to sensory input, the consequences are readily apparent with decreased motor function. Thus, the next section will focus on oral sensory approaches to feeding.

■ ORAL SENSORY APPROACHES TO FEEDING

Intervention for sensory problems may involve adaptions to the sensory environment, specific physical handling techniques, or modifcations of sensory qualities of food and feeding utensils. Sensory therapy goals and procedures should be designed to meet the needs of each individual child.

Children may have specific oral sensory problems or more commonly a combination of oral motor and oral sensory impairments. Hyporeactive responses, hyperreactive responses, or sensory defensive responses to oral input can be demonstrated (Table 9–2). A whole-body sensory impairment can occur in addition to problems that are primarily associated with the oral facial region. Feeding problems may range from a limited repertoire of tastes and textures in the diet to total deprivation of oral feeding experiences. In the latter instance, nutrition needs are met via nonoral tube feedings (Chapter 5).

Management of Oral Sensory Deficits

Oral Sensory Management for Hyporeactive Responses

Children with hyporeactive responses to oral input often have diminished responses to all sensory experiences. They commonly demonstrate poor sucking and chewing because of reduced oral discriminative abilities. These children may benefit from a sensory environment that tends to "wake up" or "alert" the nervous system to allow them to focus on meal time (Klein & Delaney, 1994). The room should be well lit. Furnishings and utensils can

Table 9–2. Types of Abnormal Sensory Responses in Children with Oral Sensory Disorders

Type of Response	Signs and Symptoms
Hyporeaction	Diminished response to sensory input Craving foods with increased oral input Drooling Inclination to overstuff mouth with food
Hyperreaction	Excessive reactions to sensory input resulting in abnormal reflex patterns and increased postural tone
Sensory defensiveness	Emotional responses to sensory input Sensory input perceived as a threat Aversion to toothbrushing Texture avoidance

be brightly colored. Food of strong and contrasting flavors can be presented to help the child have increased sensory feed back. Some children respond to foods with increased oral input (e.g., tart and spicy flavors, extreme temperatures, crunchy or lumpy textures). Such children may benefit from animated feeders who use body language and voice to engage children and to increase overall responses. In addition, sensory awareness of mandible, lips, and cheeks may be enhanced in some children by tapping and stroking with the middle finger from midcheek to the mouth, around the lips, and to the mandible. A drop of liquid placed at the corner of the lip or in the cheek pocket may encourage increased activity of the lips and cheeks (Morris & Klein, 1987), usually pursing of lips and "tightening" of cheeks. Functional activities should follow immediately to include nipple, cup, or spoon for feeding.

Oral Sensory Management for Hyperreactive Responses

Children with hyperreactive responses demonstrate an exaggerated response to oral input. These children often benefit from an inhibitory approach to sensory input in an environment that is modified to decrease sensory input. For example, dim lighting, muted colors, bland tastes, and neutral temperatures may be appealing to such children. The feeder may move slowly and calmly, use a quieter voice, and should verbally prepare the child for what to expect during the feeding process, (e.g., "are you ready for another bite?"). In addition, these children typically need positioning that promotes stability.

Management of Oral Sensory Defensiveness

Children with oral sensory defensiveness demonstrate an emotional response to sensory input. They take only a limited variety of tastes and textures orally. Food refusal is frequent. Caregivers need to develop a trusting relationship with these children, who need to be verbally prepared for what to expect. Treatment is explicitly child focused, and the caregiver must anticipate the child's cues carefully. These children are more defensive about the face and mouth than any other parts of the body. Thus, a whole-body approach to sensory input is recommended. Children will likely respond to carefully graded approaches to tactile input that are designed to alter input in incremental steps as they tolerate.

A physical-handling approach to sensory defensiveness incorporates techniques that can be used during and apart from mealtimes (Case-Smith & Humphry, 2000; Glass & Wolf, 1998). Firm-pressure tactile input is given to the face, lips, or inside the mouth. Caution is advocated, particularly for the invasive process of intraoral stimulation. Children should not become stressed with any intervention procedures.

A treatment approach that addresses sensory defensiveness should not be time-consuming. It should be easily incorporated into the child's typical daily routine and be acceptable to caregivers. They may not have time for complex home programs with many demands in the care of children with feeding problems, who also may need time-consuming medical appointments and other therapies. Programmatic integration into daily routines emerges as an obvious approach, given that children who are orally defensive often resist caregiver's attempts at toothbrushing, which results in poor oral hygiene. Thus, oral sensory programs that are incorporated into the daily toothbrushing regimen are encouraged. Similarly, treatment recommendations that can be incorporated into the mealtime routine are sought. Caregivers can incorporate proprioceptive input by placing spoons or cups with firm but gentle pressure at midtongue during mealtimes. Oral sensory experiences may be graded by modifying the taste, temperature, or texture of foods one at a time in small steps, so as not to overwhelm the child. Oral sensory experiences can be considered in a heirarchy that systematizes gradual changes. Children may be seen individually with their parents with guidelines for follow-up at home. Some children with relatively mild sensory deficits may benefit from a group program where parents are involved as they help each other with suggestions and insights.

Desensitization Hierarchy Example

Children from 18 months and older whose primary feeding difficulty relates to sensory deficits are frequently good candidates for a group program (e.g., Haas & Creskoff, 2000). This approach requires that children be able to self-feed, follow simple directions, learn group routine, and observe others in a group (other than parent), and be part of a stable environment (eg., parent without serious psychopathology). The goals are described for children and their caregivers for group intervention; however, these goals are the same for the child in individual intervention with minimal modifications to the goals for caregivers (Table 9–3). These children typically do not have obvious oral–motor deficits. They may have oral sensory problems due to sensory deprivation, although it is difficult, but important, to separate motor and sensory components in many instances (see Table 7–4). They are likely to be transitioning from tube to oral feeding; have low-volume oral intake, poor weight gain, limited variety of tastes and textures in the diet, and difficulty in transitioning from one texture to another; or demonstrate food refusal. A desensitization heirarchy has the following steps (Toomey, 2000):

1. Tolerating—child moves from being in the same room with food to looking at it when food is directly in front of the child;

Table 9–3. Goals for Oral Sensory Approach to Feeding Young Children With Relatively Mild Problems in a Group Program

Goals for Children	Goals for Caregivers
Positive experiences with mouth and food	Provide opportunity to tell the child's story
Teach mealtime routines and cues to eating	Listen to other parents and provide support
Increase comfort with touching, tasting, and swallowing food	Understand ways children learn how to and how not to eat
Increase range of foods with which children will interact	Learn the cues to eating and the steps involved in eating
Increase volume of food children will eat	Gain additional knowledge to manage child's nutritional needs
	Create a feeding program for home follow-up

Adapted from *The S.O.S. Approach: Sequential Oral Sensory Approach to Feeding,* by A. Haas & N. Creskoff, November 2000. Handout from seminar presented at the annual convention of the Speech-Language-Hearing Association, Washington, D.C.

2. Interacting—child uses utensils; may stir food, but not put into mouth;
3. Smelling—child tolerates the odor of food in the room to picking up food to smell it;
4. Touch—child tolerates food on fingers, hand, upper body, chin and cheek, nose, lips, teeth, and tongue;
5. Taste—child licks lips or tongue, bites then spits out, bites and holds in mouth before spitting out, chews and partially swallows, chews and swallows with drink, chews and swallows independently;
6. Eating—gradual changes throughout the steps lead the child to functional eating without any specific focuses by caregivers, except the expected monitoring of young children at mealtimes.

As with any set of guidelines or protocols for programs, individual variations need to be considered. Collaboration with physicians, dietitians, daycare or school professionals, other therapists, and all caregivers is an integral part of any program. All persons involved in the child's care must be consistent in the mealtime approach and in the ways they give encouragement and feedback.

Infants and children with complex feeding and swallowing problems are not likely to have sensory deficits in isolation. They frequently present with abnormal muscle tone and are unable to attain or maintain appropriate positions for efficient feeding. Oral sensorimotor function can be examined and treated only in the context of the total child. Motor development is strongly related to sensory input. As stated in the principles for management, tone and movement patterns throughout the body must be optimal to expect improved function of the oral mechanism. Adequate posture and position are basic to oral feeding. The next section discusses management of posture and position problems.

■ POSITION AND POSTURE MANAGEMENT

Positioning Goals

The general goal of positioning is the same as for all interventions: to promote a safe and pleasant mealtime experience for the child and the family. Caregivers need to be included in the development of a positioning and seating plan. The many different mealtime environments include home, daycare center, school, restaurant, and other places where the child regularly eats. The goals of the child and family need to be included in the selection process. In a home-based study of children with significant feeding problems, only 6 out of 12 families used the adaptive seating system that was provided for them. The parents considered the equipment a nuisance and found it easier to position the child on the couch (Reilly & Skuse, 1992). This highlights the need for clinicians to consider the practical use of a chair within the mealtime environment.

Seating and Positioning Requirements

The establishment of central alignment is basic for coordination of the body and mouth for effective oral sensorimotor and feeding activities. Adjustments are made to attain neutral head, neck, and trunk position (essentially a straight line). The neck and trunk are elongated, pelvis is stable and symmetrical, shoulder girdle stable and depressed, hips at 90° with neutral base of abduction and rotation, and feet in neutral with slight dorsiflexion and never plantar flexed. Clinicians must keep in mind that there may be exceptions to these "rules." When children appear to resist the midline position, other considerations need to be made. For example, a child may hyperextend the neck as a means of keeping the airway open and functional. Thus, postural modifications would be made, and the child would be seen by the appropriate physicians to examine the airway. Children communicate their needs in a variety of ways even when they are nonverbal. Clinicians and parents have an obligation to figure out the message and give them the respect they deserve. Hypertonic children usually require inhibition of increased muscle tone to promote proximal stability and distal mobility (Figure 7–3). Hypotonic children need overall postural stability and alignment and midrange control (Figure 7–2).

Several factors need to be considered in recommendations for an adaptive seating device for mealtime. These factors include family and school environment as mentioned above and ease of use, because a busy caregiver may not have the time necessary to secure many belts, buckles, and snaps. The seating system should be light-weight, attractive, easy to use, and washable. Seating systems that can fit easily under a kitchen table or a school cafeteria table will allow the child to be included more fully in the family mealtime and the school lunch experience.

Optimally, a chair should be used for a variety of purposes. Seating that can be used for meal time, transport, and support for fine motor activities may be the most cost-effective option. Typically, developing children have a wide variety of seating options available to them. In some cases where challenging seating and posture issues are present, a clinician may need to advocate for a child to have a chair for mealtime in addition to a chair for transport to allow him or her to be more fully included in the mealtime environment.

Positioning for Infants

Infants are generally held by caregivers during nipple-feeding. Caregivers must be comfortable with positioning recommendations because holding an infant is one of the most important experiences in the bonding process. Positions that promote good eye contact and close physical contact, as well as a safe and functional feeding position for the infant are suggested. A semireclined position with a neutral head and neck posture and flexion at the hips and knees may be achieved in a variety of ways. The classic posture is achieved by holding the child with the caregiver providing support for midline neutral posture. The child's knees and ankles are flexed over the caregiver's leg (Figure 9–1). An infant or young child can be held with head and neck supported by the caregiver's upper arm while the child's back rests against the arm (Figure 9–2).

Parents can provide an ergonomic feeding posture with an angled bottle (Figure 7–9) that encourages physiologic flexion of the infant and promotes increased comfort for the feeder (Farber, Van Fossen, & Koontz, 1995). A caveat must be considered: as a feeding progresses, the liquid is below the angle of the bottle, and one has an essentially straight bottle. Feeders must monitor closely to make sure the entire nipple end is covered with liquid so that the infant does not take in excessive air.

Positioning for Young Children

Children are ready to sit in a high chair once they have improved head and trunk control to enable them to sit independently. This transition is important

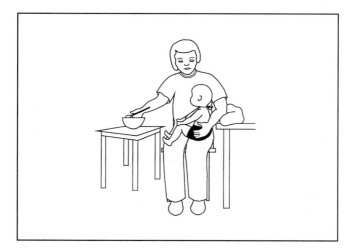

Figure 9–1. A child positioned upright on a lap for feeding. The caregiver provides support for midline neutral posture. The child's knees and ankles are flexed over the caregiver's leg, and the upper extremities are supported anteriorly. [Adapted from Finnie, N. R. (1974). *The Young Cerebral Palsied Child at Home* (2nd ed., p. 118). New York: E. P. Dutton.]

to both caregiver and child because it represents a step toward independence. Any chair modifications should be attractive, light-weight, and practical to use during busy mealtimes. Families need to be comfortable with high chair adaptations so they will use the high chair in social environments that include family parties and restaurants. Towel rolls or cushions can be added at the sides of the trunk and pelvis to promote symmetry. The Snugglebud positioning devices are examples of commercially available systems (Figure 9–3). The Snugglebud support system includes quilted materials that can be attached by Velcro to a variety of infant toddler equipment including carseats, high chairs, and strollers.

Caregivers may be more comfortable using adaptable commercially available seating equipment designed for typically developing infants and toddlers than with "special" seats. Fabric covered foam or towel rolls can be added to infant seats to promote symmetry. Carseats may be adapted for use during mealtime. Feeding in laps or high chairs may be practical only for infants and toddlers with mild postural impairment. The Tumbleforms feeding seat is a seating system that offers minimal support, but it is practical for mealtime use because it is easy to adjust and clean. It offers nonadjustable support at the head, trunk, and pelvis. It includes a lap belt and chest harness. It has a curved back, and this may promote less extensor thrusting in a child with high muscle tone and a tonic labyrinthine reflex.

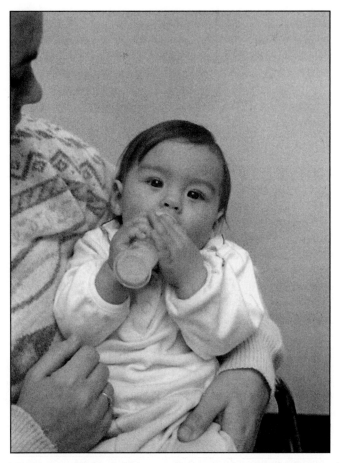

Figure 9–2. Young child is held in a well-supported position, allowing for eye contact between feeder and child. This child has just learned to hold a small bottle independently, and she likes being in control of the feeding process.

On the other hand, it may be inadequate for children with a kyphotic posture and low muscle tone because the curved back may promote a bent, kyphotic posture.

Commercially made strollers are adaptable for preschool children and may be used for mealtime with children who have moderate impairments. The Kid-Kart system is an adjustable seating system that offers multiple ways to support the head, trunk, and pelvis (Figure 7–4). It includes a lap tray and foot rest, chest harness, and lap belt. It has a tilt-in-space option that allows it to be reclined. This option is recommended for reclining the

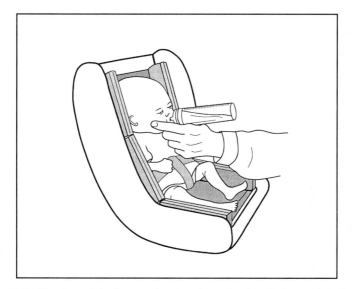

Figure 9–3. The Snugglebud support system is made of quilted materials that can be attached by Velcro to seating devices that include carseats, high chairs, and strollers.

whole body. Some children feed better when they are in a slightly reclined position. This is particularly true for those with poor head control and those with poor lip closure and tongue thrusting. Children with kyphotic posture may also benefit from a reclined chair that can help reduce pressure on the abdomen. The head and neck should remain neutral. Clinicians and parents must be aware that these children may be at higher risk for aspiration in that slight reclined posture because they may have difficulty controlling the bolus in the oral cavity, although maintenance of a neutral head and neck posture may reduce the risk.

Options for Adaptive Seating for Older Children

The seating support needed to promote the optimal position for children must take into account the severity of the postural abnormalities (Table 9–4). For children with mild impairment, adaptive seating options may be added to chairs that are used by typically developing children. Children with moderate and severe impairments usually need customized seating systems. These seating systems may be wheelchairs that include a variety of seating options needed to control posture. The Zippie wheelchair is a seating system that may be used for mealtime as well as transport.

Table 9–4. Classification of Children by Degree of Abnormal Muscle Tone (Hypertonic or Hypotonic) With Seating Options for Each Group

Degree of Abnormal Tone	Characteristics	Seating Options
Mild	Good head control Fair trunk control Symmetrical posture	Standard system (e.g., Tumbleform) Modifications to regular chairs for typical children

Moderate	Fair-to-good head control
	Fair-to-poor trunk control
	Fair-to-poor motor skills
	Mild-to-moderate orthopedic
	  deformities
		Multi-adjustable system
		  (e.g., Snug Seat, Safety
		  Travel Chair, Kid Kart)

Severe	Fair-to-poor head control
	Poor trunk control
	Poor fine motor skills
	Severe orthopedic deformities
		Custom-contoured system
		  (e.g., Pindot, Foam-in-Place,
		  Zippie wheelchair)

Trunk and pelvic symmetry may be promoted by lateral supports and a chest harness. Chest straps can be of various types, from an H pattern with minimal support to a butterfly harness that promotes a flexion pattern by putting pressure on the sternum and a neutral shoulder position with a snug fit across the shoulder girdle (Figure 7–4). Flexion at the hip, knees, and ankles can be achieved through a hip strap and a foot rest.

Optional support for the head and neck range from a backrest for minimal support to a multiadjustable system, such as the Whitmeyer headrest, that offers maximal support (Figure 9–4). The Whitmeyer headrest grasps a child at the occiput and includes a multiadjustable lateral support and a strap that may be placed across the forehead. The Headmaster Collar for head and neck assists midline neutral posture for neck and head (Figure 9–5).

Children vary considerably in their tolerance for seating systems, even when a system is custom designed and meets all specifications considered important in relation to the complexities of the disability. Children also change over time. They outgrow their seats as they get taller or heavier or develop scoliosis or kyphosis. Thus, regular monitoring with adaptations as needed is necessary. Occasionally, a child seems to refute all basic principles for positioning and seating. Clinicians are urged to consider all possible options, and variations within those options. Some children will not require direct oral sensorimotor treatment once posture and postion are maximized; however, many children with complex feeding and swallow problems do have oral sensorimotor problems that are amenable to treatment.

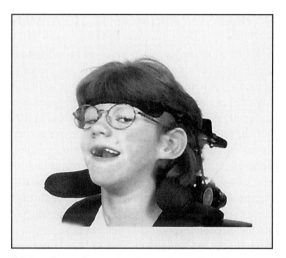

Figure 9–4. Child with a Whitmeyer Biomechanix head support, SOFT PRO-3, three piece head support system, with an optional PRO-DF53 (Dynamic Forehead Strap). This head support offers support to the child to maintain neutral midline head posture.

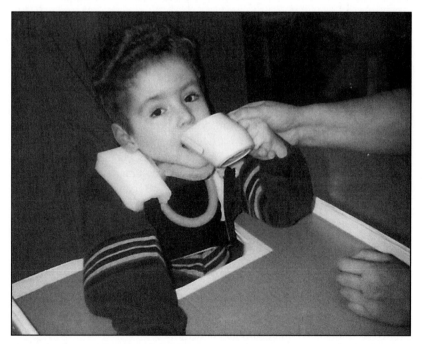

Figure 9–5. Headmaster collar for head and neck support. It can be used in radiology during videofluoroscopic swallow studies, as well as at home and school.

■ DIRECT ORAL SENSORIMOTOR TREATMENT

Oral sensorimotor therapy frequently is recommended for children with a variety of types of swallowing and feeding problems. Some children tolerate direct oral sensorimotor stimulation and treatment well, but others find it aversive and stressful as described in the Oral Sensory section of this chapter. Thus, careful analysis of the child's responses to this kind of approach to motor function is important, so that changes can be made accordingly. This treatment approach is appealing because the structures of the oral cavity are accessible to a clinician for stimulation. These structures under voluntary and stimulatable control are those primarily involved in bolus formation or the oral preparatory phase of swallowing. Thus, oral sensorimotor treatment should be feasible. That such treatment has a direct positive role in helping the child reduce the effects of motor impairment is still open to question.

This section discusses treatment focused on improving jaw, lips, cheeks, tongue, and palate function (Table 9–5). These oral–motor treatment suggestions may be adapted for oral secretion control in older children who drool (Chapter 11). This discussion offers a sampling of procedures that may aid in improving oral–motor function. All persons working with the child for oral stimulation should carry out proper hand-washing techniques. Clinicians are reminded that universal precautions regarding human fluids should always be followed when working in and around a child's mouth. Gloves that are latex free should be used routinely because of the high incidence of allergies to latex.

The following treatment guidelines can be adapted for infants and children of all ages. Direct work at the mouth should be done only when the stimulation does not cause or increase undesired tone and movement in the rest of the body. Thus, the positioning concerns must be considered in every instance as described in the previous section. Effective changes in mouth function can occur only when consideration is also given to alignment of the neck and head, integrity of the anatomic structures, and development of sensory orientation within the mouth (Nelson & de Benabib, 1991).

Table 9–5. Oral Sensorimotor Treatment for Anatomic Structure Problems

Structure/Problem	Treatment
Jaw thrust (increased tone)	Mouth play with fingers and toys Assisted toothbrushing Soft object held between teeth to promote jaw closure
Jaw retraction (increased tone)	Prone positioning Forward pull under jaw

(continues)

Table 9–5. *(continued)* Oral Sensorimotor Treatment for Anatomic Structure Problems

Structure/Problem	Treatment
Jaw clenching (decreased tone)	Mouth play to get gradual opening Pleasurable stimulation on face
Jaw instability (decreased tone)	Activities to encourage jaw closure
Tonic bite reflex (not related to tone)	Pressure at temporomandibular joints Sensory stimulation Coated flat spoon to protect teeth
Lips—retraction (increased tone)	Finger tapping or vibration to cheeks and lips Jaw stability procedures
Limited upper-lip movement (increased and decreased tone)	Varied food textures and temperatures Tapping and stroking Straw drinking with low tone
Cheeks—reduced tone	Stroking and tapping on cheeks, especially at temporomandibular joint
Reduced sensory awareness	Varied food textures and temperatures Drop of liquid at the corner of the lip
Tongue thrust (increased or decreased tone, or respiratory stress)	Jaw stabilization Thickened liquid released at lip Food placed at sides on molar tables (or gums) Exercises for lateral tongue movement Spoon placed at midtongue with downward pressure
Tongue retraction (increased or decreased tone)	Prone position Tongue stroking from back to front Chin tuck position when upright (older child) Upward tapping under chin
Tongue hypotonia (decreased tone)	Varied textures and tastes to increase sensory input Food or liquid added gradually
Tongue deviation	Maintenance of head midline Stimulation of less active side with finger, toys, toothbrush
Tongue—limited movement	Varied textures, temperatures, tastes Vibration
Soft palate (nasopharyngeal reflux)	Upright or prone position Angled bottle used for prone position Cheek and tongue function activities Thickened liquids (if normal swallow)

Programs to Enhance Coordinated Movements of Oral Structures

Jaw

Mandibular stability is basic for bolus formation, swallowing, and speech motor control. Jaw control assistance may be needed for infants and children who demonstrate either hypertonicity or hypotonicity. Suggestions for treatment related to specific jaw problems follow (Table 9–5). Jaw thrust and retraction are more common with hypertonicity. Jaw clenching and instability occur more often with hypotonicity. Tonic bite reflex does not appear directly related to either hypertonicity or hypotonicity.

Problem: Jaw thrust

Jaw thrust is characterized by sudden forceful jaw opening or by exaggerated up-and-down movements; it is a common abnormality that is usually associated with increased tone. The jaw thrust can be precipitated by poor posture, overstimulating environment, hypersensitivity, and, in some instances, dislocation of the temporomandibular joint that may cause pain upon jaw opening (Swigert, 1998).

Recommendation

Mouth play with the child's fingers and soft toys, as well as assisted toothbrushing, may aid in reducing jaw thrust. For example, a finger toothbrush–gum massager that slips on a caregiver's finger has soft bristles and can be used to massage tender gums gently and clean teeth easily and effectively. Sustained jaw closure can be encouraged by having the child hold a cloth or similar soft object between the teeth. However, caution is urged because the maneuver may precipitate jaw clenching.

Problem: Jaw retraction

Jaw retraction may be a part of excessive muscle tension that limits the range of movement, particularly with overall increase in body extension. This type of jaw retraction must be differentiated from the retrognathic mandible that is characteristic of Pierre Robin sequence and other craniofacial anomalies (Chapter 12).

Recommendation

Prone position may be helpful for feeding some children because gravity assists the tongue and jaw to move into a more forward position, thus enlarging the pharyngeal airway and reducing the jaw retraction. The hand can be placed under the child's jaw with a slight forward pull to enlarge the airway further (Morris & Klein, 1987) and to improve feeding efficiency.

Problem: Jaw clenching and teeth grinding

Jaw clenching and teeth grinding may be compensatory attempts to keep the mouth from sagging open when there is postural instability and low tone in the trunk. Jaw clenching may also be an attempt to prevent invasion of the mouth because of past negative experiences with invasive procedures. Jaw clenching obviously restricts oral activity for feeding. Teeth grinding may be one part of both tactile and auditory sensations employed for exploration and play by the child. The sound of the teeth grinding often is irritating to adults.

Recommendation

The best response by an adult usually is to pay no attention to the activity at all because any attention may be perceived by the child as a way to gain control and even more attention. Jaw clenching and teeth grinding can be replaced by pleasurable mouth play. This is encouraged by the clinician or parent who uses fingers to effect a gradual opening of the jaw. Meaningful activities are then facilitated by helping the child get fingers, toys, tooth-brush, and feeding utensils to the mouth more independently. Food is used functionally at mealtime.

Problem: Jaw instability

Jaw instability is characterized by a shift of the jaw to one side or forward. This instability usually results from a generalized hypotonia in the body and face, which is focused at the temporomandibular joint.

Recommendation

Activities that encourage jaw closure are usually helpful with this problem. Jaw stability may be enhanced by placing the middle finger under the chin and the index finger between the chin and lower lip (Figure 9–6). Support can be given from the front or from the side. The degree of pressure is deter-mined by the response of the child, who may indicate displeasure by turn-ing the head, trying to push the hand away, or fussing. Pressure maintained throughout a feeding may be more accepted than frequent changes in hand placement. Maintenance of jaw closure can be encouraged by having the child hold a terry cloth or a small soft toy that can be moved back and forth gently by the clinician or caregiver. The goal is to maintain jaw closure with an object in the mouth (e.g., Hall, 2001).

Problem: Tonic bite reflex

A tonic bite reflex can interfere with feeding. This reflex can be caused by or exacerbated in multiple ways from postural tension to oral hypersensi-tivity to purposeful clenching of teeth to keep something out of the mouth. The tonic bite reflex occurs when the jaw moves upward into a clenched position on presentation of a nipple, a spoon, or another object into the

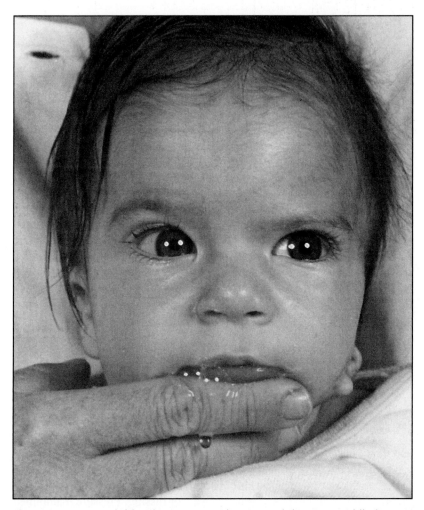

Figure 9–6. Young child with parent providing jaw stabilization. Middle finger is placed under the chin and index finger is placed between the chin and the lower lip.

mouth when contact is made to the biting surfaces of the side gums (molar tables) or teeth. Once the tonic bite occurs, release is usually quite difficult. Any attempt to pull against a tonic bite reflex typically increases the strength of the bite.

Recommendation
Release of the bite may be achieved with pressure applied at the temporomandibular joint on both sides of the face. An inhibitory sensory environ-

ment (e.g., dim lights and quiet voices) may reduce the frequency of occurrence. Well-graded oral tactile stimulation may aid in prevention, or at least reduction in strength, of the bite reflex. A coated, fairly flat spoon may prevent harm to the teeth in some children.

Lips

Lip closure is necessary for keeping food in the mouth and also assists tongue action for moving a bolus of food posteriorly. Common problems that affect the function include lip retraction and limited upper-lip movement.

Problem: Lip retraction
Lip retraction is commonly observed in children with hypertonicity. In attempting to counter the lip retraction, a child may end up with exaggerated lip pursing.

Recommendation
Finger tapping or vibration to the cheeks may reduce the hypertonicity, which in turn reduces the lip retraction. Lip closure can be facilitated by the jaw control procedures described above that, in turn, may encourage an effective spontaneous swallow. The stroking or tapping may be repeated several times in a rhythmic way. A functional activity should follow immediately. Examples of functional activities include nonnutritive sucking on a pacifier, nutritive sucking on a nipple, cup-drinking, or spoon-feeding. In addition to tapping, firm and sustained pressure can be applied to the face with a finger, palm of the hand, or a warm cloth in a direction to move the cheeks and lips into a more normal nonretracted position. These actions of "facial molding" may help the child feel a more normal, less retracted position (Morris & Klein, 1987). Tart flavors and cold temperatures may also facilitate lip closure.

Problem: Limited upper lip movement
Limited upper lip movement may result from either hypertonicity or hypotonicity or from specific cranial nerve damage (CN V or CN VII). Tapping at the cheeks and drawing cheeks forward may reduce hypertonicity in cheeks and lips, which should then result in increased upper lip movement.

Recommendation
Treatment to help reduce hypotonicity and to increase sensory input consists of stimulation with varied food textures and temperatures, as well as tapping and stroking. Similar tapping and stroking activities may be used with both hypertonicity and hypotonicity. Straw drinking may be useful with low tone and limited movement in the cheeks and lips. A straw with a large diameter coupled with a physical assist can help a child close the lips around the straw.

Cheeks

Children need adequate tone in the cheeks to assist lip closure and to keep food from falling into the lateral sulci. Adequate tone in the cheeks indirectly assists the tongue as it forms a bolus.

Problem: Reduced tone
Common problems include reduced tone in the cheeks and reduced sensory awareness. Reduced tone in the cheeks has a direct effect on reduced movement of lips. The mouth may hang open, and excessive drooling can be seen. Food may fall into the lateral sulci in the buccal cavity so that bolus formation is difficult.

Recommendation
Treatment consists of stroking and tapping the cheeks, especially around the temporomandibular joint, which may aid jaw stability. A functional activity, such as sucking on a nipple, cup-drinking, or spoon-feeding, should follow immediately.

Tongue

Coordinated tongue action is fundamental to functional swallowing and speech production. Incoordinated tongue action does not automatically mean that aspiration will occur with swallowing, however. All problems with tongue strength and coordination have direct implications for the oral phase of swallowing and, thus, indirectly for the pharyngeal phase of swallowing. Oral–motor stimulation for facilitation of improved tongue action is often a major focus in therapy with children. The problems most often are characterized by tongue thrust, tongue retraction, or hypotonia of the tongue and less frequently by tongue deviation and limited tongue movement.

Problem: Tongue thrust
Tongue thrust may be exaggerated in some children so that the tongue moves forward beyond the border of the gums and may even stick out between the lips. This forceful protrusion often makes it difficult to insert a nipple or a spoon into the mouth, and may even cause liquid and food to be pushed right back out of the mouth. The tongue thrust may be one aspect of an overall increased extensor tone in the body and may compensate for low tone or movement related to stressful respiratory patterns. A lack of tongue lateralization also can lead to exaggerated tongue protrusion.

Recommendation
Postural modifications should be made as needed. Treatment consists of imposing jaw stability with fingers between the lower lip and the chin to assist lip closure, changes in food texture, and placement of food on the tongue. When up–down sucking movements are not habitual, thickened liquid can be

released from a cup placed on the lower lip. Simultaneously, jaw stability is used to encourage the upper lip to come down on the cup. A sucking motion should get started at the lips as they come together, which in turn helps the tongue to stay behind the lips. In addition, food placed at the side of the gums or posteriorly on the molars can stimulate a munching or chewing action, which in turn, may encourage lateral tongue action, thus reducing the thrusting motions. Lateral tongue action also can be attempted without any food having to be swallowed.

The spoon can be used to create gentle downward pressure at the middle of the tongue (Morris & Klein, 2000). This stimulation can activate a downward movement of the upper lip that helps lips to close around the spoon, and in turn assists with removal of food from the spoon. If immature suckling with in–out tongue actions is predominant, thinner pureed food may help reduce the amount of tongue action needed to move the material posteriorly for a swallow. Feeding should never be done by scraping the food off the spoon at the hard palate or upper gums. This will not facilitate desired tongue movements and lip closure, but instead will reduce the efficiency of moving a bolus posteriorly for a swallow and may precipitate a tonic bite reflex.

Problem: Tongue retraction

Tongue retraction may accompany either excessively low or high tone, may be seen with neck hyperextension, and is common with mandibular hypoplasia (Chapter 12). An infant or child may press the tongue against the hard palate for stability or to prevent the tongue from moving into the airway (Morris & Klein, 1987).

Recommendation

Prone positioning for infants, with the shoulder girdle and head elevated and in good alignment with the trunk, should help to increase the forward movement of the tongue when it is stroked from back to front. With uncoordinated suck along with the tongue retraction, these infants may also benefit from a rhythmic stroking of the tongue with finger moving from midtongue to front (see Stimulation of Nonnutritive Sucking). The prone positioning facilitates oral feeding with some infants. An angled bottle may be helpful for some of these infants in a semiprone position.

When the older child is in an upright position, the chin tucked down toward the chest helps keep the neck elongated, so that tapping upward under the chin at the base of the tongue may provide greater tongue stability, which can assist in forward movement of the tongue. Chin tuck is not advocated for young infants.

Problem: Tongue hypotonia

A hypotonic tongue frequently reflects overall hypotonia. It also can be a flaccid tongue that is directly related to cranial nerve XII damage.

Recommendation
Treatment consists of vibration to the tongue for those children who do not find that aversive. Oral sensory stimulation by objects with a variety of textures and temperatures to the mouth may result in increased tongue movement. Older children may be able to attempt to imitate movements of the tongue. Whether cold objects, warm objects, or food in the mouth encourage more effective tongue action is as yet unknown. Therapy should include cautious trial and error for individual patients.

Problem: Tongue deviation
Tongue deviation to one side of the mouth may be noted as the child attempts to protrude the tongue. It also can be observed as the child attempts to manipulate food in the mouth when both sides of the tongue do not move equally well. Deviation of the tongue may result from ipsilateral cranial nerve damage (CN XII), or it may be due to the presence of an asymmetric tonic neck reflex (ATNR) in which the tongue pulls to the side toward which the head is turned.

Recommendation
Maintaining the head at midline using position or head support may aid significantly with an ATNR. Stimulation of the less active side of the tongue can be done with a finger, a toothbrush, or selected toys.

Problem: Tongue—Limited movement
This may occur because of increased tension in the tongue due to hypertonicity, insufficient tension of the tongue due to hypotonicity, or from damage to CN XII.

Recommendation
Treatment options include, but are not limited to, increased stimulation by varying textures, temperatures, and tastes. Vibration to the tongue may help to increase awareness and discrimination and, in turn, increase movement.

Soft Palate

The soft palate plays an integral role in normal swallowing. It elevates and retracts to close off the nasal passage at the onset of the pharyngeal phase.

Problem: Nasopharyngeal reflux
Velopharyngeal insufficiency is a common occurrence with a posterior cleft of the palate, submucous cleft palate, or a short soft palate, and nasopharyneal reflux may occur during swallowing (Chapter 12). Nasopharyngeal reflux also may occur as a result of incoordination in the pharyngeal phase of the swallow, even when there is no structurally based

velopharyngeal insufficiency. The risk for nasopharyngeal reflux increases when the child is fed in a reclined or semireclined position with the neck in hyperextension.

Recommendation
Feeding may be more successful if the child is fed in an upright position; for some children an angled bottle and semi-prone position may facilitate feeding. Videofluoroscopic or endoscopic swallow study findings may be necessary for definitive management decisions when nasopharyngeal reflux is noted with neurologically based incoordination. An angled bottle may be needed for an infant to suck while in prone position. If swallowing is coordinated and the child is in an upright position, improved cheek and tongue function should also aid in bolus formation, which, in turn, may result in swallowing with less nasopharyngeal reflux. Thickened liquids may be helpful in cases where thin liquids are refluxed and the swallow pattern is basically adequate.

■ ORAL SENSORIMOTOR THERAPY IN CHILDREN WITH TUBE FEEDINGS

A major disadvantage of all feeding tubes that start from nose or mouth to the gastrointestinal tract is a high probability for a negative effect on oral sensorimotor stimulation. The infant may resist any contact with the face because of the association with tube insertion, which is invasive and uncomfortable. Overall, the infant develops many unpleasant associations in and around the mouth.

Children who cannot meet nutritional needs safely by oral feeding alone can get their nutritional needs met by a range of nonoral methods that include both enteral and parenteral feeding. Alternative feeding routes are described in Chapter 5 and types of formulas in Chapter 6.

Feeding tubes (orogastric [OG] or nasogastric [NG]) may be used up to several weeks or a few months while infants are in a hospital. The majority of premature infants, children with neurologic impairments, or those in post-surgical periods who get tube feedings for no longer than 15 to 20 days, transition to oral feeding without difficulty (e.g., Bernbaum, Pereira, Watkins, & Peckham, 1983; Dellert, Hyams, Treem, & Geertsma, 1993; Field et al., 1982). Some recommend that tubes be replaced at 3- to 4-day intervals (Moore & Greene, 1985). NG and OG tubes may have multiple negative effects (Chapter 7). These include inhibition of previously used sucking or swallowing movements because of the discomfort (Morris, 1989), reduction of a protective gag due to sensory adaptation to a tube over time, nasal and pharyngeal irritation (Dobie, 1978), emesis, gastroesophageal reflux, and delayed gastric emptying (Chapter 5), and a generalized disorganization of oral function.

A gastrostomy tube (GT) is preferred when tube feedings are anticipated for longer than 2 to 3 months. A major advantage of gastrostomy tube feedings is that the area of invasion of the tube is separated from the mouth, which may permit the infant to discover pleasurable oral sensation more quickly. Criteria and procedures for gastrostomy are discussed in detail in Chapter 5. The risks for anesthesia are considered carefully in children. The percutaneous endoscopic gastrostomy (PEG) is being used more frequently with children (Kutiyanawala, Hussain, Johnstone, Everson, & Nour, 1998; Benkov, Kazlow, Waye, & Lelieko, 1986). These procedures have made it possible to minimize the number of infants who go home on NG tube feedings. Elimination of NG tubes is highly desirable for safety and for potential oral sensorimotor gains toward oral feeding. Caregivers are trained in the management of the GT. They also are given techniques for oral sensorimotor stimulation as discussed in following sections and reminded that oral stimulation must be pleasurable and nonstressful to help children accept touch to the cheeks and lips (Figure 9–7A&B). The child should be an active participant (Figure 9–8A&B).

■ INFANT ORAL FEEDING

Most term infants take oral feeding sufficient to meet nutritional needs from birth. Other infants may require tube feedings for some time before oral feeding can be considered. Even in the healthiest preterm infant (i.e., a gestational age usually at least 32 to 34 weeks), respiratory stability, alertness, and a coordinated suck/swallow/breathe pattern are all prerequisites to successful oral feeding. High-risk premature infants mature in their sucking behaviors and in their ability to maintain a more alert behavior state from 34 weeks postconceptional age (PCA) to term. At 34 weeks PCA, the preterm infant state of alertness may not enhance sucking skills (Medoff-Cooper, McGrath, & Bilker, 2000). These infants may be too stressed to manage feeding, the work of breathing, and response to stimulation from the environment that is unavoidable when they are alert. It is desirable for tube-fed infants to tolerate bolus feedings before oral feedings are seriously considered.

Readiness for Oral Feeds

Extended and early contact between mother and infant leads not only to more interaction, but also more touching by the mother for term infants as well as for premature infants. Rooming-in opportunities should be

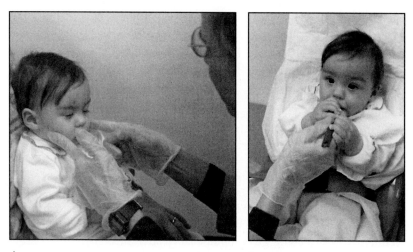

A   B

Figure 9–7.   A. A 9-month-old child, whose nutritional needs are met via GT feeds, accepts firm but gentle touch on her cheeks with stroking toward her lips in preparation for a "taste" as part of oral sensorimotor stimulation. **B.** She eagerly reaches for the spoon and helps get it to her mouth.

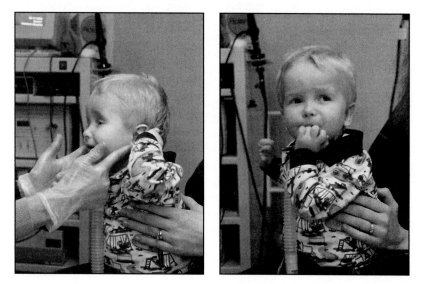

A

Figure 9–8. A. A toddler who has a tracheostomy, is on a ventilator, and is at risk for aspiration with oral feeding. He gets nutritional needs met by GT feeds. He accepts touch and stroking to his face. **B.** He prefers doing his own intraoral stimulation over someone else "invading" his mouth.

encouraged for all stable newborn infants (Prodromidis et al., 1995). Prolonged nurturing contact from mother to infant assists in readiness for successful oral feeding.

An awake, alert infant should be able to ingest a full feeding in less than 30 min, whether it is an oral feeding or a bolus tube feeding. Tolerance for bolus feedings is one indicator for oral feeding readiness. Gradually the infant develops the internal cues related to hunger and subsequent satiation in relation to time intervals between feedings. The infant needs to be alert at feeding time. One cannot feed a sleeping or lethargic infant.

The shift to oral feedings may be gradual for infants who can tolerate small amounts of liquid with the oral sensorimotor practice just before or during a tube feeding. The amount given by tube can be reduced relative to the amount taken orally. Some infants may signal displeasure with the oral feeding. The oral feeding practice should then be separated from the tube feeding. A tube feeding given immediately after an oral feeding during which the infant has shown negative behavior would be a reinforcer for that behavior. At best, the result would be a delay in attaining oral feeding; at worst it could set up a cycle of food refusal and behavioral complications.

Infants with sucking and swallowing problems present special challenges to caregivers and professionals in the establishment of oral feeding. The introduction of liquid with nipple-feeding attempts must be done cautiously and carefully. Varied nipples and containers can be tried so the optimal rate of flow can be found (Mathew, 1991, 1988; Mathew, Belan, & Thoppel, 1992) (Figure 7–9). A flow that is too fast will exacerabate incoordination problems, and a flow that is too slow may create frustration and fatigue. Collapsible containers have been found to shorten the duration of feedings significantly without negatively affecting ventilation for healthy preterm infants (Duara, 1989). Infants improve efficiency and reduce duration of nipple feedings with a self-pacing system and vacuum-free bottles (Lau & Schanler, 2000). Ventilated bottles have been found to reduce the incidence of otitis media with effusion in infants (Brown & Magnuson, 2000). The negative pressure created inside a conventional bottle may cause the infant to suck excessively, causing intraoral pressure to be transmitted to the middle ear via the eustachian tube, which leads to otitis media with effusion and the accompanying negative consequences. These negative pressures were not recorded in the middle ear with a fully ventilated bottle that showed positive pressure throughout the feeding procedure, similar to normal breast-feeding.

Stress Signals During Oral Feeding

Infants communicate stress in a variety of ways. These signals include irregular breathing or breath holding, gagging, choking, yawning, or hiccuping. Whole-body changes may occur, such as arching, squirming, facial grimacing, and increased hypotonicity or hypertonicity (Morris & Klein, 1987). Inner stress can also be communicated by staring, averting gaze, roving the eyes, showing a worried expression, and falling asleep. Inconsolable crying and a rapidly changing behavioral state may be other means of communicating stress. These signals mandate that caregivers reconsider the manner of sensory input. Effective stimulation allows for smooth respiration at appropriate rates, a healthy skin color, visual attentiveness and an animated facial expression, a more normal postural tone, and self-quieting after crying.

Two types of infants have been described as having difficulty in becoming functional nipple feeders (Harris, 1986): "lackadaisical" and "aversive." The lackadaisical infant sucks well on a finger or a pacifier but has a weak and dysrhythmic suck when presented with liquid. This infant may show an adequate suck-and-swallow sequence when assessed with very small amounts of formula, but in a real feeding situation, he or she appears disinterested, frequently falls asleep, or pushes the nipple away after taking only a very small amount of liquid. The aversive infant appears resistant to nippling attempts and may or may not do coordinated nonnutritive sucking on a finger or pacifier. This infant usually takes a few sucks when liquid is presented, then squirms, squeals, hyperextends, and arches the body. Both types of behavior patterns may represent oral–motor, sensory, and behavioral problems, or they may relate to a more fundamental physical or physiologic distress.

Management of Specific Oral Sensorimotor Problems

Guidelines for management of sucking and swallowing problems differ according to the underlying problem areas (Table 9–6). Suggestions are made below for management of a weak and dysrhythmic suck, suck-and-swallow incoordination, sensory problems, resistance to feeding, appetite considerations, and gastroesophageal reflux.

Weak and Dysrhythmic Suck

Modification of a weak and dysrhythmic suck can be tried in several ways. During feeding, firm but gentle pressure can be applied to the lips, specifically to the orbicularis oris. Jaw stabilization may improve efficiency of sucking (Hill, Kurkowski, & Garcia, 2000) and increased volume consumed (Einarsson-Backes, Deitz, Price, Glass, & Hays, 1994). Once a suck pattern has been initiated, a tug on the nipple may smooth out the suck pattern and strengthen the suck (Harris, 1986). Thickened liquid allows for greater resistance to the suck and may facilitate improved

Table 9–6. Management of Sensorimotor Suck and Swallow Problems

Problem Area	Management Suggestions
Weak, dysrhythmic suck	Pressure to assist lip closure Jaw stabilization (upward pressure to chin) Tug at nipple as though pulling it out of mouth (may smooth out and strengthen the suck) Thicken liquid (rice cereal) Adjust nipple opening
Suck-and-swallow incoordination	Stroking hyoid muscle toward sternum Gradual introduction of liquid (finger, pacifier, cotton swab, or cheesecloth dipped in liquid and placed into mouth) Nipple changes to get optimal flow Bypassing nippling to spoon and cup
Sensory problems: Hyposensitivity Hypersensitivity	 Firm but gentle stroking around mouth and on tongue Deep, sustained pressure in and around mouth by caregiver's or infant's hand
Resistance to feeding: Aversive Lethargic Fussy	Position change: Prone with head supported in extension More upright and away from caregiver's body, with back, neck, and head support Swaddling and holding close to caregiver's body
Limited to no hunger or appetite	Feeding when infant is hungry Demand schedule may help With tube feedings, reduce during daytime and supplement at night for some
Gastroesophageal reflux	Thickening of liquid Head elevated prone positioning (not clearly supported) Medical or surgical treatment probable

timing. Thickening is usually done with rice cereal. Nipple openings need to be adjusted accordingly.

Nipples come in a variety of shapes, sizes, and textures (Figure 7–9). Premature infants usually respond better to a fairly soft nipple that allows a steady liquid flow as these infants tend to tire more easily. A larger hole, more holes, or a cross-cut in the nipple will increase the liquid flow. Fewer holes or smaller cross-cuts can be used as the sucking improves. Caution must be used so that the flow does not become so fast that it causes coughing or choking. On the other hand, if the hole is too small or there are too few holes, the infant has to work too hard and may fatigue before taking a sufficient quantity of liquid.

Suck and Swallow Incoordination

Incoordination between sucking and swallowing may be a greater management challenge because it is difficult to evaluate directly. Infants frequently show aversion to feeding because of negative experiences with coughing or choking. Liquid can be introduced gradually by dipping the pacifier or a finger into formula and then placing it into the infant's mouth. A clean piece of cheesecloth may be twisted over the finger and dipped into formula, then placed into the infant's mouth. This gives the infant experience in sucking, but with such a small amount of formula that the risk for choking is minimized and the probability of a safe swallow is maximized.

If the infant accepts a nipple and continues rhythmic tongue action without tongue retraction, nipple-feeding may be possible with careful monitoring of the rate of flow. The flow rate should be steady and even to reduce potential for excessive air that can lead to gastrointestinal discomfort. The infant needs an optimal balance of easy sucking and appropriate flow for functional feeding. The flow rate can be monitored readily with standard bottles because the bubble flow can be seen. Bubbles are noted with each suck when feeding is efficient. This monitoring is not possible with collapsible or fully ventilated containers or in breast-feeding.

Infants with severe oral–motor incoordination and prolonged periods of nonoral feeding may bypass the breast-feeding or bottling stage. Infants with a tonic bite reflex who elicit a clamping bite with a touch to the gums will produce a bite, not a suck, on presentation of a nipple. Using a nipple will be ineffective when stimulation to the tongue results in retraction or disorganized movement of the tongue. Some caregivers have erroneously encouraged the use of a larger nipple hole, a long lamb's nipple, or a cleft palate nipple for infants with incoordinated swallowing patterns. This may be dangerous because the increased flow of liquid could threaten health and sometimes survival. The infant's most common response is to try to stop the suck to slow down the liquid flow. The tongue may be pulled into stronger retraction as an attempt to block the entrance of liquid into the oropharynx. The compensatory actions that develop may be more detrimental to oral feeding than the underlying neurophysiologic incoordination.

Resistance to Feeding

When infants show resistance to oral feeding attempts, whether "lackadaisical" or "aversive," the first step is to change the position. Prone position with the head supported in extension may facilitate feeding for some infants. Harris (1986) suggests that the airway is opened by ventral displacement of the pharyngeal structures, allowing for increased pharyngeal diameter and separation of the routes of feeding and respiration. The postural demands are on the posterior musculature, the neck extensors, that may permit greater dissociation of feeding and postural functions (Takagi & Bosma, 1960). Level of alertness may also be increased and will facilitate feeding.

Drowsy infants may be stimulated by position changes to get them more upright and further away from the caregiver's body, although with good back, neck, and head support. A fussy infant may respond favorably to swaddling and being held close to the body.

Appetite Considerations

Infants should be hungry at feeding time and in a quiet alert behavioral state. Infants on tube feeding supplements frequently are on specific schedules, and they never demand to be fed. Infants who have been fed on demand have been found to fare as well as those on scheduled feedings. They also have been discharged to home earlier than similar infants on scheduled feedings (Collinge, Bradley, Perks, Rezny, & Topping, 1982). Thus, close cooperation with nursing and physician staff in the intensive care nursery may lead to the flexibility required to achieve oral feeds on demand.

Some infants on oral and tube feedings may make more rapid progress if they can be given oral feedings during the daytime at appropriate intervals with supplemental tube feedings at night. This procedure can be useful as a transition stage to work toward discharge from the hospital in essentially the same manner.

■ STIMULATION AND INTERVENTION WITH PREMATURE INFANTS

Neonates at risk for prolonged feeding problems in infancy should be identified so that appropriate intervention and follow-up can be implemented as soon as possible. These problems can be more persistent than caregivers and professionals would like. At 6 months corrected for gestation, premie graduates with ongoing feeding difficulties are characterized by inconsistencies in oral–motor skill development, fewer readiness behaviors for solids, fewer self-feeding and biting skills, more aversiveness, and poor attention (Mathisen, Worrall, O'Callaghan, Wall, & Shepherd, 2000). Compared with premature neonates with normal initial feeding assessments, premature neonates with disorganized or dysfunctional feeding are 6 times more likely to vomit and 3 times more likely to cough when offered solid food at 6 months of age. At 12 months, these same children have difficulty tolerating lumpy food and enjoying mealtimes (Hawdon, Beauregard, Slattery, & Kennedy, 2000).

Developmental Care Before Readiness for Oral Feeding

Early intervention for very-low-birth-weight premature infants is encouraged as a means of facilitating dimensions of neurobehavioral development: autonomic, motor, behavioral state, attention and interaction, and self-regulation. The National Association of Neonatal Nurses (NANN) (1995) guidelines suggest consideration of "skin-to-skin" contact between the infant and parent as early as possible when the premature infant is in medically stable condition. Kangaroo Care (KC) is a synonym for skin-to-skin contact in which the infant, wearing only a diaper, is placed upright chest-to-chest with a parent. KC is found to provide a milieu that supports autonomic stability and fosters improvements in basic physiologic functions (Ludington-How & Swinth, 1996). Stability in these physiologic functions and rhythmic nonnutritive sucking are prerequisites for oral feeding. Nonnutritive sucking opportunities can be given by providing access to the breast well before the infant is ready to attempt oral feeding. KC satisfies in part handling, self-consoling/soothing, nonnutritive sucking, and parenting interventions that promote closeness and confidence in the parents (Zaichkin, 1996).

Stimulation of Nonnutritive Sucking

The term *nonnutritive sucking* (NNS) is used here to refer to either suckling or sucking (defined in Chapter 2) on any object, such as a pacifier, finger, or toy. This contrasts with nutritive sucking, which is sucking on a nipple containing liquid by breast or some other nipple. Rhythmic NNS appears to be an underlying skill necessary for successful oral feeding, although in and of itself the skill is not sufficient to guarantee success for nutritive sucking. NNS is not necessarily followed by a swallowing response, and thus caution must be used in interpreting the infant's performance with NNS as a basis for readiness to feed orally.

The low-birth-weight premature or sick infant has lacked the opportunity to build positive associations between sensations in the mouth and the contrasting feelings of hunger and satiation. Infants who get slow and continuous tube feeds do not develop hunger or appetite and likely do not get feelings of satiation either. Thus, multiple complicating factors are at work as these infants become medically stable for oral feeding. Once medical conditions are under control, oral feeding does not necessarily follow immediately as most physicians and parents would like to see happen. This lack of awareness of a relationship between learning to handle food in the mouth and the satisfying inner feelings of satiation may be as big a factor in later attempts to establish oral feedings as any underlying oral sensorimotor problem(s). Thus, early oral sensorimotor stimulation may be a preventive measure for some infants as pleasurable sensation is experienced along with the rhythmic sequencing of sucking.

Normalization of oral sensorimotor function, not immediate oral feeding, is the first goal. Some infants may demonstrate such degrees of oral hypersensitivity that they resist touch and taste experiences. They require systematic approaches to establish readiness for sucking or for tastes. Stimulation of NNS can include stroking the face and the tongue, providing taste experiences, and reducing sensory stimuli (Table 9–7). Parents, other primary caregivers, and nurses follow-up with guidelines to provide the stimulation several times each day. Oral–motor feeding specialists monitor and alter suggestions as gains are made and situations change. The infant's tolerance of bolus feeds via tube rather than continuous feeds is desirable as a basis for establishing appetite, interest in sucking, and knowledge that the gastrointestinal tract can handle appropriate size volumes in an expected oral feeding time frame, usually less than 30 min.

A meta-analysis of randomized controlled trials in 19 studies reveals that NNS is found to decrease significantly the length of hospital stay in preterm infants (Pinelli & Symington, 2000). NNS did not consistently correlate with weight gain, energy intake, heart rate, oxygen saturation, intestinal transit time, and age at full oral feeds. No short-term negative impacts were found. Limitations in these studies included designs, outcome variability, and lack of long-term data. Based on the available evidence, NNS in preterm infants would appear to have some benefit. Future research in this area should include outcome measures.

Stroking the Face and Tongue

By 32 weeks gestation, infants with stable respiratory status can tolerate brief periods of rhythmic stroking around and in the mouth. The infant may be most receptive to stroking if the initial firm, but gentle, touch is made with the palm of the hand (Field, 1986; White & Labarba, 1976) or a finger (Rausch, 1981) at the periphery of the face. The caregiver starts the movement at the ears, goes to the cheeks and chin, and gradually moves toward the mouth using a circular pattern around it. As the infant tolerates the stroking at the lips, the little finger can be used to ease into the mouth

Table 9–7. Nonnutritive Oral Sensorimotor Stimulation for Common Problems

Problem	Technique	How Used
Oral hypersensitivity	Stroke face	Palm of hand or finger rhythmically from periphery to mouth; firm but gentle
Inconsistent sucking	Stroke tongue	Stroke with gloved finger from middle to tip of tongue at 1 stroke per sec for 4 to 6 times; hold to give infant chance to suck; repeat process for 5 to 10 min total if tolerated
	Tap lips and tongue	Tap 2 times per sec, which is nonnutritive rate, firm but gentle
Mild sucking incoordination or limited sucking Reduced cheek tone	Offer pacifier (or finger)	Pacifier or finger placed in mouth and held in place by caregiver if infant tends to push it out or simply does not keep it in mouth
Incoordinated suck/swallow/ breathe sequencing; not safe for oral feeding but taste experience desired	Use cotton swab dipped in water, formula, or breast milk	Swab placed at midtongue with downward pressure to release minimal amount of liquid; stroke as with little finger; repeat as tolerated in pleasurable way
Inability to integrate competing sensations	Reduce sensory stimulation	Reduce noise and light levels Rocking, walking, rhythmic tapping; music with regular rhythm; swaddling

to midtongue region to encourage nonnutritive sucking. Light touch tends to be ticklish, and strong pressure may yield an aversive reaction.

Stroking the tongue may help to stimulate a rhythmic suck, although there is no way to impose a sucking pattern directly. The infant can be held in a comfortable position before or during a tube feeding, so that a connection is made with oral stimulation and satiation. The caregiver's little finger can be moved from middle of the tongue to the front with slight downward pressure or upward on the palate at a rate of 1 stroke (nutritive sucking rate) per second for six to eight strokes. The finger is then held in the infant's mouth for several seconds with the fingertip at about the middle of the tongue to approximate nipple placement, but not so far as to trigger a gag response. If the infant begins to suck, the finger can be left in place on the tongue as a pacifier. If no sucking is noted after several seconds, the stroking can be repeated for six to eight strokes with the finger again held in the mouth. Caregivers may carry out this process several times each day for 5- to 10-min sessions, especially in connection with tube feedings. The caregiver monitors for signs of fatigue or stress. The infant's mother or other primary caregiver should provide this stimulation as much as possible because the infant associates the caregiver's smell, touch, and voice along with the actual oral facial stimulation that strengthen all aspects of bonding, interaction, and communication.

A pacifier may be sufficient stimulation for some infants. NNS on a pacifier alone is shown to be more effective in bringing preterm infants to optimal states for feeding than stroking and NNS with rocking (McCain, 1992). In terms of heart rate, the stroking was not only ineffective for feeding readiness, but less calming than no intervention at all. The observer can only make inferences about the suckling patterns when the infant has a pacifier, whereas when the caregiver uses the little finger as a pacifier, she can tell whether the infant is using "stripping" action for sucking, has grooving or cupping around the finger/nipple, and the strength and consistency of sucking.

These sucking experiences associated with feeding time have been found to provide positive gains in a variety of ways to include (a) increased transcutaneous oxygen tension between 32 and 35 weeks gestation (Paludetto, Robertson, Hack, Shivpuri, & Martin, 1984), (b) enhanced growth and maturation (Bernbaum et al., 1983), (c) reduced number of tube feedings needed before oral feedings (Field et al., 1982), (d) improved digestion by simulating the natural way nutrients are ingested (Measel & Anderson, 1979), (e) reduced amount and degree of fussing and crying during invasive procedures (e.g., heelsticks) (Field & Goldson, 1984), and (f) higher transcutaneous oxygen tensions (tcPO2s) after crying was induced by a heelstick (Treloar, 1994).

Premature infants lack sucking pads that provide the cheek and jaw stability found in term infants, and NNS experiences may help them strengthen oral musculature. Caregivers can provide jaw stability and draw the cheeks forward, which may be helpful for some infants to get a better seal around a pacifier or a nipple.

Providing Taste Experiences

Taste experiences may be helpful in stimulating a swallow, because swallowing does not occur as often with NNS compared with oral nipple-feeding. Liquid must be introduced cautiously and in very small amounts when an infant demonstrates incoordination of sucking and swallowing with risk for aspiration. Premature infants can be given water, breast milk, or formula. In addition, older infants and children may be given juice or small amounts of pureed fruit or vegetables. The pacifier or finger can be dipped into liquid. A single drop of liquid may be presented via cotton swab, a plastic medicine dropper, or a syringe (Morris, 1989). The infant should maintain rhythmic tongue movements of sucking. A drop of liquid may be sufficient to stimulate a swallow but not to increase the risk for aspiration. Gradually, sucking experiences may become linked with a sensation of satiation. The amount of liquid or food is increased in small steps to keep the infant unstressed and to maintain a rhythmic sucking pattern.

Reducing Sensory Stimuli

The neonatal intensive care unit (NICU) often is noisy and brightly lit, as are many other hospital and home environments. As emphases are placed on neurodevelopmental care, more attention is paid to the infant's environment. The importance of allowing the infant to be in a calm state cannot be overstated. Premature and neurologically impaired infants may not be able to sort through competing sensations of bright lights, noises, and temperatures to achieve an integrated organization of the nervous system. They frequently become irritable or they fall asleep as a means of coping with competing stimuli. These infants may be calmed by rocking, walking, rhythmic tapping on the infant's lips, or having instrumental music with a regular rhythm at a slow tempo playing in the background. Music with a tempo of 50 to 70 beats per minute, that is, a similar tempo to the pattern of one suck–swallow per second, has been associated with enhanced learning and retention (Schuster & Mouzon, 1982). Some children feed with better coordination when baroque music is played in the background (Morris, 1985). Swaddling in cotton blankets seems to provide a constant firm tactile input to the nervous system of some infants, who in turn show reduced irritability and increased organization of responses (Morris & Klein, 1987).

Early oral sensorimotor stimulation may be a cost-effective means of intervention that can aid in prevention or reduction of more extensive feeding problems later. Field (1986) stressed that infant intervention may be effective in the long run only if "the tools of the trade are left with the primary interventionist—the parent" (Field, p. 190).

Special Concerns for Infants With Neurologic Impairment

An infant with neurologic impairment may have significantly greater incoordination of suck/swallow/breathe patterns or weaker suck than the neurologically intact infant. A congenital incapacity to swallow is a life-threatening condition in neonates and infants and is usually a marker of broader neurologic deficits. A transitory dysphagia lasting a few days or even a few weeks may relate to immaturity of suck/swallow/breathe sequencing and is not uncommon in premature infants with very low birth-weight and occasionally may be evident in a term infant. A prolonged inability to take oral feeds is unusual and can be due to variable causes (Chapter 3).

One should be suspicious of a neurogenic dysphagia when the pregnancy has been complicated by polyhydramnios, which can reflect a swallowing defect in utero. The fetus swallows about 500 ml amniotic fluid during later stages of gestation, and about the same amount is excreted in urine (Ogundipe, Kullama, Day, & Ross, 1994). As the severity of polyhydramnios increases, so does the likelihood of detecting congenital malformations (Ross & Nijland, 1997). As clinicians work with infants for stimulation, they need to keep reminding themselves about underlying etiologies of problems and continue to search for answers, likely requiring collaboration with multiple disciplines. It is widely accepted that generalized stimulation of an infant influences maturation (McBride & Danner, 1987), although it is not clear how much of what type stimulation is optimal.

Massage therapy is reported to result in positive outcomes for infants and children with various medical conditions (Field, 1995). Preterm infants with more complications appear to benefit more from massage therapy than those with fewer complications (Scafidi & Field, 1996a). Preterm and term neonates born to HIV-positive mothers show gains in multiple developmental measures and also greater daily weight gain with massage therapy (Scafidi & Field, 1996b). Diffuse central nervous system dysfunction results in immature behavioral and motor response patterns. Therefore, premature infants with neurologic impairment may need to remain on nonoral feeding programs longer than their neurologically intact peers.

Children with significant neurologic impairment have a higher probability of need for a gastrostomy than healthy premature infants. The oral sensorimotor functional gains may be slow. The duration for nonnutritive stimulation needs, and thus for nonoral feeds, is difficult to predict for infants with neurologically based suck/swallow/breathe problems when there is likely to be at least some risk for aspiration with oral feeding. Some infants will become full oral feeders within a few weeks, and others may need a GT for several months or even a lifetime. Some of these children may bypass the nipple stage of oral feeding and go directly to spoon-feeding and cup-drinking. Nonetheless, it must be anticipated that not all children will become total oral feeders.

Children with GTs are discharged to home once the they are stable with feeding. Guidance and encouragement are important for caregivers so they will follow through in adapting the tube feeding to parent–infant needs for physical contact and interpersonal interaction, along with continued oral sensorimotor stimulation. As children increase the oral feeding, the tube feedings are decreased in proportion so the total volume meets the daily needs per nutrition guidelines (Chapter 6). Tolerance of bolus feedings by tube is an important variable in weaning children from tube to oral feeding. Gastrointestinal systems need to tolerate bolus feeds without stress. Children have particular difficulty if they experience gagging, retching, or other physiologic discomfort from the tube feeds. Many children who are given bolus feeds during the day without stress but continue with a slow night feed (e.g., 8–10 hours) do not develop hunger and appetite and sufficient self-interest in feeding to make the transition until the night feed can be eliminated.

One example of a data-based protocol for tube weaning is from Senez and colleagues (1996) who reported on two groups of children: (a) neonates and infants who have never taken oral feeds from birth and (b) older children in posttraumatic or postsurgical periods, who have had normal feeding before becoming ill. They emphasized the importance of not stressing the children, and not feeding by force. The infants became oral feeders through a protocol of intermittent bolus feeds with stimulation provided during the tube feedings: nursing, tactile stimulation, and olfactory and taste stimulation. Children in group two were also on an intermittent tube feeding schedule. Cryotherapy stimulation was the first step to obtain muscular relaxation and combat trismus (difficulty in opening mouth), followed by tactile stimulation, and olfactory and taste bud stimulation. Principles of swallowing neurophysiology and biologic rhythm are basic considerations to reestablishing oral feeding.

Parents typically want to remove the GT once a child takes full oral feedings, but many physicians encourage parents to keep it in place, even though it is not being used, for at least a few months after the child has started taking full oral feedings. The GT can be considered a safety valve because infectious illness can put these delicately balanced children at risk for acute malnutrition and dehydration (Chapter 5, 6). Thus, the tube is kept in place until recovery from at least one fairly significant upper respiratory illness. Parents then have assurance that the infant can continue to take oral feedings sufficient to meet nutritional needs even when not feeling well. Children with GTs are followed closely by the interdisciplinary feeding and swallowing team so that guidelines can be modified as the child changes over time.

Breast Feeding of Premature and Term Infants

Breast-feeding is encouraged for numerous reasons beyond nutritional superiority over infant formulas. Some of the advantages include species specificity of the milk, host-resistance factors, immunologic protection, and allergy protection. Other important factors include, but are not limited to, close interaction between mother and infant at the breast, the semiupright position of the infant during breast-feeding helps eliminate entry of milk into the middle ear, and sucking at the breast minimizes intake of air (Lawrence, 1995). Lactation and feeding/oral–motor specialists can work together when problems relate not only to the mother, but also to the infant's abilities to latch on to the breast and maintain coordination. Breast-feeding through the 1st year of life is associated with toddlers taking greater amounts and variety of food at age 18 months (Fisher, Birch, Smiciklas-Wright, & Picciano, 2000). One of the hypotheses is that the longer term breast-feeders have more exposure to odors and flavors in the breast milk that facilitates the transition to solid food compared with bottle-fed infants. Thus, the breast-fed group accepts solid foods more readily.

Questions related to the feasibility of breast-feeding are asked frequently. Low-birth-weight infants have demonstrated that they can learn to feed at the breast and to gain weight as readily as bottle-fed infants (Meier & Pugh, 1985; Pearce & Buchanan, 1979). Breast milk can be given to the premature infant by tube feedings while the mother pumps her breasts regularly to establish and maintain the milk supply. Nonnutritive oral–motor stimulation can be done as described above, and in addition, the infant can be given the opportunity for nonnutritive sucking at the nearly empty breast just after pumping. Nonnutritive sucking at the breast is most desirable to avoid the potential confusion with different stimuli, such as a pacifier or finger (McBride & Danner, 1987). Cup-feeding is an option with premature infants when the mother is planning to breast-feed, although her constant presence in the NICU for all feeds is nearly impossible (Lang, Lawrence, & Orme, 1994). An open cup is tilted so the milk just touches the infant's lips. The infant then "laps" the milk onto the tongue, produces suckle tongue actions, and swallows.

When the infant is ready for oral feedings, breast-feeding can be tried. As with other nipple feedings, jaw and cheek stability can be provided by the feeder as the infant is maintained in a flexed position. Infants who have an incoordinated or weak suck but are not at high risk for aspiration can suck at the breast and at the same time get additional assistance from a supplemental nursing system. As the infant sucks at the breast, an additional regulated amount of liquid flows through tubing placed next to the breast nipple but does not interfere with the nursing process. As an infant gets more milk directly from the breast, the supplemental tubing can be fazed out.

To summarize the nipple feeding process, it is desirable that all nipple feedings be completed within 30 min. The infant must take an appropriate quantity so that feeding intervals commonly are from 3 to 5 hours with a satisfied (happy) infant in the interim. Growth and development should occur appropriately and be monitored at regular intervals by primary care physicians. The feeding team may assess at intervals so that recommendations and guidelines can be modified as changes occur.

■ TRANSITIONAL FEEDING

Typical infants are ready for transition feeding by age 4 to 6 months, although these time frames may vary in different cultures. The American Academy of Pediatrics has stated that children should be at least 6 months of age before spoon-feeding is initiated. This guideline was established primarily because of digestive immaturity, not ability to eat by spoon. At 4 to 6 months, children maintain their balance while sitting in a high chair and are putting fingers and toys into their mouths. Parents begin offering a spoon and a few weeks later a cup for drinking (Chapter 2). Children with sucking and swallowing problems may be delayed in reaching these milestones, but the same order of skill acquisition is desirable for both typically developing children and for those with dysphagia. The developmental quotient or global developmental level is a useful indicator of readiness for transition feeding. The treatment suggestions given for oral structure problems are applicable in this section that examines specific skills needed and the expected ages for introduction of spoon-feeding, cup-drinking, straw-drinking, and chewing. The risk for aspiration is monitored closely throughout all phases of oral sensorimotor treatment. Again, the importance of the complex issues involved in children with feeding and swallowing problems cannot be overemphasized. The requirements are described for each task and suggested guidelines appear in Table 9–8. Special behavioral concerns are present when weaning children from tube to oral feeding (Chapter 13).

Spoon Feeding

Spoon-feeding initially is a kind of sucking of soft or pureed foods from the spoon, but it requires different skills from those used to suck liquid from the breast, bottle, or cup. Spoons should be fairly flat and made of a hard, rounded plastic (Figure 9–9A), with adaptations as children need them (Figure 9–9B). Differences are evident in the amount of cupping of the tongue, the cheek activity, and the manner of collection of food on the tongue to form a bolus. Heavier food provides increased touch and pressure cues in the mouth. Many clinicians are concerned about spoon-feeding techniques, but the bigger question about spoon-feeding relates to whether a child is ready for spoon-feeding and whether it is safe, not how many maneuvers the clinician or caregiver has to perform to get the child to accept the spoon.

Table 9–8. Developmental Age for Introduction of Transition Feeding and Necessary Skills

Function	Age of Introduction	Necessary Coordination
Spoon-feeding	4 to 6 months	Initially sucking off spoon Opening mouth in anticipation Tolerance of spoon pressed down at midtongue Closing lips around spoon Lateral tongue movements minimal Minimal loss of food around lips Jaw stability (external control as needed)
Cup-drinking	1 month after spoon	Suckling at first Cup with no spout Wide-lipped cup with narrow base Mouth closure around cup crucial Jaw closure on rim of cup lip Slightly thickened liquid at first
Straw-drinking	2–3 years, may be as early as 12–18 months	Cup-drinking is a prerequisite Lip mobility may be improved Useful when child cannot lift cup Thick-walled polyethylene tube is helpful
Chewing	6–7 months	Munching at first—vertical jaw action and limited lateral tongue movements Lateral tongue and rotary jaw action gradually developed Placement of food at sides on gums or molar tables Food that breaks down readily for bolus formation, not flaking apart Consistent texture for each bite, not mix of liquid and pieces Gradual increase in thickness and lumpiness

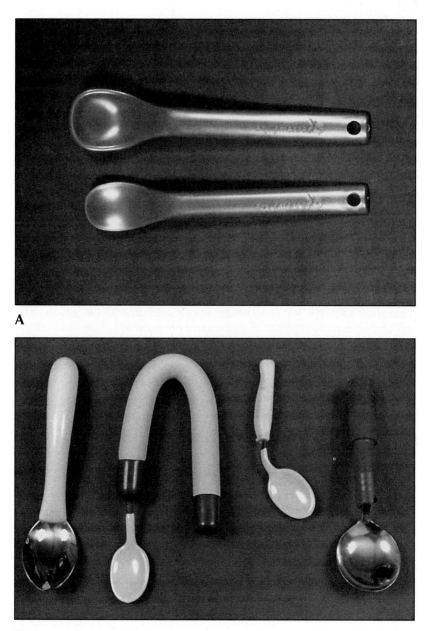

Figure 9–9. Sample of spoons useful for children. **A.** Spoons with flat bowl and smooth hard plastic coating of two sizes. **B.** Spoons with built up and curved handles are useful for children with special needs as they learn to do self- or assisted-feeding.

The immature suckling movements (to differentiate from sucking in this instance) of the tongue are expected if spoon-feeding is introduced before 4 months in normal infants. The infants appear to anticipate the spoon by these suckling tongue movements. The upper lip is moved slightly forward, but it does not yet move downward toward the bowl of the spoon. Therefore, because the infant does not use the upper lip to assist in removing food from the spoon, a typical scenario is as follows. The feeder usually scrapes the food off the palate or upper gums. The infant then pushes the food out of the mouth by the in–out tongue movements typical of suckling. The feeder tends to scrape the chin and put the food back into the mouth. This pattern is repeated until the feeder feels that enough food has been consumed for a meal. This sequence is fairly common with older handicapped children who have retained the immature suckling tongue movements and who may have a tongue-thrust pattern because of the developmental delay. In most instances, this sequence will lead to more and larger problems as time passes.

In contrast, effective spoon-feeding occurs when the infant opens the mouth far enough for the spoon to be placed easily at midtongue. Slight downward pressure will encourage lip closure around the spoon. The feeder then removes the spoon and should not need to scrape food off the palate. The food is on the tongue at a location that encourages bolus formation and a swallow with appropriate timing and coordination. There should be minimal loss of food as the infant begins to use some lateral tongue and up–down sucking movements, not the in–out primitive suckling. This is the desired pattern for all spoon-feeding and needs to be the goal for all children, including those with significant oral–motor incoordination.

Treatment also may include jaw control procedures, gradual texture and taste changes, and reduction of oral hypersensitivity. Adequate jaw control is necessary for effective spoon-feeding and especially for children with oral dysfunction. External jaw control is frequently needed to improve the ability to eat from a spoon. As oral functioning improves, the external jaw control can gradually be reduced.

Transition from smooth foods to lumpy solids is often more successful if the transition is made gradually. The child should not be confused by a taste change introduced at the same time as a texture change. It is helpful first to introduce one new taste, while keeping the texture familiar. The next single change can be made after several days to maximize the acceptance by the child. This transition can be illustrated by an example of how to shift from commercially prepared baby food to table food. A child who has been eating Stage II carrots (commercially prepared food in the United States) is more likely to accept cooked carrots put through a blender to reach the same consistency as the familiar Stage II texture. In this way, only the taste is changed. Gradually the carrots can be blended less to approximate a mashed consistency. The mashed texture can then be left with small lumps, gradually to larger lumps, and finally bite-size pieces for chewing. Sufficient time between each step allows the child to be ready for the next step. Some foods can be thickened with wheat germ, rice cereal, dehydrated potatoes, and similar foods that are not strongly flavored. In contrast, children who appear orally defensive or who have been on prolonged nonoral tube feedings may have greater success with spicier foods that they seem to prefer.

Foods with multiple consistencies in the same spoonful, such as cereal with milk or soup with pieces of vegetables, require significantly finer motor coordination than that needed for a consistent texture per spoonful. Foods with mixed textures per spoonful should be avoided until the child demonstrates good motor coordination for each desired texture individually. The mixed type of food is often difficult for children with even relatively mild incoordination of oral phase functioning and thus should not be pushed.

Children with oral hypersensitivity may resist food with small lumps more than they resist a larger piece of food of uniform consistency that can be chewed. Smaller pieces presented independently may not stimulate chewing immediately. Pieces may get scattered in the mouth, causing the child to gag or spit out the food. Caregivers may need to experiment to determine the optimal bite size for specific food items. Either too large or too small bites will make it more difficult to form a bolus. Appropriate bite sizes may differ depending on the particular food. Foods that must be chewed and are apt to cause choking (e.g., peanuts, popcorn, hotdogs, raw vegetables, and mixed textures) should be avoided in young children less than 3 to 4 years of age. By this age, children are usually consistent in their chewing with rotary jaw and lateral tongue action. They also have molars needed for grinding these types of solid food.

Children communicate their food preferences to caregivers, but these communications are not always clear. For instance, when a child spits out a bite of food, it may be related to temperature, texture, taste, or smell, but the caregiver may not be able to discern the reason immediately. It is important for caregivers to attempt to sort out the reasons for certain behaviors and responses, so the entire process of oral–motor function and feeding can proceed in a systematic way that is pleasurable to the child and appropriate for the developmental skill level.

Cup Drinking

Most children revert to a more primitive motor pattern when they are introduced to a new task. For example, in typical infants approaching 6 months of age, a gradual change has occurred from the in–out tongue action in suckling to the up–down suck movements with nipple feeding. The movements are likely to be predominantly suckling when cup-drinking is first introduced prior to 6 months of age because that is the familiar pattern for a child who has been taking liquids via nipple. With children who have oral–motor difficulties, it is important not to use a cup with a spout like those commonly available in the United States called "sippy cups." Some tend to persist with a primitive in–out tongue action of the suckling pattern, which can actually delay attainment of functional cup-drinking skills.

The feeder holds the cup in the early stages of cup drinking for all children. The choice of the first cup should be made by taking into account the child's needs for improved coordination of oral movements and the swallow (Figure 9–10). A transparent plastic cup with a wide lip is useful for many children (e.g., Solo 9-oz wide lipped cup). The narrow base permits the child to maintain good posture with head and neck in midline even when there is only a small amount of liquid in the cup. These cups can be found in the picnic section of most supermarkets in the United States. Criteria for cup selection include wide lip and narrow base permitting it to be tipped without the child's head extending back, a rolled rim that allows for a stabilized bite during drinking, and flexibility so that it will not crack if a child has a bite reflex. A transparent or clear cup is preferable when the feeder initially holds the

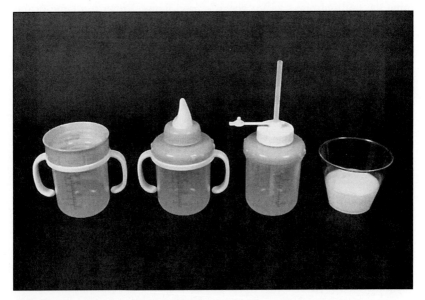

Figure 9–10. Sample of cups from left to right: the MagMag training cup system (cup with opening in the lid that allows for controlled release of liquid, cup with modified nipple that may be the first used by a child in transitioning from bottle feeding, and a straw arrangement that minimizes spills) and a Solo open cup that may be one of the most useful to cargiver and child for practice in early stages of cup drinking.

cup for the child. The feeder can see to place the lip of the cup with the child's tongue underneath. The wide lip allows the cup to be placed into the corners of the mouth. This reduces spillage and allows the feeder to see exactly how much liquid is going into the mouth. Cups with a "cut out" on one side allow for tipping the cup while the child holds the head straight and makes a space for the nose. Some children may need gradual changes (e.g., the MagMag training-cup system from modified nipple, to straw, and finally to regular cup with a recessed slot (Figure 9–10).

The feeder can assist jaw control and head positioning. It is desirable to let the cup rest on the lower lip between swallows rather than removing the cup completely after each swallow. In this way, head and jaw control may be maintained more consistently than if the cup is removed completely from the lips. Typical 6-month-old children begin to move the lower lip actively upward and outward to stabilize under a cup. The active lower lip stability aids in limiting the range of up–down and forward–backward jaw movements, as well as in–out tongue movements. The lower lip stability also provides a base, so that downward upper lip movement can be used when liquid is being drawn into the mouth from a cup (Alexander, 1987). By about 10 months, tongue protrusion with upward–forward lower lip movement under the cup rim is used for stability as jaw movement continues to range through up–down and forward–backward directions. At 12 to 15 months of age, biting on the cup with active lip closure is common as a means of attempting jaw stabilization. According to Alexander, cordinated jaw stabilization during cup-drinking may not be consistent until 24 months of age.

As a child gains coordination skills for taking liquid and swallowing without risk for aspiration, self-feeding can become a goal. Parents usually prefer a cup with a lid to reduce spillage. A cup with a recessed lid is preferable to a lid with a spout, because it allows the child to feel the cup rim on the lip. The child's jaws must remain closed while the rim of the cup is resting between his or her lips for swallowing to occur without gulping air. Straight and narrow cups may encourage undesirable neck hyperextension.

At first, slightly thickened liquid (e.g., formula with rice cereal or strained pears thinned slightly with water) may be easier as the child learns the necessary coordination for this new combination of movements. The child may accept the cup more readily if the feeder presents the spoon, then eases directly to the cup (Figure 9–11). Acid liquids may be more difficult, because they tend to increase the flow of saliva (Mueller, 1987). The ability to stabilize the jaw in both open and closed positions is a prerequisite skill in development of graded movements for control during drinking. This coordination gradually improves at 6 to 12 months of age in typical children and the equivalent developmental period in children with developmental delays. Gains are likely to be significantly slower in children with

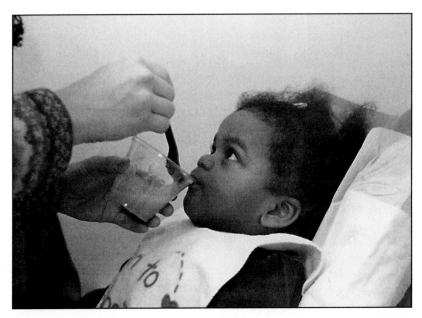

Figure 9–11. Feeder is presenting thickened liquid by spoon to prepare child for cup drinking which will follow immediately.

neurologic impairment, and external assistance for jaw control may be needed for prolonged periods of time.

Straw-Drinking

Efficient sucking through a straw usually develops later than regular cup-drinking. There is considerable variability in the age of initial exposure to straw-drinking among typical children. Children as young as 12 months may drink through a straw, but it is not uncommon for children up to the age of 3 years to lack the skills for use of a straw. At first, a child will usually draw several inches of straw into the mouth, then curl the tongue around it and use a sucking motion to draw the liquid up through the straw. With practice, a small portion of straw is placed between the lips such that the lips and cheeks play a larger role in creating the negative pressure necessary to draw the liquid through the straw.

As with most normal children, children with cerebral palsy or other neuromuscular problems should have coordinated cup-drinking skills before attempting a straw. Straw- or tube-drinking may help some children improve lip mobility. Straw-drinking may also be helpful for children whose lip mobility is adequate but athetoid or ataxic movement problems prevent lifting a cup. Mueller (1987) suggested that a thick-walled polyethylene or polyester tube with a small inner diameter be used so that one suck admits a limited amount of liquid and minimal air. The tube is held and sucked by the lips while the jaws remain closed. The tube can be inserted and held in place if a cup with a lid and spout is used. The child can put both hands on the table around the cup. This will help to stabilize the child further while sucking in the liquid through the tube. Several other techniques available for teaching straw drinking are described by Morris and Klein (1987, 2000).

Chewing

Normal infants begin to munch by 6 to 7 months of age. Oral control should have developed so that gagging is not a problem. Chewing skills may be encouraged by placement of chewable food between the gums or teeth (if present) at the side of the mouth. Choices of food become important at this stage, because it is vital that the entire experience be pleasant. Therefore, the risk for gagging or choking must be kept to a minimum. Gum chewing is never encouraged with young children because of the risks for choking by accidental swallowing.

Foods that readily break down for bolus formation and do not require extensive chewing should be tried first. For example, one small piece of graham cracker or sugar cookie, in a strip shape that is approximately the length of a thumb nail, can be placed on one side of the mouth on the molars or the gums. Foods that flake apart should be avoided (e.g., saltine crackers, pretzels, and some kinds of cereal). Bread may be difficult at first because it becomes "gummy" once saliva is mixed with it. The feeder may be able to estimate potential usefulness of a food item by taking a bite size amount into the mouth and noting carefully how that texture breaks down when he or she munches in a vertical way two times. Food items with an outer shell, such as peas or corn, are usually more difficult and should be avoided in the early stages of chewing practice. Mixed textures also should be avoided until skills are refined. The general guideline is to increase texture in small steps, going from a thin, smooth texture to a gradual change in thickness and graininess, but not to a mixture of particles in a smooth base. The change from pureed to ground texture then requires increased lateral tongue action and rotary jaw movement. Morris and Klein (1987) stated that all children should experience the textural variations of ground foods before solids (which require chewing) are added to the diet.

There are differences of opinion regarding the expected age for well-coordinated rotary chewing in normal children, ranging from 24 to 36 months. The development of rotary chewing requires tongue lateralization that, in turn, requires jaw stability. This sequence of development reinforces the need to accomplish the underlying skills ncessary as a basis for introducing more difficult tasks. Chewing practice without having the child swallow food can be conducted by wrapping some food in a piece of gauze and tying it with a string. This "food ball" can then be moved between the teeth to stimulate chewing (Morris & Klein, 1987, 2000). Some children may respond to the use of long, thick licorice sticks (or "Twizzlers") moved from one side of the mouth to the other with the tongue. These are stiff enough that it is unlikely a child will bite through the sticks. The adult should watch closely, however, because as the licorice softens, a portion should be cut off to keep the practice safe. To encourage tongue lateralization, the food placement can be alternated from one side of the mouth to the other.

Gradually as chewing improves, food with a long, thin shape can allow the child to continue a biting and chewing pattern while the strip of food is moved slowly between the teeth. Some food items that can be cut or broken into strips include graham crackers, cheese, French fries, bread sticks, and partially cooked carrots or potatoes. As skills increase for tongue lateralization and intermittent rhythmic chewing, other foods can be added. Foods that do not dissolve provide a challenge.

Once the ability to move food from side to center or from center to side has been mastered, a child at 18 to 24 months developmental age is ready to work on cross-midline transfer of food (Morris & Klein, 1987). Children often respond to turn-taking activities, and at this developmental stage, they can understand that each side of the mouth also "wants" to take turns.

Although some treatment options are listed in Table 9–8, evidence-based data are needed through clinical trials to establish the efficacy for any specific form of treatment in children. Specific concerns in the pediatric population may complicate the treatment of impaired swallowing. Two major problems involving cognition and posture have been delineated by Tuchman (1988). First, the limited cognitive skills of children with mental retardation prevent therapeutic instruction-following. Second, children with neuromuscular disorders or cerebral palsy may exhibit poor control of the head and neck, that, in turn, interferes with the ability to position the oropharynx properly during swallowing. Abnormal motor and reflex functions may also affect all phases of swallowing (Jones, 1989).

■ GASTROESOPHAGEAL REFLUX DISEASE (GERD)

GERD is often seen in infants and children with oral sensorimotor and feeding problems. Detailed discussion regarding etiology, assessment, and management is found in Chapter 5. Effective management of GERD is primarily by medical and surgical methods. Conservative approaches include thickening formula for infants, elevating the head of the bed, and changing diet to reduce caffeine and other highly spiced foods in older children. Thickening of formula and head-elevated prone positioning are often recommended with GERD (Meyers & Herbst, 1982; Orenstein & Whitington, 1983). The head-elevated prone positioning has come into question, however (Orenstein, 1990).

It is important to differentiate GERD from emesis and gagging that can be produced for other reasons. Some infants (and older children) produce a gag reflex and induce emesis because of oral hypersensitivity or response to aromas, tastes, and textures. These children can be managed with techniques that help to reduce oral hypersensitivity. The oral sensorimotor swallow specialist needs to be alert to the possibility of gastroesophageal problems or some other medically based diagnosis that may include or be masked by oral–motor and swallowing incoordination. Appropriate diagnosis is a critical basis for optimal management.

■ TREATMENT OF CHILDREN WITH SPECIFIC DIAGNOSES

The following section presents specific diagnostic groups of children who commonly present with dysphagia. The previous treatment suggestions are applicable to most of these groups. Unique aspects for treatment in each group are highlighted.

Cerebral Palsy (CP)

Children with CP are heterogeneous, and they make up the largest single "group" with neurogenic dysphagia. In general, children who have quadriplegia and are dependent on others to feed them have the most severe dysphagia. They show three major abnormalities of swallowing: poor lingual function, delayed swallow production, and reduced pharyngeal motility (Jones, 1989). These three characteristics result in pharyngeal phase timing and coordination dysfunction. Patterns of oral sensorimotor dysfunction include tongue thrust, prolonged and exaggerated bite reflex, abnormally strong gag reflex, tactile hypersensitivity in the oral area, and drooling (Casas, McPherson, & Kenny, 1995; Mueller, 1987). These problems do not occur in isolation to the oral and pharyngeal mechanism but are often associated with problems of trunk, shoulder, and head control. The safety of oral feeding is dependent on proper postioning of the head, neck, and trunk (Larnett & Ekberg, 1995). In addition, some children with CP are on anticonvulsant medication. Some have frequent coughing with meals, aspiration marked by choking, and a history of pneumonia (Waterman, Koltai, Downey, & Cacace, 1992).

Drooling is a problem in many children with CP. In-depth discussion can be found in Chapter 11. For oral sensorimotor therapy to have a positive effect, most children need to have a cognitive level high enough so they can follow 1 to 2 step simple requests (Table 9–9). After approximately 6 months of intensive therapy, reevaluation is needed to determine other options for intervention (Chapter 11).

All of the above-mentioned abnormalities are considered when making management decisions. Attention must be paid to (a) poor bolus formation, with food getting into the pharynx while the airway is still open, leading to aspiration and gagging before a swallow is produced; (b) slow oral transit time resulting in extended feeding times and poor nutrition, and (c) slow pharyngeal transit time resulting in residue in the pharynx after a swallow, with possible aspiration through the open larynx. The incidence of silent aspiration is high in these children (Arvedson, Rogers, Buck, Smart, & Msall, 1994). The aspiration of specific food textures appears more common than aspiration on all textures (Rogers, Arvedson, Buck, Smart, & Msall, 1994). Children who aspirate are found to have poorer oral–motor skills in spoon-feeding, biting, chewing, and swallowing than those who do not aspirate (Gisel, Applegate-Ferrante, Benson, & Bosma, 1996). Improvement in oral–motor skills should help these children take food more competently with less spillage, but the weight in the children

Table 9–9. Conservative Intervention for Children With Drooling

Goal	Recommendations
Improve sensory awareness	Experience contrast: (vary texture and temperature of food and objects in or near the mouth)
	Help child know when chin is wet or dry
Improve jaw, lip, and cheek control	See recommendations in Table 9–5
	Chin strap may assist jaw closure during meals for children with hypotonia; caution: strap should not force jaw closed
	Lip closure activities
	Straw drinking may increase lip and cheek activity
Keep face dry	Wiping reminders
	Wrist bands may aid spontaneity for wiping
	"Secret signals" between child and caregiver may offer reminder without others knowing

studied by Gisel and colleagues remained at the lowest level of age norms. Gisel (1994) found that children with CP and moderately impaired feeding skills need to combine oral–motor therapy with calorie supplementation as they reach adolescence. Clinicians working with these children for oral sensorimotor intervention must be vigilant about potential chronic health problems, such as chronic lung disease. Children's airway status and nutritional well-being must never be jeopardized by interventions to improve oral skills.

The interaction of oral skills and body posture seems logical. Postural adjustments have been discussed in relation to facilitation of oral feeding. Likewise, oral postures have an effect on overall body posture. For example, the open mouth posture with drooling and tongue thrust is common in children with CP, is often interpreted as facial distortion, and is difficult to change with tranditonal oral–motor therapy. An intraoral applicance (ISMAR) therapy for 1 year has shown significant improvement in jaw stability in some children that results in better lip closure, facilitating chewing and oral manipulation of food (Gisel, Schwartz, & Haberfellner, 1999; Gisel, Schwartz, Petryk, Clarke, & Haberfellner, 2000). This type therapy also results in significant improvement in functional feeding skills in children with moderate dysphagia (Haberfellner, Schwartz, & Gisel, 2001).

Children with CP or other neuromuscular difficulties often appear unable to chew. These children make tongue thrusting motions that push the food back out of the mouth. Sometimes they hold the tongue tightly to the hard palate, resulting in food getting squashed but not chewed. Thus, when the food gets to the back of the oral cavity, it has not been formed into an effective bolus for swallowing. Gagging and choking result. When the oral phase is characterized by incoordination and delay, the child's potential for aspiration and choking is greater with thin liquids than with thickened liquids and thick semisolid foods. The thicker textures provide greater sensory information and do not tend to fall back in the oral cavity as quickly as thinner textures. Alexander (1987) suggested that many children get more active tongue and jaw movements when soft solids, such as graham crackers, are presented on the side gums or teeth. As some solid foods that mix with saliva remain in a more solid state for a longer time, the child with significant hypotonicity of the oral area may get increased lateralization of tongue, more cheek activity, and up–down jaw movements. The early introduction of solid foods aids in reducing the strength of the gag response; it also helps in the development of more active tongue, jaw, and cheek–lip movements in chewing and biting (Alexander, 1987).

In contrast to oral phase incoordination, children with reduced pharyngeal motility and persistent residue after a swallow are most likely to aspirate on paste-consistency foods, because these firmer, sticky foods are harder to clear from the pharynx with subsequent swallows. Children also may experience considerable irritation and discomfort, which can lead to food refusal and behavioral problems related to feeding. Food texture modifications often help.

Efficacy studies of oral sensorimotor, swallowing and feeding treatment programs for children with CP are limited. Weight gain lacks sufficient sensitivity as a measure of functional improvement in feeding patterns (Ottenbacher, Hicks, Roark, & Swinea, 1983; Ottenbacher et al., 1981). The relationship of increased weight gain to improved health needs to be established in severely handicapped nonambulatory persons.

Neurophysiologic facilitation of orofacial muscles by stretching, brushing, vibrating, icing, and stroking areas of the face and mouth is reported effective in some children with CP (Sobsey & Orelove, 1984; Gallender, 1979, 1980; Farber & Huss, 1974). However, regression occurred when facilitation was withdrawn. If there is no long term carryover beyond a treatment period, clinicians need to make critical reviews about the use in their programs.

The importance of individualized treatment programs that employ both clinical and videofluoroscopic assessments has been stressed because of the high incidence of silent aspiration with no cough or other visible signs to the feeder (e.g. Griggs, Jones, & Lee, 1989; Helfrich–Miller, Rector, & Straka, 1986). Questions are raised frequently about these children who demonstrate aspiration on VFSS and do not contract severe aspiration pneumonia. Helfrich-Miller and colleagues suggested that the relative young age of their group, resiliency of respiratory membranes and lungs in young persons, and aggressive use of antibiotics must have been factors in their survival. Fatal upper respiratory infections have been reported in many of these persons as they age (Carter & Jancar, 1983). Thus, it is important to prevent respiratory complications to attain positive outcomes. Instrumental examinations may be needed at times to delineate pharyngeal phase status. Clinicians and families may need to make changes in textures, timing, and in determining whether oral feeding can be continued safely for persons with multiple handicaps whose status may change over time.

Children who live in residential settings usually have multiple caregivers, which may complicate the feeding program (Korabek, Reid, & Ivancic, 1981). Increased intake at the expense of prolonged mealtimes (1 hour) is not feasible for the caregiver, or for the safety of the child, because fatigue and thus the risk for aspiration increases with the length of feeding time. For children who consistently require lengthy mealtimes, nonoral supplemental feedings may need to be considered. Future research should be directed toward the need for effective yet practical staff management procedures, acceptability of such procedures, and efficiency for the children as they strive for participation in social and communicative activities.

Children with Multiple Handicaps: Food Refusal and Selectivity

Dietary inadequacies are common among handicapped children and may occur in as much as one-third of that population (Palmer & Horn, 1978). Artificial feeding methods may be used in crisis situations but are undesirable as long-term solutions because the methods do not actively promote effective feeding behavior and may actually be associated with additional health risks (Raventos, Kralemann, & Gray, 1982). Behavioral mismanagement is found to be the primary factor associated with more than 21% of all feeding problems in handicapped children referred to their nutrition clinic over a 4-year period (Palmer & Horn).

Eating behavior has been examined in children with multiple handicaps who showed either low overall or highly selective oral food intake (Riordan et al., 1980; Riordan, Iwata, Finney, Wohl, & Stanley, 1980). Use of preferred foods as a reward for a bite of nonpreferred food was found to have potential, but the authors concluded that it is not possible to generalize behavioral guidelines for food refusal and selectivity.

Head Trauma

Head trauma in children has multiple causes: trauma during delivery, nonaccidental trauma due to abuse or neglect (e.g., shaken baby syndrome), traumatic brain injury from falls or other accidents (e.g., bicycle, motor vehicle), penetrating wounds (e.g., drive-by shootings), and brain tumors.

Shaken Baby Syndrome (SBS)

Infants who are victims of SBS demonstrate diffuse brain damage with signs of acceleration–deceleration trauma, usually with no external signs of head trauma. There are an estimated 1,000 to 1,500 cases each year in the United States. More than half the cases are under 1 year of age, and perhaps 80% are under 2 years of age; none are over 4 years (Alexander, Sato, Smith, & Bennett, 1990). Abusive head trauma is responsible for a portion of CP and other developmental problems. The reported incident is not usually the first. A high index of suspicion is important. For example, a new onset of seizures in a young, healthy infant should suggest a diagnosis of abuse.

In the acute phase, nutrition needs are likely met via nonoral routes. With severe brain damage, a GT is often necessary. Once the acute phase is past, oral–motor stimulation can facilitate oral intake as tolerated on the basis of clinic and instrumental examinations. Feeding and swallowing deficits relate closely to alertness, sensory, and motor function (Alexander

& Smith, 1998). The long-term outcome relates closely to the underlying neurologic status. Prevention programs warning of the dangers of shaking children are in place in all states of the United States. The goal for all children is prevention of such injuries.

Traumatic Brain Injury in Older Children

Older children with head injuries appear to have similar physiologic disorders of feeding and swallowing as adults with head injury (Ylvisaker and Weinstein, 1989). The research literature does not include reports specific to pediatric outcomes, however. The most common problems include reduced tongue control and bolus manipulation in the oral cavity, delayed production of the pharyngeal swallow, and inefficient transport of food through the mouth and pharynx. Gastroesophageal reflux also is relatively common and may become evident following placement of a gastrostomy tube in a child with a head injury or any other kind of neurologic impairment.

Management decisions are based on accurate determination of cognitive levels of functioning. The ability or lack of ability to follow commands and to learn new procedures will directly impact intervention procedures. Although many children with head injuries recover enough sensory and motor function for safe oral feeding, they remain at risk because of behavioral problems that necessitate one-to-one monitoring of eating (Ylvisaker, Feeney, & Feeney, 1999). Food refusal may be a function of confusion and agitation, discomfort, conditioned responses to feeding, or the absence of sensations of hunger and thirst. Conditioned dysphagia may be a reasonable hypothesis if other explanations for resistance to oral feeding have been ruled out through a careful differential diagnostic process (Ylvisaker, 1998).

Emphasis in treatment is focused on changes in positioning, method of food presentation, and food textures. Treatment usually proceeds in a systematic way from tube feeding to oral feeding. Initial treatment is likely to be integrated into a sensorimotor or coma-stimulation program carried out in an interdisciplinary framework. Interventions may include improving awareness and alertness; normalizing muscle tone, head and trunk control, and movement patterns; and increasing appropriate responses to sensory stimulation.

Overall, a cautious approach is urged in the early stages of recovery from head injury. Children should perceive a pleasurable feeding and eating experience to whatever degree possible. As with all persons, regardless of underlying diagnosis, oral–motor and feeding practices should not be forced.

Thickened liquids may be helpful as the child works toward improved coordination of oral sensorimotor functioning. Improved oral sensorimotor patterns must occur as a necessary general underlying skill for oral feeding. As oral intake increases, careful monitoring of nutritional status is done so a formula for reducing tube feedings relative to the oral intake can be determined. Parents are included in the oral–motor and feeding stimulation program. Techniques vary according to the specific combination of symptoms and are similar to those used with other children who have neurologic impairments. As with all aspects of rehabilitation of children, family involvement is an integral aspect of recovery.

Brain Tumors in Children

In the United States, approximately 1,400 infants and children are diagnosed with brain tumors each year, with the poorest survival in children diagnosed at less than 24 months of age (Duffner et al., 1993). Diagnoses are often late because the signs and symptoms of irritability, projectile vomiting, and somnolence are initially seen as related to possible gastrointestinal tract problems. In some instances, a rapidly enlarging head circumference is noted by parents, which leads to neuroimaging and diagnosis. Posterior fossa tumors are common in young children (Freeman et al., 1996). The increased intracranial pressure produces headache, nausea, and vomiting. Feeding and swallowing issues usually relate to changes in appetite in relation to treatments. Nausea and emesis have negative impact on appetite. With cranial nerve involvement, children experience oral sensorimotor deficits and pharyngeal phase deficits that place them at risk for aspiration. As in other diagnoses related to head injury, the prognosis relates closely to underlying neurologic status. Intervention related to swallowing is likely to be intermittent with information and guidelines to parents as they adapt to the child's changing neurologic status.

Tracheotomy

Children with tracheotomy vary significantly in the frequency and degree of feeding difficulty. The differences relate most closely to the underlying cause(s) for the tracheotomy (Singer, Wood, & Lambert, 1985) (Chapter 4) and in some instances to the levels of oral–motor functioning prior to the tracheotomy (Simon & McGowan, 1989). It is therefore difficult to make general management suggestions.

Long-term tracheotomy is shown to affect swallowing and speech in infants (Rosingh & Peek, 1999) and toddlers' swallowing physiology (Abraham & Wolf, 2000). Parents of the four toddlers studied by Abraham & Wolf did not report swallowing difficulties at home, but clinical examination and videofluoroscopic swallow studies revealed pharyngeal phase dysfunction marked by pharyngeal penetration (76%) and aspiration in one swallow.

Children with tracheotomies are also susceptible to behavioral feeding difficulties. Refusal of food may occur with forced feedings, because caregivers try to meet the caloric needs orally to avoid tube feedings. Children who experience long-term hospitalizations frequently demonstrate negative behaviors because of multiple caregivers, time constraints for feeding, and a distracting environment.

Oral–motor stimulation done in a pleasurable way can be initiated as soon as physicians give clearance, which may be after the first tracheotomy tube change (Arvedson & Brodsky, 1992). Children with documented aspiration may benefit from a nonnutritive focus. Other children can be managed with careful considerations for possible variations in seating and head position, texture changes, and timing of food presentations. Communication skills must also be maximized in this group of patients.

Undernutrition

Undernutrition (failure to thrive) usually describes an individual whose weight is consistently below the 3rd percentile for age or is less than 80% of ideal weight for age (see Chapter 5 and 6 for detailed discussion). It is estimated that 3 to 5% of admissions to pediatric academic hospitals are made for children with poor weight gain or other nutrition-related feeding difficulties (Herman, 1991). Fewer than 25% of the hospital referrals have an identifiable organic etiology, such as endocrine deficiencies, chronic disease, enzymatic defects, or congenital or genetic anomalies (Berwick, Levy, & Kleinerman, 1982). Given that the first 2 years of life are crucial for brain growth, infants with undernutrition in this time period are at high risk for lasting deficits in growth, cognition, language, and socioemotional functioning.

Children with oral sensorimotor dysfunction are at risk for receiving inadequate nutrition for numerous reasons (Herman, 1991). These children are often difficult to feed. One must consider that oral–motor dysfunction may be at least one factor in combination with other problems (Mathisen, Skuse, Wolke, & Reilly, 1989), such as poor mother–infant interactions, the infant's behavioral state, psychosocial issues, environmental deprivation, child abuse, nutritional neglect, and poor feeding practices. Heptinsall, Puckering, Skuse, Dowdney, & Zur-Szpira (1987) found that in socioeconomically disadvantaged inner-city families, nearly 50% of neurologically normal 4-year-olds with chronic growth retardation had some form of oral–motor dysfunction. Specific treatment guidelines are developed on the basis of the degree and nature of oral–motor function with close attention to the multiple interacting factors that underlie undernutrition. The importance of an interdisciplinary team approach to evaluation and treatment processes and, in turn, improved outcomes is stressed by Accardo (1982).

Acquired Immune Deficiency Syndrome (AIDS)

Dysphagia has been found to be a prominent problem in children with AIDS, with estimates from about 20 to 45% (Pressman, 1992; Pressman &

Morrison, 1988). Seventy-six percent showed some improvement with treatment (Pressman & Morrison, 1988). Identification and treatment by an interdisciplinary team can make a significant contribution to the quality of life and total health care. Nutritional management of this group of children is a high priority because malnutrition predisposes them to further infection and malabsorption (Bentler & Stanish, 1987).

Presenting problems include poor weight gain, refusal to feed, inability to tolerate specific consistencies, and choking when feeding. Oral preparatory, oral, and pharyngeal phase problems are common. Recommendations relate to changes in position, nipples or utensils, textures of food, and strategies to introduce new foods.

A major goal for children demonstrating an aversion to eating is desensitization. The children are encouraged to eat food they like and to eat with other family members. Clinicians need to be aware of the possibility of oral candidiasis that is a common problem and is treated with local oral hygiene and topical antifungal agents. Candida esophagitis is another possibility that may require more aggressive medical therapy extending over the course of several weeks (Pressman & Morrison, 1988). Children who experience odynophagia in conjunction with oral or esophageal candidiasis have been found to do well with cold liquids, pureed foods, and puddings. Avoidance of juice and food with citric acid is helpful (Pressman, 1992).

Children who lose feeding skills because of progressive encephalopathy need to have texture modification in their diets (e.g., soft foods, pureeds, and thickened liquids). Clinical monitoring and videofluoroscopic swallow studies can assist in determination of best textures for optimizing safety. Positioning and utensil changes may help to maximize intake. Increased caloric intake can be achieved through high-concentration liquid or pudding supplements.

In this population, the symptoms vary over the course of time, and thus the treatment of feeding varies accordingly. Complications of respiratory status, fever, abdominal pain, infections, and fatigue all have direct effect on the feeding program.

Fetal Alcohol Syndrome (FAS)

Children exposed to alcohol in utero have multiple craniofacial anomalies that include a thin upper lip, short palpebral fissures and smooth philtrum. Other characteristic findings include growth retardation, CNS neurodevelopmental deficits, congenital heart defects, hearing loss, and cleft palate (Smith, 1979, 1980; Thackray & Tifft, 2001). Neurologic findings include microcephaly, mental retardation, and abnormal behaviors.

Significant feeding problems are common in some of these children (Van Dyke, Mackay, & Ziaylek, 1982). Alcohol exposure can continue postnatally if the infant is breast feeding. Problems of breast- and bottle-fed infants include limited sucking patterns, easy fatigue, irritability, and distractibility. Some children may need nonoral feeding supplements even extending beyond 12 months of age.

Normalization of oral sensitivity and tolerance for nipples with nonnutritive stimulation are initial goals when nonoral feedings are the major source for meeting nutritional needs. Given the limited sucking patterns, appropriate nipples that allow for easy flow, but not so fast as to result in choking, must be used. Frequent small feedings may be necessary because of the tendency for fatigue. In the presence of a cleft palate, adaptations appropriate for feeding infants with clefts may be needed (Chapter 12).

Rett Syndrome

Rett syndrome is included as an example of a progressive neurologic disorder in which feeding skills regress and management guidelines must be adjusted accordingly. Rett syndrome affects primarily female infants who are apparently normal until 6 to 12 months of age, and then lose both motor and cognitive skills (Budden, Meek, & Henighan, 1990). They develop inappropriate social interactions, decelerated head growth in some, and severe language deficits. Abnormal chewing associated with tongue thrusting and involuntary, undulating tongue movements have been described (Budden, 1986). Prominent symptoms include difficulty in chewing and swallowing, choking, and emesis. Respiratory patterns are immature in all stages of Rett syndrome. The severe hypertonicity in the later stages of the disease signal a regression to total abdominal respiration, with restricted movement and limited expansion of the thoracic rib cage. At this stage, pureed or soft foods become the major texture in the diet because of difficulties in chewing and tongue manipulation for solid foods (Budden et al.).

Pervasive Developmental Disorder (e.g., Autism or Psychosis)

These children do not usually show swallowing problems, but may have significant feeding problems. The common types of eating abnormalities include (a) automatic, mechanical eating; (b) shoveling food, gulping, stuffing; (c) not chewing; (d) avoiding touching food with the lips, not looking at food; (e) spitting or regurgitating; (f) throwing food; (g) scavenging, grabbing food from other people's plates; (h) excessive fads or refusals; (i) patterning of food; and (j) holding food in the mouth for long periods (Stroh, Robinson, & Stroh, 1986).

The child's communicative signals need to be well understood because such awareness may be an aid to clinicians and caregivers to develop more effective intervention. These children may work through the feeding difficulties in conjunction with their global program. Home carryover with the family or institutional caregivers is critical because that is where the child's functional social and cultural events take place.

■ REGRESSION WITH FEEDING

Over time, regression can occur with a number of progressive neuromuscular conditions, brain tumors, acquired neurologic disorders, and in some static conditions, such as CP. Children receiving oral feeds show symptoms of increased respiratory distress, aspiration, incoordination, lengthy feeding times, weight loss or lack of weight gain, and decreased alertness, so a recommendation may be necessary to reduce or discontinue oral feeding. A gastrostomy may be needed for some children who have been oral feeders for several years. Frequently these children have severe motor disabilities as part of their cerebral palsy and severe-to-profound mental retardation. Parents may find this recommendation difficult to accept, but when information is provided that stresses the importance of adequate respiratory and nutritional status, the parents and other caregivers usually come to realize that the child's safety is most important. Parents need to realize that oral sensorimotor stimulation will continue to be a part of the total program. Small amounts of oral feeding may be continued for practice, pleasure, and to experience taste and texture. Keeping the oral sensorimotor mechanism as coordinated as possible may reduce the risk for aspiration of secretions.

■ NONORAL FEEDERS AT RISK FOR ASPIRATION ON SECRETIONS

Children who get no food or liquid orally continue to have risk for aspiration on their own saliva because they typically do not swallow frequently. These children need some type of oral stimulation to encourage production of purposeful swallows, unless such stimulation actually results in increased salivation, which could then increase aspiration risks. Tastes in some minuscule way may help to keep the child swallowing. For example, a drop of cold cranberry juice on the tongue is less liquid than in saliva, but it may provide sensory cues that in turn would be the impetus for the child to produce a swallow. In general, it is desirable to have short (a few minutes) and frequent practice sessions. The potential for carryover is greater than with one session per day. A person may tolerate 5 to 10 min of stimulation four to six times each day much better than 60 to 90 min one time each day. In many instances, the most effective practice sessions are those carried out just before and during the first part of the nonoral feeding session, which can also be part of the family's social mealtime. All oral sensorimotor treatment programs for children with swallowing problems must be carried out with close communication between the oral sensorimotor specialist and physicians overseeing the child's health status. The day-to-day management may be primarily under the responsibility of parents and other caregivers, but the periodic monitoring by highly trained professionals is crucial with these high-risk children.

■ CASE STUDIES

Case Study 1

"Rosa" presented to feeding clinic at age 9 months with parental concern that "she is not feeding by mouth, has been on GT feeds since she was 2 weeks old, but everything else is fine." History revealed meconium aspiration immediately after a vaginal delivery. Apgars were 8 at 1 min and 8 at 5 min. Apnea and bradycardia were associated with all feeding attempts. She was put on orogastric tube feedings. Magnetic resonance imaging (MRI) was interpreted as normal. She had evidence for patent ductus arteriosus and patent foramen ovale, but the murmur was no longer evident at 12 days of life. Chromosome analysis revealed normal female karyotype. Neurologic examination was most notable for poor suck and poor airway protection. Videofluoroscopic swallow study (VFSS) revealed multiple episodes of silent aspiration. She underwent a gastrostomy procedure at 2 weeks of age, without a fundoplication because parents decided they wanted to delay that procedure. She was placed on metoclopramide. After a few weeks, her mother stopped the medication because Rosa seemed sleepy most of the time. She was given some bottle feedings, but nutrition needs were met via GT.

Follow-up VFSS at 4 months of age was essentially unchanged, and Rosa was kept NPO ("Nothing per oral"). She came to the children's hospital from out-of-state because parents were seeking answers to their questions about why she was having this swallowing problem. A detailed history revealed halitosis, intermittent spitting up, excessive drooling, hoarse voice, reduced frequency of swallowing, and recurrent hiccups. Flexible fiberoptic nasopharyngolaryngoscopy revealed a larynx that was classic for extraesophageal reflux: severe vocal fold edema, hypopharyngeal cobblestoning, posterior glottic swelling, and loss of arytenoid architecture. Findings of that nature are indicative of severe gastroesophgeal reflux. She was seen to aspirate on her saliva.

Gastroenterology consult resulted in an upper gastrointestinal (UGI) study with small bowel follow through and 24-hour dual-channel pH monitor. She had one brief episode of GER on UGI and normal anatomy, consistent with prior studies. She was found to have severe GER with 139 acid refluxes in the distal probe and 18 acid refluxes to the proximal probe. Neurodevelopmental examination revealed no focal neurologic deficits. Developmental delays in gross and fine motor skills and communication skills were noted at about 50% of expected level. Cognitive skills appeared several months delayed.

Rosa's mother administered a GT feed at the feeding clinic in her usual routine (Figure 9–12). The 8-oz (240 ml) formula was given by gravity in less than 5 min. This prompted a discussion about timing for GT feeds, with the recommendation that the feeding should take about 20 to 30 min. Repeat VFSS revealed multiple aspiration events during and after consecutive swal-

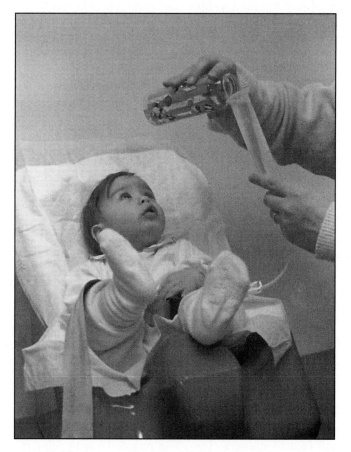

Figure 9–12. Child is in a seated position as she watches her mother put formula into the gastrostomy tube right after her oral sensorimotor practice with tastes.

lows via nipple due to pharyngeal incoordination and reduced motility, which in turn resulted in nasopharyngeal reflux. She was eager to take tastes.

Interdisciplinary consultation resulted in several recommendations: (a) Begin medical therapy for the underlying medical condition—start reflux medications. (b) Refer to early intervention program for physical and occupational therapy, as well as oral sensorimotor stimulation with tastes. Demonstration was given to parent for ways to present minuscule tastes (e.g., spoon dipped into juice with minimal amount that would cling to the spoon, not even a true drop). Rosa was eager to take the spoon, used her hands to help bring it to her mouth, closed her lips around it immediately, made suckle movements with her tongue, and appeared to produce swallows without obvious delay (Figure 9–7B). (c) Alter regimen of GT feeding.

Telephone call from parent a week after she returned home: She was so pleased to find her child without bad breath! She was following through to slow down the GT feeds. Rosa had decreased the emesis frequency and amount. She was eager for the oral stimulation and tastes. She will return in 6 months to monitor progress and make further recommendations.

Comment

This is an excellent example of how what appears to be a focal problem of pharyngeal phase swallowing in the neonatal period has implications for broader developmental problems over time. The importance of diagnosis and management of GERD/EERD cannot be overstated. The ramifications with lack of treatment for GERD/EERD are significant and have effects on aspiration risks, airway status, appetite, and overall development. Pleasurable oral stimulation with tastes is needed to whatever degree is considered safe. Children are at risk for aspirating on their own secretions, and they may not swallow as frequently when they are strictly NPO. Risks need to be weighed in relation to quality of life and overall function.

Case Study 2

"Carrie" was an alert, active child until she suffered a skull fracture with a left parietal contusion at age 13 months. A ventriculo-peritoneal shunt for hydrocephalus was placed 2 weeks later. As she gradually became alert by 6 weeks postonset, she was noted to have a breathy and somewhat "gurgly" voice quality. Flexible fiberoptic laryngeal examination revealed a mild erythema, but no pooling of secretions and no vocal fold paralysis.

She was assessed a few days later by the oral–motor and feeding specialist with videofluoroscopic swallow study (VFSS) recommended before major oral feeding attempts. The VFSS revealed a mild delay in the oral phase, no major pharyngeal dysmotility, and no aspiration. Recommendations were to begin liquid and soft food. She was not able to take sufficient amounts to maintain an adequate nutritional status, so a GT was placed at 12 weeks after her initial injury. She was discharged to the custody of her grandmother after a 4-month hospital stay. She was fed orally as tolerated for approximately 20 min at each feeding time, and supplemented via GT to meet nutritional needs.

Carrie was followed by the interdisciplinary feeding team at periodic intervals, and she was also in an early intervention program where she received physical, occupational, and speech–language therapy. Oral sensorimotor practice, which included strained food by spoon, was a part of the therapy program. Carrie was positioned in a Tumbleforms seat for the oral–motor and feeding practice.

Although Carrie had always shown a mild degree of irritability, this increased approximately 2 months after discharge. At that same time increased drooling, a tonic bite reflex, and very limited tongue action appeared. Excessively increased weight gain, which is not unusual with GT feedings, was also noted. The amount of Pediasure was adjusted by the dietitian. The feeding team raised the question of possible shunt malfunction as the regression in oral–motor function and increase in irritability were evident. Indeed, that was the situation. A shunt revision was accomplished immediately.

Oral sensorimotor stimulation continued, primarily nonnutritive, but with some limited taste and texture experiences incorporated with pureed textures via spoon. In this time period, she had frequent illnesses, usually upper respiratory infections, which interfered with the oral sensorimotor gains because it was more difficult for family to keep the regular practice routine when Carrie did not feel well. Practice continued regularly when Carrie's health was stable. The feeding team continued to monitor with the program and the family. Although gains seemed inconsistent, overall gradually it was felt that Carrie was ready for more oral feeding. When changes in management could be considered with possible increase in amounts of food and liquid, a repeat VFSS was recommended.

A swallow study was repeated at age 37 months. At that time, Carrie showed primarily an oral phase delay with only mild dysmotility in the pharyngeal phase of the swallow. She appeared safe for small amounts of food via spoon for oral–motor practice. As Carrie continued to make gains in the amount of food and liquid being taken orally, the GT feedings were adjusted accordingly by the dietitian and nurse.

Comment

This child exemplifies the complexities of some children with neurologic impairments when the total needs become almost overwhelming to caregivers because of multiple concerns. It is important for professionals to be aware that relatively sudden regression in oral–motor and feeding skills, other motor skills, and communication levels may be related to shunt malfunction. Thus, appropriate medical and surgical assessment and follow-up are needed. Regular and on-going communication among professionals can help in the provision of coordinated services to meet the changing circumstances of the child.

Case Study 3

"Annie" was delivered at 29 weeks gestation, with birth weight at 1,329 g. Apgars were 7 at 1 min and 9 at 5 min. Diagnoses included prematurity, laryngomalacia, right grade I intraventricular hemorrhage, bronchopulmonary dysplasia (BPD), GER, and hyperbilirubenimia. She was on mechanical ventilation for 19 days and nasal continuous positive airway pressure (CPAP) for 5 days, followed by supplemental oxygen via nasal cannula. She underwent 2 days of phototherapy for the hyperbilirubinemia. The Grade I IVH had resolved on the basis of ultrasound at 6 weeks of life. Hearing screening was passed.

By 33 to 34 weeks gestation, she had been given trial nipple feeds but demonstrated respiratory stress. She was examined at the bedside on day 28 of life. Oral peripheral examination revealed no structural basis for any feeding difficulty. At that time, she showed functional nonnutritive sucking with appropriate strength and rhythm. She did not appear at high risk for aspiration on the basis of the feeding observation with a "standard" nipple. Suck, swallow, and respiration appeared coordinated initially. She became disorganized with desaturation events as low as 85% noted by pulse oximetry as the feeding progressed. Given her history of underlying respiratory problems and findings on the bedside examination, she was taken to VFSS the following day. Although she showed intermittent trace nasopharyngeal reflux while she was sucking and swallowing, it appeared within acceptable levels for a premature infant. She had no other pharyngeal phase deficits. She was still on caffeine and reflux medications at that time.

Recommendations included oral feeding as tolerated with close monitoring of respiratory status, supplementing by NG tube as needed. She made gains while in the NICU and was discharged home as a full oral feeder. She was gaining weight well. She went home on oxygen by nasal cannula (1/4 liter at 100%). Prognosis for successful and safe oral feeding appeared positive and related closely to her airway status.

Comment

This infant is a good example of the need for a stable airway as a requirement for successful oral feeding. She met the criteria for a diagnosis of BPD as she was on supplemental oxygen for at least 28 days. In general, these infants weigh < 2,000 g and are < 34 weeks' gestation at birth. Once she was able to manage the work of feeding superimposed on the work of breathing, she continued to show weight gain with improved timing and coordination of nipple feeding. The laryngomalacia and GERD tend to interrelate, and aggressive management of reflux is needed. As caregivers became familiar with her and could interpret her communication related to stress, they helped Annie attain functional oral feeding status. They were cautioned to allow Annie to set the pace and not to push hard to increase volume of feedings because of the risk for food refusal that can make it more difficulty for an infant to reach full oral feeding status.

All infants in the NICU are followed at periodic intervals for their neurodevelopmental progress. At age 24 months, Annie had mental and motor performance within normal limits. She was growing well.

Case Study 4

"Tammy" was born at 36 weeks gestation with a birthweight of 2,400 g. She had no spontaneous respirations following vacuum extraction. She appeared hypotonic and was intubated immediately. Apgars were 2 at 1 min, 5 at 5 min, and 6 at 10 min. An OG tube was placed with moderate difficulty after an NG tube could be passed only 6 cm. She was transferred to the regional perinatal intensive care nursery during the 1st day of life. The next day, an otolaryngologic examination revealed stridor and supraglottic edema probably secondary to intubation. Both true vocal folds appeared ulcerated but with normal mobility. She showed nasopharyngeal reflux of her own secretions and with oral feeding attempts. A scintiscan showed evidence of gastroesophageal reflux. A dysmorphology examination did not result in a recognizable syndromic diagnosis. Neurodevelopmental examination report stated, "mild peripheral hypotonia, otherwise normal."

At 3 days of life, Tammy was assessed by the oral–motor and feeding specialist. She appeared alert and readily initiated a nonnutritive rhythmic sucking pattern on the examiner's little finger and a pacifier. By that time an NG tube had been placed. Because she appeared well-coordinated for nonnutritive sucking, she was given the opportunity for nutritive sucking, which she initiated with appropriate timing and coordination; however, nasopharyngeal reflux of large quantity was noted. Therefore, oral feeding attempts were eliminated, except for test purposes in the next few days.

VFSS at 10 days of life revealed no aspiration and appropriate timing of oral and pharyngeal phases of the swallow, but with some incoordination of the pharyngeal phase and significant nasopharyngeal reflux. By that time, she was showing increased respiratory distress and could not be fed orally. Neurodevelopmental reexamination revealed mildly abnormal findings, placing her at risk for developmental problems. Direct laryngoscopy and bronchoscopy revealed subglottic stenosis. An anterior cricoid split procedure was performed. After several weeks, she still could not be extubated successfully, and thus a tracheotomy was performed. The nasopharyngeal reflux continued and aspiration of feeds was noted around the tracheotomy tube. Oral feeds were discontinued. A GT was placed. She was discharged to home with parents trained to care for the tracheotomy tube, to administer GT feedings, and to provide nonnutritive oral sensorimotor stimulation. Recommendations included dipping the pacifier or finger into very small amounts of 5% glucose solution, water, or formula to give Tammy taste experiences and to attempt to encourage specific swallowing. Parents communicated with the oral sensorimotor feeding specialist by telephone to report status. She was not a candidate for a speaking valve because of the degree of subglottic stenosis.

Tammy eagerly sucked on a pacifier with appropriate nonnutritive rate and rhythm. Parents and home care nurses incorporated small amounts of formula or water via nipple every few days to test for potential for oral feedings as suggested by the interdisciplinary team. Evidence of aspiration in her secretions continued when she was suctioned. She appeared safer with the tastes when pacifier or finger was dipped into liquid. Thicker textures were gradually introduced as the caregiver dipped a finger into thickened liquid or strained fruit. Tammy was followed closely by the pediatric otolaryngologist and the oral–motor and feeding specialist during the first several months while nutritional needs were met by GT feeds.

At age 5 months, aspiration was still noted during the "tests" with thin and thickened liquid, and thus no advances could be made for oral feeding. By age 7 months, evaluation by the feeding team revealed that oral phase of the swallow appeared appropriate for nipple attempts and for spoon-feeding, but the practice had to be limited to 3 to 4 small swallows because of aspiration noted in the tracheal secretions. Growth had been appropriate with her GT feeds. Head control and mobility had improved significantly. Cognitive and receptive language skills appeared age appropriate. Tammy made "raspberries" with her lips and seemed to enjoy mouth play, although she produced no phonation. Guidelines included continued nonnutritive mouth play focus with small tastes as tolerated.

Tammy was followed closely for medical and developmental monitoring. Aggressive management for GER was carried out. She made appropriate developmental gains and gradually began to improve in phonation with speech–language intervention. As she increased her repertoire of speech sounds along with the increased phonation around the tracheotomy tube, she was able to take increased quantity of food, although it took longer for her to take thin liquids safely. Eventually by age 5 years, the GT was removed in the springtime once she had demonstrated the capability of full oral feeding through one upper respiratory infection in the winter. She was decannulated successfully at the same time because airway growth resulted in resolution of clinically significant subglottic stenosis.

Comment

Given that it is impossible to do any direct "exercises" for the pharyngeal phase of the swallow, the practice can consist of a variety of ways to encourage oral–motor function for rhythmic sucking and mouth play with toys and fingers. This mouth play is also a preliminary skill for speech production even when no vocalizations can be produced. During the direct oral practice, changes in positioning and in food textures may indirectly enhance the pharyngeal phase of swallowing.

Close monitoring is necessary to determine when a repeat VFSS may provide useful information. Indications for repeat VFSS study usually are to document safety status of swallow or to assess swallow when changes in management are considered. Ongoing problem solving by parents, other caregivers, and professional team members is needed when obvious solutions are not readily available. This child also demonstrates that adequate airway protection is necessary for oral feeding, but it is not clear as to how much and what kinds of food or liquid can be taken for purposes of "practice" when aspiration is noted. As clinicians ponder the range of options for aspiration, they must regularly consider possibilities of GERD/EERD, as well as aspiration, with swallowing.

■   REFERENCES

Abraham, S. S., & Wolf, E. L. (2000). Swallowing physiology of toddlers with long-term tracheostomies: A preliminary study. *Dysphagia, 15,* 206–212.

Accardo, P. (1982). Growth and development: An interactional context for failure to thrive. In P. Accardo (Ed.), *Failure to thrive in infancy and early childhood* (3–18). Baltimore: University Park Press.

Alexander, R. (1987). Oral-motor treatment for infants and young children with cerebral palsy. *Seminars in Speech and Language, 8,* 87–100.

Alexander, R., Sato, Y., Smith, W., & Bennett, T. (1990). Incidence of impact trauma with cranial injuries ascribed to shaking. *American Journal of the Disabled Child, 144,* 724–726.

Alexander, R. C., & Smith, W. L. (1998). Shaken baby syndrome. *Infants and Young Children, 10,* 1–9.

Arvedson, J. C. (1993). Management of swallowing problems. In J. C. Arvedson, & L. Brodsky, (Eds.), *Pediatric swallowing and feeding:*

Assessment and management (327–387). San Diego, CA: Singular Publishing Group.

Arvedson, J. C., & Brodsky, L. (1992). Pediatric tracheotomy referrals to speech-language pathology in a children's hospital. *International Journal of Pediatric Otorhinolaryngology, 23,* 237–243.

Arvedson, J., Rogers, B., Buck, G., Smart, P., & Msall, M. (1994). Silent aspiration prominent in children with dysphagia. *International Journal of Pediatric Otorhinolaryngology, 28,* 173–181.

Benkov, K., Kazlow, P. G., Waye, J. D., & Lelieko, N. S. (1986). Percutaneous endoscopic gastrostomies in children. *Pediatrics, 77,* 248–249.

Bentler, M., & Stanish, M. (1987). Nutrition support of the pediatric patient with AIDS. *Journal of the American Dietetic Association, 87,* 488–491.

Bernbaum, J. C., Pereira, G. R., Watkins, J. B., & Peckham, G. J. (1983). Nonnutritive sucking during gavage feeding enhances growth and maturation in premature infants. *Pediatrics, 71,* 41–45.

Berwick, D. M., Levy, J. C., & Kleinerman, R. (1982). Failure to thrive: Diagnostic yield of hospitalization. *Archives of Disease in Childhood, 57,* 347–351.

Brown, C. E., & Magnuson, B. (2000). On the physics of the infant feeding bottle and middle ear sequela: Ear disease in infants can be associated with bottle feeding. *International Journal of Pediatric Otorhinolaryngology, 54,* 13–20.

Budden, S. (1986). Rett syndrome: Studies of 13 affected girls. *American Journal of Medical Genetics, 24,* 99–109.

Budden, S., Meek, M., & Henighan, C. (1990). Communication and oral-motor function in Rett syndrome. *Developmental Medicine and Child Neurology, 32,* 51–55.

Carter, G., & Jancar, J. (1983). Mortality in mentally handicapped: Fifty-year survey at Stoke Park Group of Hospitals. *Journal of Mental Deficiency Research, 27,* 143–156.

Casas, M. J., McPherson, K. A., & Kenny, D. J. (1995). Durational aspects of oral swallow in neurologically normal children and children with cerebral palsy: An ultrasound investigation. *Dysphagia, 10,* 155–159.

Case-Smith, J., & Humphry, R. (2000). Feeding intervention. In J. Case-Smith (Ed.), *Occupational therapy for children* (4th ed.; 453–488). St. Louis: Mosby.

Collinge, J. M., Bradley, K., Perks, C., Rezny, A., & Topping, P. (1982). Demand vs scheduled feedings for infants. *Journal of Obstetric and Gynecologic Neonatal Nursing, 11,* 362–367.

Dellert, S. F., Hyams, J. S., Treem, W. R., & Geertsma, M. A. (1993). Feeding resistance and gastroesophageal reflux in infancy. *Journal of Pediatric Gastroenterology and Nursing, 17,* 66–71.

Dobie, R. A. (1978). Rehabilitation of swallowing disorders. *American Family Physician, 27,* 94–95.

Duara, S. (1989). Oral feeding containers and their influence on intake and ventilation in preterm infants. *Biology of the Neonate, 56,* 270–276.

Duffner, P. K., Horowitz, M. E., Krischer, J. P., Friedman, H. S., Burger, P. C., Cohen, M. E., Sanford, R. A., Mulhern, R. K., James, H. E., Freeman, C. R., Seidel, F. G., & Kun, L. E. (1993). Postoperative chemotherapy and delayed radiation in children less than three years of age with malignant brain tumors. *New England Journal of Medicine, 328,* 1725–1731.

Einarsson-Backes, L. M., Deitz, J., Price, R., Glass, R., & Hays, R. (1994). The effect of oral support on sucking efficiency in preterm infants. *American Journal of Occupational Therapy, 48,* 490–498.

Farber, S., & Huss, A. J. (1974). *Sensorimotor evaluation and treatment procedures for allied health personnel.* Indianapolis: Indiana University Foundation.

Farber, S. D., Van Fossen, R. L., & Koontz, S. W. (1995). Quantitative and qualitative video analysis of infants feeding: Angled- and straight-bottle feeding systems. *Journal of Pediatrics, 126,* S118–S124.

Field, T. (1986). Interventions for premature infants. *Journal of Pediatrics, 109,* 183–191.

Field, T. (1995). Massage therapy for infants and children. *Journal of Developmental and Behavioral Pediatrics, 16,* 105–111.

Field, T., & Goldson, E. (1984). Pacifying effects of nonnutritive sucking on term and preterm neonates during heelsticks. *Pediatrics, 74,* 1012–1015.

Field, T., Ignatoff, E., Stringer, S., Brennan, J., Greenberg, R., Widmayer, S., & Anderson, G. C. (1982). Nonnutritive sucking during tube feedings: Effects on preterm neonates in an intensive care unit. *Pediatrics, 70,* 381–384.

Fisher, J. O., Birch, L. L., Smiciklas-Wright, H., & Picciano, M. F. (2000). Breast-feeding through the first year predicts maternal control in feeding and subsequent toddler energy intakes. *Journal of American Dietetic Association, 100,* 641–646.

Freeman, C. R., Bourgouin, P. M., Sanford, R. A., Cohen, M. E., Friedman, H. S., & Kun, L. E. (1996). Long term survivors of childhood brain stem gliomas treated with hyperfractionated radiotherapy. Clinical characteristics and treatment related toxicities. The Pediatric Oncology Group. *Cancer, 77,* 555–562.

Gallender, D. (1979). *Eating handicaps: Illustrated techniques for feeding disorders.* Springfield, IL: C. C. Thomas.

Gallender, D. (1980). *Teaching eating and toileting skills to the multi-handicapped in the school setting.* Springfield, IL: C. C. Thomas.

Gisel, E. G. (1996). Effect of oral sensorimotor treatment on measures of growth and efficiency of eating in the moderately eating-impaired child with cerebral palsy. *Dysphagia, 11*, 48–58.

Gisel, E. (1994). Oral-motor skills following sensorimotor intervention in the moderately eating-impaired child with cerebral palsy. *Dysphagia, 9*, 180–192.

Gisel, E. G., Applegate-Ferrante, T., Benson, J., & Bosma, J. (1995). Effect of oral sensorimotor treatment on measures of growth, eating efficiency and aspiration in the dysphagic child with cerebral palsy. *Developmental Medicine and Child Neurology, 37*, 528–543.

Gisel, E., Applegate-Ferrante, T., Benson, J., & Bosma, J. (1996). Oral-motor skills following sensorimotor therapy in two groups of moderately dysphagic children with cerebral palsy: Aspiration vs nonaspiration. *Dysphagia, 11*, 59–71.

Gisel, E. G., Schwartz, S., & Haberfellner, H. (1999). The Innsbruck sensorimotor activator and regulator (ISMAR): Construction of an intraoral appliance to facilitate ingestive function. *Journal of Dentistry for Children, 66*, 180–187.

Gisel, E. G., Schwartz, S., Petryk, A., Clarke, D., & Haberfellner, H. (2000). "Whole body" mobility after one year of intraoral appliance therapy in children with cerebral palsy and moderate eating impairment. *Dysphagia, 15*, 226–235.

Glass, R. P., & Wolf, L. S. (1998). Feeding and oral-motor skills. In J. Case-Smith (Ed.), *Pediatric occupational therapy and early intervention* (2nd ed.; 127–163). Boston: Butterworth-Heinemann.

Griggs, C. A., Jones, P. M., & Lee, R. E. (1989). Videofluoroscopic investigation of feeding disorders in children with multiple handicap. *Developmental Medicine and Child Neurology, 31*, 303–308.

Haas, A., & Creskoff, N. (2000). *The S.O.S. Approach: Sequential oral sensory approach to feeding.* Seminar presented at annual convention of the American Speech-Language-Hearing Association. Washington, D.C.

Haberfellner, H., Schwartz, S., & Gisel, E. G. (2001). Feeding skills and growth after one year of intraoral appliance therapy in moderately dysphagic children with cerebral palsy. *Dysphagia, 16*, 83–96.

Hall, K. D. (2001). *Pediatric dysphagia: Resource guide.* San Diego, CA: Singular, Thomson Learning.

Harris, M. (1986). Oral-motor management of the high-risk neonate. *Occupational Therapy in Pediatrics, 6*, 231–253.

Hawdon, J. M., Beauregard, N., Slattery, J., & Kennedy, G. (2000). Identification of neonates at risk for developing feeding problems in infancy. *Developmental Medicine and Child Neurology, 42*, 235–239.

Helfrich–Miller, K. R., Rector, K. L., & Straka, J. A. (1986). Dysphagia: Its treatment in the profoundly retarded patient with cerebral palsy. *Archives of Physical Medicine and Rehabilitation, 67*, 520–525.

Heptinsall, E., Puckering, C., Skuse, D., Dowdney, L., & Zur-Szpira, S. (1987). Nutrition and mealtime behaviour in families of growth-retarded children. *Human Nutrition: Applied Nutrition, 41a*, 390–402.

Herman, M. J. (1991). Comprehensive assessment of oral-motor dysfunction in failure-to-thrive infants. *Infant-Toddler Intervention, 1*, 109–123.

Hill, A. S., Kurkowski, T. B., & Garcia. J. (2000). Oral support measures used in feeding the preterm infant. *Nursing Research, 49*, 2–10.

Jones, P. M. (1989). Feeding disorders in children with multiple handicaps. *Developmental Medicine and Child Neurology, 31*, 404–406.

Klein, M. D., & Delaney, T. A. (1994). *Feeding and nutrition for the child with special needs: Handouts for parents.* Tucson, AZ: Therapy Skill Builders.

Klein, M. D. & Morris, S. E. (1999). *Mealtime participation guide.* San Antonio, TX: Therapy Skill Builders.

Koontz-Lowman, D., & Lane, S. J. (1999). Children with feeding and nutritional problems. In S. M. Porr & E. B. Rainville (Eds.), *Pediatric therapy: A systems approach* (379–423). Philadelphia: F. A. Davis.

Korabek, C. A., Reid, D. H., & Ivancic, M. T. (1981). Improving needed food intake of profoundly handicapped children through effective supervision of institutional staff. *Applied Research in Mental Retardation, 2*, 69–88.

Korner, A. F. (1990). Infant stimulation: Issues of theory and research. *Clinics in Perinatology, 17*, 173–184.

Kutiyanawala, M. A., Hussain, A., Johnstone, J. M. S., Everson, N. W., & Nour, S. (1998). Gastrostomy complications in infants and children. *Annals of the Royal College of Surgery England, 80*, 240–243.

Lang, S., Lawrence, C. J., & Orme, R. L. E. (1994). Cup feeding: An alternative method of infant feeding. *Archives of Disease in Childhood, 71*, 365–369.

Larnett, G. & Ekberg, D. (1995). Positioning improves the oral and pharyngeal swallowing function in children with cerebral palsy. *Acta Pediatrics, 84*. 689–692.

Lau, C., & Schanler, R. J. (2000). Oral feeding in premature infants: Advantage of a self-paced milk flow. *Acta Paediatrica, 89*, 393–398.

Lawrence, R. (1995). The clinician's role in teaching proper infant feeding techniques. *Journal of Pediatrics, 126*, S112–S117.

Letts, L., & Bosch, J. (2001). Measuring occupational performance in basic activities of daily living. In M. Law, C. Baum, & W. Dunn (Eds.), *Measuring occupational performance: Supporting best practice in occupational therapy.* Thorofare, NJ: SLACK.

Ludington-How, S. M., & Swinth, J. Y. (1996). Developmental aspects of kangaroo care. *Journal of Gynecologic and Neonatal Nursing, 25*, 691–703.

Mathew, O. P. (1988). Nipple units for newborn infants: A functional comparison. *Pediatrics, 81*, 688–691.

Mathew, O. P. (1991). Science of bottle feeding. *Journal of Pediatrics, 119,* 511–519.

Mathew, O. P., Belan, M., & Thoppil, C. K. (1992). Sucking patterns of neonates during bottle feeding: Comparison of different nipple units. *American Journal of Perinatology, 9,* 265–269.

Mathisen, B., Skuse, D., Wolke, D., & Reilly, S. (1989). Oral-motor dysfunction and failure to thrive among inner-city infants. *Developmental Medicine and Child Neurology, 31,* 293–302.

Mathisen, B., Worrall, L., O'Callaghan, M., Wall, C., & Shepherd, R.W. (2000). Feeding problems and dysphagia in six-month-old extremely low birth weight infants. *Advances in Speech-Language Pathology, 2,* 9–17.

McBride, M. C., & Danner, S. C. (1987). Sucking disorders in neurologically impaired infants: Assessment and facilitation of breastfeeding. *Clinics in Perinatology, 14,* 109–130.

McCain, Gail C. (1992). Facilitating inactive awake states in preterm infants: A study of three interventions. *Nursing Research, 41,* 157–160.

Measel, C. P., & Anderson, G. C. (1979). Nonnutritive sucking during tube feedings: Effect on clinical course in premature infants. *Journal of Obstetric, Gynecologic and Neonatal Nursing, 8,* 265–272.

Medoff-Cooper, B., McGrath, J. M., & Bilker, W. (2000). Nutritive sucking and neurobehavioral development in preterm infants from 34 weeks PCA to term. *MCN, 25* 64–70.

Meier, P., & Pugh, E. J. (1985). Breastfeeding behavior of small preterm infants. *American Journal of Maternal and Child Nursing, 10,* 396–401.

Meyers, W. F., & Herbst, J. J. (1982). Effectiveness of positioning therapy for gastroesophageal reflux. *Pediatrics, 69,* 768–772.

Moore, M. C., & Greene, H. (1985). Tube feeding of infants and children. *Pediatric Clinics of North America, 32,* 401–417.

Morris, S. E. (1985). Developmental implications for the management of feeding problems in neurologically impaired infants. *Seminars in Speech and Language, 6,* 293–315.

Morris, S. E. (1989). Development of oral-motor skills in the neurologically impaired child receiving non-oral feedings. *Dysphagia, 3,* 135–154.

Morris, S. E., & Klein, M. D. (1987). *Pre-feeding skills: A comprehensive resource for feeding development.* Tucson, AZ: Therapy Skill Builders.

Morris, S. E., & Klein, M. D. (2000). *Pre-feeding skills: A comprehensive resource for feeding mealtime development* (2nd ed.). San Antonio, TX: Therapy Skill Builders.

Mueller, H. (1987). Feeding. In N. Finne (Ed.), *Handling the young cerebral palsied child* (7th ed.). New York: E.P. Dutton.

National Association of Neonatal Nurses. (1995). *Infant and family centered developmental care guidelines.* Petaluma, CA: Author.

Nelson, C. A., & de Benabib, R. M. (1991). Sensory preparation of the oral–motor area. In M. B. Langley and L. J. Lombardino (Eds.), *Neurodevelopmental strategies for managing communication disorders in children with severe motor dysfunction* (131–158). Austin, TX: PRO-ED.

Oetter, P., Richter, E., & Frick. S. (1995). *M.O.R.E.: Integrating the mouth with sensory and postural functions* (2nd ed.). Hugo, MN: PDP Press.

Ogundipe O. A., Kullama L. K., Day L., & Ross M. G. (1994). Assessments of fetal swallowed volume: Tracer disappearance vs esophageal flow. *Journal of Sociology and Gynecology Investigations, 1,* 37–44.

Orenstein, S. R. (1990). Prone positioning in infant gastroesophageal reflux: Is elevation of the head worth the trouble? *Journal of Pediatrics, 117,* 184–187.

Orenstein, S. R., & Whitington, P. F. (1983). Positioning for prevention of infant gastroesophageal reflux. *Journal of Pediatrics, 103,* 534–537.

Ottenbacher, K., Hicks, J., Roark, A., & Swinea, J. (1983). Oral sensorimotor therapy in the developmentally disabled: A multiple baseline study. *American Journal of Occupational Therapy, 37,* 541–547.

Ottenbacher, K., Scoggins, A., & Wayland, J. (1981). The effectiveness of a program of oral sensory-motor therapy with the severely and profoundly developmentally disabled. *Occupational Therapy Journal of Research, 1,* 147–160.

Palmer, M. M., & Heyman, M. B. (1993). Assessment and treatment of sensory motor-based feeding problems in very young children. *Infants and Young Children, 6,* 67–73.

Palmer, S., & Horn, S. (1978). Feeding problems in children. In S. Palmer & S. Ekvall (Eds.), *Pediatric nutrition in developmental disorders.* Springfield, IL: Charles C. Thomas.

Paludetto, R., Robertson, S. S., Hack, M., Shivpuri, C. R., & Martin, R. J. (1984). Transcutaneous oxygen tension during nonnutritive sucking in preterm infants. *Pediatrics, 74,* 539–542.

Pearce, J. L., & Buchanan, L. F. (1979). Breast milk and breastfeeding in very low birthweight infants. *Archives of Disabled Children, 54,* 897–899.

Pinelli, J., & Symington, A. (2000), Non-nutritive sucking for promoting physiologic stability and nutrition in preterm infants. *Cochrane Database System Review, 2,* CD001071.

Pressman, H. (1992). Communication disorders and dysphagia in pediatric AIDS. *Asha, 35,* 45–47.

Pressman, H., & Morrison, S. H. (1988). Dysphagia in the pediatric AIDS population. *Dysphagia, 2,* 166–169.

Prodromidis, M., Field, T., Arendt, R., Singer, L., Yando, R., & Bendell, D. (1995). Mothers touching newborns: A comparison of rooming-in versus minimal contact. *Birth, 22,* 196–200.

Rausch, P. B. (1981). Effects of tactile and kinesthetic stimulation on premature infants. *Journal of Obstetric and Gynecologic Neonatal Nursing,* 34–37.

Raventos, J. M., Kralemann, H., & Gray, D. B. (1982). Mortality risks of mentally retarded and mentally ill patients after a feeding gastrostomy. *American Journal of Mental Deficiency, 86,* 439–444.

Reilly, S. & Skuse, D. (1992). Characteristics and management of feeding problems of young children with cerebral palsy. *Developmental Medicine and Child Neurology, 34,* 379–388.

Riordan, M. M., Iwata, B. A., Finney, J. W., Wohl, M. K., & Stanley, A. E. (1984). Behavioral assessment and treatment of chronic food refusal in handicapped children. *Journal of Applied Behavior Analysis, 17,* 327–341.

Riordan, M. M., Iwata, B. A., Wohl, M. K., & Finney, J. W. (1980). Behavioral treatment of food refusal and selectivity in developmentally disabled children. *Applied Research in Mental Retardation, 1,* 95–112.

Rogers, B., Arvedson, J., Buck, G., Smart, P., & Msall, M. (1994). Characteristics of dysphagia in children with cerebral palsy. *Dysphagia, 9,* 69–73.

Rosingh, H. J., & Peek, S. H. G. (1999). Swallowing and speech in infants following tracheotomy. *Acta Oto-Rhino-Laryngologica Belgium, 53,* 59–63.

Ross, M. G., & Nijland, M. J. (1997). Fetal swallowing: Relation to amniotic fluid regulation. *Clinical Obstetrics and Gynecology, 40,* 352–65.

Scafidi, F., & Field, T. (1996a). Factors that predict which preterm infants benefit most from massage therapy. *Journal of Pediatric Psychology, 14,* 176–180.

Scafidi, F., & Field, T. (1996b). Massage therapy improves behavior in neonates born to HIV-positive mothers. *Journal of Pediatric Psychology, 21,* 889–897.

Schuster, D. H., & Mouzon, D. (1982). Music and vocabulary learning. *Journal of the Society for Accelerative Learning and Teaching, 7,* 82–108.

Senez, C., Guys, J. M., Mancini, J., Paz Paredes, A., Lena, G., & Choux, M. (1996). Weaning children from tube to oral feeding. *Child's Nervous System, 12,* 590–594.

Simon, B., & McGowan, J. (1989). Tracheostomy in young children: Implications for assessment and treatment of communication and feeding disorders. *Infants and Young Children, 1,* 1–9.

Singer, L. T., Wood, R., & Lambert, S. (1985). Developmental follow-up of long-term infant tracheostomy: A preliminary report. *Developmental and Behavioral Pediatrics, 6,* 132–136.

Smith, D. W. (1979). The fetal alcohol syndrome. *Hospital Practice, 14,* 121.

Smith, D. W. (1980). Fetal drug syndromes: Effects of ethanol and hydan-
toins. *Pediatric Revue, 1,* 165.

Sobsey, R., & Orelove, F. P. (1984). Neurophysiological facilitation of eating skills in children with severe handicaps. *Journal of the Association
for Persons With Severe Handicaps, 9,* 98–110.

Stroh, K., Robinson, T., & Stroh, G. (1986). A therapeutic feeding pro-
gramme: Theory and practice of feeding. *Developmental Medicine and
Child Neurology, 28,* 3–10.

Swigert, N. B. (1998). *The source for pediatric dysphagia.* East Moline, IL:
LinguiSystems.

Takagi, Y., & Bosma, J. F. (1960). Disability of oral function in an infant
associated with displacement of the tongue: Therapy by feeding in the
prone position. *Acta Paediatrics Scandinavia Supplement, 123,* 62–69.

Thackray, H. M. & Tifft, C. (2001). Fetal alcohol syndrome. *Pediatrics in
Review, 22,* 47–55.

Toomey, K. A. (2000). Steps to eating. Colorado Feeding Consortium.
Unpublished handout from A. Haas, & N. Creskoff, (2000). *The S.O.S.
Approach: Sequential oral sensory approach to feeding.* Presented at
annual convention of the American Speech-Language-Hearing Association. Washington, D.C.

Treloar, D. M. (1994). The effect of nonnutritive sucking on oxygenation
in healthy, crying full-term infants. *Applied Nursing Research, 7,*
52–58.

Tuchman, D. (1988). Dysfunctional swallowing in the pediatric patient:
Clinical considerations. *Dysphagia, 2,* 203–208.

Van Dyke, D. C., Mackay, L., & Ziaylek, E. N. (1982). Management of
severe feeding dysfunction in children with fetal alcohol syndrome.
Clinical Pediatrics, 21, 336–339.

Waterman, E. T., Koltai, P. J., Downey, J. C., & Cacace, A. T. (1992).
Swallowing disorders in a population of children with cerebral palsy.
International Journal of Pediatric Otorhinolaryngology, 24, 63–71.

White, J., & Labarba, R. (1976). The effects of tactile and kinesthetic stimulation on neonatal development in the premature infant. *Developmental Psychobiology, 9,* 569–577.

Wilbarger, P. & Wilbarger, J. L. (1991). *Sensory defensiveness in children
aged 2-12.* Santa Barbara, CA: Avanti Educational Programs.

Wolf, L. S. & Glass, R. P. (1992). *Feeding and swallowing disorders in
infancy: Assessment and management.* Tucson, AZ: Therapy Skill
Builders.

Ylvisaker, M. 1998. (Ed.). *Traumatic brain injury rehabilitation: Children
and adolescents* (2nd ed.). Boston: Butterworth-Heinemann.

Ylvisaker, M., Feeney, J., & Feeney, T. J. (1999). An everyday approach to
long-term rehabilitation after traumatic brain injury. In B. S. Cornett

(Ed.), *Clinical practice management for speech-language pathologists* (117–162). Gaithersburg, MD: Aspen.

Ylvisaker, M., & Weinstein, M. (1989). Recovery of oral feeding after pediatric head injury. *Journal of Head Trauma Rehabilitation, 4*, 51–63.

Zaichkin, J. (1996). *Newborn intensive care: What every parent needs to know*. Petaluma, CA: NICU INK Book Publishers.

■ PART II ■

Special Topics in Pediatric Swallowing and Feeding

■ CHAPTER 10

Aspiration

Linda Brodsky and Joan Arvedson

■ SUMMARY

Aspiration is defined as the entry of foreign material below the true vocal folds into the tracheobronchial tree. Children with neurologic impairment are at greatest risk for both acute and chronic aspiration. Aspiration of orally ingested material (usually food or liquid), saliva, sinonasal mucous secretions (1° aspiration), and gastroesophageal refluxate (2° aspiration) can compromise the lower airways in a variety of ways.

Recognition of aspiration may be difficult from clinical examination alone. A high index of suspicion and the use of a variety of imaging studies are required. Coughing with swallowing, postprandial wheezing, laryngeal gurgling, and recurrent pneumonia are strong clinical indicators of aspiration. Nonetheless, in many patients, aspiration is without signs or symptoms (i.e., "silent") and diagnosis may be aided with one or more of the following studies: chest X-ray, computerized tomographic (CT) scan of the chest, flexible fiberoptic nasopharyngolaryngoscopy[1] (FFNL), flexible endoscopic examination of swallowing (FEES), videofluoroscopic swallow study (VFSS), and rigid airway endoscopy including evaluation of bronchial secretions.

Treatment varies with the severity of the problem, overall health of the patient, and attitudes of the family and other caregivers. Adjustments in food textures, feeding patterns, patient position, and feeding routes are tried first. Medical therapy may be directed at reducing saliva or mucous

---

[1]The terms flexible fiberoptic nasopharyngoscopy, flexible fiberoptic nasopharyngolaryngoscopy, and flexible fiberoptic laryngoscopy are used interchangeably.

secretions or treating gastroesophageal reflux disease and extraesophageal reflux disease[2] (GERD/EERD). Surgical options may include management of GERD/EERD with fundoplication, salivary gland surgery to reduce secretions, laryngeal closure or separation procedures, and gastro-esophageal separation procedures. This chapter will describe the pathology and pathophysiology of chronic aspiration, clinical evaluation, imaging and other laboratory studies, and treatment principles and options. Case studies highlight salient points.

■ INTRODUCTION

The larynx has three major functions: protection of the lower airways, respiration, and phonation. The most important is protection of the lower airways. Structural and functional neuromuscular abnormalities of the upper aerodigestive tract can result in swallowing dysfunction (dysphagia). When dysphagia occurs, the finely timed, synchronized, and highly coordinated series of events that constitute a normal and safe swallow are disrupted, placing the protective function of the larynx at great risk (Loughlin & Lefton-Greif, 1994). Varying degrees of laryngeal penetration occur in individuals with dysphagia, and thus the risk of aspiration varies. The potential of pulmonary contamination from aspiration poses life-threatening risks to the airways and the vital function of respiration.

Aspiration, strictly defined as the passage of foreign materials below the level of the true vocal folds, can be acute or chronic. Acute aspiration is an event marked by cough, tachypnea, fever, and wheezing. Chest X-ray demonstrates infiltrates indicative of a pneumonitis. The severity of the pulmonary response is determined by aspirate amount and contents and by the age and general health of the patient. The remainder of this chapter will focus on chronic aspiration.

---

[2]Gastro-esophageal reflux disease (GERD) refers to the abnormal regurgitation of acid into the esophagus causing symptoms. When the acid and other stomach contents emerge from the upper esophageal sphincter in the pharynx, larynx, mouth, and nasal cavities, the most commonly accepted term is extra-esophageal reflux disease or EERD (Sasaki & Toohill, 2000).

■ PATHOPHYSIOLOGY OF CHRONIC ASPIRATION

Chronic aspiration may be much more insidious in its presentation than acute aspiration, but no less dangerous to the health of the child. Direct (or 1°) pulmonary aspiration occurs when saliva, oral flora, mucous, and ingested food enters the tracheobronchial tree. Indirect (or 2°) pulmonary aspiration occurs when GER/EER (containing gastric acid, enzymes, bacteria, and partially digested food) spill over into the larynx and into the tracheobronchial tree. Children with swallowing dysfunction and neuromuscular disease are the most prone to chronic aspiration. Unfortunately, clinical indicators may be scarce. Chronic or intermittent cough is often absent, and the presence of recurrent pulmonary infections often signifies aspiration with advanced pulmonary complications. Thus, a high index of suspicion and vigilant monitoring of all children with oral sensorimotor dysfunction will help the clinician to promptly recognize and appropriately treat chronic aspiration in children.

The term *aspiration* is often confused with the term *laryngeal penetration*. Laryngeal penetration refers to secretions or food entering the laryngeal inlet, which can be divided into two parts, the upper and the deep. The upper laryngeal inlet starts at the tip of the epiglottis and extends to the top of the arytenoids. Deep laryngeal penetration refers to aspirate penetrating below the level of the plane defined by the top of the arytenoids to the top of the thyroid cartilage but above the true vocal folds (Figure 10–1). Deep laryngeal penetration is not uncommon in neurologically normal children (Delzell, Kraus, Gaisie, & Lerner, 1999) in whom it is not a predictor of aspiration. Neurologically impaired children who have deep laryngeal penetration are at risk for aspiration (Friedman & Frazier, 2000).

Aspirated materials include ingested food and liquids, oral secretions, mucous, and regurgitated gastric contents (acids, enzymes, bacteria, and partially digested food). Aspiration of these materials endangers the airway by producing mechanical obstruction, bacterial pneumonia, chemical tracheobronchitis, and pneumonitis. Mucosal desquamation of the cells of the trachea and bronchi is accompanied by damage to the cells and capillaries in the alveoli. First neutrophils, and then monocytes invade these areas causing a foreign body reaction and granuloma formation. Long-term complications can include tracheal and bronchial granuloma formation, stenosis, recurrent pneumonia, bronchitis, bronchiectasis, and lung empyema.

Life-threatening physiologic alterations associated with aspiration can be severe. Arterial oxygenation is reduced, pulmonary capillary membrane permeability increases with a decreased intravascular volume, increase in hematocrit, and extravasation of plasma into the lungs (Kush & Sanders, 1988). In chronic aspiration, a lower arterial oxygen level results in an increase in cardiovascular resistance. An effective swallow is the best

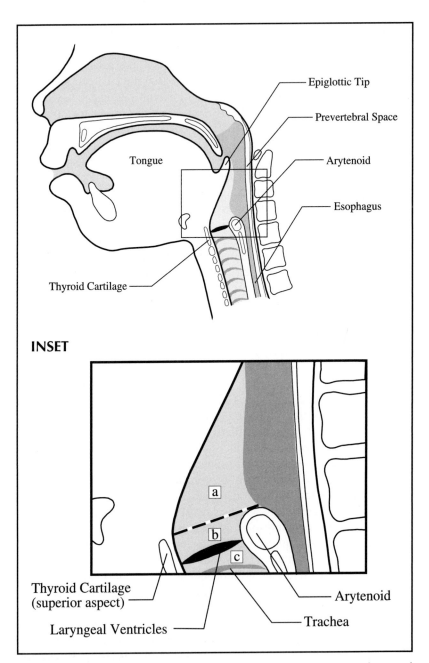

INSET

Figure 10–1. Inset of endolarynx. (a) Laryngeal penetration into upper laryngeal inlet, (b) deep laryngeal penetration, and (c) aspiration (penetration below the vocal folds and laryngeal ventricles).

protection from aspiration. The physiology of a normal swallow in relation to airway protection is described in Chapter 2.

Underlying pulmonary disease and an increased respiratory rate present a special challenge to infants with dysphagia. Swallowing to clear secretions before a breath is much more difficult, and aspiration is thus more likely.

Aspiration may occur before, during, or after a swallow. The time sequence may have clinical importance in predicting etiology and treatment. When aspiration occurs before a swallow, a delay in pharyngeal swallow initiation or abnormal tongue movements may prove to play a role. Aspiration during a swallow usually indicates ineffective laryngeal closure or timing incoordination. Aspiration after a swallow is from residue in the larynx and hypopharynx being drawn through the larynx with the next breath. Decrease in tongue-base movement, incoordination of the pharyngeal constrictors, reduced sensation, decrease in laryngeal excursion, and structural or functional deficits of the esophagus may all play a role (Logemann, 1993).

After a normal swallow, the cough reflex is the best protector of the lungs. The cough reflex is highly redundant in its neurologic connections (Holinger & Sanders, 1991). Other protectors of the lungs are gag reflex, mucociliary clearance, phagocytosis by alveolar macrophages, and lymphatic drainage. Although cough is an important protection against aspiration, it is not reliable even in infants who have normal swallows. Only 25% of preterm infants and between 25 and 50% of term infants have a well-functioning cough reflex (Loughlin & Lefton-Greif, 1994). By 1 month of age, 90% of children have a well-developed cough reflex (Holinger & Sanders).

Associated medical conditions that place the child at greater risk for aspiration are developmental anomalies, anatomic defects of the upper aerodigestive tract (congenital and acquired), and neurologic and neuromuscular diseases. When multiple areas of dysfunction are present simultaneously, the risk of aspiration markedly increases (Arvedson, Rogers, Buck, Smart, & Msall, 1994; Loughlin & Lefton-Greif, 1994). The presence of assistance with feeding seems to have a predictive value for aspiration—90% of aspirators are dependent feeders, either partially or totally. Combined oral and pharyngeal deficits are found in 98% of aspirators (Arvedson et al.). Children with endotracheal, nasogastric, or orogastric tubes also face an increased risk for aspiration.

The complexity of patients who are at risk for aspiration makes it difficult for one clinician to have the expertise to sort out the various problems contributing to aspiration in children. Thus, interdisciplinary evaluation is mandatory. Specialists from developmental pediatrics, dysmorphology, gastroenterology, pulmonology, otolaryngology, speech–language pathology, occupational therapy, and radiology are usually involved. Steps in interdisciplinary diagnosis and management are diagrammed in Figure 10–2.

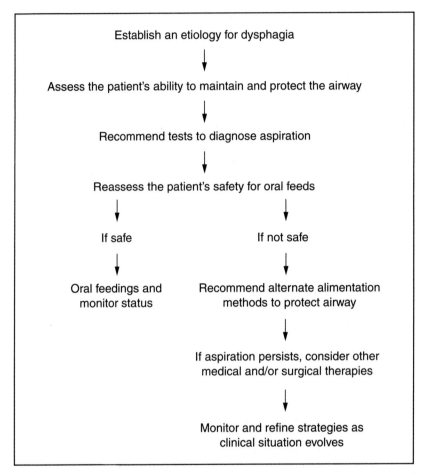

Establish an etiology for dysphagia

Assess the patient's ability to maintain and protect the airway

Recommend tests to diagnose aspiration

Reassess the patient's safety for oral feeds

If safe

Oral feedings and
monitor status

If not safe

Recommend alternate alimentation
methods to protect airway

If aspiration persists, consider other
medical and/or surgical therapies

Monitor and refine strategies as
clinical situation evolves

Figure 10–2. Diagrammatic representation of interdisciplinary management of patients with suspected aspiration.

■ CLINICAL PRESENTATION

The first step in evaluating for chronic aspiration is a detailed history. Any child who has swallowing dysfunction should raise the clinician's index of suspicion for aspiration. Cough during a swallow, choking with feeds, vomiting and choking, and recurrent pneumonia are all strong indicators of chronic aspiration (Bauer, Figueroa-Colon, Georgeson, & Young, 1993). Aspiration may elicit a vigorous cough response or may be asymptomatic (i.e., silent aspiration). Wheezing, recurrent bronchitis and recurrent croup are also seen. A past medical history of neuromuscular disease, airway compromise, GI dysmotility, previous surgery on the digestive tract (e.g., pyloric stenosis, tracheoesophageal fistula, gastrostomy tube, colon inter-position, esophageal stricture repair), or treatment for GERD/EERD is often found. When the child has multiple problems, requires assisted feeding, or is neurologically impaired, aspiration is even more likely. A history of frequent gagging or choking, especially during or immediately following feeds, can be helpful in diagnosis. Children with intractable seizures who are treated with vagal nerve stimulation may be at increased risk for aspiration (Lundgren, Ekberg, & Olsson, 1998). The differential diagnosis of the presentation for aspiration is found in Table 10–1.

The physical examination usually provides limited information. Nonetheless, direct observation of the infant or child feeding or eating is critical. An excess of saliva may drool anteriorly out of the mouth or posteriorly into the hypopharynx and larynx. (For a complete discussion of anterior drooling, see Chapter 11.) Posterior drooling (also known as hypopharyngeal pooling) is highly correlated to aspiration and sometimes produces laryngeal gurgling at rest. A wet cough and ineffective throat clearing are other indicators of secretions partially obstructing the larynx. To protect the airway, the child may sit with the neck in extreme extension. This posture brings the larynx into a protected anterior position under the tongue base and opens the esophageal inlet for freer flow of saliva and mucous secretions into the esophagus. Auscultation of the neck may reveal gurgling, wet respiration, laryngeal "wheezing," and increase in airway resistance. The lungs may be clear or have transmitted sounds from the larynx. Wheezes and rales on auscultation are found in more advanced cases of chronic aspiration with pulmonary complications.

Table 10–1. Differential Diagnosis for Chronic Aspiration

Upper airway
   Acute life-threatening events
   Recurrent croup
Lower airway
   Pneumonia
   Asthma
   Chronic pulmonary disease
   Recurrent bronchitis
   Interstitial lung disease
   Cystic fibrosis
Other
   Congestive heart failure
   Failure to thrive/malnutrition/undernutrition

Most children who aspirate have severe neuromuscular abnormalities (e.g. muscular dystrophy), cerebral palsy, and mental retardation. Occasionally, a seemingly neurologically normal child will present with difficulty handling secretions. When this occurs, a detailed neurologic examination may reveal isolated or multiple cranial nerve palsies as is seen in Mobius syndrome (Cohen & Thompson, 1987) or extremity weakness seen with an occult Arnold Chiari malformation, best diagnosed using MRI (Loughlin & Lefton-Greif, 1994). Pulmonary problems such as asthma, recurrent bronchitis, and pneumonia may be due to microaspiration of secretions or refluxate in the absence of other symptoms, even in neurologically normal children (Bowrey, Peters, & DeMeester, 2000; Orenstein, 2000).

■ DIAGNOSTIC EVALUATIONS

Many different diagnostic studies are available to provide information about the presence and severity of aspiration (Table 10–2). Each test has its usefulness, as will be described in this section. The evaluation and treatment possibilities are depicted in Figure 10–3. (Decision trees can be useful to the less experienced clinician in gaining some understanding of a complex clinical problem. Most patients do not follow a precise path, and often, simultaneous evaluations and variations in treatment will occur.) The choice of diagnostic procedure is dependent on the setting for the evaluation (inpatient vs. outpatient), the severity of the illness, comorbidities (e.g., tracheotomy), and the availability of equipment and personnel with expertise in a given procedure (e.g., VFSS, FEES). Chest X-ray is useful if it shows lower lobe or upper lobe, posterior segment infiltrates.

Table 10–2. Diagnostic Studies Useful in the Evaluation of Aspiration

Diagnostic Study	Information Gained
For all aspiration	
Chest X-ray	Presence of infiltrates consistent with aspiration
	Other pulmonary pathologies
Computerized tomographic scan of chest	Ground glass appearance of aspiration
	Other thoracic or airway abnormalities
For 1° aspiration	
Flexible fiberoptic nasopharyngolaryngoscopy (FFNL)	Structure of upper aerodigestive tract
	Function of larynx
	Handling of secretions, including aspiration

(continues)

Table 10–2. *(continued)*

Diagnostic Study	Information Gained
Videofluoroscopic swallow study (VFSS)	Bolus of contrast from oral preparatory phase or bolus formation phase
	Oral phase of bolus transport
	Timing for swallow initiation in relation to other events
	Pharyngeal phase of swallow
	Evidence and location of residual secretions
	Function of cricopharyngeus muscle
Fiber-optic endoscopic evaluation of swallow w/ sensory testing (FEES/ST)	Everything seen on flexible nasopharyngolaryngoscopy
	Events before and after a swallow in the larynx and hypopharynx
	Laryngeal adductor reflex when air blast used to test sensation
Scintiscan for GERD/EERD	Reflux
	Aspiration in delayed sequence at about 6 hours
Salivagram	Evaluate the aspiration of salivary secretions
Direct laryngoscopy/ bronchoscopy/esophagoscopy	Structural view of at larynx not attainable w/flexible scope
	Evaluation of structure of tracheobronchial tree
	Evaluation of tracheobronchial secretions
	• Amylase
	• Lipid laden macrophages
	• Glucose (enteral feeds)
	• Pepsin
	Evaluation for esophagitis or strictures
For 2° Aspiration:[a]	
Flexible fiberoptic nasopharyngolaryngoscopy (FFNL)	Changes associated with GERD/EERD:
	• Lingual tonsils filling vallecula
	• Posterior glottic swelling/pachyderm appearance
	• Loss of arytenoid architecture
	• True and false vocal fold swelling
	• Hypopharyngeal cobblestoning

[a]Other tests for GERD/EERD, a potential contributor to aspiration, are the upper gastrointestinal series and 24-hour dual channel pH probe. These do not demonstrate aspiration per se and are discussed more fully in Chapter 5.

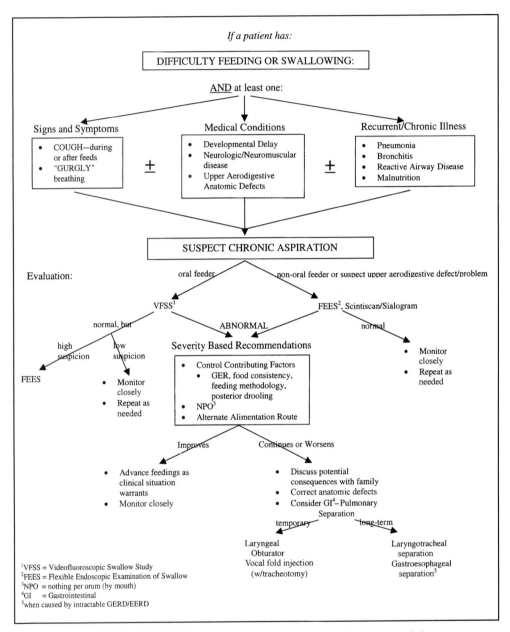

Figure 10–3. Suggested decision tree for the diagnosis and treatment of chronic aspiration.

CT scan of the chest is useful in the identification of chronic changes in the lung parenchyma. A ground glass appearance is classic for chronic aspiration (Figure 10–4). Other changes may be seen such as increase in pulmonary vasculature, peribronchial thickening, bronchiectasis, and pulmonary abscesses. When several investigations might be useful, judicious use of resources should be encouraged.

All children with a potential for aspiration should undergo FFNL, which allows the clinician to evaluate the airway for both structural and functional abnormalities. Normal appearance of the larynx at endoscopy is shown in Figure 10–5. Evidence of GERD/EERD can be diagnostic (Carr et al., 2000; Kaye, Zorowitz, & Baredes, 1997). Pooling of secretions with frank aspiration might be seen directly and obviate the need for more invasive study (Figure 10–6; Case Study 1). Structural changes such as vocal fold paralysis and absent epiglottis (Bonilla, Pizzuto, Brodsky, & Brody, 1998) are important to delineate because in some cases the swallow may not be safe. Identification of functional changes, such as severe laryngomalacia or glossoptosis, may be invaluable in the diagnosis and management of aspiration. Although aspiration, pharyngeal residue, and decreased laryngeal sensation at FFNL correlate to VFSS, the absence of these findings does not indicate the absence of aspiration. Thus, FFNL is only a screening tool for aspiration.

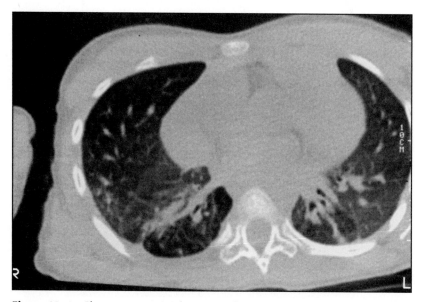

Figure 10–4. Chest computerized tomographic (CT) scan showing ground glass appearance of lungs consistent with chronic aspiration.

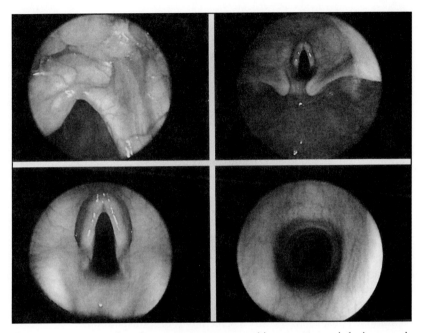

Figure 10–5. Normal endoscopic appearance of larynx. Upper left shows vallecula and epiglottis with small amount of lingual tonsils. Upper right shows sharply defined arytenoids and absence of posterior glottic selling. Lower left is magnified view of vocal folds, well defined ventricles, and normal interarytenoid mucosa. Lower right depcts normal subglottic region.

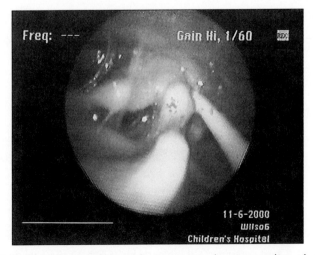

Figure 10–6. Flexible nasopharyngolaryngoscopy showing pooling of secretions and aspiration. Note presence of NG tube and wide open vocal folds.

VFSS is a radiologic evaluation of the swallow that uses contrast to highlight the swallow from oral preparatory phase (bolus formation) to the esophageal phase. VFSS is the mainstay of instrumental evaluation for aspiration; all other diagnostic studies are measured against this "gold standard" (see Chapter 8). An extensive literature exists on the subject (e.g. Arvedson & Lefton-Greif, 1998; Arvedson et al., 1994; Lefton-Greif & Loughlin, 1996). In children with cerebral palsy and feeding problems, VFSS demonstrated aspiration to be "silent" in 94% of the aspirators. Certain findings on VFSS are highly predictive of aspiration risk. These include delay in swallow initiation, presence of laryngeal residue after the swallow, laryngeal penetration (traces of bolus in the vestibule), and deep laryngeal penetration (residue left on the true vocal folds) (Friedman & Frazier, 2000). Friedman and Frazier found that in 125 dysphagic children, 60% had laryngeal penetration, 31% with deep laryngeal penetration. When deep penetration occurred, 85% had associated aspiration, most inducible with liquids and after prolonged feeding times.

Radionuclide studies that are useful in the diagnosis of aspiration include the scintiscan and the salivagram (Cook, Lawless, Mandell, & Reilly, 1997). Both are performed using technecium colloid to follow the course of secretions. The scintiscan follows the course of refluxate from the stomach into the hypopharynx and sometimes the lungs (2° aspiration). The salivagram follows the course of saliva from the mouth into the lungs (1° aspiration). The scintiscan is used primarily for evaluation of GERD/EERD, but delayed scanning from 4 up to 24 hours after the ingested radioactive material may reveal radioactivity in the lungs. Similarly, the salivagram uses radionuclide tracer placed in the mouth and mixed with saliva. Detection of tracer in the lungs 1 hour later is diagnostic (Cook et al., 1997; Cook, Lawless, & Kettrick, 1996). Interested radiologists and special equipment are necessary.

FEES utilizes FFNL (with direct visualization of the larynx and hypopharynx) combined with contrast highlight of secretions using food dye during a swallow (Hartnick, Miller, Hartley, & Willging, 2000; Kaye et al., 1997; Liu, Kaplan, Parides, & Close, 2000; Willging, 2000). Saliva, food, and liquids are enhanced, usually using green food coloring. A team of an otolaryngologist who passes the scope and a speech–language pathologist, who does the feeding, is most effective. When sensory testing is desired, a side port on the flexible scope may deliver a blast of air to the arytenoid area. This is known as flexible endoscopic evaluation of swallow with sensory testing (FEES/ST) (Liu et al.; Link, Willging, Miller, Cotton, & Rudolph, 2000). During FEES, swallowing function parameters most often measured include pooling of secretions, laryngeal penetration, aspiration, laryngeal adductor response (sensory testing), vocal fold mobility, and presence of a gag reflex. Aspiration correlates best to observation of frank aspiration, pooled secretions (Figure 10–6), and laryngeal penetration (Link et al.). A more complete discussion of the procedure is found in Chapter 8.

Direct visualization of the larynx, tracheobronchial tree, and esophagus can yield important information not available using other studies. Rigid laryngoscopy affords detailed evaluation of the interarytenoid area to assess for the presence of a laryngeal cleft. Excessive lingual tonsillar tissue may support the diagnosis of GERD/EERD (Figure 10–7). Bronchoscopy may uncover a tracheoesophageal fistula (TEF) (Chapter 4) or evidence of chronic aspiration. The normal tracheobronchial tree is shown in Figure 10–8. Chronic aspiration associated with GERD/EERD reveals severe mucosal cobblestoning (Figure 4–5), loss of tracheal rings secondary to mucosal edema, and blunting of the carina (Carr et al., 2000). Evaluation of secretions or washings often reveals markedly elevated amylase levels (greater than 500 u/ml), lipid laden macrophages (Figure 10–9) (Bauer & Lyrene, 1999; Colombo & Hallberg, 1987; Delzell et al., 1999; Nussbaum, Maggi, Mathis, & Galant, 1987), glucose from enteral feeds (Metheny, St. John, & Clouse, 1998), and, available in some tertiary care settings, traces of pepsin, a gastric enzyme. Lipid laden macrophages are nonspecific and can be found in other clinical conditions (Colombo & Hallberg, 1999). Esophagoscopy may identify esophagitis or esophageal strictures, both potential contributors to dysphagia and aspiration.

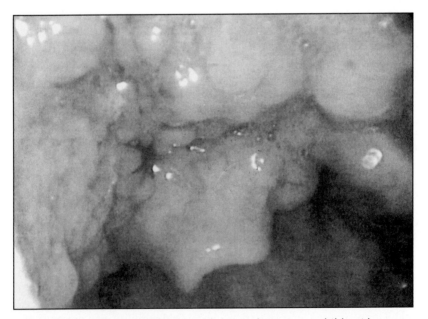

Figure 10–7. Excessive lingual tonsil hyperplasia in a child with severe GERD/EERD and tracheobronchial aspiration.

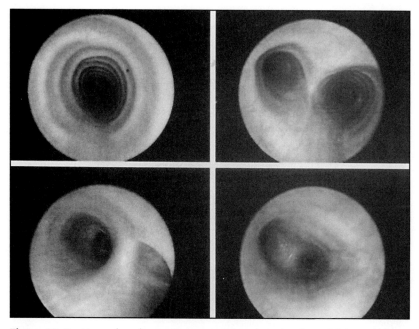

Figure 10–8. Normal endoscopic appearance of tracheobronchial tree. Upper left: note sharply defined tracheal rings at mid-trachea. Upper right: sharp carina, no secretions; Lower left and right: well defined bronchi. No cobblestoning seen.

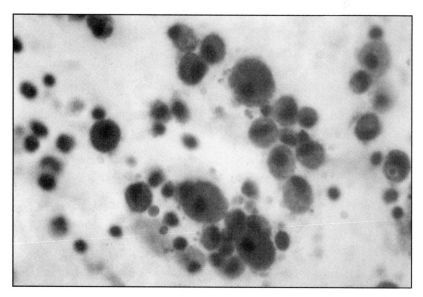

Figure 10–9. Red Oil stain of bronchial secretions positive for large numbers of lipid-laden macrophages.

■ TREATMENT OPTIONS

Treatment of aspiration is highly dependent on the etiology and severity of underlying problems and whether aspiration is 1° or 2°. Ideally, the treatment of aspiration should stop the aspiration, allow normal swallowing, preserve vocalization to communicate, be minimally invasive, and be reversible (Eliachar, Roberts, Hayes, & Tucker, 1987). Unfortunately, no single approach or procedure fulfils all these criteria or is applicable in most cases (Table 10–3) (Baron & Dedo, 1980; Eisele, Seely, Flint, & Cummings, 1995; Eliachar et al.; Krespi, Pelzer, & Sisson, 1985; Laurian, Shvili, & Zohar, 1986;

Table 10–3. Management Options for Chronic Aspiration

Noninvasive
- Swallow therapy
- Alterations in food texture, presentation, rate of eating
- Oral–motor therapy
- Posture therapy for swallowing
- Pulmonary toilet

Medical
- Treat GERD/EERD
- Treat drooling (anticholinergics)

Surgical
- Salivary gland surgery (saliva reduction procedures)
- Gastrostomy tube/patient nonoral (useful only if secretions are not a problem)
- Tracheotomy (for pulmonary toilet)
- Aspiration procedures[a] (voice sparing):
    Vocal fold medialization for unilateral adductor vocal fold paralysis
    Vocal fold injection (gelfoam, fat, or collagen)
    Vented laryngeal stent (endoscopically placed)
    Subperichondrial cricoid resection
    Cricopharyngeal myotomy
    Nerve muscle reinnervation for adductor vocal fold paralysis
- Complete separation—potentially reversible:
    Epiglottic flap
    Laryngeal diversion
    Laryngotracheal separation (Figure 10–10A–D)
    Glottic/subglottic closure
    Gastroesophageal separation
- Complete separation—irreversible:
    Laryngectomy[b]

[a]Almost all require a tracheotomy to maintain the airway.
[b]Rarely performed today.

Sasaki, Milmoe, Berry, & Kirchner, 1980; Tucker, 1993; Weisberger, 1991). Cessation of oral alimentation is recommended until both aspiration context and severity are identified. For patients with mild degrees of neuromuscular impairment and trace or mild aspiration, noninvasive techniques should be tried and are described in detail in Chapter 9. Briefly, change in bolus volume, texture, temperature and rate of bolus delivery, posture manipulation, swallow therapy, and exercises to enhance oral sensation may prove to be useful. Vigorous pulmonary toilet can also be helpful to elicit a more effective

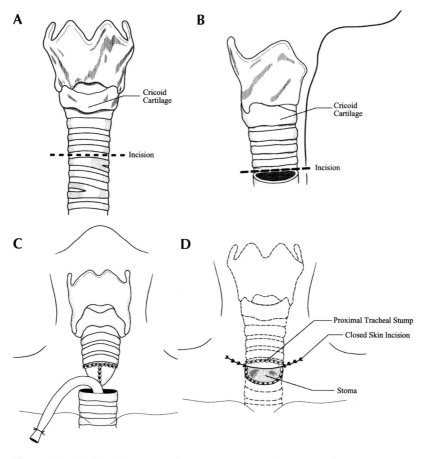

Figure 10–10A–D. Diagrammatic representation of laryngotracheal separation. A. Incision in neck is made low over the third to fourth tracheal rings. B. The larynx and trachea are incised. C. An endotracheal tube is used to secure the airway. The proximal stump is closed. Note that the strap muscles are used to secure the proximal anastamosis to prevent fistula formation (not shown in this drawing). D. The trachea is sutured to the skin incision which is closed in layers.

cough response. Underlying medical problems that need to be treated include poor oral hygiene and GERD/EERD (see Chapter 5).

Medical treatment of secretions using anticholinergic pharmacologic agents is usually ineffective in the treatment of posterior drooling with associated aspiration (see Chapter 11); however, salivary gland surgery to reduce the amount of (and not merely redirect) secretions, consisting of ligation of the submandibular ducts or submandibular gland excision along with parotid duct ligation, can be helpful in secretion reduction (Gerber, Gaugler, Myer, & Cotton, 1996; Kelm & Mair, 1999). Careful attention must be paid to hydration to prevent constipation and development of GERD/EERD (Sullivan, 1997).

When long-term treatment is anticipated, alternate routes to meet nutritional needs must be considered. Prolonged, outpatient use of orogastric or nasogastric tubes is not recommended because these tubes are uncomfortable, may irritate mucosal linings, and increase the risk for aspiration. Feeding gastrostomy or jejunostomy tubes are preferred, each having its own advantages and disadvantages (Chapter 5). Feeding gastrostomy tubes have been found by some to increase the incidence of GERD/EERD, particularly in the neurologically impaired child (Jolley, Tunell, & Hoelzer, 1986; Launay et al., 1996). Thus, preoperative evaluation for simultaneous fundoplication should be undertaken when the reflux is moderate to severe and uncontrolled by medical therapy (Putnam, 1998; Sullivan, 1997).

When aspiration continues despite the above recommendations, surgical intervention for airway protection is considered. A tracheotomy is necessary for the maintenance of airway patency. Tracheotomy is not sufficient to prevent or treat the aspiration; in some instances, tracheotomy exacerbates the problem further. Even when a cuffed tube is utilized in older children, the aspirate sits above the cuff and can invade the airway, especially when cuff deflation is undertaken, as should be done every 1–2 hours.

Surgical management of chronic aspiration is reserved for medical failures and choice of procedure ultimately depends on the underlying etiology for the aspiration. In such instances, the prognosis for survival and the patient's quality of life are weighed against the patient's and family's wishes. When a unilateral adductor vocal fold paralysis underlies an incompetent larynx, vocal fold medialization may be helpful, temporarily with gelfoam injections, more permanently with fat or collagen injections or medialization with cartilage, such as described in thyroplasty techniques (Carrau, Pou, Eibling, Murry, & Ferguson, 1999). Subperichondrial partial cricoidectomy has been described to collapse the subglottic airway and facilitate swallowing (Eisele et al., 1995). A vented laryngeal obturator may also be useful (Eliachar et al., 1987). These are voice-saving procedures and therefore have an appeal in selected cases.

Other surgical procedures for aspiration endeavor to completely separate the air and food passages (Cook et al., 1996; Hensel et al., 1997;

Laurian et al., 1986; Sasaki et al., 1980; Tucker, 1993). Except for gastroe-sophageal separation (Bianchi, 1997), loss of vocalization for communica-tion invariably accompanies such procedures,. Thus, separation procedures involving the airway are reserved for patients with no oral communication or for those in extreme life-threatening situations (Case Study 2). If any pos-sibility of oral communication exists, procedures that are potentially reversible should be considered. The wide variety described here indicates that no single procedure meets the need of every patient. Each situation demands careful, individualized assessment to ensure the most conservative but effective approach to the vexing problems of chronic aspiration.

■ CASE STUDIES

Case Study 1

"Kathy" is a 17-year-old young woman who has cardiomyopathy and a degenerative muscular disorder of unknown etiology. She was ambulatory and eating normally until she suffered a cerebrovascular accident, which left her with a left-sided hemiparesis. Subsequently, she was admitted to the intensive care unit in respiratory failure. Inability to be weaned from the ventilator led to the placement of a tracheotomy.

After the tracheotomy, Kathy was weaned from the ventilator. While on a ventilator, she had been fed by nasoduodenal tube feedings; however, she had lost quite a bit of weight and was now malnourished. Once off the ventilator, oral feeds were resumed, but it soon became apparent that food and liquid were coming out of her tracheotomy tube, indicating that aspi-ration was a problem. Oral feeds were stopped, and a VFSS was ordered. The patient's medical condition did not allow for completion of the study. FFNL was performed and showed glottal incompetence and a right, adduc-tor vocal fold paralysis. Aspiration of secretions was readily apparent, and no further evaluation of swallow was warranted at that time.

Kathy became depressed over her inability to eat; however, she did not want to lose function of her voice. After lengthy discussions with Kathy and her family, microlaryngoscopy with gelfoam injection was offered to achieve glottal competence. Despite her compromised cardiac status, the procedure was performed under general anesthesia without complications. One week later, FFNL revealed good glottic closure with phonation and no aspiration of secretions. FEES showed reasonable swallow function for solids, with lit-tle to no residue. Drinking single sips of liquids slowly had no adverse effect; however, faster rates (gulps and consecutive swallows) of ingestion of liquid resulted in hypopharyngeal pooling without aspiration. This failed to clear after several swallows, thus keeping her at some risk for aspiration.

Recommendations were made for solid and pureed textures, eaten slowly, with close monitoring of pulmonary status. Liquids would be thickened for single sips initially. Nutritional needs were supplemented by a feeding gastrostomy tube inserted using the percutaneous endoscopic gastrostomy (PEG) technique (see Chapter 5). She was transferred to cardiac rehabilitation where she is gaining strength and awaiting a heart transplant. It is anticipated that reevaluation of her larynx will be necessary in 6 to 8 weeks to assess the need for another vocal fold injection. It is hoped that eventually, as she gains strength, muscle mass, and swallowing abilities, that further vocal fold injections or permanent medialization will not be necessary. If after 9 months, glottal incompetence and swallowing dysfunction with aspiration persists, further surgery will be offered to this patient.

Comment

Kathy represents an unusual presentation of cerebrovascular accident in a teenager. The needs to treat her malnutrition, preserve her voice for communication, provide the pleasure of oral feeding, and treat her severe aspiration challenged the clinicians to work closely and creatively with the patient and family. Long-term, close follow-up will be necessary to optimize the final outcome.

Case Study 2

"Robin" is a $3\frac{1}{2}$-year-old girl who presented to the otolaryngology service for tracheotomy. She had suffered bacterial meningitis at the age of 12 months and was left with severe neurologic impairment. Robin was completely dependent on her family for feeding and all other care. Since the meningitis, she had been hospitalized 12 times in $2\frac{1}{2}$ years for aspiration pneumonia, spending 1 to 2 months in the intensive care unit with several of these episodes.

Robin's past medical history included a feeding gastrostomy and Nissen fundoplication for severe gastroesophageal reflux. No oral feedings were given because of severe oral defensiveness. She received medication for reactive airway disease. The family denied snoring, gagging, choking, or laryngeal gurgling sounds except when she had a pneumonia. Robin had no functional oral communication.

Physical examination revealed a 3-year-old, well-nourished child with copious oral secretions. There were no spontaneous movements of her extremities. She had a social smile for her mother and was otherwise minimally aware of her surroundings. Respiratory efforts were increased, but no frank stridor or stertor was noted. Cough and gag reflexes were absent. Auscultation of the larynx revealed laryngeal gurgling; auscultation of the lungs revealed diffuse wheezing.

Flexible nasopharyngolaryngoscopy revealed copious secretions in her hypopharynx. She had no sensation in her larynx. Oral secretions were flowing freely through the true vocal folds. A CT scan of the chest revealed pulmonary changes consistent with chronic aspiration (Figure 10–4).

Although the parents were expecting tracheotomy to be recommended, laryngotracheal separation was recommended instead (Cook et al., 1996). Extensive discussions ensued to explain why the tracheotomy was not sufficient and separation was required. Their concerns about reversibility were genuine, although somewhat unrealistic. A low tracheotomy was created to have sufficient trachea superiorly for potential reversal. The recurrent laryngeal nerves were exposed and preserved. Postoperatively, Robin continued to have pulmonary problems and occasional pneumonia. These were thought to be secondary to her chronic lung disease from years of aspiration. Vigorous pulmonary toilet, judicious use of oral and inhaled antibiotics, and bronchodilators have been useful. She has been hospitalized only once in the past 2 years. At age 5, she continues to live at home, has less oral defensiveness, and has been tasting foods for pleasure. She has been joined by a new baby sister and obviously gives and receives great pleasure from her family.

Comment

Advances in medicine have allowed patients to survive from a once-fatal disease; however, and unfortunately, these individuals suffer devastating effects on neurologic function. Despite these terrible tragedies, many families are confronted with children with limited abilities and enormous care requirements. Robin's family had come to expect a tracheotomy but the physicians caring for her had to work with them to accept the separation procedure. Robin is doing well and has enjoyed significant improvements in the quality of her own life, as well as that of her family.

■ REFERENCES

Arvedson, J., & Lefton-Greif, M. A. (1998). *Pediatric videofluoroscopic swallow studies: A professional manual with caregiver guidelines.* San Antonio, TX: Communication Skill Builders.

Arvedson, J., Rogers, B., Buck, G., Smart, P., & Msall, M. (1994). Silent aspiration prominent in children with dysphagia. *International Journal Pediatric Otorhinolaryngology, 28,* 173–181.

Baron, B., & Dedo, H. (1980). Separation of the larynx and trachea for intractable aspiration. *Laryngoscope, 90,* 1927–1932.

Bauer, M., Figueroa-Colon, R., Georgeson, K., & Young, D. (1993). Chronic pulmonary aspiration in children. *Southern Medical Journal, 86,* 789–795.

Bauer, M., & Lyrene, R. (1999). Chronic aspiration in children: Evaluation of the lipid-laden macrophage index. *Pediatric Pulmonology, 28,* 94–100.

Bianchi, A. (1997). Total esophagogastric dissociation: An alternative approach. *Journal of Pediatric Surgery, 32,* 1291–1294.

Bonilla, J. A., Pizzuto, M., Brodsky, L., & Brody, A. (1998). Absent epiglottis—a rare congenital anomalie. *Ear, Nose and Throat Journal, 77,* 51–55.

Bowrey, D., Peters, J., & DeMeester, T. (2000). Gastroesophageal reflux disease in asthma: Effects of medical and surgical antireflux therapy on asthma control. *Annals of Surgery, 231,* 161–172.

Carr, M., Nguyen, A., Nagy, M., Poje, C., Pizzuto, M., & Brodsky, L. (2000). Clinical presentation as a guide to the identification of GERD in children. *International Journal of Pediatric Otorhinolaryngology, 54,* 27–32.

Carrau, R. L., Pou, A., Eibling, D. E., Murry, T., & Ferguson, B. J., (1999). Laryngeal framework surgery for the management of aspiration. *Head & Neck Surgery,* 139–145.

Cohen, S., & Thompson, J. (1987). Variants of Mobius syndrome and central neurologic impairment: Lindeman procedure in children. *Annals of Otology, Rhinology and Laryngology, 100,* 93–100.

Colombo, J., & Hallberg, T. (1987). Recurrent aspiration in children: Lipid laden alveolar macrophage quantitation. *Pediatric Pulmonology, 3,* 86–89.

Colombo, J., & Hallberg, T. (1999). Pulmonary aspiration and lipid-laden macrophages: In search of gold (standards). *Pediatric Pulmonology, 28,* 79–82.

Cook, S. P., Lawless, S. T., & Kettrick, R. (1996). Patient selection for primary laryngotracheal separation as treatment of chronic aspiration in the impaired child. *International Journal of Pediatric Otorhinolaryngology, 38,* 103–113.

Cook, S., Lawless, S., Mandell, G., & Reilly, J. (1997). The use of the salivagram in the evaluation of severe and chronic aspiration. *International Journal of Pediatric Otorhinolaryngology, 41,* 353–361.

Delzell, P., Kraus, R., Gaisie, G., & Lerner, G. (1999). Laryngeal penetration: A predictor of aspiration in infants? *Pediatric Radiology, 29,* 762–765.

Eisele, D., Seely, D., Flint, P., & Cummings, C. (1995). Subperichondrial cricoidectomy: An alternative to laryngectomy for intractable aspiration. *The Laryngoscope, 105,* 322–325.

Eliachar, I., Roberts, J. K., Hayes, J. D., & Tucker, H. M. (1987). A vented laryngeal stent with phonatory and pressure relief capability. *Laryngoscope, 87,* 1264–1269.

Friedman, B., & Frazier, J. B. (2000). Deep laryngeal penetration as a predictor of aspiration. *Dysphagia, 15,* 153–158.

Gerber, M. E., Gaugler, M. D., Myer, C. M. III, & Cotton, R. T. (1996). Chronic aspiration in children. When are bilateral submandibular gland excision and parotid duct ligation indicated? *Archives of Otolaryngology Head and Neck Surgery, 122,* 1368–1371.

Hartnick, C., Miller, C., Hartley, B., & Willging, J. (2000). Pediatric fiberoptic endoscopic evaluation of swallowing. *Annals of Otology, Rhinology and Laryngology, 109,* 996–999.

Hensel, M., Haake, K., Vogel, S., Flugel, W., Krausch, D., & Kox, W. (1997). Management of swallowing disorders and chronic aspiration by glottic closure procedure. *Journal of Neurosurgical Anesthesiology, 9,* 273–276.

Holinger, L., & Sanders, A. (1991). Chronic cough in infants and children: An update. *Laryngoscope, 101,* 596–605.

Jolley, S. G., Tunell, W. P., & Hoelzer, D. J. (1986). Lower esophageal pressure changes with tube gastrostomy: A causative factor of gastroesophageal reflux in children? *Journal of Pediatric Surgery, 21,* 624–627.

Kaye, G. M., Zorowitz, R. D., & Baredes, S. (1997). Role of flexible laryngoscopy in evaluating aspiration. *Annals of Otology, Rhinology, & Laryngology, 106,* 705–709.

Kelm, C., & Mair, E. (1999). Four-duct ligation: A simple and effective treatment for chronic aspriation from sialorrhea. *Archives of Otolaryngology Head and Neck Surgery, 125,* 796–800.

Krespi, Y., Pelzer, H., & Sisson, G. (1985). Management of chronic aspiration by subtotal and submucosal cricoid resection. *Annals of Otology Rhinology and Laryngology, 94,* 580–583.

Kush C. M., & Sanders, A. (1988). Aspiration pneumonia. Medical management. *Otolaryngologic Clinics of North America, 21,* 677–689.

Launay, V., Gottrand, F., Turck, D., Michaud, L., Ategbo, S., & Farriaux, J. P. (1996). Percutaneous endoscopic gastrostomy in children: Influence on gastroesophageal reflux. *Pediatrics, 97,* 726–728.

Laurian, N., Shvili, Y., & Zohar, Y. (1986). Epiglotto-Aryepiglottopexy: A Surgical Procedure for Severe Aspiration. *The Laryngoscope, 96,* 78–81.

Lefton-Greif, M. A., & Loughlin, G. L. (1996). Specialized studies in pediatric dysphagia. *Seminars in Speech and Language, 17,* 311–330.

Link, D. T., Willging, J., Miller, C. K., Cotton, R., & Rudolph, C. D. (2000). Pediatric laryngopharyngeal sensory testing during flexible endoscopic evaluation of swallowing: Feasible and correlative. *Annals of Otology, Rhinology, and Laryngology, 109,* 899–905.

Liu, H., Kaplan, S., Parides, M., & Close, L. (2000). Laryngopharyngeal sensory deficits in patients with laryngopharyngeal reflux and dysphagia. *Annals of Otology, Rhinology, and Laryngology, 109,* 1000–1006.

Logemann, J. A. (1993). Noninvasive approaches to deglutitive aspiration. *Dysphagia, 8,* 331–333.

Loughlin, G. M., & Lefton-Greif, M. A. (1994). Dysfunctional swallowing and respiratory disease in children. *Advances in Pediatrics, 41,* 135–161.

Lundgren, J., Ekberg, O., & Olsson, R. (1998). Aspiration: A potential complication to vagus nerve stimulation. *Epilepsia, 39,* 998–1000.

Metheny, N. A., St. John, R. E., & Clouse, R. E. (1998). Measurement of glucose in tracheobronchial secretions to detect aspiration of enteral feedings. *Heart and Lung: Journal of Acute and Critical Care, 27,* 285–292.

Nussbaum, E., Maggi, C., Mathis, R., & Galant, S. (1987). Association of lipid-laden alveolar macrophages and gastroesophageal reflux in children. *Journal of Pediatrics, 110,* 190–194.

Orenstein, S. R. (2000). Update on gastroesophageal reflux and respiratory disease in children. *Canadian Journal of Gastroenterology, 14,* 131–135.

Putnam, P. E. (1998). Gastroesophageal reflux. In Bailey, B. (Ed.), *Head & Neck Surgery Otolaryngology* (1144–1156). Philadelphia: Lippincott.

Sasaki, C., Milmoe, G., Berry, K., & Kirchner, J. (1980). Surgical closure of the larynx for intractable aspiration. *Archives Otolaryngology, 106,* 422–423.

Sasaki, C. T., & Toohill, R. J. (2000). Ambulatory pH monitoring for extraesophageal reflux—introduction. *Annals of Otology, Rhinology, & Laryngology, 109* (Suppl.10), 2–3.

Sullivan, P. B. (1997). Gastrointestinal problems in the neurologically impaired child. *Bailliere's Clinical Gastroenterology, 11,* 529–546.

Tucker, H. (1993). Double Barreled Tracheostomy: Long Term Results and Reversibility. *The Laryngoscope, 103,* 212–215.

Weisberger, E. (1991). Treatment of intractable aspiration using a laryngeal stent or obturator. *Annals of Otology, Rhinology and Laryngology, 100,* 101–106.

Willging, J. (2000). Benefit of feeding assessment before pediatric airway reconstruction. *The Laryngoscope, 110,* 825–834.

■ CHAPTER 11

Drooling in Children

Linda Brodsky and Joan Arvedson

■ SUMMARY

Drooling is the abnormal and unintentional spillage of saliva from the mouth onto the face and clothing. Primarily affecting patients with neuromuscular impairments and mental retardation, the need to treat these individuals has become increasingly recognized because greater numbers of children are living beyond early childhood with this condition. Medical problems, social isolation, increased caregiver time, and limited employment opportunities—all of which are associated with drooling—highlight the need for effective control of oral secretions.

The evaluation of drooling begins with an assessment of the severity and impact of the problem on each individual patient. A thorough search for underlying etiologies and other contributing factors is made. Particular attention is devoted to severity of neurologic impairment, posture, medications, airway obstruction, and oral and dental health. The environmental impact on self-image, family, friends, school, and other caregivers is considered. Treatment recommendations may include elimination of situational factors, improved seating, oral–motor therapy, behavioral modification, pharmacotherapy, and surgery. Team assessment results in comprehensive therapeutic recommendations, which are tailored to the unique needs of each patient.

■ INTRODUCTION

Drooling (salivary incompetence, sialorrhea, hypersalivation, ptyalism[1]) is the abnormal, unintentional spilling of saliva from the mouth onto the

---

[1]Although these terms are all used to describe drooling (or sialorrhea), technically speaking they have different meanings. Hypersalivation refers to the excessive production of saliva; ptyalism includes both hypersalivation and drooling.

lips, chin, neck, clothing, and environmental objects. *Posterior drooling* is the term used for secretions that pool in the hypopharynx and contribute to aspiration (see Chapter 10). Gagging, choking, dysphagia, and breathing difficulties are characteristic symptoms found in patients who have trouble with aspiration (Blasco et al., 1992). Most notably, drooling affects children and adults with neuromuscular incoordination, cerebral palsy, mental retardation, learning problems, and structural problems that cause inadequate lip closure or poor oral, oropharyngeal, and hypopharyngeal sensorimotor function. Rarely, otherwise healthy children will have troublesome drooling after the age of 5 years, when most normal children are able to control their secretions.

The magnitude of the problem is difficult to estimate. Cerebral palsy affects approximately 1 in 200 to 300 newborns; 10 to 15% of whom will have severe drooling that requires some type of intervention (Brundage & Moore, 1989; Crysdale, 1989; Crysdale, Greenberg, Koheil, & Moran, 1985; Hussein, Kershaw, Tahmassebi, & Fayle, 1998; Weiss-Lambrou, Tetreault, & Dudley, 1988). Many other disease entities (Hussein et al., 1998; Walker, Hutchinson, Cant, Parmeter, & Knox, 1994) may be associated with drooling (Table 11–1), however.

Drooling is a distressing problem, and its presence may have significant negative effects on the physical, social, and psychological well-being of

Table 11–1. Diseases Associated with Drooling

Neurologic
    Cerebral palsy
    Cranial nerve palsies—VII, IX, and XII
    Global developmental disorder
    Stroke
    Amyotrophic lateral sclerosis
    Down syndrome
    Motor neuron disease
    Parkinsonism
    Congenital suprabulbar palsy

Other
    Head trauma
    Encephalitis
    Heavy metal intoxication
    Grave's disease
    Rabies
    Extra-esophageal reflux disease
    Nasal and/or pharyngeal obstruction
    Major surgical resection of structures in the oral cavity/pharynx/hypopharynx

affected children, their families, and other caregivers. Physical problems associated with excessive drooling include facial chapping, chilling from facial wetness in cold weather, dental caries, lip cracking and fissures, and the possibility of transmission of infectious diseases. Parents and caregivers may have to change the child's clothing or bib 10 to 20 times each day (Figure 11–1). Frequent clothing or bib changes may result in decreased physical contact that then may lead to social isolation and, at times, depression. Furthermore, saliva may be dribbled on the desk, computer keyboard, and

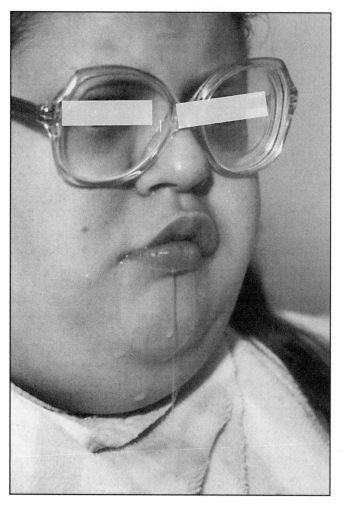

Figure 11–1. Patient with severe drooling onto clothes that occurs continually throughout the day and requires many clothing changes and constant caregiver attention.

other educational and vocational materials, resulting in decreased educational and employment opportunities, particularly for those who are cognitively aware of their environment and social interactions. The increasing inclusion of persons with disabilities in all facets of routine life mandates that we endeavor to correct problems such as drooling so as to facilitate their successful integration into mainstream society.

This chapter first discusses the relevant anatomy, physiology, and pathophysiology of drooling. The evaluation in an interdisciplinary team setting is then described. The range of management options, their rationale, and efficacy are discussed through relevant case studies.

■ ANATOMY, PHYSIOLOGY, AND PATHOPHYSIOLOGY

Approximately 1 liter of saliva per day is produced (0.2 to 2.75 ml/min) in large part (90%) by the three pairs of major salivary glands. The parotid glands are responsible for about 30% of the volume, producing mostly thin, serous secretions. The parotids are located deep in the soft tissues of the cheek, anterior to the ear. The facial nerve, which is intimately associated with the parotid gland, exits the stylomastoid foramen and courses through the parotid gland to animate the muscles of the face. Production of saliva occurs in the acini of the gland; the saliva then drains via smaller ducts into the main duct (Stenson's duct) that empties into the oral cavity after piercing the buccal mucosa opposite the second upper molar.

The submandibular glands produce between 50 and 70% of the saliva. The quality of the secretions is more viscous because of increase in the mucoid component. The submandibular gland is located in the submandibular triangle in the neck and can be palpated below the angle of the mandible. Its secretions drain into the floor of the mouth via Wharton's duct.

The sublingual glands account for about 5% of the saliva and produce predominantly mucoid secretions. These glands are located submucosally in the floor of the mouth and drain through several duct openings there. The remaining saliva is secreted by the minor salivary glands that are located throughout the mucosa and submucosa of the palate and oral cavity.

The innervation that controls the flow of saliva is from the autonomic nervous system and is primarily under parasympathetic control. Sympathetic stimulation may also occur but is thought to be a synergistic effect that results in an increase in the flow of saliva primarily through smooth muscle contraction at the duct level. The neuroanatomy is important for both medical and surgical therapeutic considerations and is therefore described in detail.

Preganglionic parasympathetic fibers to the parotid gland originate in the inferior salivary nucleus in the brain stem (Figure 11–2). They travel

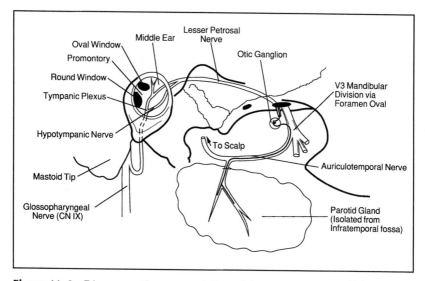

Figure 11–2. Diagrammatic representation of the neuroanatomy of the parotid gland.

with the tympanic branch (Jacobsen's nerve) of the glossopharyngeal nerve (CN IX) through the middle ear, where the nerve is covered only with mucosa or it may lie in a bony canal on the promontory of the middle ear. After receiving a branch from the lesser superficial petrosal nerve, it then goes to the otic ganglion, where it synapses with postganglionic fibers travelling to the parotid gland via the auriculotemporal nerve.

Preganglionic parasympathetic fibers to the submandibular and sublingual glands originate in the superior salivary nucleus in the brain stem (Figure 11–3). They travel with the nervus intermedius of the facial nerve (CN VII) through the geniculate ganglion and into the mastoid portion of the facial nerve. As the chorda tympani, these fibers exit from the mastoid portion of the facial nerve (just above the stylomastoid foramen) and then course anteriorly in the middle ear between the incus and malleus and then anteriorly through the petrotympanic fissure, where they join with the lingual nerve to go to the submaxillary ganglion. After synapsing in the submaxillary ganglion, the postganglionic fibers are distributed to the submandibular and sublingual glands.

Saliva has many functions (Table 11–2). Saliva is important for the digestive system in facilitating chewing and swallowing, as well as initiating the enzymatic breakdown of proteins and carbohydrates in the process of digestion. It provides protection from dental disease and oral infection. Finally, saliva has a role in speech by enabling ease of movement of the

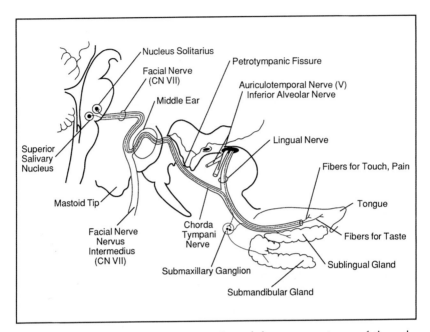

Figure 11–3. Diagrammatic representation of the neuroanatomy of the submandibular and sublingual glands.

Table 11–2. Functions of Saliva

Domain	Function
Digestive	Facilitates chewing
	Initial enzymatic breakdown of food (proteins and carbohydrates)
	Facilitates swallowing
	Enhances taste
	Decreases breath odor
	Protects lower esophageal sphincter from acid
Protective	Maintains oral health—contains gingival crevicular fluid
	Prevents caries/periodontal disease
	Buffers as an antibacterial agent
Speech	Lubricates—facilitates articulation by moistening surface of tongue, lip, and palate

tongue and lips for proper articulation. Thus, any treatment plan that changes the amount, consistency, or flow of saliva in the oral cavity must consider all of these functions.

The amount of saliva produced is not usually the problem in children with drooling. Incoordination and a reduction in the rate of the highly complex, sequential patterns of swallowing are the predominant pathophysiologic mechanisms. Normally, almost 600 swallows per 24 hours are initiated; the number and efficiency, both awake and asleep, are decreased in patients who drool (Hussein et al., 1998; Sochaniwskyj, Koheil, Bablich, Milner, & Kenny, 1986). Inefficient swallow results from the incoordination of the lips, tongue, palate, jaws, pharynx, larynx, and respiratory muscles (described in Chapter 2). Children who are unable to control their saliva have been found to have the greatest difficulty in the oral/voluntary phase of swallowing. More recently, the role of sensory innervation has received substantial attention (Blasco, et al., 1992; Weiss-Lambrou, Tetreault, & Dudley, 1988). Recognition and identification of the role of afferent innervation is particularly important in the assessment of posterior drooling (Hussein et al.).

Although hypersalivation is rarely the cause of severe drooling, certain dental diseases, such as dental caries and gingivitis, can result in increased production of saliva. Medications such as tranquilizers (i.e., clozapine [Hinkes, Quesada, Currier, & Gonzalez-Blanco, 1996], compazine [Twigg, 1996], and the anticonvulsant nitrazepam [Wyllie, Wyllie, Cruse, & Rothner, 1986]) also may result in an increase in the amount of saliva produced or a decrease in the swallow frequency. Other factors that may influence the severity of drooling include: poor body posture and tone; upper airway obstruction from large tonsils, adenoids or a deviated septum; emotional state; and ability to concentrate (Koheil, Sochaniwskyj, Bablich, Kenny, & Milner, 1987) (Table 11–3).

Table 11–3. Situational Factors Operant in Drooling

- Posture—head and trunk
- Medications
- Dental health
- Upper airway obstruction
- Extra-esophageal reflux[a]
- Psychological health

[a]Extra-esophageal reflux is the term for acid reflux that ascends out of the esophagus and adversely affects the upper aerodigestive tract with inflammation and edema, resulting in decreased swallowing, thereby leading to potential for pooling of saliva and subsequent oral incompetence and drooling.

Recognition of the multifactorial nature of drooling is important in guiding the practitioner to evaluate drooling patients carefully. An interdisciplinary assessment and management approach is recommended. The following section describes this evaluation as it is practiced in a tertiary care setting at the Children's Hospital of Buffalo.

■ INTERDISCIPLINARY EVALUATION OF DROOLING

Interdisciplinary refers to an approach in which a patient is evaluated and treated by interactive coordination among several specialists, each with specific expertise to offer in solving a complex problem. Evaluation and subsequent treatment recommendations are made based on the input and shared ideas of a group of people who include not only the specialists involved, but also the children and their parents (or other caregivers). Using an interdisciplinary approach, the treatment plan is reached by consensus and does not rely on a single opinion. Creative problem solving, synergistic innovation, improved collegiality, and protection for the practitioner can result. The family, who may feel pulled among many, often disparate opinions, is thus offered a united, wholistic, coordinated approach. Drooling has the greatest effect on "quality of life" issues, and therefore therapeutic choices may be less obvious. A deliberate and thoughtful consensus approach is highly effective and greatly appreciated by families.

Many approaches to the child with drooling have appeared in the literature over the past 30 years, which indicate that no single approach is suitable for every patient (Becmeur et al., 1996; Blasco, Allaire, et al., 1992; Brundage & Moore, 1989; Camp-Bruno, Winsberg, & Green-Parsons, 1989; Cotton, 1981; Dunn, Cunningham, & Backman, 1987; Fear, Hitchcock, & Fonseca, 1988; Harris & Purdy, 1987; Koheil et al., 1987; Maisel, 1982; Moulding & Koroluk, 1991; O'Dwyer, Timon, & Walsh, 1989; Shott, Myer, & Cotton, 1989; Trott & Maechtlen, 1986; Wilkie, 1967; Wilkie & Brody, 1977; Hussein et al., 1998). The concept of team evaluation and management was first introduced by Crysdale and co-workers in 1985 (Crysdale et al., 1985). The model described here is based on their work with modification based on 12 years of experience and more than 400 patients treated.

First, a detailed characterization of the drooling helps to classify its severity, functional impairment, and impact on patient and family. Both the speech–language pathologist (SLP) and the otolaryngologist obtain separate histories to characterize fully and corroborate the drooling problem. Oral, oropharyngeal, and hypopharyngeal sensorimotor functions and swallowing evaluations are performed at the same time by the SLP. The pediatric dentist performs a thorough assessment of the level and effectiveness of dental care, including the gingiva, teeth, and maxillary and mandibular occlusal relationships as affecting production and control of saliva. The occupational therapist evaluates the contribution that posture, particularly control of head and trunk, have on drooling. The pediatric otolaryngologist is responsible for the overall medical evaluation, as well as a detailed evaluation of the upper aerodigestive tract. Neurologists, physiotherapists, psychologists, pediatric gastroenterologists, and developmental pediatricians are consulted as needed.

The family is prepared beforehand for a lengthy first visit so that each team member has enough time to complete the evaluation. The team discusses each patient before making final recommendations. A conference with the family and other caregivers is held to discuss the rationale for the recommendations made and to implement the treatment plan. Sometimes the team must reconsider initial recommendations, and the family must be consulted again before a treatment plan is implemented. This process is described in detail below, and examples are presented in the case studies at the end of the chapter.

Assessment of Drooling and Oral Sensorimotor Function—Role of the Speech-Language Pathologist

The role of the SLP is to assess the impact of the drooling in qualitative and quantitative terms. This includes an in-depth interview with the caregivers to focus on the amount, timing, extent, contributing habits, and untoward social and psychologic effects of the drooling. A classification system to quantify the disability has been proposed by Crysdale and White (1989) and is presented in modified form in Table 11–4. The number of clothing or bib changes, child's neurologic function, educational setting, and communication modalities are also assessed. Some investigators advocate quantifying the amount of saliva (Heine, Catto-Smith, & Reddihough, 1996; Sochaniwskyj et al., 1986). We do not advocate precise quanitification because the effects of varying amounts of drooling on more or less cognitively aware individuals are not taken into account with this approach. Our preferred approach is to address qualitative issues as a whole in a framework of the child, the family, and the day-to-day interactions that are affected.

The intellectual/cognitive level, speech production efficiency, and language function are assessed. It is rare that speech production is normal in a child who drools. The strength and coordination of the lips, jaw, and tongue are determined; perioral and intraoral sensitivity, gag reflex, and swallowing function are assessed (Chapter 7). Special attention is given to the presence of dysphagia, particularly if aspiration has been a problem in the past or if symptoms that raise the level of suspicion are uncovered. Approximately 15% of patients presenting to the interdisciplinary team,

Table 11–4. Functional Classification of Drooling[a]

Description	Severity	Frequency	Functional Effects
0—Absent	Dry, never drools	Never	None
1—Mild	To lips only	Not every day, on occasion	Minimal except in individuals with high cognitive and social function
2—Moderate	Lip and chin	Every day with some dry periods	Moderate to severe, depending on functional and cognitive level and associated physical problems
3—Severe	Clothing soiled	Constant	Severely limiting and isolating
4—Profuse	Clothing, hands, and table wet	Constant	Severely limiting and isolating

Note. Modified from "Submandibular Duct Relocation for Drooling: A 10-year Experience with 194 Patients" by W. S. Crysdale and A. White, 1989, *Otolaryngology—Head and Neck Surgery, 101,* pp. 87–92.
[a]In addition to drooling severity classification, the neurologic status of the patient and an impact analysis on the life of the child and/or caregivers is determined and used in treatment recommendations. In general, those patients with more profound neurologic impairment will require multiple therapeutic interventions, one of which usually includes surgery.

will undergo videofluoroscopic swallow study to assess the presence of microaspiration or silent aspiration (unpublished data, Brodsky & Gillihan) (Chapter 10).

Previous management of the drooling is explored in depth to assess exactly which treatments were employed and how each was performed. In particular, an oral–motor program may have been initiated in the past, but the exact content, frequency of administration, and techniques used may need to be reassessed and then reapplied. The attitudes of the patient, if possible, and all those concerned with his or her care are recorded and utilized in making treatment recommendations.

The Role of the Pediatric Dentist

The pediatric dentist evaluates the condition of the teeth, gingiva, and maxillary and mandibular occlusal relationships. Dental caries are a common and treatable cause for increased salivation. Repair is mandatory not only for the drooling, but also for the general well-being of the patient (Figure 11–4). Developmentally disabled persons tend to receive less frequent and vigorous dental care, the result of which is periodontal disease and chronic gingivitis (Figure 11–5). Disorders of malocclusion that may be attributable primarily to neuromuscular hypotonia or secondary to chronic nasal obstruction (see below) may also lead to an open bite posture with decreased oral sphincteric function and consequent loss of saliva.

The pediatric dentist takes an active role in counseling the family regarding fluoride use, oral hygiene habits, and dietary advice. Regular professional scaling and polishing are recommended. Procedures to seal fissures, repair caries, and restore the gingiva to health may be needed.

The Role of the Occupational Therapist

The evaluation of truncal posture and head control is the same for children who drool as it is for those undergoing any feeding evaluation. This is described in detail in Chapter 7.

The Role of the Pediatric Otolaryngologist

The pediatric otolaryngologist assesses the overall medical status of the patient, including past medical and surgical histories, review of systems,

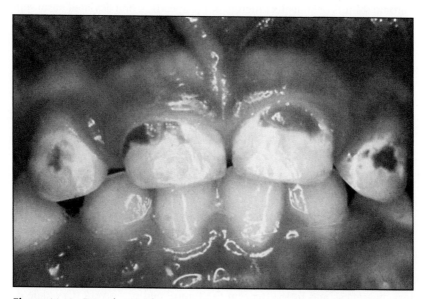

Figure 11–4. Dental caries leading to increased production of saliva.

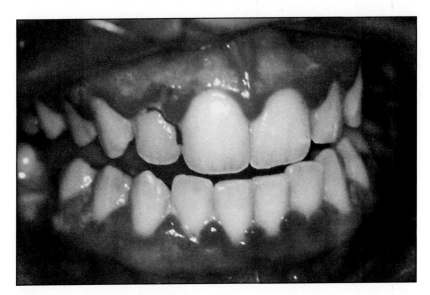

Figure 11–5. Periodontal disease.

medications, neurologic status, and, in particular, the structures of the upper aerodigestive tract. Nasal obstruction from enlarged adenoids, chronic rhinitis or sinusitis (allergic or nonspecific), or a deviated nasal septum may be contributing factors to obligate mouth breathing and an open mouth posture. These should be corrected when present before other therapy is initiated. Enlarged obstructing tonsils or an enlarged, protrusive tongue may both adversely affect the control of saliva. The otolaryngologist also does an independent assessment of the attitudes of the caregivers and reviews the previous treatment modalities. As the physician responsible for the overall treatment recommendations, his or her role as an advocate for the multiply impaired child is critical.

■ MANAGEMENT ISSUES IN DROOLING

Therapeutic recommendations are based on the severity of the drooling, previous interventions, level of neurologic dysfunction, and the attitudes of the patient and family. A child who is less affected but more cognitively aware of the problem may suffer a greater degree of social isolation and disability from the drooling than one with a greater degree of drooling with less awareness and little effect on the family and caregivers (Crysdale & White, 1989). The range of therapeutic choices is presented in Table 11–5.

Table 11–5. Treatment Options for Drooling

Reassurance
    No reassessment
    Reassessment

Eliminate situational factors
    Posture control
    Dental caries, gingivitis, severe malocclusion
    Upper aerodigestive obstruction or inflammation

Therapies
    Oral–motor therapy
    Behavior modification
    Biofeedback
    Hypnotherapy

Pharmacologic treatment
    Benztropine
    Saltropine
    Scopolamine
    Robinul

Surgery
    Wharton's duct relocation, sublingual gland excision
    Submandibular gland excision, parotid duct ligation

Miscellaneous
    Dental prostheses
    Radiation

Multimodal therapy may be most successful and should be considered as needed. A suggested treatment algorithm is shown in Figure 11–6.

In general, the optimal therapy should be minimally invasive, of substantial benefit for the majority of severe droolers, safe, and cost-effective. Side effects should be few, and the therapy should have no permanent adverse sequelae even if it is successful (Camp-Bruno, Winsberg, & Green-Parsons, 1989). The range of therapies listed in Table 11–5 presents clear evidence that no one therapy satisfies all of these requirements (Harris & Purdy, 1987). It is incumbent on clinicians to entertain the many options available and to keep an open mind when recommending a treatment plan.

Reassurance

Some normal children will continue to have occasional drooling up to the age of 5 years. Conversely, continued drooling may be symptomatic of a

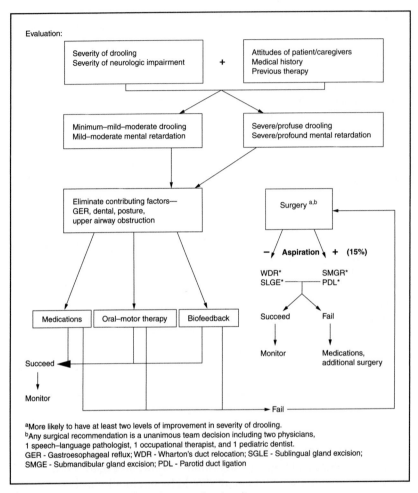

Figure 11–6. Treatment flow diagram for drooling.

child with as-yet-unrecognized focal or global neurologic impairment. Even children with severe developmental disabilities may have significant improvement of their drooling through these early childhood years; therefore, caution must be exercised in making recommendations for this group. Most will have been receiving speech–language therapy that usually, but not always, includes an oral–motor program (see below). It is recommended that before determining the success or failure of a particular modality, a 6- to 9-month plateau in the status of the drooling is observed so that further spontaneous improvement is not encountered, particularly in younger patients. As with all patients who drool, contributing factors should be identified and treated, no matter the age.

Some severely affected children may have other significant medical problems that make the drooling problem very low on the priority list. In addition, if the available options present significant medical risk, no treatment may be the wisest course of action.

Eliminate Situational Factors

Certain situational factors may lead to increased drooling (Table 11–3). Treatment of dental problems, chronic nasal obstruction with obligate mouth breathing, enlarged tonsils, extra-esophageal reflux disease, and poor posture may lead to a significant decrease in the drooling and obviate the need for further therapy (Case Study 1). The dentist is helpful in improving the oral health and, in some cases, the orthodontic correction of malocclusion or in extreme cases orthognathic surgery. Prosthetic management with a lip plumper prosthesis (Moulding & Koroluk, 1991) may be useful in select cases.

An assessment of the medications may reveal one that stimulates salivary secretion; in such cases, consultation with the primary care physician or neurologist may result in a medication change. Correction of a deviated septum, enlarged tonsils or adenoids, chronic hypertrophic rhinitis (both allergic and nonallergic), and, in rare instances, macroglossia may be effective if related to the drooling problem.

Nonmedical and Nonsurgical Options

Oral–Motor Programs

Oral–motor therapy is intended to increase coordinated muscle function in the oral cavity and to improve swallowing and control of secretions. These programs are the mainstay of nonmedical/nonsurgical therapy for neurologically impaired patients who drool and are usually initiated at a very early age as part of a total rehabilitation program (Blasco et al., 1992; Harris & Purdy, 1987; Hussein et al., 1998; Walker et al., 1994). The particulars of such a program are discussed in detail in Chapter 9. The efficacy for persons who drool is as yet unknown.

Speech–language pathologists, with their expertise in the related acts of speech and swallowing, are best qualified to carry out these programs. The position, mobility, strength of the tongue, lips, jaw, and head control are the most important aspects of an oral–motor program. An occupational therapist, a physical therapist, or both can be helpful in some settings, particularly in positioning issues, wheelchair design, and adaptive feeding tools. Carryover into the home and classroom is highly desirable for optimal results. When combined with behavioral modification, these techniques may be particularly helpful for those who have higher intellectual function and some voluntary control over oral sensorimotor function.

Behavioral Programs

Behavior modification (Dunn et al., 1987; Trott & Maechtlen, 1986) and biofeedback (Koheil et al., 1987) are applicable for a small group of patients who are highly motivated (along with the families and other caregivers) and who have the intellectual capacity to perform these techniques. The intention of these therapies is to increase the sensory awareness and voluntary swallowing rate. Timing devices with auditory signals (Rapp, 1980), chin cups combined with oral–motor therapy (Harris & Dignam, 1980), and auditory feedback using electromyography (EMG) in training the orbicularis oris muscle (Koheil et al., 1987) are a few examples. Overcorrection with the use of praise for a dry face and tissue-pressing to the lower lips has been recommended (Trott & Maechtlen). Hypnotherapy also has been suggested.

These management approaches are all time-consuming and labor intensive, and when used alone, the reduction in drooling is modest at best. Approximately 30% of patients treated with a 9-month course of oral–motor therapy, behavior modification, or both will have a modest improvement (17%) or totally resolve their drooling (6%) after completion (Brodsky & Gillihan, unpublished data). Regression may occur once the stimulants for behavioral change are removed. The use of biofeedback and behavior modification should be considered in select patients before or in concert with other treatments, such as chronic medication or posture control. Relapse is common, especially as the patient ages.

Miscellaneous

Prosthetic devices are helpful in some patients and are usually made by the dentist (Hussein et al., 1998). Radiation therapy may be safe and effective but is limited to the elderly (Borg & Hirst, 1998) in which the potential for radiation-induced malignancy is less of a concern.

Pharmacologic Therapy

Those patients who come to the attention of a salivary management/drooling team usually require additional treatment above and beyond oral–motor therapy and behavior modification. Pharmacotherapy alone may have a useful role in many patients, especially those with mild to moderate drooling and mild to moderate mental retardation. However, added benefit may be gained from medications when some drooling persists after oral–motor therapy, behavior modification, or surgery (Case Study 2).

Several different medications with anti-cholinergic activity are available and thereby provide the opportunity for combination therapy. The anticholinergics benztropine, saltropine, glycopyrrolate, and scopolamine have received the most attention for use in this population (Talmi, Zohar, Laurian, & Finkelstein, 1988; Luetje & Pharm, 1996; Wilkinson, 1987; Camp-Bruno et al., 1989; Klein, Reed, & Ashenburg, 1985; Spivack et al., 1997; Stern, 1997; Bachrach, Walter, & Trzcinski, 1998; Blasco & Stansbury, 1996). Response rates are unpredictable and highly variable (Camp-Bruno et al.). Of patients treated, 45% can expect no change in their drooling, 30% minimal to modest improvement, and 20% complete resolution. Some have maintained an excellent result for more than five years (Brodsky and Gillihan, unpublished data).

Anticholinergic medications inhibit salivary secretion by a reversible blockade of the cholinergic receptors that control salivary secretion. Side effects such as dry mouth, pupilary dilation, blurred vision, urinary retention, constipation, confusion, and disorientation have been reported and were found in 5 to 15% of our population necessitating discontinuance of the medication. Drug interactions with other medications must also be considered. Commonly used medications, mechanism of action, dosing, route, and potential side effects are listed in Table 11–6.

Surgical Treatment Options

Historic Perspective

Surgery for severe drooling was first described in 1967 when Wilkie popularized the use of parotid duct transposition to reroute salivary flow more posteriorly in the oral cavity. When submandibular gland excision was added to this procedure, 85% success rate was reported (Wilkie & Brody, 1977).

During the 1960s and 1970s, interruption of the innervation for salivary flow was often undertaken for drooling (Benedek-Spat & Szekely, 1985; Chilla, de Paula Lima, Droese, & Aglebe, 1985; Golding-Wood, 1962; Grewal, Hiranandani, Rangwalla, & Sheode, 1984;). The rationale for nerve section is based on the parasympathetic innervation of all three salivary glands. The chorda tympani section disrupts fibers going to the submandibular and sublingual glands (Figure 11–3), and the tympanic neurectomy disrupts the fibers of the tympanic branch of CN IX

Table 11–6. Medications Used to Decrease Drooling

Medication	Chemical Makeup	Mechanism of Action	Dose	Route	Additional Side Effects
Benztropine mesylate (Cogentin)	Synthetic compound similar to antihistamine and tertiary ammonium compound	Antimuscarinin Antihistaminic	0.5–2 mg twice daily	Oral	Listlessness Heat intolerance
Glycopyrrolate (Robinul)	Quaternary ammonium compound with limited crossing of blood–brain barrier	Anticholinergic	0.02–0.07 mg/ kg/dose three times daily	Oral or parenteral	Irritability Skin flushing Headaches
Scopolamine (Transderm Scopolamine patch)	Tertiary ammonium compound	Anticholinergic	1 patch every 3 days	Transdermal	Skin irritation
Atropine sulfate (Sal-Tropine)	Tertiary ammonium compound	Anticholinergic	0.1 mg (7–16 lbs) 0.15 mg (17–24 lbs) 0.2mg (24–40 lbs) 0.3 mg (40–65 lbs) 0.4 mg (65 lbs and over) three times daily	Oral	Tachycardia Skin flushing

Jacobsen's nerve (that goes to the parotid) as it passes over the promontory in the middle ear (Figure 11–2).

The technique requires a middle ear approach and is relatively straightforward. The success rate has been reported to be between 47 and 100% (Friedman & Kaplan, 1975; Goode & Smith, 1970; Michel, Johnson, & Patterson, 1977; Toremalm & Bjerre, 1976; Townsend, Morimoto, & Kraleman, 1973). However, long-term efficacy is questionable as it is believed that these crossed fibers tend to regenerate (Crysdale, 1989a, 1989b; Parisier, Blitzer, Binder, Friedman, & Marovitz, 1978; Shott, Myer, & Cotton, 1989). Disadvantages include the loss of taste, possible caries, and an operative procedure in the middle ear in a population with a high incidence of otitis media. However, the use of nerve section may be helpful in augmenting a less than optimal response from salivary gland surgery (see below) (Sellars, 1985).

Modern Surgical Approaches

In general, surgery is reserved for patients who continue to drool after correction of contributing factors, who experience failure with nonsurgical therapy, or in whom the severity of the mental retardation and the drooling is so great that it is unlikely other therapies will be successful. No single surgical procedure is appropriate for all patients. Surgical options are divided into two categories: those that reduce the amount of saliva produced and those that divert the saliva posteriorly so that spontaneous swallowing may occur more readily. However, in patients who are at risk for aspiration, reduction in production of saliva is preferred. A summary of the surgical options most commonly in use, success rates, advantages, and disadvantages are listed in Table 11–7.

Parotid Duct Transposition/Ligation

Wilkie (1967) popularized the use of parotid duct transposition to reroute the flow of saliva more posteriorly in the oral cavity for easier swallowing. Wilkie and Brody (1977) advocated the addition of submandibular gland excision to improve results. A high success rate (85%) has been cited; however, the tedious nature of the surgery and possible stenosis of the duct make this approach less popular, although still advocated by some today (Becmeur et al., 1996).

Ligation of the parotid duct when combined with submandibular gland excision (see below) has been reported to have an 88 to 100% success rate (Glass, Nobel, & Vercchione, 1978; Shott et al., 1989). Recently, intraductal laser photocoagulation of the parotid ducts has been suggested as a single procedure for drooling; however, reporting of results and long-term follow-up was not available (Wong, Chang, Chen, & Chen, 1997).

Table 11–7. Surgical Options for Drooling

Procedure	Rationale (Physiology)	Efficacy	Advantages	Disadvantages	Other
Chorda tympani section	Disrupts parasympathetic innervation to sublingual and submandibular glands	47 to 100% short term; ? long term	Technically easy	Loss of taste Possible caries Middle ear surgery	Usually bilateral and combined with tympanic neurectomy
Tympanic neurectomy	Disrupts parasympathetic innervation to parotid gland	47 to 100% short term, ? long term	Technically easy	Possible caries Middle ear surgery Late failures	Usually bilateral and combined with chorda tympani section
Parotid duct transposition	Redirects saliva from parotid gland to posterior oral cavity for easier swallowing	80%	Highly successful Physiologically acceptable	Stenosis/fistula Tedious surgery	May be combined with other procedures
Parotid duct ligation	Eliminates salivary flow from parotid gland	80%	Highly successful	Loss of saliva with possible caries Chronic parotid sialadenitis	May be combined with other procedures

(continues)

Table 11–7. *(continued)* Surgical Options for Drooling

Procedure	Rationale (Physiology)	Efficacy	Advantages	Disadvantages	Other
Submandibular gland excision	Eliminates salivary flow from submandibular gland	?	Eliminates 50% of saliva	External incisions Loss of saliva with possible caries	Usually done in combination with other procedures
Wharton's duct relocation	Redirects saliva from submandibular gland to posterior oral cavity for easier swallowing	80 to 100%	Highly successful Technically easy Physiologically acceptable	Possible ranula Intraoral dissection	Efficacy improves with removal of sublingual gland
Sublingual gland excision	Eliminates salivary flow from sublingual gland	85 to 100%[a]	Technically easy Eliminates ranula	Intraoral dissection	Usually done in combination with Wharton's Duct relocation

[a]In combination with submandibular (Wharton's) duct relocation.

Complications from both procedures include decreased saliva production with loss of protective and digestive functions, dental caries, and chronic parotid sialadenitis.

Submandibular Gland Excision
This procedure is almost always recommended in conjunction with either parotid duct transposition or ligation. It effectively eliminates all salivary secretion from the submandibular gland. External incisions are one possible disadvantage; the decrease in the amount of saliva is another disadvantage. Complications of the surgery itself may include hypoglossal nerve (CN XII) injury with decreased tongue mobility and lingual nerve injury (CN V) with decreased sensation to the tongue. Both of these complications may be of additional concern in the neurologically impaired population.

Submandibular (Wharton's) Duct Relocation
Repositioning of the submandibular duct so that saliva flows to the posterior pharynx where it may be more easily swallowed by reflex (rather than voluntary) control is the underlying principle of this operation. The efficacy of this operation has been reported to be between 80 and 100% (Bailey & Wadsworth, 1985; Cotton, 1981; Crysdale et al., 1985; Crysdale & White, 1989; Dwyer, Timon, & Walsh, 1989; Guerin, 1979). This procedure is theoretically most acceptable, physiologically speaking, as it should not decrease the absolute amount of saliva. Reduced function of at least one gland, as shown by postoperative technetium scanning (Hotaling, Madgy, Kuhns, Filipek, & Belenky, 1992), and an increase in dental caries (Arnrup & Crossner, 1990) have been noted. An aggressive program of dental care postoperatively has helped to reduce the latter.

An intraoral dissection is used (Crysdale, 1982). Ranula formation (sublingual gland cyst) was a common complication after surgery, and therefore, sublingual gland excision is carried out simultaneously by most practitioners (Ethunandan & Macpherson, 1998; Fear, Hitchcock, & Fonseca, 1988). Tonsillectomy may need to be performed simultaneously if the tonsils are hyperplastic and would interfere with duct placement in the inferior pole of the tonsillar fossa. Improvement of the drooling may be seen immediately postoperatively or not until up to four months after the procedure (O'Dwyer & Conlon, 1997).

Occasionally the relocated duct will become obstructed and chronic submandibular sialadenitis will occur which necessitates the removal of the gland (1% of patients). Long-term follow-up is very encouraging even 15 years after the procedure (O'Dwyer & Conlon, 1997).

Sublingual Gland Resection
The sublingual glands may be resected during the submandibular duct rerouting (Crysdale, 1982; Fear et al., 1988). This can be accomplished

through the same intraoral incision. This results in a decrease in the amount of saliva secreted onto the floor of the mouth where it pools and then is dribbled. Ranula formation is also eliminated.

■ CASE STUDIES

Case Study 1

"Alex" is a 4-year-old boy with Down syndrome, who presented to otolaryngology with a 6-month history of chronic profuse drooling and facial chapping. His mother was concerned about the child's chin being constantly chapped, most severely in the winter. Alex's clothes were changed several times each day. Upon further questioning, mother reports that the child had new onset dysphagia within the previous 3 months.

Past medical history was significant for laryngoscopy, bronchoscopy and esophagoscopy with biopsy 1 year before that showed severe esophagitis. The child had been treated for extra-esophageal reflux disease for the past year, using dietary control, head elevation at night, and maximally dosed medical regimen. Reflux symptoms of vomiting and stridor had been under good control, according to the mother. Adenoidectomy and insertion of pressure equalization tubes for recurrent otitis media was performed as an infant.

An interdisciplinary salivary management team evaluation was done to assess the need for further therapy. The SLP's evaluation revealed profuse drooling and an appropriate, well-executed oral–motor program along with Alex's speech–language therapy. The parents were anxious to address the problem because it made his social interactions quite difficult. There were no additional concerns with aspiration.

The occupational therapist found Alex's posture and head position to be normal.

The pediatric dentist found adequate oral hygiene and recommended a program of regular dental care, which had not yet been implemented.

The otolaryngologist found massively enlarged tonsils with an open mouth posture, anterior tongue placement, and severe posterior pharyngeal cobblestoning.

Recommendations

The child underwent tonsillectomy and repeat endoscopy to evaluate the upper aerodigestive tract for reflux changes. The drooling completely resolved immediately after surgery. The endoscopy showed continued esophagitis and laryngotracheobronchitis. Further treatment for the reflux is under consideration.

Comment

This case illustrates the effectiveness of identifying and treating situational factors.

Case Study 2

"Katie" is a 12-year-old girl with Kabuki make-up syndrome[2] who presented to the salivary management team with mild to severe drooling since birth. She was attending public middle school in an inclusion educational setting. Katie was aware and quite upset about her inability to control her drooling. Her family and peers were also aware and disturbed by the drooling. Katie is described as a friendly and outgoing adolescent who enjoys social interaction. Past medical history was significant for multiple sets of pressure equalization tubes and three hip reconstructive procedures. She was allergic to morphine, sulfa, and reglan (taken as an infant).

Interdisciplinary Evaluation

Speech–language pathology: Katie is in middle school in an inclusion classroom educational setting and doing well. She uses oral communication that is quite advanced. She receives speech services three times weekly and physical therapy and occupational therapy twice weekly. A formal oral–motor program to address the drooling had been tried on more than one occasion without success, according to the mother. Behavior modification using swallowing and wipe reminders were effective only for a limited time. Drooling onto the lips and chin were noted. Katie's mother reported that her shirt had to be changed twice daily.

Occupational therapy: Katie was ambulatory and had excellent head control. Her drooling was not affected by positional changes.

Dental: Katie was under regular dental care every 3 months with good results.

Otolaryngology: Katie was able to breathe readily through her nose. She had some problems with chronic sinusitis, but these were inactive at the time of evaluation. No enlargement of the tonsils and adenoids was noted. The intranasal and intraoral examinations revealed moderately severe velopharyngeal insufficiency. Referral for further evaluation and treatment was made.

---

[2]Kabuki make-up syndrome is distinguished by facial features that mimic the make-up worn by Kabuki actors in Japan. Mental retardation is universal and may range from mild to severe.

Recommendations

Katie was diagnosed with mild to occasionally severe drooling. Her high level of cognitive functioning made the drooling functionally disabling. Saltropine at a dose of 0.3 mg twice daily was prescribed. Two months later, she returned with a good response. She had minimal drooling, which became problematic only in the midafternoon. Her dose was adjusted to 0.4 mg three times daily. Two months later, she returned and had no drooling and no side effects from the medication. Katie returned to the salivary management team 8 months later to reveal that over the past month (5 months after the increase in dose of saltropine), the drooling had returned to its original level of severity. She discontinued the saltropine and began Robinul. A fair response to Robinul lasted for several months. Combination therapy was implemented with saltropine and Robinul.

Medical therapy again failed, and Katie underwent bilateral Wharton's duct relocation and sublingual gland excision. Her response was excellent for 2 years. She then started to have some mild drooling to the lower lip, which was effectively managed in the subsequent year with a transderm scopolamine patch. Her velopharyngeal insufficiency was treated adequately with speech therapy.

Comment

This patient illustrates the use of combination therapy to adequately control even mild drooling in a highly functioning patient.

Case Study 3

"Rachel," an 18-year-old young woman, presented to the salivary management team with a long history of profuse drooling (Figure 11–1). She had cerebral palsy and severe mental retardation. Rachel lived at home and attended the Association for Retarded Citizens (ARC) program. She had a history of an atrial septal defect and a seizure disorder treated with phenobarbitol and tegretol. Previous surgeries included endoscopy for "laryngomalacia" as an infant and multiple sets of middle ear ventilation tubes.

Interdisciplinary Evaluation

Speech–language pathology: Although Rachel attends ARC, she is at home most of the winter with upper respiratory infections. She receives speech–language, occupational, and physical therapy services ARC. She has profuse drooling. She sits with a head forward, open-mouth posture. She is unable to follow one-step verbal commands. Her mother is concerned about the drooling, but more so about three hospitalizations in the past 6 months for pneumonia.

Dental: Rachel's dental evaluation revealed the presence of several supernumerary deciduous teeth, as well as multiple dental caries. No evidence of malocclusion or periodontal disease was noted.

Otolaryngology: Rachel's family had been told in the past that her drooling was secondary to an esophageal blockage. She has had several episodes of aspiration pneumonia requiring hospitalization. Review of Rachel's sleep patterns revealed loud snoring with possible episodes of apnea. She had recurrent ear infections as well. Physical examination revealed an obese teenager with profuse drooling. No intranasal pathology was evident, and neither the tonsils nor adenoids were enlarged. The ears revealed right ear adhesive otitis with a right retraction pocket and impending cholesteatoma.

Recommendations

Team members concurred that Rachel's problems were quite complex. In addition to addressing the drooling problems there were several other concerns:

1. The question of sleep apnea would first be addressed by an audio tape of her sleep at home, possibly followed by a polysomnogram. This would help the otolaryngologist assess for upper airway obstruction.
2. A videofluoroscopic swallow study (VFSS) was ordered to evaluate the swallow mechanism and possible presence of aspiration.
3. Plans were made to correct the dental caries and attend to the otitis media with an ear examination under anesthesia and possible insertion of middle ear ventilation tubes.

Treatment Course

The sleep tape and subsequent sleep polysomnogram revealed some snoring but no evidence of obstruction or apnea. VFSS revealed abnormal oral and pharyngeal phases of swallowing with piecemeal deglutition during the oral phase and multiple swallows required to complete the swallow. Pooling of liquids in the vallecula and pyriform sinuses was evident. Silent, trace aspiration was noted before and during swallowing of liquid.

Surgical attention to the ears and teeth came approximately 6 months later. Recurrent upper respiratory infections and poor seizure control delayed the surgery on three occasions. The teeth were repaired and long-term middle ear ventilation tubes were inserted; no cholesteatoma was found.

The drooling did not change after the teeth were repaired. A surgical option was offered to the family that would consist of bilateral submandibular gland excision and parotid duct ligation. It was believed that this would best reduce the drooling and perhaps the risk of aspiration as well. Rerouting of Wharton's ducts was considered inappropriate because of the patient's history of aspiration. The surgery was scheduled, but it was cancelled by the family due to Rachel's continued poor health and marginal seizure control. No further therapy is planned at present.

Comment

This case illustrates the complexity of the patient with a drooling problem and how each consultant may have specific concerns. An alternate surgical procedure was felt to be appropriate in this situation; however, severe medical problems have prevented further treatment of Rachel's drooling.

■ REFERENCES

Arnrup, K., & Crossner, C. (1990). Caries prevalence after submandibular duct retroposition in drooling children with neurological disorders. *Pediatric Dentistry, 12(2),* 98–101.

Bachrach, S. J., Walter, R. S., & Trzcinski, K. (1998). Use of glycopyrrolate and other anticholinergic medications for sialorrhea in children with cerebral palsy. *Clinical Pediatrics, 37,* 485–490.

Bailey, C. M., & Wadsworth, P. V. (1985). Treatment of the drooling child by submandibular duct transposition. *The Journal of Laryngology and Otology, 99,* 1111–1117.

Becmeur, F., Horta-Geraud, P., Brunot, B., Maniere, M. C., Prulhiere, Y., & Sauvage, P. (1996). Diversions of salivary flow to treat drooling in patients with cerebral palsy. *Journal of Pediatric Surgery, 31,* 1629–1633.

Benedek-Spat, E., & Szekely, T. (1985). Long-term follow-up of the effect of tympanic neurectomy on sialadenosis and recurrent parotitis. *Acta Otolaryngol, 100,* 437–443.

Blasco, P. A., Allaire, J. H., et al. (1992). Drooling in the developmentally disabled: Management practices and recommendations. *Developmental Medicine and Child Neurology, 34,* 849–862.

Blasco, P. A., & Stansbury, J. C. (1996). Glycopyrrolate treatment of chronic drooling. *Archives of Pediatrics and Adolescent Medicine, 150,* 932–935.

Borg, M., & Hirst, F. (1998). The role of radiation therapy in the management of sialhorrea. *International Journal of Radiation Oncology Biology Physiology, 41,* 1113–1119.

Brundage, S., & Moore, D. (1989). Submandibular gland resection and bilateral parotid duct ligation as a management for chronic drooling in cerebral palsy. *Plast. Reconstr. Surg, 83(3),* 443–445.

Camp-Bruno, J. A., Winsberg, B. G., & Green-Parsons, A. R. (1989). Efficacy of benztropine therapy for drooling. *Developmental Medicine and Child Neurology, 31,* 309–319.

Chilla, R., de Paula Lima, F. J., Droese, M., & Aglebe, C. (1985). The effects of tympanic neurectomy and chorda tympanectomy on experimentally induced parotid duct fistulae in rabbits. *Arch Otorhinolaryngol, 241,* 295–301.

Cotton, R. (1981). The effect of submandibular duct rerouting in the treatment of sialorrhea in children. *Otolaryngology Head Neck Surgery, 89,* 535–541.

Crysdale, W. (1982). Submandibular duct relocation for drooling. *The Journal of Otolaryngology, 11(4),* 286–287.

Crysdale, W. (1989a). Drooling in children. *Pediatric Otolaryngology,* 323–328.

Crysdale, W. (1989b). Management options for the drooling patient. *Ear Nose Throat J, 68,* 820–830.

Crysdale, W., Greenberg, J., Koheil, R., & Moran, R. (1985). The drooling patient: Team evaluation and management. *International Journal of Pediatric Otorhinolaryngology, 9,* 241–248.

Crysdale, W. S. (1982). Submandibular duct relocation for drooling. *The Journal of Otolaryngology, 11,* 286–288.

Crysdale, W. S., & White, A. (1989). Submandibular duct relocation for drooling: A 10-year experience with 194 patients. *Otolaryngology and Head Neck Surgery, 101,* 87–92.

Dunn, K., Cunningham, C., & Backman, J. (1987). Self-control and reinforcement in the management of a cerebral-palsied adolescent's drooling. *Developmental Medicine and Child Neurology, 29,* 305–310.

Dwyer, T., Timon, C., & Walsh, M. (1989). Surgical management of drooling in the neurologically damaged child. *The Journal of Laryngology and Otology, 103,* 750–752.

Ethunandan, M., & Macpherson, D. W. (1998). Persistant drooling: treatment by bilateral submandibular duct transposition and simultaneous sublingual gland excision. *Annals of the Royal College of Surgeons of England, 80,* 279–282.

Fear, D. W., Hitchcock, R. P., & Fonseca, J. (1988). Treatment of chronic drooling: A preliminary report. *Oral Surg Oral Med Oral Pathol, 66,* 163–166.

Friedman, W., & Kaplan, B. (1975). Tympanic neurectomy: Correction of drooling in cerebral palsy. *New York State Journal of Medicine, 75,* 2419–2422.

Glass, L., Nobel, G., & Vercchione, T. (1978). Treatment of uncontrolled drooling by bilateral excision of submaxillary glands and parotid duct ligations. *Plast Reconst Surg, 62,* 523–526.

Golding-Wood, P. H. (1962). Tympanic neurectomy. *Journal of Laryngology, 76,* 683–692.

Goode, R., & Smith, R. (1970). The surgical management of sialorrhea. *The Laryngoscope, 80,* 1078–1089.

Grewal, D. S., Hiranandani, N. L., Rangwalla, Z. A., & Sheode, J. H. (1984). Transtympanic neurectomies for control of drooling. *Auris Nasus Larynx, 11,* 109–114.

Guerin, R. (1979). Surgical management of drooling. *Archives of Otolaryngology Head and Neck Surgery, 105,* 535–537.

Harris, N., & Dignam, P. (1980). A non-surgical method of reducing drooling in cerebral-palsied children. *Developmental Medicine and Child Neurology, 22,* 293–299.

Harris, S. R., & Purdy, A. H. (1987). Drooling and its management in cerebral palsy. *Developmental Medicine and Child Neurology, 29,* 805–814.

Heine, R. G., Catto-Smith, A. G., & Reddihough, D. S. (1996). Effect of antireflux medication on salivary drooling in children with cerebral palsy. *Developmental Medicine and Child Neurology, 38,* 1030–1036.

Hinkes, R., Quesada, T., Currier, M. B., & Gonzalez-Blanco, M. (1996). Aspiration pneumonia possibly secondary to clozapine-induced sialorrhea. *Journal of Clinical Psychopharmacology, 16,* 462–463.

Hotaling, A., Madgy, D., Kuhns, L., Filipek, L., & Belenky, W. (1992). Postoperative Technetium Scanning in Patients with Submandibular Duct Diversion. *Arch Otolaryngol Head Neck Surg, 118,* 1331

Hussein, I., Kershaw, A. E., Tahmassebi, J. F., & Fayle, S. A. (1998). The management of drooling in children and patients with mental and physical disabilities: A literature review. *International Journal of Pediatric Dentistry, 8,* 3–11.

Klein, B., Reed, M., & Ashenburg, C. (1985). Transdermal scopolamine intoxication in a child. *Pediatric Emergency Care, 1(4),* 208–209.

Koheil, R., Sochaniwskyj, A. E., Bablich, K., Kenny, D. J., & Milner, M. (1987). Biofeedback techniques and behaviour modification in the conservative remediation of drooling by children with cerebral palsy. *Developmental Medicine and Child Neurology, 29,* 21–29.

Luetje, C. M., & Pharm, J. W. (1996). Clinical manifestations of transdermal scopolamine addiction. *ENT Journal, 75 (4),* 210–214.

Maisel, R. (1982). Peritonsillar abscess tonsil antibiotic levels in patients treated by acute abscess surgery. *The Laryngoscope, 92,* 80–87.

Michel, R., Johnson, K., & Patterson, C. (1977). Parasympathetic nerve secretion for control of sialorrhea. *Archives of Otolaryngology Head and Neck Surgery, 103,* 94–97.

Moulding, M., & Koroluk, K. (1991). An intraoral prosthesis to control drooling in patient with amytrophic lateral sclerosis. *Special Care Dentistry, 11-5,* 200–202.

O'Dwyer, T. P., & Conlon, B. J. (1997). The surgical management of drooling—a 15 year follow-up. *Clinical Otolaryngology, 22,* 284–287.

O'Dwyer, T. P., Timon, C., & Walsh, M. A. (1989). Surgical management of drooling in the neurologically damaged child. *The Journal of Laryngology and Otology, 103,* 750–752.

Parisier, S., Blitzer, A., Binder, W., Friedman, W., & Marovitz, W. (1978). Tympanic neurectomy and chorda tympanectomy for the control of drooling. *Archives of Otolaryngology Head and Neck Surgery, 104,* 273–277.

Rapp, D. (1980). Drool control: Long-term follow-up. *Developmental Medicine and Child Neurology, 22,* 448–453.

Sellars, S. L. (1985). Surgery of sialorrhoea. *The Journal of Laryngology and Otology, 99,* 1107–1109.

Shott, S. R., Myer, C. M., & Cotton, R. T. (1989). Surgical management of sialorrhea. *Otolaryngology Head and Neck Surgery, 101,* 47–50.

Sochaniwskyj, A., Koheil, R., Bablich, K., Milner, M., & Kenny, D. (1986). Oral motor functioning, frequency of swallowing and drooling in normal children and in children with cerebral palsy. *Archives of Physical Medical Rehabilitation, 67,* 866–873.

Spivack, B., Adlersberg, S., Rosen, L., Gonen, N., Mester, R., & Weizman, A. (1997). Trihexyphenidyl treatment of clozapine-induced hypersalivation. *International Clinical Psychopharmacology, 12,* 213–215.

Stern, L. (1997). Preliminary study of glycopyrrolate in the management of drooling. *Journal of Pediatrics and Child Health, 33,* 52–54.

Talmi, Y., Zohar, Y., Laurian, N., & Finkelstein, Y. (1988). Reduction of salivary flow with scopodern TTS. *Annals of Otorhinology Laryngology, 97,* 128–130.

Toremalm, N., & Bjerre, I. (1976). Surgical elimination of drooling. *The Laryngoscope, 86,* 104–112.

Townsend, G., Morimoto, A., & Kraleman, H. (1973). Management of sialorrhea in mentally retarded patients by transtympanic neurectomy. *Mayo Clin Proc, 48,* 776–779.

Trott, M., & Maechtlen, A. (1986). The use of overcorrection as a means to control drooling. *American Journal of Occupational Therapy, 40(10),* 702

Twigg, J. (1996). Unrecognized drug reaction. *Nursing, 26,* 6–9.

Walker, P. J., Hutchinson, M., Cant, J., Parmeter, R., & Knox, G. (1994). Chronic drooling: A multi-disciplinary approach to assessment and management. *Aust. J. Otolarnyngology, 1,* 542–545.

Weiss-Lambrou, R., Tetreault, S., & Dudley, J. (1988). The relationship between oral sensation and drooling in persons with cerebral palsy. *American Journal of Occupational Therapy, 43-3,* 155–161.

Wilkie, T. (1967). The problem of drooling in cerebral palsy: A surgical approach. *The Canadian Journal of Surgery, 10,* 60–67.

Wilkie, T., & Brody, G. (1977). The surgical treatment of drooling. *Plast Reconst Surg*, *59*, 791–796.

Wilkinson, J. (1987). Side effects of transdermal scopolamine. *Journal of Emergency Medicine*, *5*, 389–392.

Wong, A., Chang, C., Chen, L., & Chen, M. (1997). Laser intraductal photocoagulation of bilateral parotid ducts for reducing drooling of cerebral palsied children: A preliminary report. *Journal of Clinical Laser Medicine & Surgery*, *15*, 65–69.

Wyllie, E., Wyllie, R., Cruse, R., & Rothner, A. (1986). The mechanism of nitrazepam induced drooling and aspiration. *New England Journal of Medicine*, *314(1)*, 35–38.

■ CHAPTER 12

Feeding With Craniofacial Anomalies

Joan Arvedson and Linda Brodsky

■ SUMMARY

Infants with cleft palate (CP) ± cleft lip (CL) and other craniofacial anomalies are likely to require at least some modification of feeding strategies that are used with infants who have no clefts of lip or palate. Feeding problems vary from minimal for an infant with an isolated cleft of the lip to major for infants with airway and neurologic complications with a cleft of the palate. It is vital that infants get adequate nourishment in nonstressful ways beginning with the first oral feeding. During the first few months of any infant's life, parents and other caregivers find that most interactions involve feeding and communication. Parents' concerns are magnified when they see that there is no closure between the oral and nasal cavities. Strategies to optimize growth and development are important regardless of the specific nature of the cleft or other complex craniofacial anomalies. Feeding problems related to structural and functional differences exist in these infants and children. Specific needs differ when these infants and children undergo surgical procedures. Parents want guidelines and information that will help them to help their infant feed efficiently (Oliver & Jones, 1997). Interestingly, infants with clefts, despite their special needs and care-giving requirements, seem not to have elevated risk for insecure attachments at the end of their 1st year (Speltz, Endriga, Fisher, & Mason, 1997). Management of these special feeding problems depends on a detailed evaluation, patience on the part of caregivers, and, in some instances, creativity and innovation in the search for ways to maximize nutrition status (Arvedson, 1992).

■ INTRODUCTION

Craniofacial anomalies are congenital deformities of the soft tissue and skeleton of the face. The most common anomalies involve cleft palate with or without cleft lip. Concomitant problems are not uncommon, however, especially airway and neurologic deficits. Major advances have been made in recent years in management of feeding, speech, hearing, malocclusion, gross facial deformity, and associated psychologic problems. The effects of many of these anomalies on feeding, regardless of whether airway or neurologic involvement occurs, can be substantial. The focus in this chapter is on diagnostic and management strategies of oral feeding for infants and children with CP ± CL. Strategies will be discussed for pre- and postoperative periods. Feeding problems related to other craniofacial anomalies will be discussed briefly.

The topics in this chapter are organized in the following order:

1. General background
2. Sucking with cleft palate compared with intact palate
3. Craniofacial center interdisciplinary team
4. Oral sensorimotor and feeding assessments
5. Management of feeding preoperatively,
6. Preparation for and management of feeding postoperatively
7. Feeding problems with other craniofacial anomalies

Case studies are presented to illustrate some of the complexities in management for this special group of patients.

■ GENERAL BACKGROUND

Cleft palate and cleft lip are congenital defects that occur approximately once in every 750 births (e.g., Oka, 1981). Incidence varies among racial groups (Hook, 1988). Caucasians are affected at a rate twice that of African Americans. Asians and Native Americans are affected at a rate 1.5 times that of Caucasians. Isolated clefts of the palate occur at one in about 2,500 births with less variation among racial groups. Incidence is higher in boys than in girls by nearly 2 to 1. Unilateral, left clefts are more common. When bilateral clefts occur, the left side is often more severely affected.

Not all infants and children with CP ± CL experience significant feeding difficulties. The great variability cannot be attributed to anatomic factors alone. Multiple factors that impact on the development of feeding in all children may certainly play a role here as well. Children with other craniofacial anomalies, some of whom do not have a cleft palate as part of their anomaly, may have feeding difficulties because of a variety of anatomic, physiologic, and neurologic abnormalities.

Most infants with CP ± CL need at least minor feeding modifications to accomplish safe and efficient oral feeding in the newborn period, even without complicating factors. Some require continued modifications until after primary surgical repair of the posterior palate. Spriestersbach (1973) reported that 73% (91 of 124) of infants with palatal clefts had moderate-to-severe feeding difficulties characterized as sucking inefficiency and the inability to develop adequate intraoral negative pressure for sucking from a breast or "regular" nipples. Other feeding problems include excessive air intake, nasal regurgitation of feeds, fatigue resulting in inadequate intake, and excessively long feeding times (Jones, Henderson, & Avery, 1982; Paradise & McWilliams, 1974). These difficulties are seen most readily during the first few weeks of life but may continue for several months or years unless appropriate steps are taken to improve the overall feeding efficiency and effectiveness in the presence of significant structural abnormalities.

Infants with more complex craniofacial anomalies, especially those involving airway compromise, typically demonstrate more severe feeding difficulties. For example, infants with Pierre Robin sequence encounter feeding difficulties with the severity being proportional to the degree of airway obstruction (Tomaski, Zalzal, & Saal, 1995). The goal of feeding is to maintain optimal nutrition with a stable airway through the use of feeding techniques that are as "normal" as possible. If central or peripheral nervous system damage has occurred, the feeding problems likely relate more to the neurologic status than to any structural differences as seen in uncomplicated clefting.

■ SUCKING WITH CLEFT PALATE COMPARED WITH INTACT PALATE

Infants with an intact palate create negative intraoral pressure as their lips make a tight seal around the nipple and the tongue produces rhythmic suckling movements. An intact soft palate elevates to close off the nasopharynx. Lip seal is the least important factor. Infants with an isolated cleft lip usually feed without significant problems. In contrast, the infant with a posterior cleft palate usually has considerable difficulty developing sufficient negative pressure while nipple feeding (Table 12–1). Thus, the inability to seal off the nasal cavity and nasopharynx from the oral cavity and oropharynx contributes greatly to inefficiency. Nasopharyngeal reflux and even nasal regurgitation may occur in some instances during nipple feedings by infants with cleft palate (Figure 12–1A & B).

Successful sucking also depends on coordinated intraoral muscle movements. This coordination is often disturbed in infants with cleft palate, especially those who also have central nervous system deficits. However,

Table 12–1. Common Feeding Problems With Cleft Palate and Other Craniofacial Anomalies

Problem Area	Clinical Signs/Symptoms
Structural deficits (cleft)	
Inability to develop negative intraoral pressure	• Inefficient or ineffective suck • Excessive air intake (choke, gag may result)
Inability to seal off nasal cavity	• Nasal reflux • Inefficient or ineffective suck
Fatigue	• Lengthy feeding times
Airway deficit	
Upper airway obstruction	• Inspiratory stridor/stertor • Glossoptosis • Micrognathia
Neurologic impairment	• Incoordination of suck, swallow, and respiratory sequencing • Hypotonicity • Hypertonicity

most neurologically normal and healthy infants with a cleft palate make appropriate rhythmic sucking movements with the tongue and lips. The relative lack of negative intraoral pressure leads to excessive amounts of air being ingested with resultant bloating, choking, gagging, and fatigue because of prolonged feeding times. All of these situations may have negative impact on growth and development. Adequate nutrition and growth are especially critical during the first 2 years of life for all children.

Children with cleft palate are reported to have mean birth weights that are similar to normal infants. However, the weight gain in the first 2 years has been found to be significantly lower in children with clefts; male infants are affected more often than females (Jones, 1988; Richard, 1994; Seth & McWilliams, 1988). Infants with isolated cleft palate show the lowest weight gain even though that defect appears to be the least complex anatomically (Jones, 1988; Lee, Nunn, & Wright, 1996). Close nutrition follow-up early in infancy is advocated (Brine et al., 1994). Rapid recovery usually follows surgical repair of cleft palate as seen in a group of 83 children reported by Lee and colleagues. Children with underlying syndromes were significantly more likely to be shorter than their peers at follow-up, but type or severity of cleft was not significantly related to height.

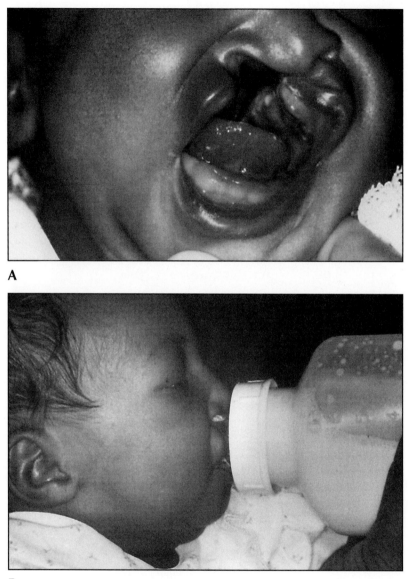

Figure 12–1. A. Infant with unilateral complete cleft of lip and palate; B. Infant with cleft feeding well with cleft palate nurser. Note formula at right nostril due to nasopharyngeal reflux, which did not interfere with success of feeding for this infant.

■ CRANIOFACIAL CENTER INTERDISCIPLINARY TEAM

In addition to professionals involved in the interdisciplinary management of oral sensorimotor and feeding problems, other specialists are generally involved with infants who have a CP ± CL and other craniofacial anomalies (Table 12–2). Since 1988, the team at the Craniofacial Center of Western New York (CFC/WNY) has stressed the importance of diagnosis based protocols for management over time. The interaction and impact of deficits in other systems on feeding cannot be overemphasized. When an infant is born with a cleft palate, cleft lip, or other craniofacial anomalies, the coordinator of the CFC/WNY is consulted. The coordinator then contacts the dysmorphologist, plastic surgeon, speech–language pathologist (who is a feeding specialist), and otolaryngologist. A dysmorphologist examines the infant in the newborn period to establish a diagnosis and to obtain evidence of other associated congenital anomalies. More than 650 syndromes may be associated with clefting (Jones, 1997). Establishment of an etiology

Table 12–2. Disciplines That May Be Involved With Infants and Children With Cleft Lip and Palate

Team Member	Functions
Dysmorphologist (clinical geneticist)	Determine diagnosis
	Detect syndrome
	Counsel family
Coordinator of Center	Coordinate appointments
(Usually RN, can be social worker,	Keep database
geneticist, psychologist, speech–	Assist in coordination of care
language pathologist)	Provide information about community resources
Speech–Language Pathologist	Feeding and swallowing
	Early communication
	Later, speech and language development
Plastic Surgeon	Surgery for cleft palate/lip
	Pharyngeal flap or other surgery
Audiologist	Identification and monitoring of hearing and middle ear status
Otolaryngologist	Airway obstruction
	Ear and hearing health status
Dental-Maxillofacial Specialist(s)	
Prosthodontist	Prosthesis: palatal, pharyngeal
Pediatric Dentist	Dental care
Oral Maxillofacial Surgeon	Orthognathic surgery (e.g., bone grafting, jaw advancement)
Orthodontist	Complex orthodontic care

and a diagnosis is critical because both prognosis and appropriate management decisions depend on accurate diagnosis. The oral sensorimotor and swallowing assessments are made for determination of the best means for meeting nutrition needs in each individual infant. The otolaryngologist examines the infant with focus on the status of the airway, hearing, and ears.

A plastic surgeon meets with the family of an infant with a cleft lip or palate within the first few days of life. The surgeon discusses timing of surgical procedures, stresses the importance of adequate weight gain, and reviews potential speech implications with the family. Primary repair of the cleft lip is generally performed between 1 and 3 months of age (Weatherley-White, 1990). There are research protocols for surgery earlier in the neonatal period and even in utero; however, common practice appears to consider the recommendation for surgery when the infant reaches a weight of at least 10 pounds (4.5 kg), has a hemoglobin of 10 g, and a white blood cell count of at least 10,000 (Wilhelmsen & Musgrave, 1966). Primary repair of a cleft palate is usually completed between the ages of 6 and 12 months. Modern anesthetic and improved surgical techniques have permitted even earlier surgery in some instances. Before 1960, palate repair was rarely performed before the age of 12 months, and most were not repaired until 18 to 24 months of age (Kernahan, 1990). Earlier surgery is favored as a means for enhancement of normal speech, the most important goal of successful cleft palate surgery. Two major surgical procedures within the 1st year of life for infants with cleft lip and palate will have at least temporary disruptions in feeding routines.

The patient-care coordinator sets up appointments and facilitates communication among specialists and the family over time. Regular communication with the primary pediatrician is important for integrated care (Paradise, 1990). Although not as common in recent years in many places, a dental–maxillofacial specialist may be consulted during the neonatal period if a palatal prosthesis is considered for feeding facilitation. They will be involved at other times for dental or bony maxillofacial procedures. Orthodontists also are involved with some children for dental issues. Other specialists consulted over time include a clinical social worker, parent support groups, speech–language pathologist (early speech and language development), and audiologist for hearing assessment within the first 3 months of life. Many infants get audiology screening prior to discharge from hospital in the newborn period. Early identification of hearing loss is advocated for all infants.

■ ORAL SENSORIMOTOR AND FEEDING ASSESSMENT

The initial oral sensorimotor and swallow examination may be carried out within a few hours of birth for a term infant with CP ± CL at an appropriate time for the first oral feeding; however, this examination may be delayed for infants with added complications, such as prematurity, airway problems, neurologic deficits, and other craniofacial anomalies. General concerns in evaluation of this group of patients are similar to those for other infants and children (Chapter 7).

The infant should be awake, alert, and calm during the examination before oral feeding is attempted. A general physical examination includes observation of posture, position, tone, state, and movement. The oral peripheral mechanism is examined as for all infants. A cleft of the lip is readily obvious. If there is no cleft lip, the face is examined for possible asymmetry of lips, tongue, jaw, and upper face. An asymmetric facial droop indicates facial muscle weakness; when no movement occurs, bilateral paralysis may be present as seen in Möbius sequence. Respiratory rate and rhythm are noted as the infant is moved into varied positions. Changes in rate and rhythm during nonnutritive sucking are noted. If inspiratory stridor or stertor is noted or if there are any other indications of airway compromise, an oral feeding assessment should be postponed until the infant's airway is examined. The otolaryngologist can perform flexible fiberoptic laryngoscopy as part of the examination before any further feeding evaluation. Occasionally, further evaluation of the airway will be needed before the feeding examination can be completed. Once the infant is given medical clearance, the clinician can proceed with an oral feeding examination.

A structural and functional evaluation of the oral cavity yields valuable information helpful for treatment planning. The location and size of a cleft have a direct relationship with options for oral feeding (Table 12–3). Infants

Table 12–3. Feeding Options With Cleft Palate and Cleft Lip

Type of Cleft	Feeding Options
Cleft lip alone	Breast-feeding
	Bottle-feeding
Cleft lip with alveolar involvement	Breast-feeding with assistance
	Bottle-feeding (may need easy flow nipple)
Cleft palate with or without cleft lip	Haberman feeder
	Mead-Johnson squeeze bottle
	Soft nipple with large cross-cut
	Assisted breast-feeding (may not be adequate alone to meet nutrition needs)

with a cleft of the lip and no cleft of the palate may show no difficulty or only temporary, minimal difficulty in becoming successful oral feeders at the breast or with regular nipples and containers. Occasionally, isolated small clefts of the hard palate are seen with an intact soft palate. The cleft in the hard palate may be covered by a nipple in such a way that the negative intra-oral pressure can be obtained. A large cleft in the hard palate is difficult to cover by any nipple. With unilateral cleft palate, tissue on the contralateral side of the palate may more than adequately serve for nipple placement and successful sucking motions may result. It is not likely that the infant will feed successfully with a regular nipple (breast or bottle), however, because of the infant's inability to build up intraoral pressure. When there are no air-way or neurologic problems, infants with complete bilateral clefts of the lip and palate usually have the most difficulty with nipple-feeding.

The greatest variability in feeding abilities is seen in infants with an isolated cleft of the soft palate. This variability relates to the specific nature and degree of the palatal deficit. This variability can range from little or no difficulty to major feeding problems with nasopharyngeal reflux, choking, prolonged feeding times, and poor weight gain.

Once the oral cavity has been examined and the infant appears safe for a trial oral feeding, various nipples and containers can be considered to minimize the impact of anatomic deficits on feeding potential (Clarren, Anderson, & Wolf, 1987). Fundamentally, the infant needs a nipple that responds to compression without the need to build up intraoral pressure. A range of options includes, but is not limited to, a "regular" nipple with a fairly large cross-cut at its tip, Mead-Johnson cleft palate nurser, and the Haberman feeder (Figure 12–2). The Haberman feeder has been proven to be useful because of the design for (a) the flow lines on the nipple so the feeder can assist in helping the infant achieve optimal flow, (b) monitoring flow without the necessity for squeezing the bottle, and (c) the valve that prevents back flow and reduces the potential for excessive air buildup (Haberman, 1988). Infants who have stable airways and are neurologically normal should be efficient and take adequate volumes of liquid within 20 to 30 min for appropriate weight gain. If an infant shows incoordination of sucking and swallowing, additional options may need to be tested. For example, a thickened liquid may be given to see if the infant appears to improve coordination of sucking and swallowing. Nonetheless, clinicians and caregivers must keep in mind that thickened feeds can increase the amount and frequency of coughing during feeds, delay gastric emptying, and increase constipation (Orenstein, Magill, & Brooks, 1987). Further evaluation of sucking and swallowing is recommended when airway con-cerns persist after oral feeds are established and incoordination of sucking and swallowing are noted, both of which should raise the clinician's index of suspicion about the possibility of aspiration risks during oral feeding.

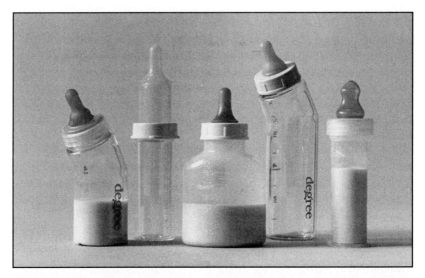

Figure 12–2. Sample of nipples and containers for feeding with cleft lip or palate. Angle and straight bottles are made by numerous manufacturers. From left to right, Degree angle bottle (Baby Products, Inc., Chatsworth, CA) with Ross standard nipple (Ross Laboratories, Division of Abbot Laboratories, Columbus, OH), Haberman feeder (Medela, McHenry, IL), Mead-Johnson cleft palate nurser (Evansville, IN), Degree bottle with Enfamil premature nipple (Mead-Johnson), Volufeed (Ross Laboratories) with Nuk nipple (Gerber, Freemont, MN manufactured in Germany).

■ MANAGEMENT OF FEEDING PREOPERATIVELY

Procedures for effective oral feeding may vary depending on the specific anatomic, airway, and neurologic factors involved for each infant. In this section, minor modifications are described first for infants who have uncomplicated cleft lip, then infants with uncomplicated cleft palate ± cleft lip, and for both types with normal swallowing and no additional complications. Breast-feeding with clefting is then detailed. Next, advantages and disadvantages with the use of palatal feeding prostheses are reviewed.

Feeding Modifications With Uncomplicated Cleft Lip or Cleft Lip With Alveolar Involvement

Basic guidelines for healthy infants with a cleft of the lip are essentially the same as for noncleft infants. These infants should be able to establish breast or bottle feeding with no major modifications required.

Breast Feeding

Breast-feeding is a viable option for infants with an isolated cleft lip (Figure 12–3). An added advantage for breast-feeding of infants with clefts, as well as in noncleft infants, is that fewer middle ear infections have been found than in exclusively formula fed infants (Paradise & Elster, 1984).

Mothers who plan to breast-feed infants with cleft lip may need to prepare and assist the infant initially, possibly with cup-feeding in preparation for breast-feeding (Lang, Lawrence, & Orme, 1994; Thorley, 1997). The healthy term infant should adapt to feeding at the breast once milk production is regular.

Guidelines for breast-feeding preparation include the following:

- Finger-feed or cup-feed to help facilitate readiness for breast-feeding during the first few days (proper technique is critical to minimize risk for aspiration; Thorley, 1997).
- Place the infant at the soft breast for practice to prepare for the transitional milk production when breasts become swollen with increased supply of blood and lymph fluid.
- Experiment with positions to find the one in which the infant gets the best seal that allows for most effective expression of milk.

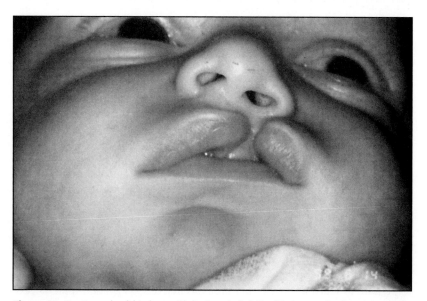

Figure 12–3. 4-week-old infant with isolated cleft lip. He breast-feeds successfully.

Cautions include the following:

- A small amount of milk may leak out around the cleft, but that does not usually interfere with sucking.
- If the lip curls under, the mother can simply lift it up.
- Pressure can be applied to the cheeks at the sides of the lips for increased lip closure around the nipple, which is likely to be needed only infrequently.

Bottle-Feeding

Guidelines for bottle feeding include the following:

- Hold the infant in an upright position with head, neck, and trunk aligned in neutral midline posture.
- Use a cross-cut nipple with a soft, thin wall for easy compression (slightly larger cross-cut may be helpful when alveolus is involved).
- Choose a nipple that may be slightly longer than a standard nipple, especially with alveolar involvement.
- Monitor flow rates carefully to assure that the infant gets adequate volume efficiently, neither working hard to get the liquid nor using additional effort to slow the flow; both are to be avoided.

Feeding Modifications With Cleft Palate ± Cleft Lip

Breast-Feeding With Cleft Palate

In some instances, infants with a mild or small submucous cleft of the soft palate become successful breast feeders (Moss, Jones, & Pigott, 1990), while some others may have feeding difficulties. These infants have the same high incidence of middle ear disease as those with overt cleft palate. It is important that a diagnosis be made early with any degree of feeding difficulty. It may be possible, but less likely, that infants with a narrow posterior cleft of the palate will meet nutritional needs for adequate weight gain from the breast alone. Infants with large clefts of the palate have the poorest prognosis for successful breast-feeding.

Infants with an isolated cleft of the palate typically have difficulty with breast-feeding. No consistent recommendations exist for breast-feeding in this situation. When an isolated palatal cleft exists, breast-feeding is discouraged by many practitioners (Davis, 1990), because of the infant's inability to build up intraoral pressure for adequate expression of the milk. Nonetheless, some infants with cleft of the soft palate have been reported to be able to learn to "milk" the breast (Grady, 1977). The nipple is protruded by the mother's finger pressure to the breast at the top and bottom edges of the areola, so it is easier for the infant to take the nipple into the mouth. The mother then holds the nipple in the infant's mouth throughout the feeding. The infant uses gums and tongue similarly to the mother's use of her fingers to pump or express the milk. This process may be assisted by a supplementary nursing system (SNS), which has several advantages over supplemental feedings from a bottle or a cup. Other mothers may pump breast milk and use that for bottle-feeding, along with some direct attachment to the breast (Crossman, 1998). The Hotz-type orthopedic plate is described as a facilitator for breast-feeding with infants, although these infants needed supplementing to meet nutritional needs (Kogo et al., 1997).

Advantages include the following:

- Infant is assured of food whether or not nursing is successful.
- No confusion about nipples, because all feeding is done at the breast.
- Infant improves the technique as the sucking urge is satisfied.
- Milk supply may be improved with more stimulation by the infant at the breast.

A nursing mother can use a breast pump to have sufficient milk for her infant at the breast with a SNS or a bottle supplement.

Infants with complicating factors, such as prematurity, sucking and swallowing coordination problems, or a micrognathic mandible, may not be successful directly at the breast. For those infants, a compromise may be reached by pumping the breast milk and feeding the infant with a bottle that has the modifications already discussed. Some infants with limited clefting may become fully successful at the breast after several weeks or even months. As with any other method of feeding, evaluation is based on an infant's growth pattern, time required for feeding, and overall success. An important aspect of success is efficient feeding with minimal or no stress to infant and mother.

Bottle Feeding With Cleft Palate

Basic guidelines for nipple oral feeding of healthy and neurologically normal infants with cleft palate are listed in Table 12–4. Infants with a unilateral (Figure 12–1) or bilateral (Figure 12–4) complete cleft of lip and palate are likely to feed successfully with a nipple that requires only compression (e.g., Haberman feeder) or a cross-cut nipple with a squeezable bottle (e.g., Mead Johnson cleft palate nurser). A squeezable bottle should improve the efficiency of the liquid flow compared to a rigid bottle (Shaw, Bannister, & Roberts, 1999). Relatively minor modifications of normal feeding procedures have been described by numerous authors (e.g., Barone

Table 12–4. Basic Oral Feeding Guidelines With Cleft Palate.

Attribute	Guideline
Position/posture	Upright with good trunk, neck, and head support to maintain a neutral posture
Nipple	Breast with supplemental nursing systems
	Haberman feeder
	Cross-cut with easy compression
	Soft with thin wall, easy compression
	Wide, flat (Nuk or orthodontic) type optional
	Strengthening of orofacial muscles without excessive effort
Container	Haberman feeder
	Flexible plastic squeeze bottle
	Rigid container cutout to allow squeeze of bag or liner
Liquid flow	Normal swallow should occur (flow not too fast)
	Easy, steady, burst-and-pause pattern
	Slowly enough to prevent choking
Timing	Frequent burping during feed (may be needed)
	20 to 30 min for total feeding
	2- to 4-hour intervals (shorter intervals may be needed initially; goal: 3 to 4 hour intervals)

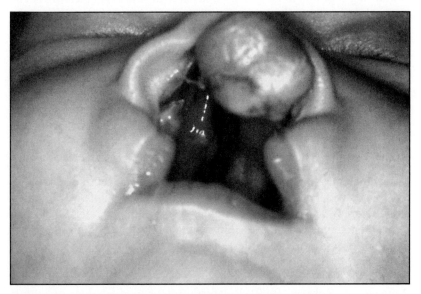

Figure 12–4. 3-week-old infant with bilateral complete cleft of lip and palate. He feeds successfully with a Haberman feeder.

& Tallman, 1998; Curtin, 1990; McWilliams, Morris, & Shelton, 1990; Morris & Klein, 1987; Richard, 1991; Suslak & Desposito, 1988). A decrease in feeding problems and remarkably improved weight gain have been described with the above procedures (Paradise & McWilliams, 1974).

Creative parents and caregivers can make adaptations with other feeding containers that are inexpensive and take advantage of materials at hand. The adaptations may include the following:

- Vary the nipple type or the size of the hole in the nipple (lengthen limbs of cross-cut nipple slightly with razor blade or similar instrument. Place extra holes or enlarge existing opening. Caution is needed).
- Consider container options (Figure 12–2).
- Provide jaw stabilization or control.
- Place infants with mild airway problems in prone position. Although this position is not likely to be sufficient for adequate oral intake when infants have major airway problems, it can be helpful with minor problems. An angle bottle may aid in appropriate nipple placement and flow of liquid if this position seems feasible.

Cautions include the following:

- Avoid continuous flow nipples for infants who could choke easily.
- Avoid lamb's nipples (frequently recommended in the past) because they are long and bulky. Liquid is released so far posteriorly in the oral cavity that most infants experience difficulty in maintaining a coordinated suck-and-swallow pattern. These infants are at high risk for gagging, emesis, and aspiration.

The Haberman feeder (Figure 12–2 and Figure 12–5A & B) was developed to overcome some of the common problems experienced in feeding infants with cleft palate (Haberman, 1988). Benefits include the following:

- One-way valve in the mouthpiece allows easy flow of liquid and prevents backflow. Thus, no vacuum is produced. The nipple must be filled completely before feeding is started (Figure 12–5A & B).
- Slit-valve opening closes between sucks, thus preventing too fast a flow.
- Nipple has three different flow rates, indicated by raised markings on the nipple itself, so feeder can adjust flow rates to aid infants.

Campbell and Trenouth (1987) reported that infants who had either craniofacial anomalies or neurologically based diagnoses fed faster and more easily with the Haberman feeder than with other nipples (Figure 12–6). The Haberman feeder was found to be the most popular feeding method by parents in their sample (Trenouth & Campbell, 1996). These

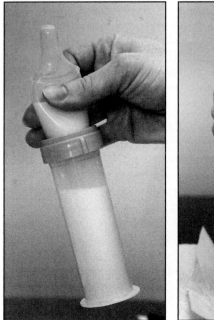
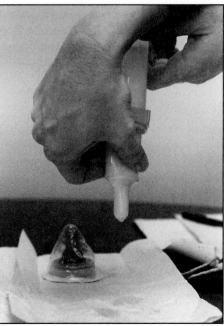

Figure 12–5A. Filling the nipple of Haberman feeder. The first step is done as feeder is held upright and nipple is compressed near the base.

Figure 12–5B. The second step in filling the Haberman feeder is to tip the feeder upside down and slowly release the compression so the liquid can flow into the nipple. Both steps are repeated several times until filling is complete.

infants had less gastroesophageal reflux and required less frequent burping than with other more conventional feeding techniques. A drawback of the Haberman feeder is the relatively high cost, which may be a problem for some families. In the United States, Haberman feeders are available directly from the manufacturer. It is possible that some pharmacies may have Haberman feeders, but they are not likely to be found in most retail shops. Families would have to check possibilities of insurance coverage by third-party payers with a prescription by physicians. Availability in other countries is not known to these authors.

Palatal Feeding Prostheses to Assist Feeding With Cleft Palate

The purpose of a feeding prosthesis, or obturator, is to provide a normal contour to the alveolar process and palate that is desirable for infants with cleft palate (Schaaf, Casey, & McLean, 1992). No consensus has been reached regarding the use of feeding prostheses for infants with clefts, however. Thus, no specific guidelines have been published for use of palate prostheses. Feeding prostheses are used less often than they were 10 to 15 years ago. In the past, some facilities would fit prostheses for all newborns with complete cleft of the lip, alveolus, and palate (Rosenstein, 1990). Other facilities would offer infants a trial period for oral feeding without any prosthesis, then recommend a prosthesis only for those who continued to have feeding difficulties (Balluff & Udin, 1986; Jones, Henderson, & Avery, 1982).

Several procedures for fitting and making prostheses have been described (e.g., Fleming, Pielou, & Sounders, 1985; Jones et al., 1982: Jones, Meade, & Edwards, 1985; Razek, 1980; Samant, 1989). Jones et al. (1985) emphasized that the prosthesis should be worn 24 hours a day and removed only 2 to 3 times per day for cleaning. Advantages and disadvantages are described below.

Advantages may include the following:

- Creates a false palate against which the infant can suck.
- Creates palatal arch stability.
- Secures molding of maxillary alveolar segments prior to surgery.
- Prevents maxillary segment collapse after lip closure (Jones et al., 1985).

Disadvantages may include the following:

- May cause irritation and edema of oral mucous membrane (Fogh-Andersen & Forchhammer, 1970).
- Replacement needed to accommodate growth (Jones et al., 1985).
- Hygiene concerns.
- May alter oral flora and increase risk of caries in the primary dentition (Bokhout et al., 1996).

Overall, palatal prostheses are used relatively infrequently, likely related to research findings. Lateral radiographs and videofluoroscopic images revealed no discernible difference in tongue placement between cleft and noncleft infants at rest or while feeding. In addition, presence or absence of a palatal prosthesis made no difference in the tongue placement for infants with cleft palate (Brogan, Foulner, & Turner, 1987; Schaaf, Casey, & McLean, 1992). Prahl, Kuipers-Jagtman, & Prahl-Anderson, (1996) failed to find any benefit on feeding frequency, food intake, or velocity of food intake during the first 24 weeks of life in a randomized trial of feeding plates for 40 infants with complete unilateral clefts of palate. Choi, Kleinheinz, Joos, & Komposch (1991) reported that the presence or

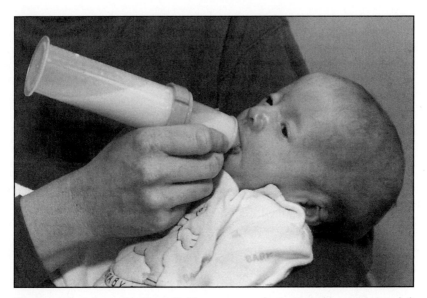

Figure 12–6. Infant with Pierre Robin sequence characterized by posterior cleft palate, micrognathia, and glossoptosis is feeding with the Haberman feeder.

absence of an intraoral orthopedic plate does not make any difference in the ability of infants with clefts to generate negative intraoral pressure. When one considers that the plate cannot be fitted for precise and direct contact of the prosthesis to the posterior pharyngeal wall to achieve closure of the nasopharyngeal port, these findings are not surprising.

Special procedures are seldom necessary because most caregivers learn to feed their infants by simply altering nipples and containers (McWilliams et al., 1990). Shaw and colleagues (1999) compared effectiveness of bottle types for oral feeding of infants with cleft lip and palate. They had planned to study two groups of infants with cleft lip and palate: infants fed with obturators and infants fed without obdurators. However, by the 24- to 36-hour period when the maxillary impression would typically be made, they found that most infants were already feeding successfully. Thus, they determined that it would be unethical to insist on use of the obturator, so they altered the study design and eliminated the obturator group. Obturators or "roofies" may be used for children who undergo repair of soft palate, and repair of hard palate is delayed for a few years because of wide clefts. In these instances, the obdurator is used for speech purposes, which involve different considerations than feeding related issues.

After review of multiple studies, Shaw et al. (1999) concluded that the evidence did not support the treatment burden and the cost of palatal obturators for feeding. Likewise, positive effects of a feeding prosthesis on tongue habits are inconclusive (Berkowitz, 1977; Finger & Guerra, 1989). Children can be creative as revealed in a case report of a 14-month-old child with a cleft palate who had learned to obturate her own cleft with her thumb as she took nipple feeds. She had not undergone prosthodontic treatment nor had her palate been repaired (Sykes & Essop, 1999). Individual needs and differences must be considered in determining the most effective feeding procedures for infants with CP ± CL.

Oral Care After Feeding

When the infant has finished oral feeding, the areas around the cleft should be cleaned. Food should not be left to accumulate because it will mix with mucous secretions from the mouth and nose to form a hard crust that becomes a potential source for infection. The areas adjacent to the cleft can be cleaned with plain water, or water with hydrogen peroxide (50%), on a wash cloth or gauze. If the cleft lip area becomes dry, it can be moistened with baby or mineral oil externally. Caregivers should make sure that no oil gets into the infant's mouth.

■ PREPARATION FOR AND MANAGEMENT OF FEEDING POSTOPERATIVELY

Feeding is a major concern for families preparing for postoperative care. The surgeon is the primary source of information for any restrictions in the immediate postoperative period. Any alterations of feeding strategies are planned to facilitate, and not to interfere, with wound healing. Surgeons differ in their recommendations for duration of time away from nipple-feeding (Skinner, Arvedson, Jones, Spinner, & Rockwood, 1997). Before surgery, parents can help prepare their children for alternative forms of oral feeding that may be needed after surgery. Children may learn to drink from a cup (Figure 12–7) or take liquid via syringe; however, recent evidence suggests that the prolonged cup-drinking or syringe feeding advocated in the past may not be necessary to maintain suture line integrity. Some centers advocate unrestricted breast- and bottle-feeding within 24 hours after lip surgery and within 48 hours after palate surgery (Cohen, Marschall, & Schafer, 1992). During the first 24 hours following surgery, feeding is by cup or syringe.

Feeding in Relation to Surgery for Primary Lip Repair

Postoperative feeding techniques for infants following primary repair of cleft lip vary considerably. Surgeons' recommendations range from immediate

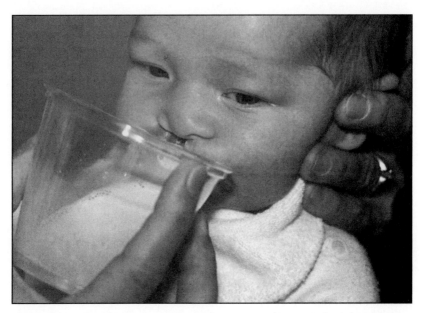

Figure 12–7. Cup drinking practice prior to primary lip repair for infant who has a unilateral complete cleft of lip and palate.

return to nipple feeding postoperatively to abstinence from nipple-feeding for up to 6 weeks (Skinner et al., 1997).

Preoperatively

The oral–motor feeding specialist works with the infant and family to facilitate successful feeding techniques that may be needed postoperatively. If cup-drinking is part of the plan, parents can practice with the infant to facilitate those skills. The child needs to be in a well-supported upright position. The feeder holds an open cup, not a spout cup, to release liquid into the mouth so that the cleft area will not be in contact with a hard surface. Although the lip repair frequently is done at an age younger than usual to begin cup-drinking, the principles of feeding in the 4-to-6-month age range are applied (Chapter 9). Initially, infants are likely to handle thickened liquids in the open cup, rather than their regular formula or juice. The practice sessions are likely to be more effective if they are frequent and of short duration, for example, 3 to 5 min five to six times per day for 7 to 10 days before the surgery date. Some infants respond to cup practice best when they are really hungry. Others want the breast or bottle, but will take small amounts of fluid by cup when they are partially satiated. It is not necessary to have the infant drinking totally by cup at the time of the surgery but with enough cup experience that parents are confident that the infant can carry out the task.

Postoperatively

Most infants will resume nipple-feedings after an interim of cup-drinking, although there may be some who will not return to bottle-feeding. There is no magic age for attaining skills for cup-drinking.

Infants with an isolated cleft of the lip are likely to return to breast-feeding after the first 24 hours following surgery (Darzi, Chowdri, & Bhat, 1996; Weatherly-White, 1990). Infants using a soft nipple (e.g., the Haberman feeder) should be able to return to nipple-feeding within a short time period following surgery. Because the nipple on the Haberman feeder requires compression and not suction, the infant typically does not use lips in a pursed position, which could place strain on the sutures that would then interfere with wound healing. The nipple arrangement on the Haberman feeder keeps the newly repaired upper lip away from a firm surface (i.e., a hard plastic ring at the base of the nipple).

Different surgeons prescribe different postoperative feeding protocols among and within centers. Some surgeons recommend unrestricted breast- or bottle-feeding immediately after cleft lip repair, stating that the potential strain on the lip from crying due to the absent, familiar nipple is greater than the strain that may be caused by the nipple itself (Cohen, Marschall, and Schafer, 1992; Johnson, 1978). Other surgeons cite established practices and protocols of mentors that recommend non-nipple-feeding techniques from 10 days up to 6 weeks following surgery (Davis, 1990; Millard, 1976; Musgrave, 1971).

Caregivers typically comply with surgeons' postoperative feeding recommendations (Skinner et al., 1997). A retrospective study from one center compared three groups of infants: (a) unrestricted return to nipple, (b) 2–3 weeks of non-nipple-feeding, and (c) 6 weeks of non-nipple-feeding. No medical or surgical complications (i.e., dehiscence) occurred that were related to feeding strategies (Skinner et al.). A survey of craniofacial–cleft palate centers in the United States and Canada (39 responses) revealed that parents used a multitude of products and techniques to feed their infants. The products included the Mead-Johnson cleft palate feeders (15%), syringe (16%), Haberman feeders (11%), rubber tubing (11%), and cross-cut nipples (11%) as the most frequently used immediately following surgery for repair of cleft lip (Deck, Steinwach, Jones, and Arvedson, 1998).

Spoon-Feeding Introduction

A child with a CP ± CL should start spoon-feeding at approximately 6 months of age just as other children without CP ± CL. The child with a repaired cleft lip is likely not to have any restrictions about utensils or other objects placed into the mouth by the time spoon-feeding is introduced. The child with a cleft palate should have no difficulty in handling thin purees by spoon. Strained foods can be diluted and should be fed by spoon to enhance normal development with spoon-feeding. Parents can avoid thickened food consistencies that may lodge in the cleft area. The nasal mucosa may be sensitive to spicy foods. Both should be avoided until after the cleft palate repair. Some children handle mashed food efficiently before the palate repair, but foods to be avoided include peanut butter, cooked cheese dishes (because of their stickiness), leafy vegetables, or other foods that are fed in small pieces. Children vary in their taste preferences as well as in their readiness for textures before and after palate repair.

Feeding in Relation to Surgery for Primary Repair of Cleft Palate

Recommendations for feeding in the immediate postoperative period appear to be based primarily on tradition and individual surgeon's preferences, rather than population-based data collection. It appears to be common practice that children do no sucking or spoon-feeding in the immediate postoperative period so as to minimize tension and thus potential dehiscence of the suture line. Surgeons typically determine the duration in relation to wound healing, with maximum time likely to be 5 to 6 weeks. Children in the 8 to 12 month age range can take soft food and liquid by cup.

Basic guidelines include the following:

- Give all food and liquid by cup (no spout).
- Keep all utensils out of the mouth (e.g., no spoon or straw).
- Give smooth and lumpy purees, or food that has been blended, that is thin enough for a cup.
- Hold off on crunchy and chewable food until wound healing is complete, per surgeon.
- Monitor nutrition and hydration, so that growth and development continue (Wellman & Coughlin, 1991).

The introduction of lumpy foods at developmental ages of 10 to 11 months is important for children with cleft palate, just as it is for other children (Illingworth & Lister, 1964). If the introduction of such textures is delayed until the child reaches 14 to 16 months of age, food refusal and negative feeding behaviors may result. Children with clefts who continue to take bottles to bed once their teeth have erupted have shown an increased risk of developing baby bottle tooth decay (Lin & Tsai, 1999). These findings suggest that oral health promotion programs should begin in infancy for children with clefts and their parents.

■ FEEDING PROBLEMS WITH OTHER CRANIOFACIAL ANOMALIES

This section features brief discussions of feeding and swallowing issues that are commonly associated with Mobius syndrome, hemifacial microsomias, Pierre Robin sequence, and velocardiofacial syndrome. These conditions represent some of the craniofacial anomalies that commonly have an impact on feeding effectiveness and efficiency. A range of difficulties can be noted. Each child is different, even within each category, and thus adaptations to enhance feeding safety will also differ.

Möbius Syndrome

Möbius syndrome is characterized by congenital facial diplegia (cranial nerve [CN] VII) and restricted horizontal eye movements (CN VI) (Mobius, 1888). The clinical spectrum can include multiple cranial nerve palsies, craniofacial defects, cardiac anomalies, and somatoskeletal dysmorphic features (Henderson, 1939). Weakness in the lower face usually affects the mandible, lips, and tongue. Weakness of the perioral musculature compromises lip closure. Thus, food and liquid tend to dribble out of the mouth. The open mouth posture makes it difficult to use the tongue efficiently to form a bolus; however, pharyngeal phase swallowing is usually safe (Arvedson & Brodsky, 1996). Furthermore, during transition feeding ineffective lip closure around a spoon occurs, which then adversely affects the tongue function. Food tends to fall out of the mouth when solid food is chewed. Accordingly, speech difficulties are common. Children typically have the most difficulty with bilabial consonants.

Hemifacial Microsomias (e.g., Facial Auriculo-Vertebral Sequence, Goldenhar Syndrome)

Hemifacial microsomia refers to a broad group of first and second branchial arch malformations that result in varying degrees of mandibular hypoplasia and facial weakness. This unilateral weakness can affect the lips and tongue as well. Successful feeding may be established by placing the food or liquid into the mouth toward the stronger side while simultaneously applying external pressure to the weaker side. These infants and children are usually able to develop compensatory tongue movements with a soft nipple allowing for an easy flow of liquid. They can feed successfully as long as the pharyngeal swallow is safe.

Pierre Robin Sequence

Pierre Robin sequence (PRS) is a common craniofacial anomaly characterized by micrognathia, glossoptosis, and a U-shaped cleft palate (see Chapter 4 for detailed description). Incidence is reported at 1 in 2,000 births. Infants with Pierre Robin sequence in isolation typically are neurologically intact. Thus, feeding difficulty relates directly to the degree of airway obstruction. The glossoptosis places the infant at high risk for airway obstruction, choking, and aspiration of liquid. Airway obstruction may result from several different physiologic factors and mechanical bases (Sher, 1992; Sher, Shprintzen, & Thorpy, 1986).

Treatment of airway obstruction varies considerably in the United States, although all agree that management of infants with Pierre Robin sequence with airway compromise is critical (Argamaso, 1992; Bath & Bull, 1997; Caouette-Laberge, Plamondon, & Larocque, 1996; Freed, Pearlman, Brown, & Barot, 1988; Frohberg & Lange, 1993; Myer, Reed, Cotton,Willging, & Shott, 1998; Smyth, 1998). Airway stability is absolutely critical for successful, safe oral feeding. One report describes early discharge of infants with nasopharyngeal tubes to home as a nonsurgical treatment (Olson, Kearns, Pransky, & Seid, 1990). Surgical procedures may include glossopexy, subperiosteal release of the floor of the mouth, and tracheostomy (see Chapter 4). Once the airway is stabilized, providing there are no other neurologic or structural deficits, most infants feed efficiently and effectively with relatively minor adjustments related to the posterior cleft palate as discussed previously (Figure 12–6). Management strategies and feeding techniques must be adapted to the specific needs of the infant (Glass & Wolf, 1999).

In cases of severe upper airway obstruction, infants may not be able to take oral feedings sufficient to meet nutritional needs. These infants may need a nasogastric tube initially (Prodoehl & Shattuck, 1995) and a gastrostomy tube to assure adequate nutrition and hydration if it appears that the infant will need supplemental feeding for several months. They may be able to tolerate only brief oral feeding times because they work so hard at feeding. Parents are encouraged to give their infants opportunity to take nipple feedings to whatever extent they tolerate in nonstressful ways, usually no more than 15 to 20 minutes per feeding time. It is more important that the infant experience pleasurable sucking and swallowing with smaller quantities than for feeders to try to increase volume. A major push for increaed volume places the infant under greater stress and increases the risk for aspiration and for airway problems. Occasionally, children with major neurologic deficits may not be safe for oral feedings at all, although that is the exception rather than the rule.

As facial growth occurs in a downward and forward direction over the 1st year of life, children do improve in airway status. Those who have undergone tracheostomy are likely to be decannulated after the posterior cleft palate is repaired. They become spoon-feeders, cup-drinkers, and learn to take chewable food when they achieve the appropriate developmental level requirements.

Velocardiofacial (VCF) Syndrome

VCF consists of multiple anomalies that include cleft palate, cardiac defects, learning difficulties, speech disorder, and characteristic facial features (Shprintzen, 1992; Shprintzen et al., 1978). Incidence is estimated at 1 in 5,000 (Pike & Super, 1997). An autosomal dominant genetic disorder involves microdeletion at chromosome 22q11.2 in most cases of VCF . The phenotype of this condition shows considerable variation because not all principal features are present in each case, and identification of the syndrome can be difficult because many of the anomalies are minor and present in the general population. Velopharyngeal insufficiency may be the primary finding, likely noted by speech–language pathologists (Carneol, Marks, & Weik, 1999).

A history of feeding difficulties is common. Findings on videofluoroscopic swallow studies suggest that the underlying problem is due to dysmotility in the pharyngoesophageal area and not gastroesophageal reflux. Nasopharyngeal reflux, esophageal dysmotility, hyperpharyngeal contraction, and diverticula of the cervical esophagus have been found in some children (Zackai et al., 1996). Pharyngeal hypotonia is found in 90% of the VCF population and correlates with generalized hypotonia (Shprintzen, Goldberg, Young, & Wolford, 1981). The pharyngeal hypotonia is found in association with swallowing and other oral–motor problems. The pharyngeal hypotonia and collapse are further accentuated by the buildup of negative pressure in the pharynx that occurs during feeding. Pharyngeal hypotonia is a major factor contributing not only to feeding abnormalities but also to obstructive sleep apnea (Arvystas & Shprintzen, 1984; Shprintzen et al.).

Fatigue may also be a factor in poor oral feeding because of cardiac involvement seen in VCF. Some infants require tube feedings for extended time periods, and thus a gastrostomy tube may be considered. Oral sensorimotor stimulation should be carried out even when food or liquid cannot be given for feedings (Chapter 9). Minimal amounts of food or liquid for taste experience and for encouraging swallows are acceptable and help prepare the child for resumption of oral feedings when the respiratory and cardiac systems stabilize.

Neurologic Factors with Some Craniofacial Anomalies

Infants with CP ± CL may have neurologic deficits in addition to or as a component of a craniofacial syndrome. Central nervous system deficits contribute to incoordination of suck/swallow/breathe patterns as discussed previously. For some infants, the CP ± CL may become almost incidental when compared with other complicating factors. Feeding strategies in these children are similar to those employed for any child with neurologic impairment. This subject is discussed in detail in Chapter 9 (intervention).

■ CASE STUDY 1

This case study provides an example of successful oral feeding in an infant with multiple cranial nerve deficits, no true suck, and no gag. This child emphasizes the need for extensive knowledge about a diagnosis and history, along with thorough clinic or bedside and instrumental examinations.

History

"Charles" was delivered at 36 weeks gestation via repeat C-section. His mother had gestational diabetes and was on insulin therapy. Birth weight was 2,644 g. Apgars were 7/8. Upon physical exam, he was found to have a micrognathic mandible, hypoglossia, and diminished facial movement, even with crying. Digital hypoplasia of varying degrees was noted bilaterally on hands and feet. Restricted eye movements were evident.

Diagnosis

The diagnosis was oromandibular-limb hypogenesis syndrome (OMLHS), which has a natural incidence of 1/175,000 live births (Alexander, Friedman, Eichen, & Buchbinder, 1992; Bush & Williams, 1983). Presumed etiology is an intrauterine insult to the fetus early in gestation (< 6th week). Pathogenesis is thought to be a vascular disruption with hyperfusion of distal structures (D'Cruz, Swisher, Jaradeh, Tang, & Konkol, 1993). Recurrence risk is small.

Features of OMLHS related to cranial nerve damage that may affect safety of oral feeding include pharyngeal incoordination, vocal fold paralysis, impaired gag reflex, nasopharyngeal reflux, and aspiration during swallows. The prognosis is variable. If cranial nerves IX and X are involved, one can expect abnormal swallowing and speech deficits. Most children have normal cognition, although approximately 15% have developmental disabilities related to the diffuse insult to the developing brain.

Examination

Oral–motor feeding exam on day 2 of life revealed the physical features of the small jaw, small tongue that appeared retracted and bunched. Charles had no true suck, absent gag reflex, and questionable swallow safety. He appeared to swallow a drop of sterile water placed on his tongue via spoon. Next, he took a drop of formula off the spoon. Then he seemed eager to take slightly bigger amounts by medicine cup. From the bedside oral–motor feeding examination, the recommendation was made for parents and nurses to help Charles practice using liquid in a cup in preparation for a videofluoroscopic swallow study (VFSS) scheduled for the next day. They were cautioned to keep volume limited and to make sure he did not get stressed.

VFSS

The VFSS revealed no delayed pharyngeal swallow onset, no aspiration, and no residue in pharyngeal recesses after swallows. Thus, Charles appeared safe for oral feeding.

Recommendations and Course

The next step was to decide what type nipple, container, and techniques could be initiated. He took formula in a well-coordinated way with a Haberman feeder that responds to compression and does not require true sucking. Within 10 days, he was a full oral feeder who was gaining weight appropriately and able to complete the feeds in less than 30 min. He was a safe oral feeder in spite of the fact that he had no true sucking ability and an absent gag reflex.

He grew well and thrived over the next several months. He spit up with most feeds, and underwent a workup for gastroesophageal reflux, which was positive. He was managed medically. He had the expected difficulties with speech production, particularly for bilabial consonants (m, p, b). When he started chewable food, he was a messy eater because of the difficulty in containing food within the oral cavity. Nonetheless, he was functional.

Comment

Charles is an excellent example of how infants and children can make adaptations for safe oral feeding in the presence of physical and physiologic findings that would be predictive of significant deficits and consideration for nonoral feeding. Charles is a major success story and demonstrates the importance of professionals having extensive knowledge of history and global etiology, careful and thorough physical bedside examination, and use of instrumental findings to assist in making optimal management recommendations. Follow-up monitoring is done periodically through the medical setting. Direct intervention is provided through an early intervention program.

■ CASE STUDY 2

This case study provides an example of feeding problems in the presence of a cleft, but in fact, the cleft was only a minor factor in the overall oral–motor and feeding decision-making process. The most obvious basis for a problem may turn out to be relatively insignificant.

History

"James" was delivered at home by precipitous vaginal delivery just a few days before term. He was transferred immediately to the Children's Hospital.

Diagnosis

Diagnoses included Down syndrome, unilateral cleft of lip and alveolus, and cardiac deficits not requiring surgery. He was fed initially by nasogastric (NG) tube because parent and nurses could not get him to take enough to meet nutritional needs.

Feeding Examination

Upon initial oral–motor feeding examination at 5 days of life, James was noted to have the Down syndrome facies, narrow left unilateral cleft of the lip and alveolus, and hypotonia. He rooted for a nipple. He initiated nonnutritive sucking weakly on the examiner's gloved little finger with appropriate rate and rhythm. He produced a gag reflex with stimulation by gloved finger over posterior tongue.

James was held in a well-supported upright posture for the oral feeding observation. He started sucking on presentation of a standard nipple with pumped mother's breast milk. Once the infant and the feeder got into appropriate rhythm, he took liquid with no obvious risk for aspiration. He showed variable efficiency, tended to suck only 3 to 4 times, then paused, and needed some stimulation to "stay on task." Overall, his suck appeared weak. He never had a firm latch on the nipple, so some liquid dribbled out.

The nipple was changed to an orthodontic type that was easier flow. He became more consistent, but never seemed to get too much liquid that could result in coughing or choking. He took a full feed within 30 min while the feeder provided support to keep him using his tongue and to keep him in a calm, alert state. Airway appeared stable, with only mildly increased work of breathing as the feeding progressed, but no indication of any airway obstruction.

Recommendations and Course

James was placed on a schedule with encouragement to maximize efficiency with oral feeding, and then supplement with NG tube, so that all feedings were given as bolus feedings. He gradually increased efficiency and volume of intake so that the NG tube was pulled after 1 week. He was discharged home on full oral feeding with the orthodontic nipple. Parent was cautioned that as he grew stronger, he might need a different nipple so that the flow would not be as fast. He should not have to work to slow down the flow of liquid.

Comment

In this instance, the oral feeding difficulties were most closely correlated to the hypotonia and weak suck pattern. The cleft was essentially incidental in terms of adjustments that had to be made for safe and efficient nipple-feeding. Close monitoring for signs of risk for aspiration is important. The neurologic and cardiac status will be the best predictors for long-term oral feeding safety and success. It is tempting to think that the cleft is the biggest factor in sorting out feeding issues in infants, but in the words of a favorite old song, "it ain't necessarily so."

■ REFERENCES

Alexander, R., Friedman, J. S., Eichen, M. M., & Buchbinder, D. (1992). Oromandibular-limb hypogenesis syndrome: Type II A, hypoglossia-hypodactylia—report of a case. *British Journal of Oral & Maxillofacial Surgery, 30*, 404–406.

Argamaso, R. V. (1992). Glossopexy for upper airway obstruction in Robin sequence. *Cleft Palate-Craniofacial Journal, 29*, 232–238.

Arvedson, J. (1992). Infant oral-motor function and feeding. In L. Brodsky, L. Holt, & D. H. Ritter-Schmidt (Eds.), *Craniofacial anomalies: An interdisciplinary approach* (188–195). St. Louis: Mosby-Year Book.

Arvedson, J. C., & Brodsky, L. S. (1996, November). Mobius syndrome: A case study of successful oral feeding with multiple cranial nerve anomalies. Paper presented at the 24th annual conference of the Society for Ear, Nose, & Throat Advances in Children (SENTAC), Cincinnati, Ohio.

Arvystas, M., & Shprintzen, R. J. (1984). Craniofacial morphology in the velo-cardio-facial syndrome. *Journal of Craniofacial Genetics and Developmental Biology, 4,* 39–45.

Balluff, M. A., & Udin, R. D. (1986). Using a feeding appliance to aid the infant with a cleft palate. *Ear, Nose and Throat Journal, 65,* 316–320.

Barone, C. M., & Tallman, L. L. (1998). Modification of Playtex nurser for cleft palate patients. *Journal of Craniofacial Surgery, 9,* 271–274

Bath, A. P., & Bull, P. D. (1997). Management of upper airway obstruction in Pierre Robin sequence. *Journal of Laryngology and Otology, 111,* 1155–1157.

Berkowitz, S. (1977). State-of-art (orofacial). III. Orofacial growth and dentistry. *Cleft Palate Journal, 14,* 288–301.

Bokhout, B., Van Loveren, C., Hofman, F. X. W. M., Buijs, J. F., Van Limbeek, J., & Prahl-Andersen, B. (1996). Prevalence of Streptococcus mutans and lactobacilli in 18-month-old children with cleft lip and/or palate. *Cleft Palate Craniofacial Journal, 33,* 424–428.

Brine, E. A., Rickard, K. A., Brady, M. S., Liechty, E. A., Manatunga, A., Sadove, M., & Bull, M. J. (1994). Effectiveness of two feeding methods in improving energy intake and growth of infants with cleft palate: A randomized study. *Journal of American Dietetic Association, 94,* 732–738.

Brogan, W. F., Foulner, D. M., & Turner, R. (1987). A videoradiographic investigation of the position of the tongue prior to palatal repair in babies with cleft lip and palate. *Cleft Palate-Craniofacial Journal, 24*(4), 336–338.

Bush, P. G., & Williams, A. J. (1983). Incidence of the Robin anomalad (Pierre Robin syndrome). *British Journal of Plastic Surgery, 36,* 434–437.

Campbell, A. N., & Trenouth, M. J. (1987). A new feeder for infants with cleft palates. *Archives of Diseases in Childhood, 62,* 1292–1293.

Caouette-Laberge, L., Plamondon, C., & Larocque, Y. (1996). Subperiosteal release of the floor of the mouth in Pierre Robin sequence: Experience with 12 cases. *Cleft Palate-Craniofacial Journal, 33,* 468–472.

Carneol, S. O., Marks, S. M., & Weik, L. (1999). The speech-language pathologist: Key role in the diagnosis of velocardiofacial syndrome. *American Journal of Speech-Language Pathology, 8,* 23–32.

Choi, B. H., Kleinheinz, J., Joos, U., & Komposch, G. (1991). Sucking efficiency of early orthopaedic plate and teats in infants with cleft lip and palate. *International Journal of Oral Maxillofacial Surgery, 20,* 167–169.

Clarren, S. K., Anderson, B., & Wolf, L. S. (1987). Feeding infants with cleft lip, cleft palate, or cleft lip and palate. *Cleft Palate Journal, 24,* 244–249.

Cohen, M., Marschall, M. A., & Schafer, M. E. (1992.) Immediate unrestricted feeding of infants following cleft lip and palate repair. *Journal of Craniofacial Surgery, 3,* 30–32.

Crossman, K. (1998). Breastfeeding a baby with a cleft palate: A case report. *Journal of Human Lactation, 14,* 47–50.

Curtin, G. (1990). The infant with cleft lip or palate: More than a surgical problem. *Journal of Perinatal Neonatal Nursing, 3,* 80–89.

Darzi, M. A., Chowdri, N. A., & Bhat, A. N. (1996). Breast feeding or spoon feeding after cleft lip repair: A prospective, randomised study. *British Journal of Plastic Surgery, 49,* 24–26.

Davis, A. T. (1990). Pediatric management of the child with a cleft. In D. A. Kernahan & S. W. Rosenstein (Eds.), *Cleft lip and palate: A system of management* (28–32). Baltimore: Williams and Wilkins.

D'Cruz, O. F., Swisher, C. N., Jaradeh, S., Tang, T., & Konkol, R. J. (1993). Mobius syndrome: Evidence for a vascular etiology. *Journal of Child Neurology, 8,* 260–265.

Deck, S. M., Steinwach, S., Jones, G. W., & Arvedson, J. C. (1998, November). Standards of care for individuals with clefts. Poster presented at American Speech-Language-Hearing Association Convention, San Antonio, TX.

Finger, I. M., & Guerra, L. R. (1989). Provisional restorations in maxillofacial prosthetics. *Dental Clinics of North America, 33,* 435–455.

Fleming, P., Pielou, W. D., & Sounders, D. F. (1985). A modified feeding plate for use in cleft palate infants. *Journal of Pediatric Dentistry, 1,* 61–64.

Fogh-Andersen, P., & Forchhammer, E. (1970). Preoperative care of cleft palate children in Denmark. *Cleft Palate Journal, 7,* 595–600.

Freed, G. F., Pearlman, M. A., Brown, A. S., & Barot, L. R. (1988). Polysomnographic indications for surgical intervention in Pierre Robin sequence: Acute airway management and follow-up studies after repair and take-down of tongue-lip adhesion. *Cleft Palate Journal, 25,* 151–155.

Frohberg, U., & Lange, R. T. (1993). Surgical treatment of Robin sequence and sleep apnea syndrome: Case report and review of the literature. *Journal of Oral and Maxillofacial Surgery, 51,* 1274–1277.

Glass, R. P., & Wolf, L. S. (1999). Feeding management of infants with cleft lip and palate and micrognathia. *Infants and Young Children, 12,* 70–81.

Grady, E. (1977). Breastfeeding the baby with a cleft of the soft palate. *Clinical Pediatrics, 16,* 978–981.

Haberman, M. (1988). A mother of invention. *Nursing Times, 84,* 52–53.

Henderson, J. L. (1939). The congenital facial diplegia syndrome: Clinical features, pathology and etiology—a review of 61 cases. *Brain, 62,* 381–403.

Hook, E. (1988). "Incidence" and "prevalence" as measures of the frequency of congenital malformations and genetic outcomes: Application to oral clefts. *Cleft Palate Journal, 25,* 97–101.

Illingworth, R. S., & Lister, J. (1964). The critical or sensitive period, with special reference to certain feeding problems in infants and children. *Journal of Pediatrics, 65,* 840–848.

Johnson, H. A. (1978.) The immediate postoperative care of a child with cleft lip: Time-proved suggestions. *Annals of Plastic Surgery, 2,* 430–433.

Jones, J. E., Henderson, L., & Avery, D. R. (1982). Use of a feeding obturator for infants with severe cleft lip and palate. *Special Care Dentistry, 2,* 116–120.

Jones, J. E., Meade, P., & Edwards, A. (1985). Treating cleft lip and palate infants. *Dental Assisting, 4,* 20–25.

Jones, K. L. (1997). *Smith's recognizable patterns of human malformations* (5th ed.). Philadelphia: W.B. Saunders.

Jones, W. B. (1988). Weight gain and feeding in the neonate with cleft: A three-center study. *Cleft Palate Journal, 25(4),* 379–384.

Kernahan, D. A. (1990). Sequence of procedures and timing. In D. A. Kernahan & S. W. Rosenstein (Eds.), *Cleft lip and palate: A system of management* (115–119). Baltimore: Williams and Wilkins.

Kogo, M., Okada, G., Ishii, S., Shikata, M., Iida, S., & Matsuya, T. (1997). Breast feeding for cleft lip and palate patients, using the Hotz-type plate. *Cleft Palate-Craniofacial Journal, 34,* 351–353.

Lang, S., Lawrence, C. J., & Orme, R. L. (1994). Cup feeding: An alternative method of infant feeding. *Archives of Diseases in Childhood, 71,* 365–369.

Lee, J., Nunn, J., & Wright, C. (1996) Height and weight achievement in cleft lip and palate. *Archives of Diseases in Childhood, 75,* 327–329.

Lin, Y-T. J., & Tsai, C-L. (1999). Caries prevalence and bottle-feeding practices in 2-year-old children with cleft lip, cleft palate, or both in Taiwan. *Cleft Palate-Craniofacial Journal, 36* 522–526

McWilliams, B. J., Morris, H. L., & Shelton, R. L. (1990). *Cleft palate speech* (2nd ed.). Philadelphia: Decker.

Millard, D. R., (1976). *Cleft craft* (Vol. 1). Boston: Little, Brown.

Mobius, P. J. (1888). Uber angeboren doppel seitige abducens-facialis Lahmung. *Munchener Med Wochenschr, 35,* 91–94.

Morris, S. E., & Klein, M. D. (1987). *Pre-feeding skills: A comprehensive resource for feeding development.* Tucson, AZ: Therapy Skill Builders.

Moss, A. L. H., Jones, K., & Pigott, R. W. (1990). Submucous cleft palate in the differential diagnosis of feeding difficulties. *Archives of Disease in Childhood, 65,* 182–184.

Musgrave, R. H. (1971). General aspects of unilateral cleft lip repair (33–36). In W. C. Grabb, S. W. Rosenstein, K. R. Bzoch (Eds.), *Cleft lip and palate: A system of management.* Baltimore: Williams and Wilkins.

Myer, C. M., Reed, J. M., Cotton, R. T., Willging, J. P., & Shott, S. R. (1998). Airway management in Pierre Robin sequence. *Otolaryngology–Head and Neck Surgery, 118,* 630–635.

Oka, S. (1981). Epidemiology and genetics of clefting: With implications for etiology. In H. K. Cooper, R. L. Harding, W. M. Krogman, M. Mazaheri, & R. T. Millard (Eds.), *Cleft palate and cleft lip: A team approach to clinical management and rehabilitation of the patient.* Philadelphia: W. B. Saunders.

Oliver, R. G., & Jones, G. (1997). Neonatal feeding of infants born with a cleft lip and/or palate: Parental perceptions of their experience in South Wales. *Cleft Palate-Craniofacial Journal, 34,* 526–532.

Olson, T. S., Kearns, D. B., Pransky, S. M., & Seid, A. B. (1990). Early home management of patients with Pierre Robin sequence. *International Journal of Pediatric Otorhinolaryngology, 20,* 45–49.

Orenstein, S. R., Magill, H. L., & Brooks, P. (1987). Thickening of infant feeding for therapy of gastroesophageal reflux. *Journal of Pediatrics, 110,* 181–186.

Paradise, J. L. (1990). Primary care of infants and children with cleft palate. In C. D. Bluestone, S. E. Stool, & M. D. Scheetz (Eds.), *Pediatric otolaryngology* (Vol. 2; 2nd ed.; pp 860–866). Philadelphia: W.B. Saunders.

Paradise, J. L, & Elster, B. (1984). Evidence that breast milk protects against otitis media with effusion in infants with cleft palate (abstract). *Pediatric Research, 18,* 283A.

Paradise, J. L., & McWilliams, B. J. (1974). Simplified feeder for infants with cleft palate. *Pediatrics, 53,* 566.

Pike, A. C., & Super, M. (1997). Velocardiofacial syndrome. *Postgraduate Medical Journal, 73,* 771–775.

Prahl, C., Kuijpers-Jagtman, A. M., & Prahl-Andersen, B. (1996). Evaluation of feeding. In *A study into the efects of presurgical orthopaedic treatment in complete unilateral cleft lip and palate patients. A three centre prospective clinical trial in Nijmegen, Amsterdam and Rotterdam. Interim Analysis.* Academisch Ziekenhuis Nijmegen.

Prodoehl, D. C., & Shattuck, K. E. (1995). Nasogastric intubation for nutrition and airway protection in infants with Robin sequence. *Journal of Perinatology, 15,* 395–397.

Razek, M. K. A. (1980). Prosthetic feeding aids for infants with cleft lip and palate. *Journal of Prosthetic Dentistry, 44,* 556–561.

Richard, M. (1994). Weight comparisons of infants with complete cleft lip and palate. *Pediatric Nursing, 20,* 191–196.

Richard, M. E. (1991). Feeding the newborn with cleft lip and/or palate: The enlargement, stimulate, swallow, rest (ESSR) method. *Journal of Pediatric Nursing, 6,* 317–321.

Rosenstein, S. W. (1990). Early maxillary orthopaedics and appliance fabrication. In D. A. Kernahan & S. W. Rosenstein (Eds.), *Cleft lip and palate: A system of management* (120–127). Baltimore: Williams and Wilkins.

Samant, A. (1989). A one-visit obturator technique for infants with cleft palate. *Journal of Oral Maxillofacial Surgery, 47,* 539–540.

Schaaf, N. G., Casey, D. M., & McLean, T. R. (1992). Maxillofacial prosthetics. In L. Brodsky, L. Holt, & D. H. Ritter-Schmidt (Eds.), *Craniofacial anomalies: An interdisciplinary approach* (137–153). St. Louis: Mosby-Year Book.

Seth, A. K., & McWilliams, B. J. (1988). Weight gain in children with cleft palate from birth to two years. *Cleft Palate Journal, 25,* 146–150.

Shaw, W. C., Bannister, R. P., & Roberts, C. T. (1999). Assisted feeding is more reliable for infants with clefts—A randomized trial. *Cleft Palate-Craniofacial Journal, 36,* 262–268.

Sher, A. E. (1992). Mechanisms of airway obstruction in Robin sequence: Implications for treatment. *Cleft Palate-Craniofacial Journal, 29,* 224–231.

Sher, A. E., Shprintzen, R. J., & Thorpy, M. J. (1986). Endoscopic observations of obstructive sleep apnea in children with anomalous upper airways: Predictive and therapeutic value. *International Journal of Pediatric Otorhinolaryngology, 11,* 135–146.

Shprintzen, R. J. (1992). The implications of the diagnosis of Robin sequence. *Cleft Palate Journal, 29,* 205–209.

Shprintzen, R. J., Goldberg, R. B., Lewin, M. L., Sidoti, E. J., Berkman, M. D., Argamaso, R. V., & Young, D. (1978). A new syndrome involving cleft palate, cardiac anomalies, typical facies and learning disabilities: Velocardiofacial syndrome. *Cleft Palate Journal, 15,* 56–62.

Shprintzen, R. J., Goldberg, R., Young, D., & Wolford, L. (1981). The velo-cardio-facial syndrome: A clinical and genetic analysis. *Pediatrics, 67,* 167–172.

Skinner, J., Arvedson, J. C., Jones, G., Spinner, C., & Rockwood, J. (1997). Post-operative feeding strategies for infants with cleft lip. *International Journal of Pediatric Otorhinolaryngology, 42,* 169–178.

Smyth, A. G. (1998). A simple nasal splint to assist the stability of nasopharyngeal tubes in the Pierre Robin sequence associated airway obstruction: Technical innovation. *Journal of Cranio-Maxillofacial Surgery, 26,* 411–414.

Speltz, M. L., Endriga, M. C., Fisher, P. A., & Mason, C. A. (1997). Early predictors of attachment in infants with cleft lip and/or palate. *Child Development, 68,* 12–25.

Spriestersbach, D. C. (1973). *Psychosocial aspects of the cleft palate prob-lem.* Iowa City: University of Iowa Press.

Suslak, L. & Desposito, F. (1988). Infants with cleft lip/cleft palate. *Pediatric Review, 9,* 331–334.

Sykes, L. & Essop, R. (1999). A feeding adaptation by an infant with a cleft palate. *South African Dental Journal,* 54, 369–370.

Thorley, V. (1997). Cup feeding: Problems created by incorrect use. *Journal of Human Lactation, 13,* 54–55.

Tomaski, S. M., Zalzal, G. H., & Saal, H. M. (1995). Airway obstruction in the Pierre Robin sequence. *The Laryngoscope, 105,* 111–114.

Trenouth, M. J., & Campbell, A. N. (1996). Questionnaire evaluation of feeding methods for cleft lip and palate neonates. *International Journal of Paediatric Dentistry, 6,* 214 –244.

Weatherley-White, R. C. (1990). Surgical timing and postoperative feeding in the cleft lip child. In D. A. Kernahan & S. W. Rosenstein (Eds.), *Cleft lip and palate: A system of management* (33–36). Baltimore: Williams and Wilkins.

Wellman, C. O., & Coughlin, S. M. (1991). Preoperative and postoperative nutritional management of the infant with cleft palate. *Journal of Pediatric Nursing, 6,* 154–158.

Wilhelmsen, H. R., & Musgrave, R. H. (1966). Complications of cleft lip surgery. *Cleft Palate Journal, 3,* 223–231.

Zackai, E. H., McDonald-McGinn, D. M., Driscoll, D. A., Feuer, J., Emanuel, B. S., & Eicher, P. (1996). Dysphagia in patients with a 22q11.2 deletion: Unusual pattern found on modified barium swallow (abstract). *American Journal of Human Genetics, 59,* A109, 600.

CHAPTER 13

Psychological Aspects and Behavioral Issues in Pediatric Feeding

Joan Arvedson, Linda Brodsky, and Bruce Bleichfeld

■ SUMMARY

Mealtimes are typically social events for adults and children, whether children are independent feeders or need assistance. "Behavioral" feeding problems often result from specific medical problems that may be related to oral sensorimotor, neurologic, gastrointestinal, or airway problems. Even when medical problems are solved, however, behavioral feeding problems may continue. Stress around mealtimes associated with feeding and swallowing may aggravate problematic caregiver–child interactions. Behavior of the child, caregiver, and caregiver–child interactions must be considered in a "total" child approach. Assessment and management decisions for children with feeding disorders will be affected by a variety of "nonorganic" or behavioral factors. Recognition of and intervention for the more common behavioral and psychologic issues encountered in this special patient population are described.

■ INTRODUCTION

Eating in most societies is a social event, and therefore, its significance is extremely important. A great deal of emphasis is placed on food and food-related activities. Parents and other primary caregivers gain much pleasure from mealtimes and frequently have a compelling need to get their infant or toddler to eat. Children with feeding difficulties may have an apparent lack of hunger or motivation to eat. After medically induced etiologies are eliminated, these problems have been attributed to (a) absence of learned patterns of eating behavior, (b) aversive consequences of eating (e.g., stomach ache due to gastroesophageal reflux or diarrhea), (c) aversive consequences of being forced to eat, or (d) some combination of the above.

This chapter reviews behavioral and interpersonal aspects of pediatric feeding disorders. The basic principles and guidelines for optimal feeding relationships between caregivers and children are presented within a developmental framework. The incidence, prevalence, and definition of behavioral feeding problems are then described. Behavioral assessment of children who present with behavioral components of feeding problems is discussed. Common problems include complaints of poor appetite, disinterest in food, and food refusal. Some of these children are simply "picky" eaters and do not demonstrate growth disturbances for any extended time periods. Many children with limited appetites refuse food frequently enough over some time period, however, so they demonstrate poor weight gain or even weight loss. Finally, management approaches are described. Case studies highlight some of the issues around psychologic factors, behavior components, and child–caregiver mealtime relationships involved in the assessment and management of feeding disorders.

■ DEVELOPMENT OF FEEDING AND CHILD–CAREGIVER INTERACTIONS

Feeding is a reciprocal process that depends on the specific abilities and characteristics of both the caregiver and the child. A give-and-take exchange is required for effective feeding. The focus of feeding should not be to get food into the child, but on helping the child to learn eating skills and positive eating attitudes and behaviors (Satter, 1999). Acquisition of these eating skills results from experience gained during normal development that also allows for adequate nutrition and growth.

Feeding is a uniquely complex process because it involves significant interaction with caregivers and other aspects of the environment. To be successful, the following hierarchical steps must occur: (a) acceptance of a wide variety of foods of developmentally appropriate textures and types (b) efficient and safe sucking or chewing, propelling, and swallowing.

Three stages of normal feeding development occur: homeostasis, attachment, and separation/individuation (e.g., Chatoor, Schaefer, Dickson, & Egan, 1984). Infant cues and caregiver behaviors that support normal behavioral development in regard to feeding are listed in Table 13–1. Optimum feeding at every stage depends on successful negotiation of the balance of communication and control in the stage before. High-quality feeding interactions assist the infant in developing physically, in acquiring cognitive and linguistic competence, and in securing strong emotional attachments with major caregivers (Barnard et al., 1989). Clinicians must

Table 13–1. Developmentally Appropriate Feeding Interactions Associated
With Infant/Child and Caregiver Behaviors During First 3 Years of Life

Stage of Development	Infant/Child Cues	Caregiver Behaviors That Support Infant/Child Cues
Homeostasis (0–2 months)	Demonstrates rooting and sucking, swallowing, breathing coordination	Follow signals for feeding times; stimulate rooting by touching cheek
	Shows interpretable and moderate feeding readiness cues	Feed promptly when infant is hungry, before prolonged crying
	Remains calm and alert during feeding	Hold infant fairly upright for mutual eye contact during feeding
	Eats enough to get full	Talk and smile, but do not overwhelm infant with attention
	Shows interpretable and positive signs of fullness	Avoid interactions that arouse infant unnecessarily
		Burp only if infant seems to need it; do not interrupt feeding with unnecessary burping or wiping mouth
		Stop the feeding when infant turns away or "shuts down" to indicate lack of interest
Attachment (3–6 months)	Reaches out, smiles, and makes noises to attract and hold attention	Maintain active state of reciprocity with infant, not overwhelming with energy of interaction
	Exerts control over nipple-feeding	Monitor readiness for appropriate developmental changes (e.g., spoon-feeding by 6 months developmental age)

continues

Table 13–1. *(continued)* Developmentally Appropriate Feeding Interactions Associated With Infant/Child and Caregiver Behaviors During First 3 Years of Life

Stage of Development	Infant/Child Cues	Caregiver Behaviors That Support Infant/Child Cues
Attachment (3–6 months) *(continued)*	Becomes more consistent in regularity of waking, eating, and sleeping periods	Develop routine mealtimes
	Becomes more social in the feeding interactions	Learn and follow cues; do not stop feeding too soon because undernutrition may result
Separation/Individuation (6–36 months)	Exerts increasing control over environment	Feed when child wants to eat, but gradually work into family mealtimes
	Gains complex sense of self	Seat child upright and facing forward; sit directly in front of the child
	Participates in family mealtimes as social events	Talk in quiet, encouraging ways, but do not overload with distracting activities
		Wait for child to pay attention and be responsive before feeding
	Initiates self-feeding	Remain present, but do not intrude into the process
		Let the child decide how fast and how much to eat
		Respect food preferences and cautious approaches to new foods

Note. Adapted from Satter, E. M. (1990). The feeding relationship: Problems and interventions. *Journal of Pediatrics, 117,* 181–189.

appreciate the sequences in normal development to be involved with assessment and management of children demonstrating disruptions that can occur in any one of these stages. These stages of homeostasis, attachment, and separation/individuation will be described.

Homeostasis

During the first 2 to 3 months of life, the infant's primary goal is to achieve homeostasis, a relatively stable state with the environment. Sleep regulation, satisfactory eating schedules, and a quiet and alert state at feeding times are the goals. Interaction with the environment requires the infant to achieve some degree of self-regulation. Responsive and attentive early feeding is important in helping infants organize their behavior (Chatoor, Dickson, Schaefer, & Egan, 1985).

A primary goal of the caregiver is to assist the infant in regaining an organized state after becoming overstimulated or upset. The supportive caregiver, typically the infant's mother, recognizes and responds promptly to the infant's hunger cues. In this way, the infant avoids becoming tense and overly aroused through long or active crying before feeding. The required skills need to be mastered for effective infant feeding. A failure to master basic feeding skills will interfere with the next developmental task of attachment. Interference with development of motor skills, language, and affective engagement is also likely to occur (Chatoor et al., 1984).

Attachment

Attachment is the primary emotional task for infants from about 3 to 6 months. This period is one in which the infant begins to love and to engage the interest of other people in active ways. Greenspan and Lourie (1981) describe attachment as "falling in love." Feeding becomes a social time (Pridham, 1990). The pauses following sucking bursts during feeding times become more apparent and may be incorrectly interpreted as a need for burping or as a sign of satiety, when instead the pauses may be cues for socialization. Incorrectly interpreted pausing is not uncommon and is associated with undernutrition in some infants (Whitten, Pettit, & Fischhoff, 1969).

If true engagement between infant and caregiver does not occur during this developmental stage, the infant is likely to indicate lack of pleasure with feeding and may show lack of appetite. Vomiting and rumination may be seen with severe dysfunction.

Separation/Individuation

By about 6 months of age, infants begin to exert increasing control over their environment. Gradually a complex sense of self is gained through differentiation among a variety of emotional states and bodily sensations

(Kopp, 1982). From 6 to 36 months of age, the child's primary behavioral developmental process is the struggle to achieve a sense of self. Caregivers try to provide boundaries, structure, and limits in which the child can explore safely. A balance between autonomy and dependency is particularly difficult to achieve in the feeding situation.

Transition feeding, beginning at about 6 months with spoon-feeding of smooth purees, coincides with the beginning of the period of separation. Rapid changes occur in the range of food textures children handle and the way in which they handle them. As young children begin self-feeding, the mealtime experience broadens from an intimate relationship with a primary caregiver to participation in the social event of the family meal (Satter, 1990). Caregivers and children typically work toward scheduled feeding times that by the end of the 1st year should coincide with family mealtimes. Effective feeding includes selection of developmentally appropriate feeding methods, as well as food types and quantities. Children need realistic opportunities for becoming more independent in the feeding process (Table 13–1).

Feeding problems in the separation/individuation stage of development can occur because of problems persisting from the attachment stage. They also may relate to new difficulties centered around issues of autonomy versus dependency (Chatoor et al., 1984). These principles are applicable to all children once they carry out some self-feeding, sit in a high chair, and have some control over what goes into their mouth.

■ MEALTIME PRINCIPLES

Some basic mealtime principles apply to all young children and their caregivers. Once children begin to experience their world through self-feeding, the mealtime experiences change significantly. Independence and self-control are to be encouraged. At 2 years of age, most children are likely to reject new foods initially but learn to like them with time and repeated neutral exposure (Birch & Marlin, 1982). The "food rules" make the mealtime principles concrete and measurable (Table 13–2) (Chatoor et al., 1985). Cultural and ethnic differences must be considered when clinicians make observations and judgments about what is expected at certain ages and stages of children (e.g., Phillips & Cooper, 1992). Children with a history of prematurity or developmental disabilities that affect feeding tend to be particularly cautious about new oral experiences. Most children with developmental delays go through the same sequence of development, albeit at a slower rate. Some children with anatomic and neurophysiologic based problems may never become total oral feeders, and others may not maintain success as oral feeders. The mealtime principles become particularly important when behavioral issues are prominent, when changes in feeding are implemented, or when weaning children from tube feedings. Children with

Table 13–2. "Food Rules" for Caregivers Applicable to Children Beyond Infancy

Aspect of Mealtime	"Rules" for Caregivers
Scheduling	Regular mealtimes, only planned snacks added
	Mealtimes no longer than 30 min
	Nothing offered between meals, except water if child is thirsty (no bottles or cups of milk or juice)
Environment	Neutral atmosphere (no forced feeding or commenting on intake)
	Sheet under chair to catch mess
	No game playing
	Food never given as reward or present
Procedures	Small portions
	Solids first, fluids last
	Self-feeding encouraged as much as possible (e.g., finger-feeding, holding spoon)
	Food removed after 10–15 min if child plays without eating
	Meal terminated immediately if child throws food in anger
	Wiping mouth and cleaning up only after meal is completed

Source. Arvedson, J. C. (1997). Behavioral issues and implications with pediatric feeding disorders. *Seminars in Speech and Language.* Adapted from "A developmental classification of feeding disorders associated with failure to thrive: Diagnosis and treatment," by I. Chatoor, L. Dickson, S. Schaefer, & J. Egan, 1985. In D. Drotar (Ed.), *New directions in failure to thrive: Implications for research and practice.* New York: Plenum Press.

behavioral components to feeding problems are variable. The next step is to examine epidemiology of feeding problems in infants and children.

■ EPIDEMIOLOGY AND DEFINITION OF FEEDING PROBLEMS

Childhood feeding problems appear to be common, although incidence and prevalence rates vary considerably. The lack of reliable, consistent diagnostic criteria to describe and classify feeding problems continues to hamper research-based progress in this area (Kedesdy & Budd, 1998).

Epidemiology

Feeding disturbances are estimated to occur in 2 to 45% of the pediatric population (Bentovim, 1970; Forsyth, Leventhal, & McCarthy, 1985; Marchi & Cohen, 1990). Feeding problems and other behavioral difficulties appear related, regardless of when feeding problems begin (Dahl & Sendelin,

1992). Prevalence figures in children with developmental disabilities show that 33% or more have feeding problems (Thompson & Palmer, 1974).

Mild or typical feeding problems are estimated to occur in 25 to 40% of healthy toddlers and early-school-age children (Mayes & Volkmar, 1993). The most frequently reported mild behavior-related problems include: not always hungry, eating only small amounts of food, picky eating, and strong food preferences. These mild problems are generally transitory and easily resolved if handled appropriately (Kerwin, 1999). Serious behavior-related feeding problems may occur in 3 to 10% of all children. These problems are more prevalent in children with physical disabilities, mental retardation, medical illness, and prematurity. In a biopsychosocial model, physiologic, behavioral, and social factors all contribute to the development of severe feeding problems. Table 13–3 has a nonexhaustive list of feeding problems. The remainder of the chapter will primarily address this patient population.

Definition and Classifications of Feeding Problems

Definition of Feeding Problem

A feeding problem can be defined as a deficit in any aspect of taking nutritional elements that results in undernutrition, poor growth, or stressful mealtimes for children and their caregivers. Etiologies, signs, symptoms, and severity can vary considerably among individuals and within an individual over time. A behavioral feeding problem is defined as one in which behaviors are prominent, although that does not negate some level of physiologic component.

Multiple classification systems have been used to categorize children with feeding problems, but a universal system is yet to be accepted. There

---

Table 13–3. Some Common Feeding Problems in Young Children

Inappropriate mealtime behaviors (e.g., temper tantrums, throwing food)
Lack of self-feeding
Food selectivity (eating only a few foods)
Failure to advance textures from puree to table food
Food refusal (not accepting any or only small quantities of food)
Oral sensorimotor immaturity or dysfunction
Aspiration or swallowing problems
Frequent gagging or vomiting

Note. Adapted from Kerwin, M. E. (1999). Empirically supported treatments in pediatric psychology: Severe feeding problems. *Journal of Pediatric Psychology, 24,* 193–214.

is a psychiatric classification; other systems tend to be descriptive, causal, or multidimensional (Kedesdy & Budd, 1998).

Psychiatric Classification

Psychiatric nomenclature in the Diagnostic and Statistical Manual-IV (DSM-IV) (American Psychiatric Association, 1994) has a new section for pediatrics titled "Feeding and Eating Disorders of Infancy or Early Childhood," characterizing eating and feeding disturbances that occur early in life. Types of disorders include those of infancy or early childhood, pica, and rumination disorder (Table 13–4).

Table 13–4. Classification of Pediatric Feeding Disorders According to DSM-IV

Type of Disorder	Characteristics
Infancy or early childhood	Persistent failure to eat adequately with significant failure to gain weight or significant loss of weight over at least 1 month Not due to associated gastrointestinal or other medical condition (e.g., gastroesophageal reflux) Not better accounted for by another mental disorder (e.g., rumination disorder) or by lack of food Onset is before age 6 years Includes many cases described as "Failure to Thrive"
Pica	Persistent eating of nonnutritive substances, at least 1 month Inappropriate to developmental level Not part of a culturally sanctioned practice If eating behavior occurs exclusively during course of another mental disorder (e.g., mental retardation [MR], pervasive developmental disorder [PDD]), it is severe enough to warrant independent clinical attention
Rumination disorder	Repeated regurgitation and rechewing food for at least 1 month following a period of normal functioning Behavior is not due to associated gastrointestinal or other medical condition (e.g., gastroesophageal reflux) Behavior does not occur exclusively during course of anorexia or bulemia. If symptoms occur exclusively during course of MR or PDD, they are sufficiently severe to warrant independent clinical attention

From *Diagnostic and statistical manual* (DSM), 4th ed., by the American Psychiatric Association, 1994. Washington, DC: Author.

Descriptive Classification

Food refusal and distress at mealtimes are indicators of feeding problems that may be closely linked to behavior by observation but also may include some aspect of physiologic underpinnings. Undernutrition is a likely consequence to at least some degree. Children who refuse food or liquid are usually communicating something about a variety of past and present experiences (Macht, 1990) (Table 13–5). Most problems in feeding, growth, and food acceptance can be attributed to the medical or physical condition of the child, inappropriate food selection, or inappropriate dynamics around feeding (Satter, 1992). In some children, what started out as a physiologically based feeding problem may evolve into a behavior-based problem (see case studies). Common in children with gastrointestinal (GI) problems who have undergone multiple surgeries is the difficulty in reestablishing oral feeds once the GI tract can tolerate enteral feedings. Strong aversions to oral feeding develop in the absence of early, positive experiences of tasting and swallowing liquid or food (Illingworth & Lister, 1964).

It is possible to have a sudden onset of food refusal. For example, food refusal has been reported as a posttraumatic eating disorder after an incident of choking (Chatoor, Conley, & Dickson, 1988). Following a severe bout of strep throat, a child may refuse to take solid food. A child who witnesses an ailing grandfather with significant swallowing problems just before death might refuse food for some weeks following the event.

Behavior Problems Stemming From Physical Problems

Children with physical problems may develop a variety of feeding disorders: oral–motor dysfunction, swallowing and digestive difficulties, and aspiration (O'Brien, Repp, Williams, & Christophersen, 1991). Conditioned food

Table 13–5. Food Refusal and What Children May Be Communicating

- No physical sensation of hunger or thirst
- Experiences of physical discomfort while eating or drinking
- Experiences of emotional discomfort resulting from prior unpleasant associations with eating or drinking
- Learned through experiences with primary feeders how to behave adaptively to get something (e.g., certain foods or specific attention)
- Need to learn that eating and drinking by mouth will produce pleasant tastes and reduction of physiologic discomfort
- Confusion of child as to what it means to eat as parents wish
- May eat sufficiently and comfortably for one adult, but not for others

Note. From Macht, J. (1990). *Poor eaters: Helping children who refuse to eat.* New York: Plenum Press.

aversion develops when actual or attempted oral ingestion occurs in a setting of real distress. When any of these medical conditions persist, food aversion is maintained, and frequently food refusal continues after the underlying medical problem is resolved (Luiselli, 2000). Chronic food refusal follows ongoing escape and avoidance of the perceived or learned feeding situation (Ahearn, Kerwin, Eicher, Shantz, & Swearingin, 1996).

Disorders Related to Abnormal Feeding Development

Two types of disorders relating to abnormal development of feeding are described: (1) disorder of attachment and (2) disorder of separation/individuation (Egan, Chatoor, & Rosen, 1980). Type 1 is a disorder of attachment that is directly related to inadequate parenting, often for multiple socioeconomic stressors. These children show severe growth failure from the first months of life. Type 2 is a disorder of separation/individuation. These children show a period of normal weight gain until about age 8 months when they fail to gain weight or start to lose weight. Affected children typically take liquid and puree foods, show definite food dislikes, throw tantrums at mealtimes, resist introduction to new tastes and textures, and are overall delayed in feeding development. Feeding disturbances can appear at each of the three major developmental stages in the first years of life. Descriptions by age of onset and associated infant/child and caregiver behaviors are listed in Table 13–6 (Chatoor, Menvielle, Getson, & O'Donnell, 1989).

Table 13–6. Classification of Feeding Disorders Based on Age at Onset and Associated Infant/Child and Caregiver Behaviors

Feeding Disorder (age at onset)	Infant Behaviors	Caregiver Behaviors
Homeostasis (0–2 or 3 months)	Cries, does not calm or nestle when held	Appears anxious or depressed
	Appears sleepy in responses	Becomes overwhelmed, easily distressed
	Is difficult to engage	Misses/overrides infant's signals
	Has poor suck, gags easily, and vomits	
	Cries during feed or falls asleep after short feed	Misreads infant's cues of hunger or satiety
	Has irregular feeding pattern	

(continues)

Table 13–6. *(continued)* Classification of Feeding Disorders Based on Age at Onset and Associated Infant/Child and Caregiver Behaviors

Feeding Disorder (age at onset)	Infant Behaviors	Caregiver Behaviors
Attachment (3–6 months)	Appears sad, withdrawn, or hypervigilant Avoids eye contact Does not vocalize or smile Does not reach out Stiffens or arches when picked up Drinks milk and eats without difficulty (per mother) Might spit up or vomit frequently Might ruminate Looks away from mother during feeding	Appears detached, depressed, agitated, or hostile Fails to engage infant visually or vocally Holds infant loosely, no physical closeness Does not respond to cues or needs Feeds mechanically or props bottle Does not talk to infant during feeding Unaware of nutritional needs and age-appropriate foods
Separation/ individuation (6–36 months)	Appears angry, defiant, and irritable around feedings Is curious and cheerful during play Alternates between seeking closeness and asserting own will in defiant manner Engages mother in frequent battle of will Appears disinterested in food or loses interest in food quickly Refuses to be fed by not opening mouth, turning away from food, or spitting food out Plays with food and eats very little	Appears anxious, insecure, worried, frustrated, discouraged, depressed Controls interactions by over-riding infant's drive for autonomy Fails to set appropriate limits Controls feeding by force-feeding or playing distracting games Fails to read child's signals of hunger or satiety Fails to facilitate self-feeding Appears bothered by messiness and cleans infant excessively during feeding

Note. From "Behavioral issues and implications with pediatric feeding disorders" by J. C. Arvedson, 1997. *Seminars in Speech and Language, 18,* 57. Adapted from I. Chatoor, E. Menvielle, P. Getson, & R. O'Donnell. (1989). *Observational scale for mother-infant interaction during feeding.* Washington, DC: Children's Hospital Medical Center.

Regulatory Disorder of Feeding

A primary regulatory-based eating disorder occurs when an eating or feeding disturbance, manifested by difficulties establishing regular feeding patterns with adequate or appropriate intake, is the presenting problem in an infant under 1 year of age (Greenspan &Weider, 1993). The diagnostic construct of regulatory disorder considers distinct behavioral patterns. These distinct behavior patterns are associated with faulty sensory, sensorimotor, or processing capacities.

Feeding Skills/Oral–Motor Disorder

Undernutrition with no obvious medical or surgical basis may also be secondary to a feeding skills disorder. The signs and symptoms of a feeding skills disorder are suggestive of a neurophysiologic deficit such as an oral sensorimotor impairment that is usually present from birth or early infancy but tends to go unrecognized (Ramsay, Gisel, & Boutry, 1993).

Oral–motor dysfunction is a common finding in infants and young children diagnosed as undernourished, malnourished, or being in a state of "failure to thrive"[1] (e.g., Heptinsall, Puckering, Skuse, Dowdney, & Zur-Szpira, 1987). Inadequate nutrition results from difficult feeding, structural or functional swallowing problems, or failure to have access to adequate nutrition (e.g., inadequate lactation) (Morton, 1992).

Dysfunction in Caregiver–Child Interactions

Caregiver and child interactions are complex and require parenting skills that are not necessarily automatically in place with the birth of a child. Contributing factors to undernutrition with no obvious organic basis include family socioeconomic status, parental nurturing skills, stress management, and a history of child abuse for the child or the caregiver.

Children from economically deprived areas (based on census data in Britain for area of residence) are smaller at all ages 18 to 30 months with a widening gap as age increases (Wright, Waterson, & Aynsley-Green, 1994). Parents of children with poor weight gain in low-income, inner-city regions have been found to be less nurturant and more neglecting than parents of children matched on age, gender, race, and socioeconomic status (Black, Hutcheson, Dubowitz, & Berenson-Howard, 1994). The relationships linking parenting styles (nurturant, authoritarian, and neglecting) and feeding dysfunction are not precise and are probably heterogeneous among high-risk families.

---

[1]Failure to thrive is not a diagnosis unto itself, but a descriptive term encompassing general poor growth and development. It is preferable to use the terms *undernutrition* or *malnutrition* for diagnostic purposes.

Maternal intolerance of physical contact with the infant or a problem with the infant's feeding competence may be suspected when mothers touch their children only infrequently during interactions (Polan & Ward, 1994). Mothers who have early and extended contact (rooming in) with newborn infants do more touching and interacting than a similar group of mothers with contact only during feedings (Prodromidis et al., 1995).

Other researchers have reported that mother–child feeding interactions are similar between children with poor weight gain and two comparison groups drawn from the same low socioeconiomic clinic population (Hutcheson, Black, & Starr, 1993). However, toddlers (13.5 to 26.0 months of age) with poor weight gain had mothers who were more hostile, intrusive, and less flexible than the mothers of infants (8 to 13.4 months of age). These mothers of toddlers with undernutrition demonstrated more tension and anger in their interactions. Maternal affect was not different in mothers of infants versus toddlers within the comparison group.

A history of abuse is considered for the child as well as a primary caregiver. Mothers abused as children are more likely to have undernourished children than are mothers of children with normal growth (Weston et al., 1993). Weston and colleagues found a surprising 80% of mothers of children with "non-organic failure to thrive" reported that they were victims of abuse. The mothers with history of abuse were also younger, but of the same socioeconomic groups as the comparison mothers.

Behavioral Feeding Mismanagement (Violation of Food Rules)

Children may demonstrate feeding problems primarily related to behavioral mismanagement. Lack of a defined organic etiology does not automatically indicate a pure behavioral feeding disorder. Current diagnostic techniques may not be sensitive or sophisticated enough to identify all problems. For example, gastroesophageal reflux disease (GERD) and extraesophageal reflux disease (EERD) may be subtle, intermittent, and mild. Identification can be elusive even with the best instrumentation available (Chapter 5). Yet, the child's appetite and interest in feeding may be negatively impacted. Caregiver stresses may not be fully appreciated by observers when an infant does not take feedings easily and at regular intervals. A vicious cycle emerges as the caregiver feels pressure to feed the child adequate nutrition under circumstances of marked irritability, seemingly constant crying or fussing, and frequently poor sleep patterns. This then leads to game playing to cajole the child into eating or to forced feeding. These approaches typically make a bad situation worse. Feeding difficulties frustrate even highly educated, experienced, and motivated parents, who are shown to alter caregiver–child relationships (Budd, McGraw, & Farbisz, 1992). Families may be in varying states of frustration when they come to professionals for help. A behavioral feeding assessment with a detailed history is the first step.

■ BEHAVIORAL-FOCUSED FEEDING ASSESSMENT

All children with behavioral concerns around feeding are examined by caregiver interview, history, and physical examination, observation of caregiver–child interactions, diet inventory, and oral–motor and swallow function for feeding (Chapter 7). These children, who typically have problems in multiple areas of function, are often served best by an interdisciplinary team for evaluation (Chapter 7). The focus here is on those aspects that delineate interactions between caregiver and child as well as the behavioral implications of the child's responses. The appendix at the end of this chapter is a detailed form to assist professionals in noting pertinent history and current feeding problems reported by caregivers and to compare that information with observation by professionals.

Three Primary Questions

Three primary questions provide the framework for the behavioral focused feeding assessment:

1. Does the child exhibit appetite or hunger?
2. What behaviors interfere with the feeding process?
3. Are there contributing physiologic factors that must be addressed?

These three questions help to determine relationships among caloric intake as a marker for appetite or hunger, skills/behavior of the child around eating, and etiology of the feeding problem. The spectrum of feeding disorders can be described by the extent to which oral intake is age and developmentally appropriate, that feeding is stressful or stress free, and that growth is impeded or unimpeded. Decision making for management will differ as children demonstrate strengths or deficits in these areas.

Interview, History, and Physical Examination

Interview

The caregiver interview yields basic information on the course of the feeding problem; present status of the child; prior strategies for intervention; food and texture acceptance and refusal; amounts consumed; typical mealtime duration; and routines, environment, behavior, and stress surrounding feeding.

History

A family and social history is included. Parent–child stressors around meal-times are usually prominent.

Physical Examination

The physical examination includes a review of medications, neurodevelopmental examination (Chapter 3), and an oral sensorimotor examination (Chapter 7). Medications for seizure control (e.g., Phenobarbitol) have side effects that include sedation, which can make a child lethargic (Chapter 3). Medications for GER (e.g., metoclopromide [Reglan]) have side effects that vary but can include irritability, drowsiness, diarrhea, and extrapyramidal reactions (Chapter 5). Poor weight gain is likely to be the first finding. Other medical testing will be carried out as needed (Babbitt, Hoch, & Coe, 1994; Babbitt, Hoch, Coe et al., 1994; Putnam, 1997). The oral sensorimotor examination is described in Chapter 7.

Observation of Caregiver–Child Interactions

Observations of interactions between child and caregiver at mealtime and in other situations are critical. They can be recorded and reported in multiple ways. There is no one standardized scale for universal use.

Objective Measures

Babbitt and colleagues (1994) described objective measures of target behaviors as part of a standard baseline assessment that lead to measurable treatment goals. The baseline condition provides a standard for comparison of data collected later during treatment to assess treatment efficacy.

The Nursing Child Assessment Feeding Scale (NCAFS) (Barnard, 1978a) and the Nursing Child Assessment Teaching Scale (NCATS) (Barnard, 1978b) may be useful during the 1st year of life. Both caregiver and child behaviors are measured on subscales that are categorically similar. Areas of focus for the caregiver include sensitivity to cues, response to distress, cognitive growth fostering, and social-emotional growth fostering. Infant behaviors are measured in regard to responsiveness to parent and clarity of cues.

The Feeding Scale (Chatoor, 1998; Chatoor et al., 1997) (Chatoor et al., 1989) is useful for mother–infant interaction (birth to 36 months) during feeding. It includes rating of behaviors by infant and mother in a number of categories: dyadic reciprocity, maternal noncontingency, dyadic conflict, bargaining about food, and struggle for control. Feeding disorders differ whether the onset occurs during the developmental stages of homeostasis, attachment, or separation/individuation (Chatoor et al., 1989; Table 13–6). Thus, the management plan will also differ.

The Behavior Focused Feeding Assessment (Appendix) is a nonstandardized detailed compilation of variables in primarily a check-list format. The information is obtained from parent reports and professional observations.

The topic areas include oral sensorimotor function, food refusal, food selectivity, disruptive behavior, meal duration, self-feeding, signals used by child, and unusual habits that include rumination, eating of nonfood items (Pica), and extreme selectivity by the child. There are questions about feeding techniques currently being used in the child's home and any other settings where mealtimes occur.

Mealtime Observation for Behavior and Diet

Observation of the child and caregiver(s) during a "typical" meal is used to define the eating habits of child and caregiver. Do caregivers eat while the child eats? Or does the child eat alone? What does the caregiver do when the child shows refusal? For example, a child who consistently turns her head away when the spoon is brought near her mouth ends up being force-fed when the caregiver holds the child's face, then puts the spoon into her mouth. In another instance, the caregiver may scold the child when she throws food on the floor or refuses the spoon. Some parents use objects as distractions. The length to which some parents go to entertain the child as a means of encouraging oral intake can be beyond belief. The bottom line is that it does not work over time.

Clinicians need to learn about parental eating habits because they are pertinent to evaluation of children who demonstrate behaviors related to eating. The readiness and willingness of caregivers to make changes in the feeding relationship with their children will differ depending on their own history. Mothers of children with behavior involvement with undernutrition demonstrate higher levels of dietary restraint themselves than a control group. Thus, maternal eating habits and attitudes may underlie or at least contribute significantly to feeding disorders in some children (McCann, Stein, Fairburn, & Dunger, 1994). Some caregivers restrict their children's intake of "sweet" foods and foods considered "fattening" or "unhealthy." Caregivers have been known to switch from infant formula to low-fat milk at 12 months of age, although children should get whole milk at least until 24 months of age.

Food preferences and nutritional deficiencies need to be identified during the comprehensive behavioral focused feeding evaluation. Pairing procedures can be used to identify food preferences (e.g., Babbitt, Hoch, Coe et al., 1994; Parsons & Reid, 1990). First, the child samples two food items and is then given an opportunity to take more of one of the two foods. Several pairs of foods within a food group are presented. Foods not initially chosen are paired again with different foods. At the end of the assessment, a list is compiled of highly preferred foods, moderately preferred foods, and nonpreferred foods. The procedure is used for a variety of food groups. These pairing procedures appear to be more reliable than parent report and can be useful in setting up treatment.

Excess fruit-juice consumption and grazing feeding patterns appear to be contributing factors to undernutrition for some children (Reau, Senturia, Lebailly, & Christoffel, 1996; Smith & Lifshitz, 1994). Food consumption is reduced when children drink liquids throughout the day, in turn lowering dietary protein, fat, and nutrient intakes. When parents are asked why the children are allowed to drink juice "all the time," they state that the children show preferences for juice and with the behavioral feeding difficulties, parents will try anything to get children to eat or drink. In some instances, the juice may even be diluted to save money, thus further reducing the caloric content. Nutritional intervention and regular mealtimes are successful with many of these children. They typically do not have the added complications of physical, medical, or developmental problems as those children who are most at risk for severe and persistent feeding problems.

After a comprehensive assessment, the feeding team should be able to formulate the problem(s) and establish treatment goals. These goals are likely to be approached through physiologic or behavioral interventions (or a combination of these). Treatment for severe feeding problems has included behavioral interventions, interactional therapy, psychotherapy, hypnosis, and family oriented interventions as reviewed by Kerwin (1999).

■ BEHAVIORAL INTERVENTION FOR FEEDING DISORDERS IN CHILDREN

Professionals with caregivers set priorities and processes for attaining the desired goals with measurable outcomes. Goals can be described in a continuum of (a) prevention with anticipatory guidance and follow-up (Satter, 1995), (b) early intervention (e.g., resolution of "low-level" difficulties such as nutrition guidelines to reduce excessive juice consumption), or (c) treatment of established problems (Satter, 1992). Prevention of poor growth is the preferred goal. Thus identification of infants and families at risk for undernutrition should occur as early as possible, with aggressive nutritional and behavioral intervention to minimize the duration and long-term consequences (e.g., Tolia, 1995).

By the time children are brought to a feeding team, prevention is not likely to be a reasonable goal. Nonetheless, it is hoped that early intervention can be a reality for many children because physicians and other adults in the community recognize the importance of children eating appropriately without stress at family, child care, or school meal settings. The majority of children are likely to have well-established behaviors during mealtimes. Goals will differ in relation to the specific problems that have been identified during the evaluation of feeding.

The following goals may be approached primarily through nutritional and medical guidance for some children, for others the goals will be met primarily through behavioral approaches, and still others through an integrated treatment package:

1. Steady weight gain or catch-up growth
2. Initiation of oral feedings with a history of food refusal
3. Weaning from gastrostomy tube feeds (e.g., Gutentag & Hammer, 2000)
4. Increased oral intake
5. Improved cooperation and reduced stress at mealtimes
6. Acceptance of a wider variety of flavors and textures

Integrated plans incorporate (a) feeding integration counseling, (b) appetite (hunger) promotion, (c) growth monitoring, and (d) nutrition counseling (Kedesdy & Budd, 1998). These integrated plans are basic to establishing a positive prognosis for functional outcomes in children with these complex feeding problems. Somehow the infant or child needs to make a connection between a behavior and its biologic consequences, e.g., sucking and satiation or eating/drinking at a mealtime with no pain or discomfort. Specific plans also need to take into account caregiver readiness and tolerance for change matched to the goal or function of the child.

A team approach with a psychologist or other behavioral specialist as a central member is desired. Treatment regimens can be described on the basis of the setting and on the basis of approach (Arvedson, 1997). A variety of treatment regimens are described for outpatient settings (e.g., Babbitt, Hoch, Coe et al., 1994; Hampton, 1993; McCann et al., 1994) and for intensive inpatient settings (e.g., Babbitt, Hoch, & Coe, 1994; Blackman & Nelson, 1985; Drotar, Malone, Negray, & Denstedt, 1981; Field, 1984; MacPhee, Mori, & Goldson, 1994; Singer, 1987). Behavioral-focused treatment regimens on the basis of approach include, but are not limited to, transactional approach (Casey, 1983; Chatoor et al., 1984; Goldson, Milla, & Bentovim, 1985; Satter, 1995, 1999; MacPhee et al., 1994), behavioral modification with motivational and skill deficit problems (Babbitt, Hoch, Coe et al., 1994; Hoch, Babbitt, Coe, Krell, & Kackbert, 1994), cognitive behavioral therapy (Singer, Ambuel, Wade, & Jaffe, 1992) plus pharmacologic treatment (Atkins, Lundy, & Pumariega, 1994). These treatment regimens are described briefly.

Outpatient and Inpatient Treatment Regimens

Treatment settings can be viewed on a continuum that often correlates with severity of the behavioral based feeding problem. Outpatient treatment generally represents the first phase, inpatient the second phase, followed by a third phase that is outpatient for maintaining progress and generalization to daily living settings (home and school). The choice of treatment is determined by type and severity of the feeding disorder and the availability of suitable treatment programs (Table 13–7).

Outpatient Approaches

Treatment should begin with the least intrusive intervention. Other treatment components can be added if needed. Outpatient treatment is the first choice of professionals when the child and caregivers appear to be appropriate candidates. A basic requirement of the caregiver is the ability to carry out the recommendations wherever the child eats. Caregivers often want to start with a home program if weight is not a major issue or if weight loss has not been chronic (e.g., likely less than 3 months) and has not negatively affected head circumference or linear growth.

Inpatient Approaches

Inpatient intervention can range from short-term, family-based intervention to long-term hospitalization. In some instances, inpatient care may be the

Table 13–7. Characteristics for Consideration of Inpatient Feeding Intervention

Child Characteristics	Family Characteristics	Facility Characteristics
Severe undernutrition	Mealtime interactions between caregiver and child are highly stressful, affect appetite and behaviors other than feeding	Trained feeding team available for consistent coverage to work with feeding of child
Dramatic decrease in weight or height	Parental incompetence or neglect	Resources available for training caregivers
Already hospitalized for another purpose and stable medically	Caregivers willing to participate and able to follow through on treatment techniques	Facility has ability to allow extended treatment, likely 1–6 weeks
Previous outpatient treatment has not been successful	Previous outpatient treatment has not been successful	Controlled environment conducive for systematic change
	Family location too far away to make regular outpatient visits	

Note. Adapted from *Childhood feeding disorders: Biobehavioral assessment and intervention* by J. H. Kedesdy and K. S. Budd, 1998, p. 120. Baltimore: Paul H. Brookes.

most efficient and effective for some children as the first phase (Table 13–7). A well-controlled environment is likely to be required when a problem is severe enough that growth has been compromised or when the behavior around feeding is disruptive or stressful to caregivers.

The neonatal intensive care unit (NICU) or newborn nursery is a setting in which inpatient care occurs during the first phase. Family-based intervention in the nursery appears to reduce maternal stress and depression and to enhance early mother–infant feeding interactions (Meyer et al., 1994). Infants who are admitted during the 1st year of life and require long-term hospitalization for undernutrition with no obvious physiologic etiology are likely to be from impoverished environments (35/36 infants), according to Singer (1987). Subsequently, 67% of Singer's sample were placed into county welfare custody.

Appetite or hunger is critically important and affects both speed and efficacy of treatment (Linscheid, Budd, & Rasnake, 1995). Knowledge of ambient level of hunger can be used to create optimal conditions for treatment. The child who demonstrates some degree of appetite or hunger is already on the way to success. Whenever the child is medically safe, treatment should begin with assessment of hunger drive and appetite. Clinicians can observe the child's approach to eating and drinking when food or nutrition has been denied for sustained periods (3 to 24 hours) to determine the extent to which the infant or child experiences hunger.

Treatment Regimens on the Basis of Approach

These approaches can be used in outpatient and inpatient settings.

Transactional Approach

A transactional approach takes into account the complex interplay of physical/physiologic, psychologic, and environmental factors (MacPhee et al., 1994). Various disciplines must pool their expertise to reach a comprehensive diagnosis of caregiver–child–environment dynamics (Casey, 1983; Goldson et al., 1985). Coping strategies of families with children who have behavioral-based feeding problems and poor weight gain often are ineffective (Drotar, 1991). These families tend to have helpless or fatalistic approaches to their situations. They must feel supported before their coping skills can be influenced (Patterson & Geber, 1991).

The major focus of the transactional approach is to effect change in the feeding relationship and interaction between the child and caregiver. Professionals train and counsel parents so they can learn to interpret the child's signals and to understand the meanings of the child's behavior. Parents are also taught to make adjustments in their behavior to promote homeostasis, attachment, or autonomy, depending on the stage the child is in at the time of the intervention (Table 13–1). The elimination of forced feedings and adherence to the "food rules" during mealtimes should result in the child showing an increase in appetite, internally regulated hunger, and age-appropriate feeding skills.

When the transactional approach is used in an inpatient setting, discharge planning works toward a comprehensive plan for interventions in the community that will foster quality interactions between child and caregiver (Drotar, 1989). The team atmosphere must convey trust and respect as the foundation on which caregivers can build their confidence in following through with the changes needed for long-term success in the mealtime interactions.

Behavior Modification With Motivational and Skill Deficit Problems

The basis for treatment decisions with motivational and skill deficit problems stems from two major organizing principles (Babbitt, Hoch, Coe et al., 1994): increasing appropriate behavior and decreasing maladaptive behavior (Table 13–8).

Behavior Modification Recommendation

Use of differential attention is described in multiple studies reviewed by Kerwin (1999). Overall, the use of positive attention for appropriate feeding behavior while ignoring inappropriate behavior results in positive changes in the child. This positive attention is often combined with other treatment components, such as rewards/tokens or time-out contingent upon eating or not eating the specified amount or type of food during the feeding session or during a specific time period.

The child who has shown capability for a certain behavior but does not demonstrate the behavior consistently (motivational problems) should respond to strategies for increasing appropriate behavior (Cooper et al., 1999). Differential attention can use both positive and negative reinforcement procedures to change behavior in children with motivational problems (e.g., Luiselli, 2000). When an undesirable behavior occurs, the goal is to reduce the frequency of the behavior by five primary methods (Babbitt, Hoch, Cole et al., 1994; Freeman & Pizaaz, 1998): antecedent manipulation, extinction, time-out, differential reinforcement of alternative behavior, and punishment.

Skill Deficit Problem Recommendation

Some children who demonstrate skill deficit problems need help in learning the necessary skills through specific strategies. Skill acquisition procedures

Table 13–8. Treatment Principles for Children With Feeding Problems Related to Motivational Problems

Behavioral Objectives	Treatment	Examples
Increase appropriate behavior	Positive reinforcement	Bite of food, then praise or access to favored toys
		Gradually reduce frequency of praise
		Inattention to inappropriate behaviors
	Negative reinforcement	Swallowing a bite of food as a condition for escape
Decrease maladaptive behavior	Antecedent manipulation	Less apt to expel a nonpreferred food if taste masked by preferred food
		Mix foods, alter texture, and presentation order or portion size
	Extinction	Terminate ongoing reinforcement contingency
	Time-out	Remove child from reinforcing situation, only if incentive to avoid removal
	Differential reinforcement	Combination: praise and program of preferred foods contingent on eating nonpreferred foods
	Punishment	Use cautiously and sparingly

Note. From "Behavioral issues and implications with pediatric feeding disorders" by J. C. Arvedson, 1997. *Seminars in Speech and Language, 18*(1), 62. Adapted from R. L. Babbitt, T. A. Hoch, D. A. Coe et al. (1994). Behavioral assessment and treatment of pediatric feeding disorders. *Journal of Developmental & Behavioral Pediatrics, 15*, 278-291.

include shaping, prompting, and modeling (Table 13–9) (Babbitt, Hoch, Coe et al., 1994). Acquisition of skills and alterations of behavior initially occur through reinforcement techniques in structured settings. The child must learn to generalize behavior to the more natural environment in which daily activities occur.

Cognitive Behavioral Therapy

Children with phobic avoidance behaviors to food are reported to respond well to cognitive-behavioral treatment (Atkins et al., 1994; Singer et al.,

Table 13–9. Acquisition Procedures for Skill Deficit Problems With Feeding Disorders

Acquisition Procedures	Techniques for Skill Acquisition
Shaping	Self-feeding reduced to small steps, gradually increasing complexity Rewarding successive approximations of targeted behaviors
Prompting (gradual fading as child learns)	Instructions Gestures Physical guidance
Modeling	Imitation skills necessary for reinforcement Caregivers and peers helpful

Note. From "Behavioral issues and implications with pediatric feeding disorders" by J. C. Arvedson, 1997. *Seminars in Speech and Language, 18*(1), 63. Adapted from R. L. Babbitt, T. A. Hoch, D. A. Coe et al. (1994). Behavioral assessment and treatment of pediatric feeding disorders. *Journal of Developmental & Behavioral Pediatrics, 15,* 278–291.

1992). In some instances, family therapy is added to enlist others to reinforce the child's situation in positive ways (e.g., Bishop & Riley, 1988). The major focus is to change faulty or distorted beliefs regarding fear of swallowing or eating.

Pharmacologic Treatment With Cognitive Behavioral Therapy

Pharmacologic treatment in conjunction with cognitive behavioral therapy is not in common use with children. However, a 7-year-old boy showed rapid improvement once alprazolam was added to a program that had previously included behavioral, family, and play therapy. He had made minimal gains before the medication (Atkins et al., 1994). Alprazolam was selected as an appropriate benzodiazepine because of its overall safety and documented effectiveness in the treatment of functional dysphagia in adults (e.g., Bishop & Riley, 1988). It also has been reported to be successful in children with panic disorder with agoraphobia (Ballenger, Carek, Steele, & Cornish-McTighe, 1989) and does not interfere with academic performance (Simeon et al., 1992). A protocol is not yet broadly accepted for a safe pharmacologic approach to stimulate appetite. Selected children on growth hormone or steroids show appetite stimulation as a byproduct (clinical observation).

Choice of focused treatment approach and setting for children with feeding problems is determined by severity of the problem, age and developmental level of the child, and caregiver insights and abilities to participate and carry over strategies in all mealtime environments. A transactional model appears particularly helpful for infants and young children, although it can be useful across all ages. Some of the behavioral approaches that involve differential attention appear to be effective once a child's cognitive and language skills permit an understanding of the rules being applied.

Interventions that are promising but need more research include extinction (e.g., nonremoval of a spoon) and swallow induction training (e.g., forward or backward chaining with elicitation of the pharyngeal swallow) (Kerwin, 1999). The use of any intervention, particularly intensive behavioral intervention, requires ethical considerations. Risk for aspiration must always be kept in mind, along with other health factors. As with all treatments or interventions, clinicians strive to minimize negative side effects in a least restrictive environment and to promote function in the broadest sense of the word.

■ CASE STUDY 1

History

"DJ" was born at 27 weeks gestation. Birth weight was 1,125 g. He spent 4 ½ months in a NICU. Diagnoses included bilateral Grade III intraventricular hemorrhage (V-P shunt), visual deficits (resection of lateral rectus muscle), severe bronchopulmonary dysplasia, and patent duct arteriosus (PDA) ligation. He had significant GERD/EERD, was treated with metoclopramide, and developed aspiration pneumonia.

Feeding problems had been evident since birth. Nutritional needs were met via nasogastric (NG) tube for the first 9 months, with limited oral feeding via nipple.

Initial Evaluation

DJ presented to the Pediatric Gastroenterology Clinic at age 15 months just after the family moved to western New York. DJ had been taking only Pediasure by bottle (20 oz or 600 cc per day) for the prior four months. Height and weight were below the 5th percentile. An upper gastrointestinal (UGI) study revealed GER, and a scintiscan revealed delayed gastric emptying at 15%. A 24-hour pH probe revealed minimal GER. He was started on metoclopramide and ranitidine.

DJ presented to feeding clinic 1 week after the GI clinic appointment. DJ's mother reported that recently the family had been spending several hours each day attempting to get DJ to eat. He was eating pureed food and minimal solids, drinking a 4-oz (120-cc) bottle within 30 min, and he frequently appeared distracted. He never gagged or choked.

Feeding Observation

The members of the interdisciplinary feeding team observed through a one-way window. DJ and his mother were set up for a typical lunch time. DJ demonstrated a strong pattern of food aversion. He appeared distressed and angry when a spoon with soft food was brought to his mouth. He refused to open his mouth and turned his head away from the food. DJ's mother also appeared extremely distressed and angry. She ignored her son's cues as she tried to force a bottle and a spoon with food into his mouth. DJ and his mother revealed problems with turn taking, caregiver–child conflict, and struggle for control (Chatoor, 1998).

Recommendation

The team agreed that several issues needed to be addressed: Food rules needed to be followed, cues needed to be respected, and there could be no forced feeding. Thus, a transactional approach seemed logical as a conservative approach to see if DJ could increase oral intake sufficiently over the next 2 to 3 months so that GT placement could be avoided.

Stage I: Initial Treatment: Outpatient

Transactional Approach Recommendations

Parents were instructed to follow the food rules (Chatoor et al., 1986). They would create a quiet, calm mealtime environment to reduce stress and anxiety for the child and parents, so that increased awareness of hunger and appetite could develop. Meals would be regularly scheduled, time limited, and parents were instructed to never force-feed, but they would follow the child's cues that can encourage independent self-feeding and autonomy.

DJ came to feeding clinic biweekly for weight monitoring and feeding observations for the next 3 months. He continued to show food aversion and limited appetite that resulted in insufficient caloric intake. Weight and height remained below the 5th percentile. DJ underwent surgery for GT placement.

GT Feeding Adjustments

DJ was started with daytime bolus feeds to promote weight gain and appetite. The bolus feeds were not well tolerated, even though he was on medical management of GERD. The GT schedule was changed to continuous slow feeds.

Gradually, he tolerated a combination of slow night GT feeds over 10 hours and daytime bolus feeds, which were scheduled to coincide with regular family mealtimes. DJ was given opportunities to take food and liquid orally for 10 to 15 min, then GT feed was given while he sat right up to the table with the rest of the family. Family members were prepared to give him additional opportunities for oral feeding as their meal progressed.

Oral Feeding Variability

Over the next 3 years, DJ's growth and oral intake were variable. He gained weight during the 1st year because he drank 20 to 25 oz Pediasure each day, which was no different from total PO intake before the GT. Parents stated that they were less frustrated and that DJ had begun to ask for food.

DJ's interest in oral feeding decreased to about 16 oz Pediasure per day as he began to experience increased GER with intermittent vomiting. Once the vomiting subsided, his oral intake increased over 4 months to 50% of the total calories he received each day. He gained an average of 5 oz (150 g) per month which paralleled the 5th percentile, but without catchup growth. He took Pediasure, cookies, graham crackers, and cheese curls by mouth, but he avoided all other foods. DJ exhibited stress and extreme avoidance to utensils (cups and spoons).

Preschool Program Focus

DJ began attending an early intervention preschool where, unfortunately, well intended, overzealous teachers and therapists focused their attention on feeding. The educational program focus was directed toward the promotion of oral feeding "to get DJ to eat" (i.e., forced feeding). DJ showed extreme avoidance to cups and spoons. The feeding clinic team encouraged DJ's teachers and therapists to use desensitization games. This approach required gradual presentation of empty spoon and cup to DJ's lips, eventually with small amounts of food and liquid touched to his lips, but with no attempt to get into his mouth.

GERD Persistence

Over the next several months, GER was persistent. Medical management included medication changes with no relief from GERD. Scintiscan showed no change in gastric emptying time. He underwent surgery for fundoplication and pyloroplasty. Over the next several months, DJ's weight steadily increased. The feeding regimen included slow nocturnal GT feeds and GT bolus feeds (5 oz, 150 cc) at scheduled mealtimes during the daytime. Initially, DJ tolerated bolus feeds only at a rate of 5 oz in a 45-minute period. Gradually, the time was decreased to 10 min for 5 oz. DJ's oral intake gradually decreased during the same period, and he continued to appear aversive to oral feeding. Parents were frustrated as they expended a lot of energy for oral feeding. Nutrition needs were deemed most important. Thus, a decision was made to "back off" the oral feeding goals.

Behavioral Approach

At the end of this period, DJ's school staff decided that they could get him to eat. They initiated a vigorous feeding program that was essentially forced feeding. DJ took only small amounts of yogurt. DJ and his parents returned to feeding clinic for guidance in a more effective approach. DJ was extremely active across all settings. Consideration was given to the possibility that movement could serve as a powerful reinforcement if DJ would perceive access to freedom as a goal. A behavioral program was initiated:

Step I: DJ was seated in a chair for each meal. To get up from the chair, he was required to place an empty spoon or empty cup to his mouth.

Step II: After 2 days, he was required to taste small amounts of food to get up from his chair.

Step III: Every 2 days, DJ had to increase volume of tastes gradually. DJ's weight reached the 5th percentile, and his height/weight ratio was at the 40th percentile 8 months later. Clearly, he was no longer malnourished. DJ took 12- to 16-oz of yogurt per day. He refused to feed himself, but he continued to gain weight over the next several months. After 4 more months, he initiated limited self-feeding and would eat 2 to 3 spoonfuls of yogurt to prove his point.

During this period, a plan was initiated to decrease GT feeds. Extreme selectivity of food persisted (he would only eat yogurt), and he no longer drank liquids. After another 3 months, DJ received a nocturnal GT feed of 24 to 32 oz of Kindercal and oral feeds of 16 to 20 oz of yogurt per day. He continued to refuse liquids and other solid food. It became clear that he needed a more intensive program than could be provided to the family while DJ was an outpatient. He was admitted to an inpatient rehabilitation unit, where a structured behavioral feeding program was set up.

Stage II: Inpatient Treatment

Transactional Approach

Upon admission, DJ was receiving a continuous overnight GT feed as his primary source of nutrition. During the day, he had inconsistent oral feeds of yogurt (smooth puree texture on the spoon). Food rules were followed by all staff and parents to neutralize conflict. DJ demonstrated the ability to self-feed at the onset of the meal, but he required assistance with feeding as the meal progressed. For the 1st week, baseline data were obtained about eating and feeding behavior. DJ showed difficulty sitting during the meal. Frequently, it would take DJ up to 45 min before he would sit at the table to start a meal. He exhibited facial grimacing each time the spoon was placed in his mouth, whether he was feeding himself or his parents were doing the feeding.

Behavioral Approach

The GT feeding schedule was changed to daytime bolus feeds to approximate a typical eating schedule. DJ was offered yogurt followed by a bolus feed at five regularly scheduled meals (breakfast, lunch, supper, and 2 snacks). Once it was established that DJ could eat 8 oz of yogurt at each meal, a plan was implemented to increase oral intake gradually and to decrease the volume received by GT.

At the start of the process to wean from GT feedings, the caloric density of the yogurt was increased by adding Kindercal and Moducal. All meals took place in his room at the child-sized table. DJ demonstrated sensory integration difficulties, characterized by hypersensitivity to light touch and noises, which compromised his ability to achieve and to maintain a quiet, regulated state (homeostasis) during meals. Deep pressure stimulation helped to calm him, and the feeding environment was controlled to minimize distractions and to ensure that boundaries were clear.

DJ was given incentives to finish the amount of yogurt he was given at each meal (positive reinforcement). He was motivated to complete the meal to have access to television viewing. Initially, meals were not time limited. Frequently, DJ engaged in lengthy and intense avoidance behavior in transitioning to the mealtime situation. A meal (feeding episode) was terminated as DJ was completing the mealtime caloric goal. In this way, the approach to eating could be reinforced, while avoidance to eating could be extinguished. The initiation of meals created such intense anxiety for DJ that the family had to be instructed to role play the transition to initiation of food intake. Also, gradual reduction was made in the time allowed to reach criteria (caloric goal) from no time limit to 20 min. Over a period of 2 weeks, DJ gradually increased his oral intake per meal and decreased the amount of time spent eating a meal. An important outcome was that DJ could not escape from the mealtime situation.

DJ appeared extremely sensitive to small changes in all dimensions of taste and texture. With a graduated hierarchy, DJ was first exposed to a variety of foods (tastes) while the texture of his yogurt (smooth puree) was held constant. Gradual changes in taste and texture were offered during occupational and speech–language therapy sessions that were scheduled between meals.

DJ continued to exhibit facial grimacing and resistance to changes in texture. Near the end of the hospitalization, the focus shifted to taste. DJ was encouraged to play with a variety of foods and to develop a list of foods that he might want to try in the future. Nevertheless, he continued to avoid texture changes in the yogurt and totally refused drinking liquids from a cup. By the time of discharge from the hospital, DJ was taking all food orally but still required liquids by tube.

Stage III: Outpatient Follow-Up

At 1 year following discharge, DJ was an independent oral feeder. GT was used only for hydration purposes. Major nutrition needs were met as DJ drank high caloric and nutritionally balanced liquid formula. Repertoire of food was limited to yogurt concoctions, also limited number of textures (e.g., cookies and crackers, some chewable food). The tube has not been used for calories. Growth parameters are appropriate.

Comment

This case study presents an extremely complex child requiring interdisciplinary coordination with parents to make decisions and modify those decisions as the child communicates readiness (or lack of readiness) for change. The approaches may vary from a transactional to a behavioral approach as a child demonstrates that he or she can understand contingencies, rewards, and consequences. Although the process was slow, the long-term outcome (1 year) was positive and stable. Long-term carryover should be positive because DJ had some control as he was gaining skills. We believe it is critical to have the child as self-motivated as possible with genuine hunger and appetite. Many parents want to start in an outpatient program, which they perceive to be a less intensive approach than an inpatient stay. The importance of ongoing information and communication with caregivers cannot be overstressed. The team members have to be anticipating needs of both child and parents. Timing of changes in feeding approaches is a critical factor.

■ CASE STUDY 2

History

"George" presented to feeding clinic at age 4 years with a diagnosis of autism and parents' concern that the repertoire of food was limited. He took only a mixture of milk and strained baby food from a bottle with a specific nipple (clear nipple with the tip bitten off) and a red rim on the cap. He refused all other foods and containers. This idiosyncratic feeding pattern developed at age 2 years after a choking incident. He had refused to eat for a period of 3 to 4 days immediately after the incident, no matter what family and teachers did to try to transition him to more age appropriate eating. The parents then let him take the bottle because all the other difficulties in coping with the autistic behavior made it impossible for them to try to get George to change his feeding patterns. By the time he presented to feeding clinic, they were worried about what would happen should this nipple and rim combination be lost. By that time, the nipple and rim were no longer manufactured, and thus it was not possible to get replacements.

Considerations for intervention were limited because of the parents' limited abilities to follow through in consistent ways to modify behavior in this child who had so many communication and behavioral related deficits. It seemed most efficient to admit George to the inpatient rehabilitation unit where a structured, consistent program could be carried out.

Behavioral Treatment Approach

The goal was to eliminate exclusive dependence on the nipple and red rim configuration. The plan was to transition George from the bottle to a cup by changing the nipple gradually.

The behavioral approach combined desensitization and successive approximation. Each day a small portion of the nipple was cut off, slowly enlarging the opening. On the 4th day, someone misplaced the bottle, so a different one had to be used. George transitioned quickly from his 8-oz bottle to a 4-oz bottle with the same nipple and rim. The process was accelerated over the next 2 days with the nipple cut down significantly. George had to drink from the remaining rim of the bottle, similar to a cup. He was then given a transitional slot cup with the insert in place, and finally the insert was removed, and he had an open cup.

Outcome

George was discharged 2 weeks after admission. He was consistently taking his mixture from an open MagMag cup. George was given a 24-hour pass with his parents to go home to assess whether he would generalize the new feeding pattern to other settings. He drank from the cup and then was discharged from the hospital. Following discharge, George continued to drink from a variety of open cups, even though a younger sibling was still using the bottle. He continued to receive occupational therapy focused on global sensory needs.

Comment

This child is an example of a complex problem, but one with a relatively "quick fix" when people put their heads together and examine all aspects of a child's behavior or performance to arrive at a functional plan. Here the team with parents figured out how to move in incremental steps from what a child accepts readily to what is desirable, especially to work toward age appropriate function.

■ APPENDIX

Behavior Focused Feeding Assessment

Interview (Information needed in following aspects)

I. General Development and Background (See Chapter 7, Appendix)

Pregnancy and birth history

Health conditions/problems (inherited conditions, chronic disease, medications, neurologic conditions, etc.)

Illness, accident, traumatic events, or hospitalizations (i.e. aversive conditioning history)

Overall development (gross and fine motor skills, language, cognition)

Variations or stresses in day-to-day living conditions (moves, job changes, sibling births, serious illness in the family, etc.)

II. Feeding History

Onset of feeding problems:

Age of onset ____

Experiences contributing to the problem in the past:

____ Pain and discomfort during feeding because of underlying anatomic or physiologic problems

____ Esophagitis secondary to gastroesophageal reflux

____ Insertion of nasogastric feeding tube

____ Endotracheal suctioning

____ Other_____

Signs and symptoms in the past:

____ Crying, gagging, or choking, while eating or at sight of bottle or food

____ Refusing to chew or swallow

____ Lack of awareness/feeling of hunger

____ Acceptance of the bottle only when falling asleep

____ Other_____

Changes in feeding problems over time:

Foods and liquids child accepted at one time, but no longer accepts. Give examples. _____

_____

Previous strategies used _____

_____

Feeding milestones achieved (✔ all that apply):

Breast feeding	_____	Cup	_____
Bottle feeding	_____	Spoon	_____
Strained foods	_____	Fork	_____
Junior foods	_____	Knife	_____
Chopped foods	_____	Straw	_____
Regular foods	_____	Pours drink	_____
Finger feeding	_____	Gets food	_____

Medical/surgical restrictions on certain foods or liquids. Give examples

_____

III. Feeding Environment Used Most Often For Meals

Feeders:
Person who regularly feeds _____
Multiple feeders _____
Is one adult more successful? _____ If yes, who? _____
Other eaters or feeders present _____

Location for feeding:

_____	lap	_____	stand or roam
_____	infant seat	_____	floor
_____	highchair	_____	couch
_____	booster seat	_____	other_____
_____	regular chair up to table		

Typical meal schedule (time of day) _____
Amount of time per meal (average min. and range)_____
Typical sequence in which food is offered_____
Best description of child's appetite _____
Proportion of daily intake outside meals _____

IV. Mealtime Habits (Current mode of receiving nourishment). Circle all that apply.

Foods and liquids child currently and regularly accepts:
fruits   meats   vegetables   breads/cereals   dairy   sweets

Textures child accepts:
liquid   strained/pureed   chopped   crunchy
blenderized/mashed   chewy

Foods and liquids child regularly rejects _____

Extent to which child feeds self:
Bottle: ____does not hold bottle ____ holds with support
____independent

Self-feeding: ___ does not feed self ___ feeds self with support
___ independent

V. Current Feeding Problems (Status of the problem) (✔ all that apply):

	Reported (parent)	Observed (professional)
Oral sensorimotor dysfunction		
fails to suck	_____	_____
fails to chew food	_____	_____
not able to swallow	_____	_____
drooling	_____	_____
gagging	_____	_____
choking/coughing	_____	_____
gurgly wet vocal quality	_____	_____
increased breathing rate/effort	_____	_____
Food Refusal		
refuses all food	_____	_____
eats too little	_____	_____
accepts bottle only when falling asleep	_____	_____
Food Selectivity		
picky eater	_____	_____
taste—narrow range	_____	_____
texture—narrow range	_____	_____
liquid only	_____	_____
soft food only	_____	_____
solid (chewable) only	_____	_____
eats the wrong food	_____	_____

	Reported (parent)	Observed (professional)
Disruptive Behavior		
easily distractable	_____	_____
cries or tantrums (thrashing)	_____	_____
gagging	_____	_____
vomiting	_____	_____
stiffens when touched, arches back	_____	_____
sways or turns head to avoid nipple or spoon	_____	_____
pushes food away	_____	_____
refuses to open mouth	_____	_____
refuses to chew or swallow	_____	_____
throws or drops food	_____	_____
spits food out	_____	_____
plays with food	_____	_____
messy eater	_____	_____
struggles to get out of chair	_____	_____
gets away from the table	_____	_____
Meal Duration		
improper pacing by child	_____	_____
eats too fast	_____	_____
eats too slow (mealtimes > 30 min)	_____	_____
eats but gives up quickly, not complete meal	_____	_____
Self-feeding		
delay	_____	_____
difficult	_____	_____
refuses to feed self	_____	_____
Signals used by child		
not signal hunger or satiety	_____	_____
ambiguous (approach/avoidance)	_____	_____
not appear hungry	_____	_____
lack of reciprocity (child not "in tune" with feeder)	_____	_____
Unusual Habits		
ruminates	_____	_____
eats non-food items	_____	_____
accepts food only from single bottle or utensil (only one caregiver, or only one location)	_____	_____
other (describe)_____	_____	_____

VI. Feeding Techniques (currently used by caregivers during meals)

Coax _____ _____
Praise _____ _____
Offer Reward/bargain _____ _____
   model desired behavior _____ _____
   distract
      with play/toys _____ _____
      use music or TV _____ _____
   must eat unfamiliar foods first _____ _____
   threaten _____ _____
   spank _____ _____
   send to room/time-out _____ _____
   other (describe) _____ _____ _____
Force feed _____ _____
   restrain arms when child flails at
      the spoon or bottle _____ _____
   force the child's mouth open _____ _____
   force the mouth to stay closed until a
      swallow occurs _____ _____
   hold the child's head still in order to
      get the spoon into mouth _____ _____
   sneak attack when child is not looking _____ _____
Limits food or liquid in hope to
   encourage hunger or thirst _____ _____
Change foods offered within a meal
   ("short order cook") _____ _____
Mini-meals ad lib that result in demand
   feeds or grazing _____ _____
Allow child to eat with fingers even
   when he could use utensils _____ _____
Respond negatively to gagging or
   vomiting _____ _____
During feeding (Affective tone by feeder)
   soft _____ _____
   patient _____ _____
   firm _____ _____
   tense _____ _____
   frustrated _____ _____
   angry _____ _____
   ignore the child _____ _____

Major sources of feeding information to family_____

Professional recommendations received in past_____

Impressions of parents for most effective techniques_____

Formulation: Hypothesize the antecedent and consequences that appear to exert stimulus control over each problem behavior. Identify the functional relationship between the feeding problem and its solution. Identify the variables that appear to maintain the problem.

■ REFERENCES

Ahearn, W. H., Kerwin, M. L. E., Eicher, P. S., Shantz, J., & Swearingin, W. (1996). An alternating treatments comparison of two intensive interventions for food refusal. *Journal of Applied Behavior Analysis, 29*, 321–332.

American Psychiatric Association. (1994). *Diagnostic and statistical manual,* 4th ed.). Washington, DC: Author.

Arvedson, J. C. (1997). Behavioral issues and implications with pediatric feeding disorders. *Seminars in Speech and Language, 18*, 51–70.

Atkins, D. L., Lundy, M. S., & Pumariega, A. J. (1994). A multimodal apporach to functional dysphagia. *Journal of American Academy of Child & Adolescent Psychiatry, 33*, 1012–1016.

Babbitt, R. L., Hoch, T. A., & Coe, D. A. (1994). Behavioral feeding disorders. In D. N. Tuchman & R. S. Walter (Eds.), *Disorders of feeding and swallowing in infants and children: Pathophysiology, diagnosis, and treatment* (pp. 77–95). San Diego: Singular Publishing Group.

Babbitt, R. L., Hoch, T. A., Coe, D. A., Cataldo, M. F., Kelly, K. J., Stackhouse, C., & Perman, J. A. (1994). Behavioral assessment and treatment of pediatric feeding disorders. *Journal of Developmental & Behavioral Pediatrics, 15*, 278–291.

Ballenger, J. C., Carek, D. J., Steele, J. J., & Cornish-McTighe, D. (1989). Three cases of panic disorder with agoraphobia in children. *American Journal of Psychiatry, 146*, 922–924.

Barnard, K. E. (1978a). *Nursing child assessment feeding scales.* Seattle: University of Washington.

Barnard, K. E. (1978b). *Nursing child assessment teaching scale.* Seattle: University of Washington.

Barnard, K. E., Hammond, M. A., Booth, C. L., Bee, H. L., Mitchell, S. K., & Spieker, S. J. (1989). Measurement and meaning of parent child interaction. In F. Morrisson, C. Lord, & D. Keating (Eds.), *Applied developmental psychology.* New York: Academic Press.

Bentovim, A. (1970). The clinical approach to feeding disorders of childhood. *Journal of Psychosomatic Research, 14,* 267–276.

Birch, L. L., & Marlin, D. W. (1982). I don't like it; I never tried it: Effects of exposure on two-year-old children's food preferences. *Appetite, 3,* 353–360.

Bishop, L. C., & Riley, W. T. (1988). The psychiatric management of the globus syndrome. *General Hospital Psychiatry, 9,* 214–219.

Black, M. M., Hutcheson, J. J., Dubowitz, H., & Berenson-Howard, J. (1994). Parenting style and developmental status among children with nonorganic failure to thrive. *Journal of Pediatric Psychology, 19,* 689–707.

Blackman, J. A., & Nelson, C. L. A. (1985). Reinstituting oral feedings in children fed by gastrostomy tube. *Clinical Pediatrics, 24,* 434–438.

Budd, K. S., McGraw, T. E., & Farbisz, R. (1992). Psychosocial concomitants of children's feeding disorders. *Journal of Pediatric Psychology, 17,* 81–94.

Casey, P. H. (1983). Failure to thrive: A reconceptualization. *Developmental and Behavioral Pediatrics, 4,* 63–66.

Chatoor, I. (1998). *The feeding scale.* Washington, DC: Children's National Medical Center.

Chatoor, I., Conley, C., & Dickson, L. (1988). Food refusal after an incident of choking: A posttraumatic eating disorder. *Journal of American Academy of Child & Adolescent Psychiatry, 27,* 105–110.

Chatoor, I., Dickson, L., Schaefer, S., & Egan, J. (1985). A developmental classification of feeding disorders associated with failure to thrive: Diagnosis and treatment. In D. Drotar (Ed.), *New directions in failure to thrive: Implications for research and practice.* New York: Plenum Press.

Chatoor, I., Getson, P., Menvielle, E., O'Donnell, R., Rivera, Y., Brasseaux, C., & Mrazek, D. (1997). A feeding scale for research and clinical practice to assess mother-infant interactions in the first three years of life. *Infant Mental Health Journal, 18,* 76–91.

Chatoor, I., Menvielle, E., Getson, P., & O'Donnell, R. (1989). *Observational scale for mother-infant-toddler interaction during feeding.* Washington, DC : Children's Hospital Medical Center.

Chatoor, I., Schaefer, S., Dickson, L., & Egan, J. (1984). Non-organic failure to thrive: A developmental perspective. *Pediatric Annals, 13,* 829–843.

Cooper, L. J., Wacker, D. P., Brown, K., McComas, J. J., Peck, S. M., Drew, J., Asmus, J., & Kayser, K. (1999). Use of a concurrent operants paradigm to evaluate positive reinforcers during treatment of food refusal. *Behavior Modification, 23,* 3–40.

Dahl, M., & Sendelin, C. (1992). Feeding problems in an affluent society. Follow-up at four years of age in children with early refusal to eat. *Acta Paediatrica, 81,* 575–579.

Drotar, D. (1989). Behavioral diagnosis in nonorganic failure-to-thrive: A critique and suggested approach to psychological assessment. *Developmental and Behavioral Pediatrics, 10*, 48–55.

Drotar, D. (1991). The family context of nonorganic failure to thrive. *American Journal of Orthopsychiatry, 61*, 23–33.

Drotar, D., Malone, C., Negray, J., & Denstedt, M. (1981). Patterns of hospital based care for infants with nonorganic failure-to-thrive. *Journal of Clinical Child Psychology, 10*, 63–66.

Egan, J., Chatoor, I., & Rosen, G. (1980). Non-organic failure to thrive: Pathogenesis and classification. *Clinical Proceedings of Children's Hospital Medical Center, 36*, 173–182.

Field, M. (1984). Follow-up developmental status of infants hospitalized for nonorganic failure to thrive. *Journal of Pediatric Psychology, 9*, 241–256.

Forsyth, B. W. C., Leventhal, J. J., & McCarthy, P. L. (1985). Mothers' perceptions of problems of feeding and crying behaviors: A prospective study. *American Journal of Diseases of Children, 139*, 269–272.

Freeman, K. A., & Pizaaz, C. C. (1998). Combining stimulus fading, reinforcement, and extinction to treat food refusal. *Journal of Applied Behavior Analysis, 31*, 691–694.

Goldson, E., Milla, P. J., & Bentovin, A. (1985). Failure to thrive: A transactional issue. *Family Systems Medicine, 3*, 206–213.

Greenspan, S., & Lourie, R. S. (1981). Developmental structuralist approach to the classification of adaptive and pathologic personality organizations: Infancy and early childhood. *American Journal of Psychiatry, 138*, 725–735.

Greenspan, S., & Weider, S. (1993). Regulatory disorders. In C. H. Zemah, Jr. (Ed.), *Handbook of infant mental health* (pp. 280–290). New York: The Guilford Press.

Gutentag, S., & Hammer, D. (2000). Shaping oral feeding in a gastronomy tube-dependent child in natural settings. *Behavior Modification, 24*, 395–410.

Hampton, D. (1993). Failure to thrive—tackling feeding problems: A community-based approach. *Health Visitor, 66*, 407–408.

Heptinsall, E., Puckering, C., Skuse, D., Dowdney, L., & Zur-Szpira, S. (1987). Nutrition and mealtime behaviour in families of growth-retarded children. *Human Nutrition: Applied Nutrition, 41a*, 390–402.

Hoch, T. A., Babbitt, R. L., Coe, D. A., Krell, D. M., & Kackbert, L. (1994). Contingency contacting: Combining positive reinforcement and escape extinction procedures to treat persistent food refusal. *Behavior Modification, 18*, 106–128.

Hutcheson, J. J., Black, M. M., & Starr, R. H. J. (1993). Developmental differences in interactional characteristics of mothers and their children with failure to thrive. *Journal of Pediatric Psychology, 18*, 453–466.

Illingworth, R. S., & Lister, J. (1964). The critical or sensitive period, with special reference to certain feeding problems in infants and children. *Journal of Pediatrics, 65*, 840–848.

Kedesdy, J. H., & Budd, K. S. (1998). *Childhood feeding disorders: Biobehavioral assessment and intervention.* Baltimore: Paul H. Brookes.

Kerwin, M. E. (1999). Empirically supported treatments in pediatric psychology: Severe feeding problems. *Journal of Pediatric Psychology, 24*, 193–214.

Kopp, C. (1982). Antecedents of self-regulation: A developmental perspective. *Developmental Psychology, 18*, 199–214.

Linscheid, T. R., Budd, K. S., & Rasnake, L. K. (1995). Pediatric feeding disorders. In M.C. Roberts (Ed.), *Handbook of pediatric psychology* (2nd ed.; pp. 501–515). New York: Guilford Press.

Luiselli, J. K. (2000). Cueing, demand fading, and positive reinforcement to establish self-feeding and oral consumption in a child with chronic food refusal. *Behavior Modification, 24*, 348–358.

Macht, J. (1990). *Poor eaters: Helping children who refuse to eat.* New York: Plenum Press.

MacPhee, M., Mori, C., & Goldson, E. (1994). Change in the hospital setting: Adopting a team approach for nonorganic failure-to-thrive. *Journal of Pediatric Nursing, 9*, 218–225.

Marchi, M., & Cohen, P. (1990). Early childhood eating behaviors and adolescent eating disorders. *Journal of the American Academy of Child and Adolescent Psychiatry, 29*, 112–117.

Mayes, L. C., & Volkmar, F. R. (1993). Nosology of eating and growth disorders in early childhood. *Child and Adolescent Psychiatric Clinics of North America, 2*, 15–35.

McCann, J. B., Stein, A., Fairburn, C. G., & Dunger, D. B. (1994). Eating habits and attitudes of mothers of children with non-organic failure to thrive. *Archives of Diseases in Childhood, 70*, 234–236.

Meyer, E. C., Coll, C. T., Lester, B. M., Buokydis, C. F., McDonough, S. M., & Oh, W. (1994). Family-based intervention improves maternal psychological well-being and feeding interaction of preterm infants. *Pediatrics, 93*, 241–246.

Morton, J. A. (1992). Ineffective suckling: A possible consequence of obstructive positioning. *Journal of Human Lactation, 8*, 83–85.

O'Brien, S., Repp, A. C., Williams, G. E., & Christophersen, E. G. (1991). Pediatric feeding disorders. *Behavior Modification, 15*, 394–418.

Parsons, M. B., & Reid, D. H. (1990). Assessing food preferences among persons with profound mental retardation: Providing opportunities to make choices. *Journal of Applied Behavior Analysis*, *23*, 183–195.

Patterson, J. M., & Geber, G. (1991). Preventing mental health problems in children with chronic illness or disability. *Children's Health Care*, *14*, 96–102.

Phillips, C. B., & Cooper, R. M. (1992). Cultural dimensions of feeding relationships. *Zero to Three*, *12*, 10–13.

Polan, H. J., & Ward, M. J. (1994). Role of the mother's touch in failure to thrive: A preliminary investigation. *Journal of American Academy of Child & Adolescent Psychiatry*, *33*, 1098–1105.

Pridham, K. F. (1990). Feeding behavior of 6- to 12-month-old infants: Assessment and sources of parental information. *Journal of Pediatrics*, *117*(2 Pt. 2), S174–S180.

Prodromidis, M., Field, T., Arendt, R., Singer, L., Yando, R., & Bendell, D. (1995). Mothers touching newborns: A comparison of rooming-in versus minimal contact. *Birth*, *22*, 196–200.

Putnam, P. E. (1997). Gastroesophageal reflux disease and dysphagia in children. *Seminars in Speech and Language, 18*, 25–38.

Ramsay, M., Gisel, E. G., & Boutry, M. (1993). Non-organic failure to thrive: Growth failure secondary to feeding-skills disorder. *Developmental Medicine and Child Neurology*, *35*, 285–297.

Reau, N. R., Senturia, Y. D., Lebailly, S. A., & Christoffel, K. K. (1996). Infant and toddler feeding patterns and problems: Normative data and a new direction. *Journal of Developmental and Behavioral Pediatrics, 17*, 149–153.

Satter, E. M. (1990). The feeding relationship: Problems and interventions. *Journal of Pediatrics*, *117*, 181–189.

Satter, E. M. (1992). The feeding relationship. *Zero to Three*, *12*, 1–9.

Satter, E. M. (1995). Feeding dynamics: Helping children to eat well. *Journal of Pediatric Health Care, 9*, 178–184.

Satter, E. M. (1999). The feeding relationship. In P. Kessler, & P. Dawson, (Eds.), *Failure to thrive and pediatric undernutrition: A transdisciplinary approach* (pp. 121–144). Baltimore: Paul H. Brookes.

Simeon, J. G., Ferguson, H. B., Knott, V., Roberts, N., Gauthier, B., Dubois, C., & Wiggins, D. (1992). Clinical, cognitive, and neurophysiological effects of alprazolam in children and adolescents with overanxious and avoidant disorders. *Journal of American Academy of Child & Adolescent Psychiatry*, *31*, 847–852.

Singer, L. (1987). Long-term hospitalization of nonorganic failure-to-thrive infants: Patient characteristics and hospital course. *Journal of Developmental & Behavioral Pediatrics*, *8*, 25–31.

Singer, L. T., Ambuel, B., Wade, S., & Jaffe, A. C. (1992). Cognitive-behavioral treatment of health-impairing food phobias in children. *Journal of American Academy of Child & Adolescent Psychiatry, 31,* 847–852.

Smith, M. M., & Lifshitz, F. (1994). Excess fruit juice consumption as a contributing factor in nonorganic failure to thrive. *Pediatrics, 93,* 438–443.

Thompson, R. J., & Palmer, S. (1974). Treatment of feeding problems—a behavioral approach. *Journal of Nutrition Education, 6,* 63–66.

Tolia, V. (1995). Very early onset nonorganic failure to thrive in infants. *Journal of Pediatric Gastroenterology & Nutrition, 20,* 73–80.

Weston, J. A., Colloton, M., Halsey, S., Covington, S., Gilbert, J., Sorrentino-Kelly, L., & Renoud, S. S. (1993). A legacy of violence in nonorganic failure to thrive. *Child Abuse & Neglect, 17,* 709–714.

Whitten, C. R., Pettit, M. G., & Fischoff, J. (1969). Evidence that growth failure from maternal deprivation is secondary to undereating. *Journal of the American Medical Association, 209,* 1675–1682.

Wright, C. M., Waterston, A., & Aynsley-Green, A. (1994). Effect of deprivation on weight gain in infancy. *Acta Paediatrica, 83,* 357–359.

Glossary

■ A

Abduction   Movement of the limbs away from the midline of the body.

Achalasia   Dysfunction of the esophagus consisting of failure or incomplete relaxation of the lower or upper esophageal sphincters or absent peristalsis of the esophagus.

Adduction   Movement of the limbs toward the midline of the body.

Adjusted chronologic age (ACA)   The age a preterm infant would be if born at term; used in assessment of developmental milestones; also called "corrected age."

Afferent   Refers to neurons that carry input toward the central nervous system.

Alveoli   Tiny sac-like spaces in the lungs. Oxygen and carbon dioxide are exchanged with the bloodstream across the alveolar lining.

Ankyloglossia ("tongue tied")   A condition that occurs when the lingual frenulum abnormally tethers the inferior surface of the anterior part of the tongue to the floor of the mouth, interfering with tongue protrusion and elevation.

Anomaly   A malformation of a part of the body.

Antigravity control   Sustained posture and movement away from gravity, requiring normal muscle tone and muscle coordination, as well as the ability to preserve or restore balance.

Apgar score   A system for evaluating an infant's physical condition at birth based on a 0–10 scale. The infant's heart rate, respiration, muscle tone, response to stimuli, and color are evaluated at 1 and 5 minutes after birth, may be continued every 5 minutes for up to 20 minutes or until two successive scores are eight or more.

Apnea   Cessation of respiratory airflow for any duration, usually deemed abnormal when > 5–8 seconds.

> **Central apnea** is caused by CNS problems and is characterized by no airflow and no respiratory effort.

> **Obstructive apnea** is caused by an anatomic problem and is characterized by continual respiratory effort but no airflow.

> **Mixed apnea** is a combination of central and obstructive apnea.

Aspiration   Secretions, food, or any foreign material in the airway below the level of the true vocal folds. Ineffective air exchange can lead to asphyxiation, tracheobronchial inflammation, and pulmonary inflammation aspiration pneumonia. Aspiration may occur before, during, or after swallowing.

> **Chronic aspiration**   Repeated or intractable episodes of aspiration.

Aspiration pneumonia   Infection of the lungs following aspiration.

Associated Reactions   An overflow of movement of one part of the body to another that occurs with physical exertion; often seen in infants or individuals with neurologic impairment.

Asymmetry   Differences in appearance and action of one side of the face or body to the corresponding part on the other side.

Atelectasis   Collapse or incomplete expansion of alveoli in lungs.

Athetosis   Fluctuating muscle tone, characterized by random movement patterns.

Atresia   A birth defect in which a passage (such as a valve, a vein, or an artery) is completely blocked or absent.

Atresia choanae   Failure of posterior nasal cavity to canalize.

Atrial septal defect (ASD)   A birth defect in which a hole is present in the wall (septum) between the two upper chambers (atria) of the heart.

Auscultation (cervical)   Use of stethoscope or microphone to listen to swallow sounds; not standardized, and thus, at best, a screening tool.

Autonomic nervous system   That part of the nervous system that innervates the visceral organs. It has two divisions, the sympathetic and parasympathetic.

Aversion, oral   A negative association with or response to anything placed in or near the mouth.

■ **B**

Barrett's esophagus   Columnar metaplasia of the esophagus. The normal squamous epithelium is replaced with specialized columnar epithelium. This may occur as a result of prolonged reflux with severe damage to the esophageal mucosa and is considered a premalignant lesion that can lead to adenocarcinoma.

Bilirubin   Substance released when the body breaks down red blood cells, converted by the liver and disposed of mainly in the stool. Buildup of bilirubin in the blood may cause jaundice.

Bolus   A volume of fluid or food given within a short time period orally or by a supplemental tube, instead of in small volumes over prolonged time periods.

Bradycardia   Slowed heart rate: For full-term neonates, heart rate (HR) typically falls between 120 and 140 beats per minute (BPM). Premature infants have higher HR, not uncommon to range 160 to 180 BPM. Individual infants have less variability within themselves. During work, such as feeding, it is common to see the HR increase 10 BPM over the at rest baseline value.

Breathing, periodic   A cyclic pattern of brief (about 5 to 10 sec) pauses in breathing in infants, without any change in heart rate or skin color. This pattern is common in preterm infants and also may be seen in some healthy term infants in the first few days of life.

Bronchial tubes   The tubes that lead from the trachea to the lungs.

Bronchiectasis   Irreversible dilation of the bronchial tree and destruction of the bronchial walls. This condition may be congenital but is generally caused by recurrent inflammation or infection of the airway, such as seen in chronic aspiration.

Bronchioles   Small airway tubes that branch off from the larger bronchial tube.

Bronchopulmonary dysplasia (BPD)   A condition marked by respirator-induced (> 28 days) lung and bronchiole damage usually seen in premature infants.

Bronchospasm   Reflex constriction of the airways in response to a variety of stimuli, often associated with cough, wheezing, and mucous production. It may be seen in asthma and BPD.

Buccal fat pads ("sucking pads") Fat pads located in the cheek above the buccinator muscles, most prominent in young infants. These are resorbed by about age 6 months.

Button gastrostomy A modification of a gastrostomy tube with a valve on the abdominal wall, which is usually done when an infant with long-term feeding problems reaches about 10 pounds (4.5 kg) or 2 to 3 months of age. This procedure allows removal of the gastrostomy tube after each feeding and closure of the abdominal opening.

■ C

Cachexia Profound and marked state of ill health and malnutrition.

Calorie A measure of the energy value of food.

Cannula, nasal A soft plastic tubing that wraps around a child's face and has openings under the nose, used to deliver humidified oxygen.

Central line An intravenous line threaded through a peripheral or central vein until it comes as close as possible to the heart.

Central nervous system (CNS) The brain and spinal cord.

Cerebral palsy (CP) An umbrella term for a group of non-progressive, but often changing, motor impairment conditions secondary to brain damage arising in the early stages of development and diagnosed before age 2 years, often accompanied by mental retardation.

CHARGE (Coloboma, Heart, Atresia Choanae, Retardation, Genitourinary, and Ear) An association of multiple congenital anomalies. Children with CHARGE have neurodevelopmental deficits that further complicate feeding issues. Tracheostomy appears to be the most effective means by which to manage the airway in many of these children.

Chewing The breaking down of solid foods for swallowing through rotary jaw movements, lateral tongue movements, posterior transit with tongue, and buccal tension that holds food between teeth and cheeks.

Choana Posterior opening of the nose into the nasopharynx.

Choanal atresia or stenosis A lesion (membranous and/or bony) in the nasal airway, resulting in a failure of the oronasal membrane to rupture completely at about 6 weeks gestation.

Cholestasis Suppression of the flow of bile.

Chronic lung disease   Long term lung damage that may relate to chronic aspiration while swallowing or from gastroesophageal reflux, or other disease processes.

Cleft lip   A congenital defect resulting from the faulty fusion of the median nasal process and the lateral maxillary processes; usually unilateral, but may be bilateral.

Contraction   Shortening of muscle fibers.

Contractures   Prolonged abnormal tightening and shortening of muscle fibers.

Co-contraction   Agonist and antagonist muscles work with the same force at the same time, resulting in either postural stabilization or proximal fixation.

Cricopharyngeus muscle   Sphincter between the pharynx and esophagus, also referred to as upper esophageal sphincter.

Cyanosis   Bluish color of skin due to reduced levels of oxygen in the blood.

∎ D

Decannulation   Removal of a tracheostomy tube, usually carried out once it is determined that a child no longer needs the tracheostomy tube to assist with breathing.

Deglutition   The act of swallowing that begins with oral preparation (bolus formation) of food and ends with esophageal transit of food into the stomach.

Dehydration   Loss of body fluids or water.

Dental caries   Cavities in the teeth.

Desaturation, oxygen   Too little oxygen bound to hemoglobin molecules in the blood stream that causes lack of oxygen in the tissues.

Desensitization (systematic)   The use of competing relaxation responses to help a person overcome fears during exposure to a graduated hierarchy of anxiety-producing stimuli.

Diaphragmatic hernia   A life-threatening birth defect caused by the fetal bowel pushing up into the chest cavity through an abnormal hole in the diaphragm that should separate the chest from the abdomen.

Diastasis   A relatively quiescent period of slow ventricular filling during the cardiac cycle. It occurs in mid-diastole, following the rapid filling phase and just prior to atrial systole.

Diffuse esophageal spasm   An esophageal motor abnormality characterized by the occurrence of multiple simultaneous contractions predominantly seen in the smooth muscle section of the esophagus. Chest pain and dysphagia are associated symptoms.

Direct swallow therapy   Therapy during which patients practice their swallow techniques with small amounts of food or liquid, usually requires high enough cognitive levels of function to follow simple directions.

Disassociation   Separation of movements in a limb or segment of the body.

Duodenal atresia   A birth defect marked by a blockage in the upper portion (duodenum) of the small bowel.

Dysgnathia   An abnormality of the oral cavity and teeth that also involves the jaws.

Dysphagia   Impaired swallowing, secondary to dysfunction in oral, pharyngeal, and/or esophageal phase, i.e., anywhere from the mouth to the stomach.

Dyspnea   Subjective difficulty or distress in breathing; frequently rapid breathing.

■ **E**

Efferent   Neurons that originate in the central nervous system and innervate a peripheral target organ such as skeletal muscles, smooth muscles, or cardiac muscle.

Embryogenesis   Development of the embryo.

Emesis   Vomiting.

Endotracheal tube (ET)   A tube placed in the trachea through the nose or mouth to assist infants and children with breathing difficulties. Insertion of the tube is called intubation and removal is extubation. An infant with an ET tube is assisted with continuous positive airway pressure (CPAP) or a ventilator.

Enteral   Within or passing through the gastrointestinal tract.

Erythema   Redness of skin or tissues produced by congestion of capillaries that may result from a variety of causes.

Esophageal atresia   Congenital failure of the esophageal tube to develop.

Esophageal spasm, also segmental or diffuse esophageal spasm   An abnormality charcterized by the occurrence of simultaneous powerful contractions predominantly in the smooth muscle segment of the esophagus. Commonly causes chest pain and dysphagia.

Esophageal strictures   Narrowing of the esophageal lumen, which leads to mechanical obstruction of the bolus passage.

Esophagitis   Inflammation of the esophagus, most commonly caused by gastroesophageal reflux of stomach acid or alkali from duodenum.

Extension   In the saggital plane, movement of a limb or body part away from the body

External rotation   In the transverse plane, twisting a limb away from the midline of the body.

■   **F**

Facial motor nucleus   One of the cranial motor nuclei with motoneurons that primarily innervate muscles of facial expression.

Failure to thrive (FTT)   A descriptive term to describe a child's abnormal growth in which weight drops below the 5th percentile. Multiple etiologies are possible. Preferred term is undernutrition.

Fistula   A passage or tract between two epithelial surfaces.

Flaccidity   Loss of tone due to central nervous system dysfunction.

Flexible fiberoptic nasopharyngolaryngoscopy (FFNL)   A flexible tube used for dynamic examination of the nasal, pharyngeal, and laryngeal areas of the upper airway. The terms flexible fiberoptic nasopharyngoscopy, flexible fiberoptic nasopharyngolaryngoscopy, and flexible fiberoptic laryngoscopy are interchangeable.

Flexion   In the saggital plane, movement of a limb or body part toward the body.

Fundoplication   Surgical procedure to treat reflux which wraps the fundus of the stomach around the area of the lower esophageal sphincter. This procedure is recommended for children with life-threatening complications related directly to GER (e.g., choking, aspiration, recurrent apnea, chronic pulmonary disease, Barrett's esophagus, esophageal strictures, or large fixed hiatal hernias) unresponsive to medical management.

■ **G**

Gastroesophageal reflux (GER)   Retrograde flow of gastric or biliary secretions from the stomach into the esophagus.

Gastroesophageal reflux disease or disorder (GERD)   Chronic reflux of gastric contents into the esophagus causing anatomic damage and symptoms.

Gastrostomy   An artificial opening made in the stomach.

Glossopharyngeal nerve   The ninth of the twelve cranial nerves; carries sensory, motor, and autonomic nerve fibers primarily to tongue and pharynx.

Glossoptosis   Tongue falling back into the airway, frequently causing at least intermittent, partial airway obstruction.

■ **H**

Haberman feeder   A special feeder to facilitate efficient nipple-feeding in infants with cleft palate and for some children with weak sucking that appears related to neurologic deficits. This feeder was developed by the parent of a child with cleft palate (Mindy Haberman).

H$_2$ receptor blocker   Histamine that mediates its effects through several different receptors. Acid secretion by gastric mucosa is mediated by type 2 histamine receptors (H$_2$). Drugs such as cimetidine and ranitidine block H$_2$ receptors and thereby reduce gastric acid secretion.

Hiatal hernia   Protrusion of part of the stomach through the diaphragm into the thorax. This condition is not necessarily associated with symptoms, although commonly present with gastroesophageal reflux.

Hirschsprung's disease   A congenital anomaly in which the rectum and sometimes the lower colon have failed to develop a normal nerve network. Contents of the bowel accumulate and distend the upper colon. Surgery is required.

Hyperbilirubinemia   A higher-than-normal level or faster-than-normal rise in the level of bilirubin in the blood.

Hypercapnia   Excessive caarbon dioxide in the blood, produced by inadequate ventilation of alveoli.

Hypertonicity   Increased resistance to passive joint movement, frequently with limitations in joint range of motion. Children may also demonstrate abnormal movement patterns and remnants of primitive postural reflexes.

Hypertrophic pyloric stenosis   The only common malformation of the stomach. A marked thickening of the pylorus (distal sphincteric region of the stomach) is noted. Both the circular and longitudinal muscles in the pyloric region are hypertrophied. Severe narrowing of the pyloric canal results in obstruction of the passage of food, with projectile vomiting likely.

Hypoglossal nerve   The 12th cranial nerve which provides motor innervation to the tongue.

Hypoglossal nucleus   One of the cranial motor nuclei with motoneurons that innervate the extrinsic and intrinsic muscles of the tongue. Only one muscle protrudes the tongue so that most motoneurons innervate muscles that retract the tongue or alter its shape.

Hypoplastic left heart syndrome (HLHS)   A congenital heart defect that is fatal without treatment. It includes a small aorta, heart valve narrowing or absent, and a small left atrium and ventricle. Improved surgical techniques and heart transplants are increasing survival rates.

Hypotonicity   Poor resistance to passive range of motion, increased joint range of motion, and a generally poor ability to move up against gravity.

Hypoxia   Deficiency of oxygen reaching tissues of the body.

■ I

Iatrogenic   Refers to an illness or adverse effect resulting from a medical or surgical test or treatment.

Indirect therapy for dysphagia   Exercise programs for swallows of saliva during which no food or liquid is given.

Internal rotation   In the transverse plane, twisting of a limb towards the midline of the body.

Intubation   Insertion of an endotracheal (ET) tube.

■ J

Jaw stabilization   Internal jaw control with minimal up–down jaw movements; important for cup drinking. Begins with the infant biting a cup at 13–15 months, through to active use of jaw muscles by 2 years of age.

■ K

Ketogenic diet   A special high fat diet for some children with uncontrolled seizure disorder.

Kwashiorkor   Severe malnutrition in infants and children characterized by failure to grow and develop. Changes in the pigmentation of the skin and hair are caused by a diet excessively high in carbohydrates and low in protein.

Kyphosis   Abnormally increased convexity in the curvature of the thoracic spine as viewed from the side.

■ L

Laryngeal cleft   A cleft in the posterior larynx that may present with cough during feeding. Stridor may be present at rest and/or with feeds. It results from incomplete closure of the tracheoesophageal septum or cricoid cartilage, or both, in the sixth to seventh week of fetal life.

Laryngeal diversion procedures   Also known as subglottic closures, designed to separate the lower respiratory tract from the upper digestive tract without affecting the glottic or supraglottic parts of the larynx.

Laryngeal penetration   Entry of oropharyngeal contents into the larynx above the true vocal folds.

Laryngeal vestibule   The structures comprising the endolarynx, bounded by the rim of the epiglottis, superior edge of the aryepiglottic folds, tips of the arytenoid cartilages, and superior edge of the interarytenoid space.

Laryngomalacia   Anatomic/physiologic abnormality in which flaccid supraglottic structures prolapse into the airway with inspiration. Stridor is common and failure to thrive is seen rarely.

Laryngospasm   Abductor spasm of true vocal folds.

Laryngotracheal separation   A type of subglottic closure in which the trachea is brought to the skin as a tracheotomy; the proximal segment is closed as a blind pouch.

Lingual nerve   One of the branches of the trigeminal nerve (cranial nerve V). It innervates the anterior part of the tongue and carries input of sensory fibers responding to taste, touch, and pressure.

Lip pursing   Cheek and lip corners are slightly retracted for abnormal stability while central portions of lips are puckered.

Lissencephaly   Agenesis of the cerebral gyri; results in a smooth brain; no convolutions on the cerebrum. Generally associated with severe mental retardation.

Low birth weight (LBW) infant   Any infant with a birth weight of less than 2,500 g (5 lb, 8 oz), regardless of gestational age.

Lower esophageal sphincter (LES)   Also known as gastroesophageal sphincter. Specialized muscles that close the gastroesophageal junction and prevent gastroesophageal reflux by their tonic contraction; relax in response to swallowing.

■ **M**

Macrophage   A type of mononuclear phagocyte found in tissue. The presence of tracheal lipid-laden macrophages may be an indicator of aspiration.

Magenetic resonance imaging (MRI)   A noninvasive diagnostic scanning technique that allows visualization of the soft tissue of the body by imaging the signal produced by the protons of soft tissues after a magnetic field in which a patient is placed has been perturbed by a second magnetic pulse. Allows scanning and reconstruction much like CT scanning but with nonionizing radiation.

Malformation, congenital   An anatomic abnormality (external or internal) present in an infant at birth.

Mandibular hypoplasia   Underdevelopment of the mandible as seen in some children with craniofacial anomalies (e.g. Pierre Robin sequence, hemifacial microsomias, Treacher Collins). Also known as micrognathia.

Marasmus   Condition of chronic undernourishment occurring especially in children and usually caused by a diet deficient in calories and proteins but may result from disease or parasitic infection.

Medium-chain triglyceride (MCT) oil   An additive for breast milk or formula that contains fats that can be digested and absorbed by immature premature infants who are not yet producing certain enzymes and bile salts.

Medulla   The lowest part of the brain stem situated immediately rostral to the spinal cord. It contains several important neuronal pathways controlling respiration, blood pressure, and swallowing.

Metabolism   All the processes carried out by and chemical reactions that occur in the cells of the body as energy is produced and used.

Microcephaly   Small head; may be associated with premature fusion of skull bones; can restrict brain growth and cause mental retardation if untreated.

Micrognathia   Abnormally small mandible (see **Mandibular hypoplasia**).

Midface hypoplasia   Underdevelopment of the midface as seen in Crouzon and Apert syndromes.

Möbius Syndrome   Condition in which cranial nerves VI (lateral abducens) and VII (facial nerve) are damaged. Children typically have difficulty keeping food in the mouth because lips cannot be closed readily.

Modified barium swallow   A diagnostic technique that uses barium contrast with food and liquid to view the oral, pharyngeal, and upper esophageal phases of swallow by dynamic, real time means. (Also videofluoroscopic swallow study—VFSS.)

Motoneurons   Neurons that innervate muscles. The motoneurons innervating skeletal muscle have their cell bodies in the central nervous system and are designated alpha motoneurons. Gamma motoneurons innervate sensory receptors in muscles labeled muscle spindles and bias their discharge; they do not directly excite muscle fibers.

Munching   Early chewing pattern in which rhythmic up–down jaw movements help to spread and flatten food; begins at about 5 to 6 months of age or with introduction of solids.

Muscle tone   The tension in a muscle in its resting state measured by the amount of resistance produced during passive range of motion.

Myelinated fiber   Neurons that have an additional sheath of cells around their axon. Myelinated neurons conduct action potentials much faster than unmyelinated neurons because depolarization actually leaps from node to node (a periodic break in the myelin along the axon of the neuron).

■ N

Nasogastric tube (NG tube)   A small, flexible tube inserted though the nose into the stomach; used to gavage-feed an infant. May be used in older child for short-term feeding supplement.

Necrotizing enterocolitis (NEC)   A serious inflammatory bowel disease, most common in preterm infants.

Neonate   A term used to describe an infant during the first 28 days of life.

Nissen fundoplication   Surgical procedure used to treat gastroesophageal reflux. The fundoplication involves a complete wrap of the fundus of the stomach around the gastroesophageal junction.

Nonnutritive sucking (NNS)   Sucking for reasons other than nutrition (e.g., pacifiers, toys, fingers, or any other object). NNS typically is at a rate of 2 sucks per second, faster than nutritive sucking (NS). Adequate NNS does not guarantee adequate NS.

Nothing per oral (NPO)   Nothing by mouth or no oral feedings.

Nucleus ambiguus (NA)   One of the cranial nerve motor nuclei of the brain stem with motor neurons that innervate laryngeal, pharyngeal, and esophageal muscles.

Nucleus of the tractus solitarius   One of the cranial nerve sensory nuclei of the brain stem that receives sensory input from the oral, pharyngeal, and laryngeal regions. Some of the sensory input is involved with taste. Interneurons within discrete subdivisions of the nucleus serve multiple functions, including controlling blood pressure, respiratory rhythmicity, swallowing, and taste.

Nutritive sucking (NS)   Sucking on a bottle or breast nipple for nutrition, typically 1 suck per second.

■ O

Obdurator   Prosthesis or appliance used to fill in some kind of gap (e.g., with a cleft palate). It typically does not prevent nasopharyngeal reflux during oral feeding of infants and young children. It is not used as commonly as in the past.

Odynophagia   Pain on swallowing.

Oral preparatory phase (bolus formation stage)   Phase of swallowing in which chewing occurs and the tongue gathers the ingested food or liquid and forms it into a centrally located globular mass (bolus) that is ready to be propelled over the back of the tongue.

Oral phase of swallowing   The voluntary phase of swallowing in which a bolus is propelled toward the pharynx through repeated contractions of the tongue.

Orogastric tube (OG tube)   A small, flexible tube inserted though the mouth into the stomach; used to gavage-feed premature infants.

Oropharyngeal transit time   The time taken between the beginning of swallowing and the time when the bolus passes out of the pharynx into the upper esophageal sphincer.

■ **P**

Parasympathetic   One of the two divisions of the autonomic nervous system, with the other being the sympathetic. Postganglionic fibers innervate target tissues close to the organ. The neural transmitter released by its postganglionic neurons is acetylcholine.

Parenteral   Means of delivering nutrition through peripheral veins when the gastrointestinal tract is nonfunctional and must be bypassed for a variety of reasons.

Percutaneous endoscopic gastrostomy (PEG)   Feeding tube placed directly into the stomach from the skin, utilizing an endoscope for guidance.

Percutaneous intravascular central catheter (PICC line)   Catheter placed via a peripheral vein but fed through to a central venous location resulting in improved access to central parenteral nutrition.

Peristalsis   Progression of contractions and relaxations.

Pharyngoesophageal sphincter (PES)   See upper esophageal sphincter.

Phasic bite reflex   A rhythmic opening and closing of the jaw when gums are stimulated; present from birth until about 3–5 months of age in typical infants; commonly retained longer with neurologic damage.

Phlebitis   Inflammation of a vein, usually with edema, stiffness, and pain in the affected part(s).

Pierre-Robin sequence   Craniofacial anomaly that consists of a triad of signs and symptoms—micrognathia, glossoptosis, and U-shaped posterior cleft palate. In about 80% of cases, it is part of a broader syndome.

Polyhydramnios A condition in which more amniotic fluid than normal is present in the mother's uterus during pregnancy, often related to lack of regular swallowing by the fetus. It is sometimes a sign of a fetal anomaly.

Postconceptual age Number of weeks following conception, approximately 2 weeks less than gestational age.

Postural control Coordinated body movements against gravity.

Postural strategies Changing of the person's head or body posture which changes the dimension of the pharynx and the direction of food flow. These are used to improve effectiveness and efficiency of the swallow without increasing the person's work or effort during swallow.

Prematurity An infant born before 36 weeks gestation is premature. Anatomic structures are all present, but with decreased lung maturity, decreased body fat, poor postural control, underdeveloped fat pads (sucking pads), and underdeveloped sensorimotor systems. These infants may have difficulty coordinating suck, swallow, and breathing. Extreme prematurity is less than 28 weeks gestation. Survival at 23 weeks gestation is possible, but infants are usually not ready to feed orally until 31 or 32 weeks at the earliest, often closer to 34 weeks gestation, and some up to 37 weeks.

Primitive reflexes Considered normal in the newborn period but should disappear over the first several months of life. Examples follow:

> **Asymmertic tonic neck reflex (ATNR)** When an infant in a supine position has its head turned laterally, the extremities on the chin side extend and those on the occiput side flex. Persistent ATNR is seen in children with severe motor deficits related to cerebral palsy.

> **Moro reflex** With infant in a supine position and the head held 3 cm off a padded surface, extension of the neck, symmetrical abduction and upward movement of the arms followed by opening of the hands occur. Adduction and flexion of the arms follows.

> **Tonic labyrinthine reflex** This reflex can be elicited in an infant in either a supine or a prone position. In supine, the infant's head is extended 45° below the horizontal and then flexed 45° above the horizontal. While the neck is extended, the limbs extend. With the neck flexed, the limbs flex.

Prostaglandins One of a group of modified unsaturated fatty acids called eicosanoids that function mainly as paracrine or autocrine substances.

Public Law (PL) 94-142 Education for All Handicapped Children Act. A 1975 United States federal law requiring special education programs for all disabled children from 6 to 21 years of age.

Public Law (PL) 99-457, part H   Education of the Handicapped Amendments. A 1986 United States federal law providing early-intervention programs for disabled or at-risk infants (from birth to age 2 years) and offering incentives for states to expand services for disabled children between ages 3 and 5 years.

Pulse oximetry   A noninvasive screening method to determine arterial oxygen saturation of peripheral tissues using a probe placed on one part of the body such as a finger, earlobe, or toe.

Pyriform sinuses   Potential spaces created by the attachment of the inferior pharyngeal constrictor muscles to the larynx and median raphe. During swallowing these spaces provide a pathway for food to enter the esophagus. Material may accumulate in the pyriform sinuses before or after swallows when there are pharyngeal phase deficits.

■ R

Radionuclides   Isotopes of elements with unstable nuclei that emit radiation at a known rate of decay and are used in scintigraphy.

Real-time ultrasound (see Ultrasound)   Ultrasound images that are reconstructed rapidly, allowing the operator to view the movement of the structures imaged at the same time the images are being taken. Ultrasound is particularly useful to observe sucking patterns in infants.

Recurrent laryngeal nerve   A branch of the vagus nerve (CN X) that provides partial sensory innervation to the larynx and motor innervation to the thyroarytenoid, lateral cricoarytenoid, interarytenoids, and posterior cricoarytenoid muscles.

Reflux, gastroesophageal   The backward flow of stomach contents into the esophagus, which may trigger apnea and/or bradycardia in infants.

Residue   Material left in the oral, pharyngeal, or laryngeal cavity after the swallow.

Respiratory distress syndrome (RDS)   A condition affecting the lungs of preterm neonates due to a lack of surfactant that makes it difficult for them to breathe. This condition has also been known as hyaline membrane disease.

Reticular formation   A region of the brain stem with cells and fibers appearing histologically like a network of intertwining cells and fibers. The reticular formation is separated into functional units and includes those interneurons that function in chewing and swallowing.

Retractions   Indentations in the infant's neck or chest during breathing that indicate increased muscle effort and difficulty breathing.

Rooting response   A reflex in which infants turn their mouths toward tactile stimuli presented on the lips or cheeks, often looking for a nipple near feeding time. This reflex occurs at around 32 weeks gestational age and should disappear around 6 months of age.

Rotary jaw motion   Mature chewing pattern that involves up–down, forward–backward, lateral–diagonal, diagonal–rotary, and circular–rotary jaw movements. Children are not expected to demonstrate rotary jaw motion until they are 3–4 years of age.

Rumination   A chronic regurgitation, chewing, and re-swallowing of previously ingested food.

■ **S**

Sandifer's syndrome   Intermittent torticollis occurring in children as a sign of gastroesophgeal reflux, esophagitis, or hiatal hernia; disappears when the underlying problem is corrected.

Santmyer swallow   A method to stimulate a swallow reflex by gently blowing a puff of air in the infant's face. This reflex is present in infants ranging from 33 weeks gestation to 11 months, but should be absent in neurologically normal children after the age of 2 years.

Saturation, oxygen   The degree to which oxygen is bound to hemoglobin (a substance in red blood cells), expressed as a percentage.

Scintigraphy   Images produced by gamma camera recording the emissions of radionuclide energy. Examination is used to assess aspiration and to measure rate of gastric emptying (usually as a percentage of radioactive contents left in the stomach after 1 hour).

Sensory neurons   The neurons that innervate peripheral tissue (i.e., oral mucosa) and communicate input from sensory receptors such as touch, taste, pain, smell, and proprioception.

Short bowel syndrome (SBS)   Any of the malabsorption conditions resulting from massive resection of the small bowel, the degree and kind of malabsorption depending on the site and extent of the resection. Some causes include necrotizing enterocolitis, midgut volvulus, multiple intestinal atresias, intestinal malrotation, and abdominal wall defects. Signs are diarrhea, steatorrhea, and undernutrition. Also called short gut.

Sleep apnea   A periodic cessation of breathing during sleep.

Small for gestational age (SGA)   Term for a newborn infant whose weight (and possibly length and head circumference) falls below the 10th percentile on a standard intrauterine growth chart; indicates small size for the length of time the infant was in utero. An SGA infant can be preterm, term, or postterm.

Spasticity   Increased tension of a weak muscle with initial increased resistance to passive stretching, followed by sudden relaxation, associated with an exaggeration of deep reflexes.

Spillage   Material that has spilled into the pharynx before the pharyngeal swallow response has been initiated.

Stability   Maintenance of equilibrium with resistance to sudden change of position, achieved through co-contraction of muscle groups so a joint remains fixed while allowing other muscles to move.

State, behavioral   Level of awareness. Infants experience six states: deep sleep, light sleep, drowsy, quiet, alert, and crying.

Steatorrhea   Excessive fat in stools.

Stenosis   Narrowed passage (e.g., trachea, vein, or artery) such that flow through that passage is limited.

Stertor   An upper airway noise that indicates turbulent airflow through a narrow airway, in the region of the nasopharynx, oropharynx, or hypopharynx.

Stimulation, oral   Sensory input, either positive or negative, to the area in and around a child's mouth.

Stridor   An upper airway noise that indicates turbulent airflow through a narrow airway, usually on inspiration, but can be on expiration, usually noted at the level of larynx. Stridor is not a diagnosis itself but rather an indication of airway abnormality.

Sucking   Begins around 6 to 9 months with pattern of increasing vertical component to tongue action, maintained throughout life span.

Suckling   Occurs from birth to 6 to 9 months with primarily "in-out" tongue action.

Subglottic stenosis   Narrowing in the trachea below the level of the glottis that may result in airway obstruction. Severe forms also can interfere with feeding.

Sudden infant death syndrome (SIDS)   The death of an infant less than 12 months of age during sleep with unidentifiable causes; also called crib death or cot death.

Superior laryngeal nerve (SLN)   One of the branches of the vagus nerve (CN X) that innervates the laryngeal (cricothyroid) and hypopharyngeal regions. It is composed of predominantly sensory fibers with a small component of motor fibers supplying the cricothyroid and upper esophageal striated muscle.

Surfactant   A complex mixture of phospholipids (chiefly lecithin and sphingomyelin) secreted by alveolar type II cells that reduce the surface tension of the pulmonary alveoli and thus reduce their tendency to collapse. Surfactant is absent or lacking in infants born prematurely. Production begins at about 24 weeks gestation, but is not well developed until about 36 weeks gestation.

Surfactant replacement therapy   Natural or artificial surfactant supplied through a tube placed into the trachea to replace the natural surfactant the infant lacks because of prematurity. It coats the inner surfaces of airways and alveoli in the lungs to keep the passages open.

Swallow apnea   The normal interruption of the respiratory cycle during expiration induced by a swallow.

Symmetrical   No difference in appearance and in movement from one side of the head and/or body to the corresponding part on the other side.

Sympathetic nervous system   Part of the autonomic nervous system responsible for reflex body functions (e.g., heart rate, blood pressure, gastric motility). Its preganglionic fibers originate from the thoracic and lumbar levels of the spinal cord and its postganglionic fibers innervating target tissues reside close to the spinal cord. The main neural transmitter released by the postganglionic neurons is norepinephrine.

Synapse   The primary connection between neurons and between neurons and muscles. Chemical synapses predominate and involve a presynaptic component that secretes transmitters such as acetylcholine to the postsynaptic component across an open cleft to a specific membrane receptor for that specific transmitter.

■ **T**

Tachycardia   Heart rate that is faster than normal.

Tachypnea   Breathing rate that is faster than normal.

Taste receptor   Specialized chemoreceptors that respond to substances dissolved in oral and pharyngeal fluids.

Technetium 99m   A radionuclide commonly used for evaluation of the gastrointestinal tract, as in scintigraphy. It is linked to food or to other ligands (i.e., for injection in the body to be taken up by various organs).

Teratogen   An environmental agent (e.g., drug, chemical, or toxin) that can cause birth defects if the fetus is exposed to it during development, especially during the first three months gestation.

Tetralogy of Fallot   A cyanotic heart defect involving four abnormalities of the heart and its vessels: a ventricular septal defect (VSD), pulmonary stenosis, an overly muscular right ventricle, and positioning of the aorta over the VSD.

Theophylline   A medication that stimulates the central nervous system and is given to reduce occurrences of apnea in some infants, particularly preterm infants.

Tongue lateralization   Side-to-side movement of the tongue to maintain and move food to the teeth during chewing; begins at about 6–7 months of age.

Tongue-tied   See ankyloglossia.

Total parenteral nutrition (TPN)   Nutritional needs provided exclusively through intravenous access as opposed to the gastrointestinal tract. It is delivered through a central line.

Tracheal intubation   Placement of a tube into the trachea either translaryngeal or through a tracheostomy.

Tracheoesophageal fistula (TEF)   Abnormal communication between the trachea and the esophagus, occurring during the 4th week of development because of incomplete division of the cranial part of the foregut into respiratory and digestive portions.

Tracheomalacia   Pathologic loss or softening of tracheal cartilage.

Tracheotomy/tracheostomy   A surgical procedure in which an incision is made in the neck through the tracheal rings, below the level of the vocal folds. A tube maintains the opening which is needed to help a person breathe.

Transient lower esophageal sphincter relaxation (TLESR)   Relaxations of the lower esophageal sphincter that occur without associated swallowing activity. These events allow for 60–80% of gastroesophageal reflux events.

Transitional feeding   A stage of eating when children move from liquid to spoon feeding, usually begins about 4–6 months developmental level.

Transposition of the great arteries   A cyanotic heart defect in which the pulmonary artery, which normally carries unoxygenated blood to the lungs, and the aorta, which carries oxygenated blood to the body, are reversed. The condition results in oxygen-poor blood being sent to the body.

Trigeminal nerve   One of the major cranial nerves (CN V) with three major sensory divisions and one motor division. It provides sensation to the face and oral cavity.

Tube feeding   Feeding using a liquid formula passed into the enteral tract via tubes placed through the mouth, nose, or directly into the stomach.

■ U

Ultrasound imaging   A method of evaluating the soft tissues using high-frequency sound waves to create images. Tissue contrast is provided by the differences in each tissue's ability to reflect sound.

Upper esophageal sphincter (UES)   (Also known as the pharyngo-esophageal sphincter) Formed primarily by the cricopharyngeus muscle; this is the top sphincter along the esophagus, responsible for opening the esophagus to allow a bolus to enter during swallowing and keeping material from flowing back up into the pharynx. Opening of the UES segment is enhanced by the pull from the hyoid ascent and the pressure exerted by the luminal bolus.

Upper gastrointestinal study (UGI)   A fluoroscopic study used to evaluate the anatomic structures in the esophagus, stomach, duodenum, gastric outlet, and proximal small bowel. It may detect gastroesophageal reflux when it occurs immediately with swallowing, but it is not a definitive study for GER.

■ V

Vagus nerve   Tenth cranial nerve (CN X), which arises from the lateral side of the medulla oblongata and innervates a wide variety of visceral organs, including the tongue (sensory), pharynx (sensory and motor), larynx (sensory and motor), esophagus (sensory and motor), lungs and heart (parasympathetic and visceral afferent).

Valleculae   The space between the base of the tongue and the epiglottis where food or liquid may accumulate prior to production of a pharyngeal swallow. This may be a trigger point for onset of the pharyngeal swallow.

Ventricular septal defect (VSD) A birth defect marked by a hole in the wall (septum) between the two ventricles (lower chambers) of the heart. In some cases, the opening closes spontaneously.

Ventriculo-peritoneal (VP) shunt The most common shunting procedure for the relief of hydrocephalus, consisting of the creation of a channel between a cerebral ventricle and the peritoneum by means of plastic tubing.

Very-low-birth-weight (VLBW) infant Any infant who weighs less that 1,500 g (3 lb, 5 oz) at birth regardless of gestational age.

Videoendoscopic examination of swallow A study which evaluates the pharyngeal swallow using an endoscope placed in the pharynx.

Videofluoroscopic swallow study (VFSS) This is a barium contrast study that evaluates the oral and pharyngeal phases of swallowing physiology. The esophagus is typically scanned to observe transit time.

■ W

Waterbrash A gush of saliva produced in response to reflux.

■ X

Xerostomia Dry mouth due to salivary gland dysfunction that can occur as a result of medication, disease, or radiation therapy.

■ REFERENCES

Dorland's illustrated medical dictionary (28th Ed.). (1994). Philadelphia: W. B. Saunders.
Stedman's medical dictionary (26th Ed.). (1995). Baltimore: Williams & Wilkins.

Index

■

nipples, 420–421
nutrient needs, 255–257, 262–266
parenteral, 196
steps, 568
sucking, 416, 426
taste experiences, 426–427
transition to oral feeding,
    303–304, 428
growth charts, 238
nonnutritive sucking, 305, 423–424,
    426
physical examination, 303–309
stroking face/tongue, 424–426
Primary protein energy malnutrition
    (PEM), 188–189, 190
Proctosigmoidoscopy, 210
Prostheses, palatal feeding, 542–545
Psychologist, 8
Psychosis, feeding treatment, 450–451
Ptyalism, 495
Public Law 99-457, 9
Pulmonologist, 8
Pyloric stenosis, 38, 199
Pyloroplasty, 219

Q

Quadriplegia
    anthropometric measurements, 250
    dysphagia, 441
    undernutrition, 268

R

Radiation exposure, videofluoroscopy,
    360–361
Radiographic assessment, 160–161, 200,
    210
Radiologist, 8, 366, 368
Ranitidine, 217
RDAs, 253, 257, 259
Reassurances, 507–509
Recommended Dietary Allowances
    (RDAs), 253, 257, 259
Reflux. *See* Gastroesophageal reflux
    disease (GERD);
    Nasopharyngeal reflux

Refluxate, 163, 202, 220
Refusal, food. *See* Food refusal
Respiratory system, 32–33, 37
Retardation, 449
    aspiration, 478
    chewing readiness, 440
    drooling, 519
    gastrostomy tube (GT), 193
Rett syndrome, feeding treatment, 450
Rickets, 269
Rooting response, 56
Rubinstein-Taybi syndrome, 133
Russell Silver syndrome, 129

S

Salivagram, 483
Saltropine, 511
Santmyer swallow, 308
School Functional Assessment, 316,
    331–332
Scintiscan, 211–213, 483
Scopolamine, 511
Seating/positioning. *See*
    Positioning/seating
Seizures, 477
Separation/individuation, 564, 567–568
Shaken baby syndrome (SBS), 445–446
Short bowel syndrome, 193, 220, 259
Sialorrhea. *See* Drooling
Sickle cell anemia, 238, 251
SIDS, 164, 217
Smith-Lemli-Optiz syndrome, 131
Snugglebud devices, 401
Social worker, 8, 533
Solo open cup, 436
SOMA: Schedule for Oral Motor
    Assessment, 316, 332–333
Speech-language pathologist (SLP), 8,
    287
    assessment and, 137
    craniofacial abnormalities, 532, 533
    drooling, 502, 503–504, 509
    ultrasound imaging, 343
    videofluoroscopy, 349, 366, 368, 483
Spoon feeding, 431–435
    assessment, 318–319